Nutrition and Alcohol

Edited by

Ronald R. Watson, Ph.D.
Research Professor and Director
National Institute of Alcohol Abuse and Alcoholism
Specialized Alcohol Research Center
Department of Family and Community Medicine
University of Arizona School of Medicine
Tucson, Arizona

Bernhard Watzl, Ph.D.
Research Associate
Department of Nutrition
Justus Liebig University
Giessen, Germany

CRC Press
Boca Raton   Ann Arbor   London   Tokyo

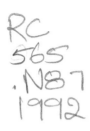

RC
565
.N87
1992

Library of Congress Cataloging-in-Publication Data

Nutrition and alcohol / [edited by] Ronald R. Watson and Bernhard
  Watzl.
      p.   cm. -- (CRC series in physiology of drug abuse)
   Includes bibliographical references and index.
   ISBN 0-8493-7933-4
   1. Alcoholism--Nutritional aspects.   I. Watson, Ronald R. (Ronald
Ross)   II. Watzl, Bernhard.   III. Series.
   [DNLM: 1. Alcoholism--complications.   2. Nutrition Disorders--
etiology.   3. Nutritional Status.   WM 274 N976]
RC565.N87   1992
616.86'1--dc20
DNLM/DLC
for Library of Congress   92-11492
                                                          CIP

PREFACE

Alcoholism affects about 10 million people in the U.S. and ranks among the world's major public health concerns. Alcohol use as well as abuse has a number of physiologic consequences including its impact on the nutritional status of the alcoholic. It is well documented that alcoholism is the most common single cause of malnutrition in developed countries.

Alcohol abuse induces malnutrition in various ways. Alcohol itself is a food that is low in micronutrients and displaces other more nutritious foods in the diet. Alcohol further affects the bioavailability of many nutrients and is toxic to almost all body tissues, especially to the brain and liver. On the other hand, there is strong evidence that the dietary composition and nutritional status of the alcoholic modify the toxicity of alcohol.

The objective of this book is to summarize the latest research data on the multiple effects of alcohol on the nutritional status of alcohol abusers. This volume further emphasizes research data on the combined effects of direct alcohol toxicity with the alterations due to malnutrition on tissue damage. This information will assist the scientist in the field of alcohol research in understanding the nutritional modulation of alcohol abuse-related disorders, as well as the clinician in preventing and treating alcohol abuse-related disorders by nutritional therapy.

CRC Series in
PHYSIOLOGY OF DRUG ABUSE
Edited by Ronald R. Watson

Published Titles:

Alcohol and Cancer

Alcohol and Neurobiology: Brain Development
   and Hormone Regulation

Alcohol and Neurobiology: Receptors, Membranes,
   and Channels

Drugs of Abuse and Neurobiology

Marijuana/Cannabinoids: Neurobiology
   and Neurophysiology

Nutrition and Alcohol

Forthcoming Titles:

Neurobiology of Opiates

Opioid Peptides in Substance Abuse

INTRODUCTION

Public attention and research efforts are being driven by an ever-increasing understanding of the problems and magnitude of alcohol abuse. Alcohol is a drug of abuse and a caloric food. It causes poorer intake and absorption of nutrients. The effects of alcohol on nutrition play major roles in many aspects of the pathology of alcohol. Two out of three high school students report that they used alcohol during the previous month. Alcohol-altered nutrition directly affects 10 million alcohol-abusing adults. It costs the people of the U.S. more than $200 billion in lost wages, health care, theft, and shortened lifespan. An intimate, detailed knowledge of the effects of alcohol on the biochemical reactions and nutritional changes is critical in preventing or treating abuse. Diets in animal studies have been used that provide ethanol. These show significant effects due to the diet composition. Their use is analyzed in detail. The progress of research over the past decade is encouraging as we begin to summarize and evaluate in detail advances in understanding changes in the nutritional biochemistry and physiology caused by ethanol. This information will assist the researcher, clinician, and student in comprehending the complex changes caused by direct and indirect effects of ethanol at the cellular level via its nutritional modification.

THE EDITORS

Ronald R. Watson, Ph.D., initiated and directs the Specialized Alcohol Research Center at the University of Arizona College of Medicine. The main theme of this National Institute of Alcohol Abuse and Alcoholism (NIAAA) Center Grant is to understand the role of ethanol-induced immunosuppression on tumor and disease resistance in animals. He has edited 24 books including 10 on alcohol abuse and 4 on other drugs of abuse. He has worked for several years on research for the U.S. Navy Alcohol and Substance Abuse Program.

Dr. Watson attended the University of Idaho, but graduated from Brigham Young University in Provo, Utah with a degree in Chemistry in 1966. He completed his Ph.D. degree in 1971 in Biochemistry from Michigan State University. His postdoctoral schooling was completed at the Harvard School of Public Health in Nutrition and Microbiology, including a 2-year postdoctoral research experience in Immunology. He was an Assistant Professor of Immunology and did research at the University of Mississippi Medical Center in Jackson from 1973 to 1974. He was an Assistant Professor of Microbiology and Immunology at the Indiana University Medical School from 1974 to 1978 and an Associate Professor at Purdue University in the Department of Food and Nutrition from 1978 to 1982. In 1982 he joined the faculty at the University of Arizona in the Department of Family and Community Medicine, Nutrition Section, and is a Research Professor. He has published 225 research papers and review chapters.

Dr. Watson is a member of several national and international nutrition, immunology, and cancer societies and research societies on alcoholism.

Bernhard Watzl, Ph.D., is a Research Associate at the Justus-Liebig University in Giessen, Germany. He holds a joint appointment as a Research Associate with the Department of Family and Community Medicine at the University of Arizona College of Medicine in Tucson, Arizona.

Dr. Watzl graduated in Human Nutrition and Home Economics at the Justus-Liebig University in Giessen, Germany in 1983, where he also received his Ph.D. degree in Human Nutrition in 1988.

From 1989 to 1991, he joined the Specialized Alcohol Research Center and the Nutrition Section of the Department of Family and Community Medicine at the University of Arizona in Tucson as a postdoctoral fellow.

Dr. Watzl's research specialities are interactions between nutrients and the immune response. His current research interest relates to the modulation of alcohol-related disorders by nutritional intervention.

CONTRIBUTORS

John P. Allen, Ph.D.
Chief
Treatment Research Branch
Division of Clinical and
  Prevention Research
National Institute of Alcohol
  Abuse and Alcoholism
Rockville, Maryland

Christiane Bode, Ph.D.
Chief
Research Laboratory
Department of Internal Medicine
  (Gastroenterology)
Robert-Bosch-Krankenhaus
and Professor of
  Pathobiochemistry
Faculty of Nutrition
University of Stuttgart-
  Hohenheim
Stuttgart, Germany

J. Christian Bode, M.D.
Chief
Department of Internal Medicine
  (Gastroenterology
  and Endocrinology)
Robert-Bosch-Krankenhaus
and Professor of Internal
  Medicine
University of Tübingin
Stuttgart, Germany

Xu Dan, M.D.
Research Scientist
Department of Biochemistry
University of Western Australia
Nedlands, Western Australia

Robert F. Derr, Ph.D.
Research Chemist
Research Service
Department of Veterans Affairs
  Medical Center
Minneapolis, Minnesota

Paul G. Drake
Research Scientist
Department of Biochemistry
University of Western Australia
Nedlands, Western Australia

John W. Erdman, Jr., Ph.D.
Professor, Department of Food
  Science
and Director, Division of
  Nutritional Sciences
University of Illinois
Urbana, Illinois

Samuel W. French, M.D.
Head, Division of Anatomic
  Pathology
Department of Pathology
Harbor-UCLA Medical Center
Torrance, California

Howard Friedman, M.P.H.
Clinical Chemistry Supervisor
Department of Chemistry
Liberty Testing Laboratory
Brooklyn, New York

Billy W. Geer, Ph.D.
Clara A. Abbott Professor of
  Biology
Department of Biology
Knox College
Galesburg, Illinois

George D. Guthrie, Ph.D.
Professor, Department of
  Biochemistry and Molecular
  Biology
Associate Director, Evansville
  Center
Indiana University School of
  Medicine
Evansville, Indiana

Charles H. Halsted, M.D.
Professor, Department of Internal
  Medicine
Chief, Division of Clinical
  Nutrition and Metabolism
University of California
Davis, California

Pieter W. H. Heinstra, Ph.D.
Research Biochemist
Department of Biochemistry
University of Leiden
Leiden, The Netherlands

**Edward J. Kasarskis, M.D.,
  Ph.D.**
Professor of Neurology,
  Toxicology, and Nutrition
Department of Neurology
University of Kentucky Medical
  Center
and Lexington VA Medical
  Center
Lexington, Kentucky

Edward C. Larkin, M.D.
Professor of Pathology and
  Medicine
Department of Pathology
Veterans Affairs Medical Center
Martinez, California
and Schools of Medicine and
  Pathology
University of California
Davis, California

Raye Z. Litten, Ph.D.
Physiologist
Treatment Research Branch
Division of Clinical and
 Prevention Research
National Institute of Alcohol
 Abuse and Alcoholism
Rockville, Maryland

Luis Marsano, M.D.
Assistant Professor of Medicine
Departments of Medicine and
 Gastroenterology
University of Kentucky Medical
 Center
and Department of Medicine
Lexington Veterans Affairs
 Medical Center
Lexington, Kentucky

Craig J. McClain, M.D.
Professor of Medicine, Nutrition,
 and Toxicology
and Director of Gastroenterology
Departments of Medicine and
 Gastroenterology
University of Kentucky Medical
 Center
and Department of Medicine
Lexington Veterans Affairs
 Medical Center
Lexington, Kentucky

**Charles L. Mendenhall, M.D.,
 Ph.D.**
Professor of Medicine
Department of Internal Medicine
University of Cincinnati Medical
 Center
and Director of Hepatic Research
Department of Veterans Affairs
 Medical Center
Cincinnati, Ohio

Robert R. Miller, Jr., Ph.D.
Visiting Research Associate
Department of Biology
Knox College
Galesburg, Illinois

Sohrab Mobarhan, M.D.
Associate Chief of
 Gastroenterology
Professor, Department of
 Medicine
Loyola University Medical
 Center
and Director, Clinical Nutrition
 Unit
Foster McGaw Hospital
Maywood, Illinois

Olakekan E. Odeleye, Ph.D.
Research Associate
Department of Family and
  Community Medicine
Arizona Health Sciences Center
University of Arizona
Tucson, Arizona

T. Norman Palmer, Ph.D.
Professor and Chairman
Department of Biochemistry
University of Western Australia
Nedlands, Western Australia

**Timothy J. Peters, Ph.D.,
  D.Sc., F.R.C.P., F.R.C.Path.**
Professor
Department of Clinical
  Biochemistry
King's College School of
  Medicine and Dentistry
London, England

**Oliver E. Pratt, D.Sc.,
  F.R.C.Path. (Deceased)**
Reader Emeritus
Department of Clinical
  Biochemistry
King's College School of
  Medicine and Dentistry
and Department of
  Neuropathology
Institute of Psychiatry
University of London
London, England

Victor R. Preedy, Ph.D.
Lecturer
Department of Clinical
  Biochemistry
King's College School of
  Medicine and Dentistry
London, England

G. Ananda Rao, Ph.D.
Senior Investigator
Department of Pathology
Veterans Affairs Medical Center
Martinez, California

Ronald C. Reitz, Ph.D.
Professor of Biochemistry
Department of Biochemistry
School of Medicine
University of Nevada
Reno, Nevada

Daphne A. Roe, M.D.
Professor of Nutrition
Division of Nutritional Sciences
Cornell University
Ithaca, New York
and Cornell University
  Medical College
New York, New York

Mikko Salaspuro, M.D., Ph.D.
Professor (Chair) of Alcohol
  Diseases
Research Unit of Alcohol
  Diseases
University of Helsinki
Helsinki, Finland

Hariharan Sankaran, Ph.D.
Research Physiologist
and Chief, Brain:Gut Peptide
  Laboratory
Department of Surgery
Veterans Affairs Medical Center
and Oregon Health Sciences
  University
Portland, Oregon

Allan D. Thomson, Ph.D.,
  F.R.C.P.(Ed.)
Director
Department of Gastroenterology
Greenwich District Hospital
London, England

Ronald R. Watson, Ph.D.
Director
NIAAA Specialized Alcohol
  Research Center
Department of Family and
  Community Medicine
College of Medicine
University of Arizona
Tucson, Arizona

Bernhard Watzl, Ph.D.
Research Associate
Department of Nutrition
Justus-Liebig University
Giessen, Germany

TABLE OF CONTENTS

1 Alcohol-Related Nutritional Derangements: Implications for Nutritional Support

INTRODUCTION

Alcohol (ethanol) abuse disrupts hepatic structure and functions. The mechanisms of drug-induced hepatotoxicity are intricately related to changes in the functional activities of enzyme antioxidant systems (superoxide dismutase, catalase, glutathione peroxidases, and the selenoenzymes) and the development of nutritional deficiencies. These inherent enzyme systems and the dietary antioxidant status of tocopherols, ascorbate, and β-carotene[5-8] protect biological systems from oxidative damage.[1-4] The ability of the hepatic cells to maintain their viability and integrity after insults from xenobiotics, including commonly used drugs of abuse, is in part dependent on antioxidant defenses. The role of xenobiotics in generating free radicals and their conversion to reactive electrophiles that generate species during cellular damage has been recently reviewed.[9,10]

Alcohol is a commonly abused drug[11] that exacts a tremendous social and economic cost. This chapter reviews alcohol metabolism as related to lipid peroxidation and its consequences for nutritional alterations, their contribution to the pathogenesis of liver disease, and the value and mechanisms of action of nutrients in interrupting and reversing the adverse effects of alcoholism.

METABOLISM AND RELATED HEPATOTOXICITY OF ALCOHOL ABUSE

METABOLISM OF ALCOHOL

Alcohol is oxidized almost exclusively in the liver by pathways located in different subcellular compartments of the hepatocyte: the alcohol dehydrogenase (ADH) pathway in the cytosol; the microsomal ethanol-oxidizing system (MEOS) in the endoplasmic reticulum; and catalase in peroxisomes.[12] The metabolism of ethanol in each of these pathways may be associated with the generation of reactive electrophiles, resulting in hepatic damage.

Alcohol Dehydrogenase Pathway

ADH catalyzes the conversion of ethanol to acetaldehyde in a series of reactions that requires nicotinamide adenine dinucleotide (NADH) as a cofactor. The overall result of ethanol oxidation is the generation of excess-reducing equivalents as free NADH in hepatic cytosol, mainly because the metabolic systems involved in NADH removal do not have the ability to fully affect its accumulation. Acetaldehyde produced in this reaction is further converted to acetate by mitochondrial ADH.[13,14] In the oxidation step NAD functions as a coenzyme and NADH is formed. The increased NADH/NAD ratio results in a major change in liver metabolism of lipids[15] and protein,[16] and consequent liver damage associated with alcohol abuse. The net result of ethanol oxidation by the hepatic ADH is acetate, which is released into the bloodstream to be further oxidized to CO_2 and water in the peripheral tissues.[17,18]

Hepatic ADH activity may be the only rate-limiting step of ethanol metabolism, although studies have reported a lack of correlation between the rates of ethanol oxidation and ADH activity.[19-21] Although chronic ethanol administration to rats decreases ADH activity in perivenous and periportal hepatocytes, the rate of ethanol elimination nevertheless increases.[22,23] Even in human subjects who have atypical ADH with a higher activity than normal, the rate of alcohol metabolism is not higher than observed in normal subjects.[24] Theorell and Bonnichsen[25] calculated that when the amount of NADH produced in the ADH reaction goes beyond immediate metabolic needs, its concentration increases with a subsequent inhibition of the ADH reaction. Other factors may also affect the rate of alcohol oxidation by ADH: the intracellular acetaldehyde concentrations, the activity of the shuttle mechanisms transporting reducing equivalents into the mitochondria, and the activity of the mitochondrial respiratory chain.[26]

Microsomal Ethanol Oxidizing System and Catalase

The cytochrome P-450 MEOS and the catalase system in peroxisomes and microsomes provide alternate pathways for ethanol oxidation.[27,28] These alternate pathways of ethanol metabolism contribute <20% of its metabolism;[29] however, the contribution of the MEOS to metabolic oxidation of ethanol increases during chronic alcohol consumption. The MEOS is localized in the endoplasmic reticulum using NADPH (reduced nicotinamide adenine dinucleotide phosphate) and oxygen, and undergoes an increase in activity after chronic ethanol consumption, which is associated with rapid growth of the smooth endothelial reticulum.[30] Compared to ADH, the MEOS requires higher ethanol levels for full saturation and maximal velocity. Therefore, at high blood ethanol concentrations, the contribution of this non-ADH pathway is markedly increased.[31]

Catalase

Catalase is also capable of oxidizing ethanol *in vivo* in the presence of an H_2O_2-generating system. H_2O_2-mediated ethanol peroxidation by catalase is limited by the rate of H_2O_2 generated. Since the physiological rate of H_2O_2 production is low, the contribution of catalase to *in vivo* ethanol elimination is not of great importance.[32]

HEPATOTOXICITY ASSOCIATED WITH ALCOHOL ABUSE

The mechanisms through which ethanol incurs hepatic injury remain a central toxicological concern. This problem has been pursued largely by following the intracellular fate of alcohol demonstrating: (1) some of the effects are caused by a direct action of ethanol or its reactive metabolites, acetaldehyde and acetate; (2) part of its effects are mediated by the hormonal changes that accompany alcohol abuse;[33] and (3) other changes are dependent on the nutritional status of the abuser,[34] the level of ethanol administered,[35] and the duration of ethanol intake.[36] Changes in immune functions may also play a role in the ultimate liver pathology.

The pathogenic mechanisms of alcohol hepatotoxicity resulting in alcoholic liver disease (ALD) is accompanied by a multitude of biologic factors, including reduced nutritional intake, improper digestion and absorption, and increased requirement for some nutrients. The complex interrelated cascade of changes result in vicious cycles leading to increasing severity of alcoholic hepatotoxicity. Alcohol abuse causes a broad spectrum of pathological, morphological, histological, and biochemical changes in the liver. Some of these changes are the subject of recent reviews,[37-41] and of other chapters in this volume. The hepatic effects of alcohol, excluding cirrhosis, are partially reversible upon cessation of alcohol ingestion. The pathological features of ALD can be divided into three broad categories: fatty liver changes, alcoholic hepatitis with or without fibrosis, and cirrhosis. This division is artificial for three major reasons: (1) the categories represent a continuum of disease; (2) at any given time, one or more combinations may be present in the liver; and (3) if a liver biopsy is performed after a period of abstinence from alcohol, the alcohol-related changes may not be seen.

The role of alcohol in the pathogenesis of fatty liver is well documented,[40-44] and the consensus of available evidence is that fatty changes alone probably have no role in the development of cirrhosis, outside of other nutritional factors.[45] The hepatic fatty changes induced by alcohol include fat cysts, lipogranuloma, megamitochondria, hepatocyte swelling, and Mallory bodies which appear after excessive alcohol ingestion — usually visible within 3 to 7 d.[46] On cessation of drinking, the changes may disappear within a few days but in severe cases, it takes 4 to 6 weeks for these changes to clear.[47] Some of these changes are not specific to ALD and are seen in many other conditions, including alimentary disorders, abetalipoprotenemia, and in prolonged steroid use.[48] Although it may appear that these nonspecific changes are unimportant, their presence in association with other more specific changes often leads to a correct diagnosis of ALD.

Alcoholic hepatitis is characterized by the presence of Mallory bodies in the hepatocyte, with a surrounding neutrophil and mononuclear cellular infiltrate. Mallory bodies are discrete collections of eosinophilic hyaline intracytoplasmic materials commonly situated around the nucleus that cause the hepatocyte to be swollen. In cirrhotic livers, hepatocytes containing Mallory bodies are most frequently found at the interphase between regenerating nodules and fibrous septa. Alcoholic hepatitis is often accompanied by or results in fibrosis. The fibrosis typically occurs as fine strands surrounding individual hepatocytes, as seen in pericellular fibrosis.

Individual hepatocytes gradually disappear and larger foci of fibrosis are formed, eventually resulting in solid, often stellate, septa of fibrosis, radiating from the central vein. A late complication of cirrhosis, immunosuppression, and dietary deficiencies is hepatocellular cancer.[49] Although it is clear that ethanol consumption is hepatotoxic, some of the other mechanisms of damage, including alterations in hepatic plasma membrane fluidity[50,51] and increased lipid peroxidation,[52,53] have yet to be fully elaborated.

Another hepatotoxic effect of alcohol is the increased susceptibility of the alcoholic to the adverse effects of various drugs. Ethanol is an inducer not only of its own metabolism but also the metabolisms of a number of other drugs. The administration of ethanol results in the inhibition or acceleration of drug detoxification, depending on the dosage and the time interval between the administration of the ethanol and the drug. *In vitro* ethanol is a competitive inhibitor of anilase, pentobarbital hydroxylases, and a mixed inhibitor of the demethylation of aminopyrine and ethylmorphine.[54] It also alters the metabolism of drugs such as 4-hydroxyphenazon and 4-aminoantipyrine from the major oxidative to the minor conjugative pathways[55] and inhibits the rates of disappearance of phenobarbital and meprobamate from the blood of humans[54] and animals.[55] The concomitant administration of ethanol and drugs such as the barbiturates and chloral hydrate results in the enhanced depression by these drugs on the central nervous system (CNS). The effect of ethanol and chloral hydrate given in combination is greater than the simple summation of the effects obtained when either drug is given alone. This potentiation of effect appears to be due to the mutual inhibition of metabolism.[56] Commonly used H_2-receptor antagonists, such as cimetidine, decrease ADH activity and enhance periportal blood levels of ethanol, precipitating liver damage.[57,58] Ethanol also interacts with narcotics to potentiate hepatotoxicity. In humans, the combined use of morphine and alcohol potentiates the effects of both drugs and increases chronic hepatic damage and death.[59] Similarly, the combined treatment of ethanol and cocaine in adult male mice potentiated cocaine-induced toxicity characterized by elevated serum transaminase activity and frank intralobular necrosis,[60] reduced hepatic glutathione (GSH),[61] and increased hepatic lipoperoxidation.[62] Chronic ethanol consumption also increased chemically induced tumors[63,64] by inhibiting the repair of alkylated DNA;[65] it also serves as a promoter of hepatocellular carcinoma.[66]

The mechanisms of increased susceptibility of alcohol abusers to the adverse effects of various drugs has been reviewed recently.[67] The mechanisms include the effect of ethanol on the rate of drug uptake, the increase in drug-plasma protein binding that thereby increases the toxicity of the drug, the interaction with hepatic blood flow and hepatic uptake of drugs and alcohol, the binding of ethanol to the cytochrome P-450 system and subsequent spectrum modification, and the alteration of the ADH system by ethanol.[66]

ENZYMES AND NONENZYME SYSTEMS INVOLVED IN ALCOHOL HEPATOTOXICITY

The morbidity and mortality associated with alcohol abuse relates to its pervasive effects on all major organ systems. Because the liver is the major site of alcohol metabolism, the increased oxidative stress and the increased formation of free radicals and enhanced lipid peroxidation occurring in this organ profoundly affect hepatic antioxidants defense systems which are designed to protect against this oxidative injury. The antioxidant system may be divided into two major groups: (1) endogenous enzymic antioxidants which include superoxide dismutase (SOD), GSH-peroxidase, catalase, uric acid, and others; and (2) the antioxidants supplied by the diet, such as vitamins E and C, the carotenoids and some vitamin A-related compounds, and selenium (Se). These antioxidant systems detoxify the hepatotoxic free radicals, reactive electrophiles, and lipid peroxides formed by the interaction of O_2 species with unsaturated lipids of the cell.

ENDOGENOUS ANTIOXIDANT ENZYME SYSTEM

Glutathione Peroxidase

GSH-peroxidase is made up of four protein subunits, each of which contain one atom of the element Se at its active site.[67] Se deficiency causes a fall in enzyme activity to very low levels, often to <5% of control activity.[68] The enzyme is found at high activity in the livers of persons who are not drug abusers.[69] An early report by McCay et al.[70] suggested that GSH-peroxidase prevented lipid peroxidation. Later reports proposed that the lipoperoxidative actions of GSH-peroxidase were due to other proteins and were not Se dependent;[71] however, recent studies by Mercurio and Combs[72] and Takahashi et al.[73] support an antioxidant defense role for Se-dependent GSH.

The depletion of GSH, one of the major defenses against oxidative stress, renders the cell more susceptible to the development of peroxidation, cell damage, and lysis.[74] Ethanol enhances GSH depletion and potentiates acute hepatotoxicity.[75] Videla and co-workers[76,77] demonstrated that the administration of a single dose of 5 g of ethanol per kilogram of body weight to rats fasted overnight induced a drastic decrease in liver GSH after 6 h of intoxication. In humans[78] and rates,[79] acute ethanol consumption leads to an increase in plasma malondialdehyde and plasma GSH, reflecting increased utilization and loss of the enzyme from the liver. The mechanisms by which ethanol exerts this effect include (1) an inhibition of hepatic GSH synthesis,[80] (2) binding of GSH to acetaldehyde produced in the degradation of ethanol,[81] (3) oxidation of GSH by lipid peroxides produced by ethanol,[82] and (4) binding of acetaldehyde to cystine, a precursor of GSH,[83] to form the 2-mTCA (N-formyl-2,2-dimethylthiazolidine-4-carboxylic acid) derivative.[84]

Catalase

In animals, catalase is present in all major organs, being especially concentrated in liver and erythrocytes.[85] Most purified catalases consist of four protein subunits, each unit containing a heme (Fe(IIII)-protoporphyrin) group bound to its active site. Each subunit also usually contains one molecule of NADPH bound ot it, which helps to stabilize the enzyme.[1]

The catalase reaction may be written as follows:

$$\text{Catalase} - \text{Fe(III)} + \text{H}_2\text{O}_2 \qquad \text{Compound I}$$
$$\text{Compound I} + \text{H}_2\text{O}_2 \qquad \text{Catalase} - \text{Fe(III)} + \text{H}_2\text{O}_2 + \text{O}_2$$

The presence of peroxidatic substrates for catalase *in vivo* decreases the concentration of compound I, causing more free catalase to be formed.[86]

The catalase activity of animals is largely located in subcellular organelles bound by single membranes called peroxisomes. The peroxisomes also contain some of the cellular H_2O_2-generating enzymes, such as glycolate oxidase, urate oxidase, and the flavoprotein dehydrogenases involved in the β-oxidation of fatty acids. Ethanol oxidation by catalase occurs in the peroxisomes. As ethanol is a substrate for the peroxidative actions of catalase, it reduces the concentration of compound I and pyridine nucleotide, a substrate for ADL.[87,88]

Superoxide Dismutases (SODs)

SODs are metalloenzymes that catalyze the conversion of O_2^- to H_2O_2 and thus prevent accumulation of the oxygen radicals generated during alcohol and drug metabolism.

ANTIOXIDANT NUTRIENTS AND LIVER DAMAGE

Chronic alcohol abuse has profound effects when depleting hepatic levels of antioxidant nutrients and thus increasing liver damage. Therefore, the high intake of nutrients may retard such toxic effects. The mechanisms of protection against alcohol-induced hepatotoxicity conferred by nutrients include: (1) decreasing localized oxygen radical concentration; (2) preventing first-chain initiation by scavenging chain-initiating radicals such as OH·; (3) binding metal ions in forms that will not generate such chain-initiating species as OH·, ferryl, or $Fe^{2+}/Fe^{3+}/O_2$ and/or will not decompose lipid peroxides to peroxy or alkoxy radicals; (4) decomposing peroxides by converting them to non-radical products such as alcohol; and (5) indurating chain breakage or scavenging intermediate radicals such as peroxy and alkoxy radicals to prevent continuing hydrogen abstraction.[89] Some are preventive antioxidants, some are chain-breaking antioxidants, and others are repairing antioxidants that diminish the rate of lipid peroxidation.

Vitamin E (Tocopherol)

Vitamin E is a closely related family of compounds called the tocopherols. There are four major tocopherols with antioxidant activity. α-Tocopherol is the most biologically important of the group,[90] and the terms α-tocopherol and vitamin E will hereafter be used interchangeably. While vitamin E, compared to a number of synthetic phenols (butylated hydroxytoluene) used industrially is a relatively poor antioxidant, it is the most important antioxidant in humans.[91]

As vitamin E is fat soluble and hydrophobic, it tends to concentrate in the interior of membranes susceptible to oxidative damage. For example, the mitochondrial membranes contain about one molecule of α-tocopherol per 2100 molecules of phospholipid in blood lipoproteins and in the adrenal glands. Both the cortex and the medulla contain high levels of vitamin E because of the high content of oxygenase enzymes in the organs which increases their susceptibility to oxidative damage.[92,93]

Vitamin E functions *in vivo* to prevent lipid peroxidation, as indicated by its decreasing ethane exhalation and hepatic malondialdehyde formation.[94] It prevents lipid peroxidation by both quenching and reacting with singlet oxygen radicals. Vitamin E is oxidized by the superoxide generating system and, like most molecules, reacts with OH˙ at an almost diffusion-controlled rate.[95] During its action as a chain-breaking antioxidant in membranes, α-tocopherol is consumed and converted to the radical form;[96] however, mechanisms exist *in vivo* for restoring the radical to α-tocopherol. A synergism between vitamins E and C in trapping the free radical has been suggested.[97] Ascorbic acid reduces the α-tocopherol radical to α-tocopherol in intact membranes.[98,99] Thus, the addition of ascorbate to membranes containing vitamin E can have anti- as well as pro-oxidant effects.[100] Furthermore, vitamin E may also protect against peroxidation by modifying hepatic lipid components,[101] thus maintaining membrane structure. In the experiment conducted by Odeleye et al.,[101] rats fed alcoholic diets supplemented with vitamin E showed hepatic lipid composition and fatty acid profiles similar to the control rats.

Vitamin A-Related Compounds

Vitamin A consists of a large group of related substances with various structural characteristics and biological activity, the most important of which are the carotenoids.[102] Excluding the *cis-trans* isomers of a given carotenoid, the number of carotenoids is estimated at 563.[103] Using singlet oxygen quenching as the biological action for classification purposes, these carotenoids may be divided into four major categories.

1.   Biologically active as antioxidants and nutritionally active (β-carotene)
2.   Biologically active but nutritionally inactive (canthaxanthin)
3.   Biologically inactive but nutritionally active (β-apo-14-carotenal)
4.   Biologically and nutritionally inactive (phytoene)

The mechanism(s) by which β-carotene exert a protective effect in biological systems has generated considerable interest. β-Carotene may deactivate reactive chemical species such as singlet oxygen and free radicals[104] which would otherwise initiate harmful reactions such as lipid peroxidation. The effectiveness of β-carotene as a quencher of both singlet oxygen and reactive triplets sensitizers has been clearly demonstrated.[105,106]

Although β-carotene does not have the structural features commonly associated with chain-breaking antioxidants,[106] its carbon-centered radical, β-car˙ react rapidly and reversibly with oxygen to form a new chain-carrying peroxyl radical, β-car-OO.[89] The role of β-carotene as an antioxidant can be summarized as shown:

$$\beta\text{-carotene} + ROO^\bullet \quad \beta\text{-car}^\bullet$$
$$\beta\text{-car}^\bullet + O_2 \quad \beta\text{-car-OO}^\bullet$$

Dietary canthaxanthin has also been shown to increase resistance to lipid peroxidation by enhancing membrane α-tocopherol and by providing antioxidant activities.[107]

Vitamin C (Ascorbic Acid)

Ascorbic acid is required *in vivo* as a cofactor for several enzymes including proline hydroxylase and lysine hydroxylase, which are involved in the biosynthesis of collagen. Analysis of rat tissues show that next to the adrenal cortex and the kidney, the liver has the highest levels of semihydroascorbate reductase activity.[108]

Ascorbate acts as a reducing agent (electron donor), and reduces Fe(III) to Fe(II),[109] which promotes iron uptake from the gut. Ascorbate inhibits the carcinogenic actions of several nitroso compounds. This has been attributed to its ability to reduce the compounds to inactive forms.[110] Ascorbate may detoxify various organic radicals *in vivo* by a similar process. Donation of one electron by ascorbate gives the semidehydroascorbate radical, which can be further oxidized to give dehydroascorbase.

Dehydroascorbate is unstable and breaks down rapidly, producing oxalic acid and threonic acids.[111] Measurement of the quantitative yield of four isomeric conjugated diene hydroperoxides using methyl linoleate as a substrate by Nikki et al.[112] showed that vitamin C scavenges the chain carrying peroxy radicals and suppresses the oxidation of the substrate.

Ascorbate is also shown to scavenge OH˙ and singlet oxygen, react with O_2^-,[113] and inhibit ethane and pentane (indices of peroxidation) in guinea pigs.[114] In addition, ascorbate regenerates the chain-breaking antioxidant α-tocopherol in biological membranes.

EFFECTS OF ALCOHOL ABUSE ON NUTRITIONAL STATUS

Alcoholism has profound deteriorating effects on nutritional status.[115] Several alcohol-induced nutrient deficiencies in turn affect the metabolism of alcohol, aggravating its hepatotoxicity and nutritional status. Alcohol depresses appetite, displaces other foods and nutrients from the diet, and decreases the value of food by interfering with digestion and absorption. Even when nutrients are absorbed, alcohol prevents them from being fully utilized by altering their transportation, storage, and excretion. Patients hospitalized for medical complications associated with alcoholism may be severely malnourished in several nutrients, including protein and energy deficiencies. Such medical complications are known to be due to the direct and indirect effect of alcoholism on nutrient availability and utilization.[116]

INTERACTIONS OF ETHANOL WITH SPECIFIC NUTRIENTS

Macronutrients

Protein

When ethanol is consumed its calories may spare nitrogen utilization, thus preventing the muscle and other organs from breaking down their proteins for use as energy sources. When ethanol replaces carbohydrate calories, an increase occurs in nitrogen losses as urea.[117] Also, the ingestion of ethanol depresses protein synthesis, inhibits hepatic and muscular mitochondrial protein synthesis,[118] depresses serum albumin fraction and total protein,[119] impairs absorption and secretion of amino acids by liver, increases serum concentration of branched-chain amino acids,[120] and inhibits the secretion of albumin and plasma glycoprotein by the liver.[121-123]

Carbohydrates and Energy Balance

The effects of alcohol on carbohydrates and energy balance in epidemiological and clinical studies in human and experimental animals has been reviewed recently.[124] The calories in ethanol are inefficiently utilized by the body, expecially when the dose is high or when the subject is an alcoholic. Even when ethanol is ingested as extra calories, it causes less weight gain than calorically equivalent amounts of carbohydrate or fat,[125] and no weight gain occurs in lean individuals.[126] The lack of energy gained from alcohol is a direct toxic effect of ethanol metabolism in the liver. The MEOS induced or activated by chronic consumption of high alcohol levels consumes NADPH-related compounds without creating new ones.[127] Consequently, the energy released from the system is dissipated as heat. Chronic ethanol consumption results in a generalized depression in hepatic mitochondria energy metabolism. It decreases both the rate and efficiency of adenosine triphosphate (ATP) synthesis via the oxidative phosphorylation system.[122] Also, hormonal imbalances leading to reduced hepatic ATP content,[128] increased ATPase activity,[129] decreased oxygen utilization,[130] and the inhibition of glucose metabolism under oxygen-poor conditions may explain the lack of weight gain commonly observed in alcohol abusers. Furthermore, ethanol, unlike carbohydrates, induces lipogenic enzymes by reducing the activity of lactate dehydrogenase and malic enzymes, increases ATP citrate lyase,[131] increases blood acetaldehyde,[132] and depresses microsomal cardiac protein synthesis.[133] Finally, ethanol consumption may affect absorption of nutrients, and hence weight gain.

Alcohol also affects carbohydrate metabolism via its regulation of pancreatic enzymes. SanKaran et al.[134] showed that the acinar content of amylase and the acinar response to cholecystokinin-octapeptide are significantly lower in rats fed diets containing 26% calories as ethanol. Human alcohol abusers with liver cirrhosis have decreased insulin sensitivity and glucose-6-phosphatase, increased hexokinase activity, low or absent glucokinase activity, and a reduced glucokinase/hexokinase ratio.[135] The resultant changes in these pancreatic enzymes lead to the glucose intolerance and insulin resistance observed in chronic alcohol abusers.

Lipids

Many biochemical abnormalities in lipid metabolism result from intoxication or chronic alcohol usage. When alcohol is present in the system, it displaces fat as the primary fuel in the liver, resulting in hepatic accumulation of fat. These lipids originate from dietary lipids that reach the bloodstream and the liver as chylomicrons, adipose tissue lipids that are transported to the liver as free fatty acids, and lipids synthesized in the liver.[3] Metabolic disturbances in the equilibrium resulting from ethanol ingestion affect hepatic lipid accumulation by increasing the amounts of precursors for hepatic lipid synthesis, increasing hepatic lipogenesis via the stimulation of lipogenic enzymes, decreasing lipid breakdown, decreasing hepatic secretion of lipids, and enhancing hepatic uptake of circulating lipids.

Ethanol interferes with the supply of precursors of lipogenesis from extrahepatic sources by providing reducing equivalents and carbon units for lipid biosynthesis.[136] The altered redox state inhibits the oxidation of fatty acids and diverts them into esterification, which is further enhanced by the increased concentration of glycerol-3-phosphate.[137,138] Ethanol also increases the amount of fatty acid transported from the adipose tissue and the small intestine into the liver where they are then deposited.[139]

Ethanol may also increase the rate of triglyceride synthesis by stimulating the enzymes catalyzing triglyceride synthesis. Both acute and chronic ethanol consumption stimulate phosphatidate phosphohydrolase in the microsomal and soluble fractions of the mitochondria,[140] and the increase in enzyme activity leads to the accumulation of hepatic triglycerides.[141] Similarly, the increased phospholipid content of the liver after chronic ethanol administration[142] is accounted for by the increased activity of two enzymes involved in the synthesis of phosphatidyl choline: choline phosphotransferase and phosphatidyl ethanolamine methyltransferase.[143]

The accumulation of esterified lipids in the alcoholic fatty liver results from an impaired capacity of lysosomal lipase and esterase to hydrolyze the glycerol esters. Chronic ethanol administration decreased or did not alter the activity of lysosomal enzymes,[144] and it decreased the activity of microsomal and cytosolic phospholipase A[145] required for the hydrolysis of hepatic cholesterol. Furthermore, the ingestion of ethanol increases the bile acids in the liver[146] while it depresses its glandular secretion.[147] This reduction in biliary secretion of bile acids is secondary to the diminution in cholesterol 7-α-hydroxylase activity and the accumulation of cholesteryl esters in the liver.[148]

Chronic alcohol exposure increases,[149] decreases,[150] or has no effect[151,152] on tissue cholesterol levels. Some authors observed little or no change in hepatic phospholipids.[142,153,154] The variations of these results may be due to differences in the species studied, the route of administration, the dose and duration of alcohol delivered, and the constituents of the administered diet. More significant effects of alcohol on tissue lipids are noted in the fatty acid redistribution. Reduced levels of arachidonic acid, a polyunsaturated fatty acid, has been observed in rat liver,[156,157] red blood cells,[158-160] platelets,[161,162] and the heart.[163] Littleton et al.[164] reported a significant decline in docosanhexaenoic acid (22:6 or 3) in mouse brain after a 2-h ethanol exposure. Similar changes in mouse brain synaptic membrane content of 22:6 or 3 in the phosphatidylserine was observed following 7 d of dietary ethanol.[155] It is, therefore, evident that ethanol metabolism exerts a degree of plasticity to the hepatic and brain polyunsaturate composition in animals.

MINERALS

CALCIUM

Alcohol abuse may directly affect Ca balance by altering water balance through its diuretic effects.[165] Negative Ca balance may also occur secondarily to fat malabsorption in human alcoholic patients[166] and in rodents.[167] However, because abnormalities of bone metabolism are prominent in alcohol abusers, some other factors distinct from reduced absorption may be involved in the negative Ca balance accompanying alcoholism.

MAGNESIUM

Severe depletion of Mg and its associated enzymatic activities is a frequent occurrence in alcohol abusers.[168] This depletion is attributed to decreased Mg intake, malabsorption, alcohol-induced Mg losses in the urine, vomiting, and diarrhea.[168] However, a positive balance occurs on withdrawal from alcohol, and Mg therapy can be used to reverse the low levels of the mineral in Mg-deficient alcohol abusers.[169]

IRON

Fe is a constituent of hemoglobin and certain enzymes involved in energy production. Alcohol abusers frequently are Fe deficient, which is a complicated physiological occurrence. Elevated serum Fe is often seen in active alcohol abusers, but this level drops quickly with abstinence.[170] Patients with alcoholic liver disease show a sevenfold increase in erythrocyte ferritin content.[171] This increase is the result of the high Fe content of the alcoholic beverages consumed, increased secretion of hydrochloric acid produced in the stomach by alcohol, and inhibition of a coenzyme (pyridoxal kinase) by ethanol which interrupts utilization and results in increased serum Fe levels.[172] In some cases, Fe deficiency may occur from increased gastrointestinal blood loss secondary to gastritis or cirrhosis.[172] Other reports[173] found increased rather than decreased Fe absorption in chronic alcoholism. This increased hepatic Fe content, resulting in siderosis, may be damaging to the liver.

ZINC

A depleted Zn status is a common finding in chronic and acute alcohol abusers.[174,175] Depletion can be as low as 60% of that of normal levels in chronic alcohol abusers with cirrhotic livers.[176,177] It is argued that reduced food intake during alcohol consumption may play a significant role in the maintenance of serum Zn levels. Thus, acute intake of ethanol in humans did not affect plasma Zn concentration anymore than that seen by the low intake of food alone.[178] Similarly, moderate doses of alcohol in rats as part of an adequate diet resulted in decreases of both serum and hepatic Zn levels similar to those caused by dietary Zn deficiency alone.[179]

Zn is a component of various enzyme systems, and is required for the maintenance of healthy skin, bones, and hair, and in the storage and mobilization of vitamin A. The impaired night vision commonly seen in alcohol abusers is a result of the derangement of vitamin A metabolism secondary to Zn deficiency.[175,180] Zn is associated with insulin in the β cells of the pancreas and for optimum humoral immune defense.[181,182] Several of the biochemical and physiological functions of Zn are affected by alcohol intake.[179] Alcohol and Zn interact to impair each other's metabolism.[179,183] Administration of a high Zn diet (10 ppm) containing 30% ethanol as calories to pregnant and lactating rats and their offspring lowered maternal Zn status to values similar to those fed low Zn diets (2 ppm) without alcohol. Furthermore, the levels of serum Zn and alkaline phosphatase were depressed in the offspring in the alcohol-fed rats.[183]

SELENIUM

In trace quantities, Se is an essential nutrient and induces antioxidant activity. Low blood Se levels are associated with abnormal liver structure and functions.[184,185] Alcohol abusers tend to be deficient in Se in the absence of severe liver disease or inadequate intake.[186] This may contribute to hepatic injuries via increased lipid peroxidation and the associated damage of liver-cell membranes.[187] Se depletion in alcohol abusers has been attributed to poor dietary intake.[185] Plasma Se also decreases in patients with nonalcoholic liver injury.[188,189] Therefore, Se deficiency may contribute to alcoholic liver injury, and low Se levels may be a consequence of liver injury.

VITAMINS

WATER-SOLUBLE

Thiamin

Although severe thiamin deficiency is uncommon in industrialized countries, an appreciable number of alcohol abusers are mildly deficient. This deficiency status results in disastrous neurological and cardiac disorders.[190] Deficient thiamin status has been found in many alcohol abusers. In a study of a drinking population, Leevy et al.[191] found that 30% of malnourished alcohol abusers had blood thiamin levels 20% lower than the lowest limit of healthy individuals. A low or deficient excretion of thiamin in the urine was found in 27% of alcohol abusers admitted to a hospital.[192] Similarly, between 20 to 73% of an alcoholic population were found to have a high risk of thiamin deficiency, as estimated by erythrocyte transketolase activity.[193] Alcoholism is a major cause of the thiamin deficiency seen in hospitals, with 43% low in B_1 status, and 65% of those were alcohol abusers. Thiamin status in alcohol abusers is partly due to impaired intestinal absorption.[195] In animal experiments, ethanol disturbs both *in vitro* and *in vivo* the active transport of thiamin across the intestinal wall.[195] Alcohol consumption-associated malnutrition also contributes to the high incidence of thiaminase deficiency observed in alcoholics.[197] Over 70% of alcohol abusers were found to have a deficient intake of thiamin estimated by the 7-d dietary recall.[198] The amount of alcohol ingested is also shown to affect the thiamin status of alcohol abusers;[192] however, the ease and safety of administration during the treatment of alcoholism revealed that thiamin reverses some of the clinical deficiency symptoms and the neurological disorders of alcohol-induced thiamin deficiency.[199,200]

Riboflavin (B_2)

Riboflavin deficiency is prevalent in alcohol abusers,[201,202] and seems to be mainly due to poor dietary intake, as ethanol has no effect on the B_2 absorption.[203a] However, riboflavin deficiency can complicate chronic alcoholism,[203] and chronic alcohol feeding can induce riboflavin deficiency when intake of the vitamin is marginal.[204,205]

Pyridoxine (B_6)

Pyridoxine (vitamin B_6) is required for normal cellular metabolism, growth, and development, particularly of the brain and CNS. In surveys of the B_6 status of alcohol abusers, lower than normal mean circulating levels have been noted.[206,207] About 50% of the alcohol abusers studied have deficient levels of the vitamin and its cofactor, 5-pyridoxal phosphate. Also, 65 of 113 alcohol abusers showed an abnormal handling of tryptophan,[208] indicative of a B_6 deficiency.

The main reason for the low circulating levels seen in alcohol abusers seems to be an abnormal handling of vitamin B_6 by alcohol abusers. Ethanol does not interfere with the passive diffusion of B_6, but it does inhibit enzymes in the intestinal lining that remove the phosphate groups of phosphorylated B_6.[173] Alcohol and acetaldehyde accelerate intracellular degradation of 5-pyridoxal phosphate,[209,210] decrease its activation by inhibiting pyridoxine kinase,[211] and reduce the availability of dietary pyridoxine.[212] Alcohol-induced vitamin B_6 deficiencies also cause depression[213] via decreased neurotransmitter synthesis and reduced brain neurotransmitter synthesis. Vitamin B_6 deficiency also reduces cellular transfer of amino acids via deficient pituitary growth hormone secretion.[212]

Folic Acid

In the U.S. folate deficiency is predominantly associated with alcoholism, poverty, and old age.[214] Folate deficiency is found in about 20 to 50% of alcohol abusers,[214,215] and the anemia seen in alcohol abusers is frequently associated with impaired folate status and activity.[216,217] Several factors contribute to these low folate levels in alcohol abusers, including decreased food intake,[217] the type and amount of alcoholic beverage consumed,[218] decreased folate absorption,[219] interference with folate storage and release, and the interference of folate utilization in the functional tissue pool by alcohol.[220] Alcohol ingestion accelerates the rate of decrease in circulating folate levels[221,222] and reduces the absorption[223] and tissue uptake[224] of folic acid, thus causing a further decrease in circulating folate levels. The reduced folate status in turn provides a malabsorption of folic acid.[219,225] This leads eventually to depletion of the body folate stores and overt signs of folate deficiency.

Cobalamin (Vitamin B_{12})

Vitamin B_{12} functions mainly as a coenzyme involved in carbohydrate and fat metabolism. The effect of chronic and acute alcoholism on B_{12} status was recently reviewed.[226] In a study of alcohol abusers, no abnormal B_{12} levels were found,[227] but impaired absorption of labeled vitamin B_{12}, as measured by the percentage of the oral dose excreted in the feces, was observed in alcoholic cirrhotic patients.[228] As most alcoholic drinks contain considerable amounts of folate which masks the gross deficiency symptoms of B_{12}, deficiency of this vitamin is not seen frequently in alcohol abusers. However, absorption is impaired in chronic alcohol abusers,[229,230] probably through interference at the site of active transport in the terminal portion of the small intestine.

Niacin

Reports conflict on the effects of alcohol on niacin levels in alcohol abusers. Some studies reported low circulating levels,[231,232] whereas others found no differences in circulating niacin levels[203,233] or in urinary excretion of n-methyl nicotinamide[192] between alcohol abusers and controls. Niacin intake did not differ greatly between alcohol abusers and abstainers,[229,234] especially when the intake of tryptophan, which can be partially converted into niacin, is also considered.

Pantothenic Acid

The few studies investigating pantothenic acid status in alcohol abusers found lower urinary excretion[235] and mean circulating levels[230,232] than in nondrinking controls; however, the mechanisms leading to these reduced levels in alcohol abusers have not been elucidated. Human alcohol abusers with liver diseases have been shown to have depleted pantothenic acid levels related to the extent of liver damage.[234] These findings could also be interpreted in terms of duration of alcoholism, and thus of duration of reduced pantothenic acid intake. Alcohol does not affect the pantothenic status of humans[236] and rats[237] fed a nutritionally adequate diet. Nevertheless, the decrease in pantothenic acid secretion found in rehabilitated alcohol abusers[235] may indicate a problem in the utilization of this vitamin.

Biotin

The role of biotin in human and animal nutrition has not yet been completely elucidated.[238] In alcohol abusers, both circulating levels and liver contents of biotin are reduced.[239] This low level is generally associated with the development of fatty liver. As no effect of ethanol per se has been noted on circulating and hepatic biotin levels, the low levels found in alcohol abusers are probably of a nutritional origin.[239]

Ascorbic Acid (Vitamin C)

Surprisingly, very few studies on the vitamin C status in alcohol abusers have been published. These investigations found not only reduced mean circulating levels but also a high frequency of deficiency levels.[206,240,241]

Vitamin C deficiency in chronically alcohol-fed guinea pigs reduced the efficiency of the microsomal ethanol oxidizing system,[240] and lowered the rate of decline of infused ethanol.[242] Ascorbic acid protects against the harmful effect of acetaldehyde on the heart,[243,244] causes weight gain,[242] and protects against toxicity[245] in alcohol-fed animals.

FAT-SOLUBLE

Vitamin A

Although dietary vitamin A deficiency is not a serious health problem in the general population, its level is adversely affected in chronic alcohol abusers.[246,247] While people who derive <20% of their daily dietary calories from alcohol ingest a normal amount of vitamin A,[248] heavier drinkers consume 75% or less of the recommended daily allowance of vitamin A.[249] Low vitamin A status has also been observed in Norwegians who consume large amounts of alcohol.[250] Ethanol and vitamin A consumption synergistically increase tracheal cancers in alcohol abusers,[251] and deficiency of vitamin A increases the susceptibility to neoplasia and carcinogenesis.[252] However, decreased nutritional intake alone does not fully explain why patients with alcoholic liver disease have very low hepatic vitamin A at all stages in the development of the disease. Experimental administration of ethanol in nutritionally adequate and even in vitamin A-supplemented diets resulted in a depression of liver vitamin A stores.[253] Thus, the low vitamin A stores of alcohol abusers may not be attributed to insufficient vitamin A consumption or to impaired absorption by the digestive system alone.[254]

Other mechanisms proposed to explain the interaction of the depletion of vitamin a status via ethanol include the increased mobilization of vitamin A from the liver to other organs. This view is consistent with the observation that after chronic ethanol consumption, vitamin A in peripheral tissue increased, even when hepatic vitamin A was depleted.[255,256] An acute, nonlethal dose of ethanol significantly increased retinyl esters in serum lipoprotein and decreased hepatic vitamin A stores.[257] These findings suggest that a shift of vitamin A from the liver to other organs through lipoprotein-bound retinyl esters occurs as a result of ethanol administration.

The second mechanism for hepatic depletion of vitamin A following ethanol consumption involves increased catabolism. Retinol is mobilized from the liver on retinol-binding protein which can be metabolized to retinal and retinoic acid via the cytosolic and retinol and retinal dehydrogenase.[258]

Retinoic acid, in turn, can be degraded through a microsomal cytochrome P-450-mediated enzyme activity. Therefore, ethanol consumption could decrease hepatic vitamin A, in part through increased metabolism in the liver. Indeed, Odeleye et al.[259] recently showed that rats fed ethanol exhibited increased lipid peroxidation and reduced vitamin A levels, while rats fed diets supplemented with vitamin E showed reduced lipid peroxidation and increased hepatic vitamin A levels. Odeleye and co-workers hypothesized that this result can be explained by the sparring action of vitamin E on vitamin A stores in alcoholism.

Vitamin D

Vitamin D metabolism is adversely affected by chronic alcohol abuse. In alcohol abusers with or without liver disease, significantly lower plasma levels of vitamin D have been reported in about 45% of the population studied.[260,261] The reasons for this depletion are multifactorial and include poor diet, reduced exposure to sunshine, malabsorption (especially in cases of fat malabsorption),[261,262] and an increased rate of vitamin D degradation.[263] The reduction in circulating vitamin D levels in alcohol abusers results in reduced bone mass and low calcium levels, arising from reduced absorption and mobilization.[165,265] Also, since vitamin D plays a vital role in glucose metabolism via a direct regulatory role in maintaining insulin levels,[265,266] alcohol-induced vitamin D deficiencies result in the impairment of insulin response by a reduced secretion and a delayed response to glucose.[267,268]

Vitamin E

Vitamin E, because of its antioxidant properties, has received tremendous attention in human nutrition. As the major antioxidant in the membrane, vitamin E is often referred to as the backbone of defense against alcohol- and drug-induced lipid peroxidation.[269,270] Studies indicate that ethanol consumption reduced the mean circulating and hepatic stores of vitamin E in rats[271,272] and in human alcohol abusers.[273-275]

Mechanism(s) leading to reduced circulating levels of vitamin E in alcohol abusers have not yet been fully explained; however, dietary intake, malabsorption and β-lipoprotein deficiency in liver disease may all contribute.[276] Feeding ethanol to rats resulted in increased hepatic α-tocopherol quinone, a metabolite of α-tocopherol by free radical reaction,[277] thus indicating that ethanol enhances the degradation of vitamin E.

Vitamin K

Vitamin K is present in a variety of foods. It is required only in relatively small amounts by man, and since part of the vitamin K requirement may be covered by intestinal syntheiss, a significant deficiency status would be very rarely encountered and very difficult to produce in humans. However, a combination of sterilization of the large intestine, pancreatic insufficiency, cholestatis, or an abnormality secondary to folate deficiency may lead to vitamin K deficiency. Nevertheless, lengthening of prothrombin time has been observed only in patients with a severe liver disease such as alcoholic and nonalcoholic cirrhosis and chronic active hepatic disease.[279] Although the prevalence of this reduced prothrombin tissue has not been compared in alcohol-induced liver disease and nonalcoholic liver disease, this reduced prothrombin time in alcoholics shows that alcohol-induced liver injury interferes with vitamin K utilization.

CONCLUSIONS

Ethanol-induced hepatotoxicity is associated with a variety of nutritional abnormalities and is multifactorial. Chronic alcohol abusers show evidence of nutritional deficiencies due to decreased intake, poor absorption, and impaired storage, utilization, and metabolism of essential nutrients. In addition, abuse of this drug depletes tissue levels and/or activities of the inherent antioxidant enzymes and dietary antioxidants that protect the biological system against reactive electrophiles generated from the oxidative degradation or metabolism of these drugs. Thus, the multifactorial effect of drug abuse on nutritional status is an undisputed factor in the pathogenesis of liver damage.

Many nutrients have been examined in humans and animals, including protein and amino acids, fatty acids, carbohydrates, folic acids, thiamin, ascorbic acid, riboflavin, Zn, Se, and Fe. Of these, protein, vitamin E- and vitamin A-related substances, and Se are the most studied. Data thus far accumulated consistently indicate that the nutritional deficiencies in the abusers clearly potentiate ethanol hepatotoxicity. Thus, when the abuser is in an adequate nutritional state the effect of the liver damage caused by ethanol may not be as severe. Nutritional support in the treatment of alcoholics with liver disease is indicated not only on the basis of the high frequency of malnutrition in these patients, but by the link between malnutrition immunocompetence, infection, and mortality. Nutrient supplementation and alteration of the dietary constituents of foods to compensate for losses in alcoholic patients may be inimical toward a complete recovery from alcoholism. However, more extensive investigations are needed, including studies of a dose-response relationship, and the effect of alcohol abuse on the nutritional status, in order to establish the beneficial effects of dietary nutrients supplementation on improving not only the nutritional status, but also the antioxidant defense systems. Results from such studies may provide necessary information in nutritional programs designed to "treat" alcohol-related diseases.

ACKNOWLEDGMENT

This review and our studies cited here are supported by NIAAA Grant 08037.

REFERENCES

1. Kirkman, H. N., Galiano, S., and Gaetani, G. F., The function of catalase bound NADPH, *J. Biol. Chem.*, 262, 660, 1987.
2. Watkins, I. A., Kawanishi, S., and Caughey, W. S., Autoxidation reactions of hemoglobin A free from other red cell components: a minimal mechanism, *Biochem. Biophys. Res. Commun.*, 132, 742, 1985.
3. Fridovich, I., Superoxide dismutases, *Adv. Enzymol.*, 58, 61, 1986.
4. Burk, R. F., Protection against free radical injury by selenoenzymes, *Pharmacol. Ther.*, 45, 383, 1990.
5. Burton, G. W., Antioxidant actions of carotenoids, *J. Nutr.*, 119, 109, 1989.
6. Kim, C., Leo, M. A., Lowe, N., and Lieber, C. S., Differential effects of retinoids and chronic ethanol consumption on membranes in rats, *J. Nutr.*, 118, 1097, 1988.
7. Nikki, E., Saito, T., and Kamiya, Y., The role of vitamin C as an antioxidant, *Chem. Lett. (Japan)*, 14, 631, 1983.
8. Burton, G. W. and Ingold, K. U., Vitamin E as an *in vitro* and *in vivo* antioxidant, *Ann. N.Y. Acad. Sci.*, 570, 7, 1985.
9. Freeman, A. B. and Crapo, J. D., Biology of disease: free radicals and tissue injury, *Lab. Invest.*, 47, 412, 1982.
10. Comporti, B., Biology of disease: lipid peroxidation and cellular damage in toxic liver injury, *Lab. Invest.*, 53, 599, 1985.
11. Gruenewald, P. J., Stewart, K., and Klitzner, M., Alcohol use and the appearance of alcohol problems among first offender drunk drivers, *Br. J. Addict.*, 85, 107, 1990.
12. Lieber, C. S. and Savolainen, M., Ethanol and lipids, *Alcohol. Clin. Exp. Res.*, 8, 409, 1983.

13. Lebsak, M. E., Gordon, E. R., and Lieber, C. S., The effect of chronic ethanol consumption on aldehyde dehydrogenase activity, *Biochem. Pharmacol.*, 30, 2273, 1981.

14. Tottman, S., Petterson, H., and Kiessling, K. H., The subcellular distribution and properties of aldehyde dehydrogenase in rat liver, *Biochem. J.*, 135, 577, 1973.

15. Lieber, C. S., Metabolism and metabolic effects of alcohol, *Med. Clin. North Am.*, 68, 3, 1984.

16. Tuma, D. S., Zetterman, R. K., and Sorrell, M. F., Inhibition of glycoprotein secretion by ethanol and acetaldehyde in rat liver slices, *Biochem. Pharmacol.*, 29, 35, 1980.

17. Watson, R. R., Mohs, M. E., Eskelson, C. D., Sampliner, R. E., and Hartman, B., Identification of alcohol abuse and alcoholism with biological parameters, *Alcohol. Clin. Exp. Res.*, 10, 364, 1986.

18. Cunnane, S. C., McAdoo, K. R., and Horrobin, D. F., Long-term ethanol consumption in the hamster: effects of tissue lipids, fatty acids and erythrocyte hemolysis, *Ann. Nutr. Metab.*, 31, 265, 1987.

19. Lieber, C. S. and DeCarli, L. M., Hepatic microsomal ethanol oxidized system: *in vitro* characteristics and adaptive properties *in vivo*, *J. Biol. Chem.*, 245, 2505, 1970.

20. Ugarte, G., Ituoriaga, H., and Pereda, T., Possible relationship between the role of ethanol metabolism and the severity of hepatic damage in chronic alcoholic, *Dig. Dis.*, 22, 406, 1977.

21. Videla, L. and Israel, Y., Factors that modify the metabolism of ethanol in rat liver and adaptive changes produced by its chronic administration, *Biochem. J.*, 118, 225, 1970.

22. Vaananen, H., Lindros, K. O., and Salaspuro, M., Distribution of ethanol metabolism in periportal and perivenous rat hepatocytes after chronic ethanol treatment, *Liver*, 4, 72, 1984.

23. Vaananen, H., Salaspuro, M., and Lindros, K. O., Ethanol metabolizing enzymes in isolated periportal and perivenous rat hepatocytes: changes after chronic ethanol injection, *Hepatology*, 4, 862, 1984.

24. Edward, J. A. and Price-Evans, D. A., Ethanol metabolism in subjects possessing typical and atypical liver dehydrogenase, *Clin. Pharmacol. Ther.*, 8, 824, 1967.

25. Theorell, H. and Bonnichsen, R., Studies in liver dehydrogenase. Equilibria and initial reaction velocities, *Acta Chem. Scand.*, 5, 1105, 1951.

26. Cedarbaum, A. I., Regulation of pathways of alcohol metabolism in the liver, *Mt. Sinai Med.*, 47, 317, 1980.

27. Koop, D. R., Morgan, E. T., Taff, G. E., and Coon, M. J., Purification and characterization of a unique isozopure of cytochrome P-450 from liver microsomes of ethanol-treated rabbits, *J. Biol. Chem.*, 257, 8472, 1982.

28. Thurman, R. G. and Brentzel, H. J., The role of alcohol dehydrogenase in microsomal ethanol oxidation and the adaptive increase in ethanol metabolism due to chronic treatment with ethanol, *Alcoholism Clin. Exp. Res.*, 1, 33, 1977.

29. Thurman, R. G., McKenna, W. R., Brentzel, J. H., and Hesse, A., Significant pathway of ethanol metabolism, *Fed. Proc.*, 34, 2075, 1975.

30. Ishii, H., Joly, J. G., and Lieber, C. S., Effect of ethanol on the amount and enzyme activities of hepatic rough and smooth microsomal membranes, *Biochim. Biophys. Acta,* 291, 411, 1973.

31. Takagi, T., Alderman, I., and Lieber, C. S., *In vivo* roles of alcohol dehydrogenase (ADH), catalase and the microsomal ethanol oxidized system (MEOS) in deer mice, *Alcohol,* 2, 9, 1985.

32. Lieber, C. S., Metabolism of ethanol, in *Medical Disorders of Alcoholism: Pathogenesis and Treatment,* Lieber, C. S., Ed., W. B. Saunders, Philadelphia, 1982, 178.

33. Lieber, C. S. and Savolainen, M., Ethanol and lipids, *Alcohol. Clin. Exp. Res.,* 8, 409, 1984.

34. Bunout, D., Gattas, V., Ituoriaga, H., Perez, C., Pereda, T., and Ugarte, G., Nutritional studies of alcoholic patients: its possible relationship to alcoholic liver damage, *Am. J. Clin. Nutr.,* 38, 469, 1983.

35. Rao, G. A., Riley, D. E., and Larkin, E. C., Dietary carbohydrate stimulates alcohol ingestion, promotes growth and prevents fatty liver in rats, *Nutr. Res.,* 7, 81, 1987.

36. Martini, G. A. and Teschke, R., Alcohol abstinence in alcoholic liver disease, *Acta Med. Scand. (Suppl.),* 703, 185, 1988.

37. Scheuer, P. J., The morphology of alcoholic liver disease, *Br. Med. Bull.,* 38, 63, 1982.

38. Desmet, V. J., Alcohol liver disease. Histological features and evolution, *Acta Med. Scand.,* 703, 111, 1988.

39. MacSween, R. N., Alcoholic liver disease, in *Recent Advances in Hepatology,* Thomas, A. C. and MacSween, R. N., Eds., Churchill Livingstone, Edinburgh, 1983, 71.

40. Popper, H., Thung, S. N., and Gerber, M. A., Pathology of alcoholic liver disease, *Semin. Liver Dis.,* 1, 203, 1981.

41. Sherlock, S., Alcoholic liver disease: clinical patterns and diagnosis, *Acta Med. Scand.,* 703, 103, 1988.

42. Szebeni, J., Eskelson, C. D., Sampliner, R., Hartman, B., Griffin, J., Dormandy, T., and Watson, R. R., Plasma fatty acid pattern including diene conjugates linoleic acid in ethanol users and in patients with ethanol related liver disease, *Alcohol. Clin. Exp. Res.,* 18, 647, 1988.

43. Mezey, E., Ethanol metabolism and ethanol-drug interaction, *Biochem. Pharmacol.,* 25, 869, 1976.

44. World, M. J., Ryle, P. R., and Thompson, A. D., Alcoholic malnutrition and the small intestine, *Alcohol Alcohol.,* 20, 89, 1985.

45. Orrego, H., Israel, Y., and Blendis, L. M., Alcoholic liver disease: information in search of knowledge, *Hepatology,* 1, 267, 1981.

46. Rubin, E. and Lieber, C. S., Early five structural changes in the human liver induced by alcohol, *Gastroenterology,* 52, 1, 1967.

47. Lieber, C. S. and Rubin, E., Ethanol — an hepatotoxic drug, *Gastroenterology,* 54, 557, 1968.

48. Patrick, R. S. and McGee, J. D., Inhibition of drug metabolism by acute ethanol intoxication: a hepatic microsomal mechanism, in *Biopsy Pathology of Liver,* Walker, F. and Neville, A. M., Eds., Chapman & Hall, London, 1980, 189.

49. Lieber, C. S., Garro, A., Leo, M. A., Mak, K. M., and Warner, T., Alcohol and cancer, *Hepatology,* 6, 1005, 1986.

50. Polokoff, M. A., Simon, T. J., Harris, R. A., Simon, F. R., and Iwahashy, M., Chronic ethanol increases liver plasma membrane fluidity, *Biochemistry,* 24, 3114, 1985.

51. Schuller, A., Moscat, J., Diez, E., Checa-Fernandez, C., Gavilanes, F. E., and Municio, A., The fluidity of plasma membrane from ethanol-treated rat liver, *Mol. Cell Biochem.,* 64, 89, 1984.

52. Dianzani, M. U., Lipid peroxidation in ethanol poisoning: a critical reconsideration, *Alcohol Alcohol.,* 20, 161, 1985.

53. Worrall, S., De-Jersey, J., Shanley, B. C., and Wilce, P. A., Ethanol induces the production of antibodies to acetaldehyde-modified epitopes in rats, *Alcohol Alcohol.,* 24, 217, 1989.

54. Rubin, E., Gang, H., Misra, P. S., and Lieber, C. S., Inhibition of drug metabolism by acute ethanol intoxication: a hepatic microsomal mechanism, *Am. J. Med.,* 49, 801, 1970.

55. Schuppel, R., The influence of acute ethanol administration on drug conjugation in the rat, *Naunyn-Schmiedeberg's Arch. Exp. Pathol. Pharmakol.,* 265, 233, 1969.

56. Kaplan, H. L., Jain, N. C., Forney, R. B., and Richards, A. B., Chloral hydrate-ethanol interactions in the mouse and dog, *Toxicol. Appl. Pharmacol.,* 14, 127, 1969.

57. Caballeria, J., Baroana, E., Rodamilans, M., and Lieber, C. S., Effect of cimetidine on gastric alcohol dehydrogenase activity and blood ethanol level, *Gastroenterology,* 97, 388, 1989.

58. Caballeria, J., Baroana, E., Rodamilans, M., and Lieber, C. S., Cimetidine and alcohol absorption, *Gastroenterology,* 97, 1067, 1989.

59. Kissing, B., Interactions of ethyl alcohol and other drugs, in *The Biology of Alcoholism, Clinical Pathology,* Vol. 3, Kissing, B. and Begleiter, H., Eds., Plenum Press, New York, 1974, 109.

60. Smith, A., Freeman, R. N., and Harbison, R. D., Ethanol enhancement of cocaine-induced hepatotoxicity, *Biochem. Pharmacol.,* 30, 453, 1981.

61. Boyer, C. S. and Petersen, D. R., Potentiation of cocaine-mediated hepatotoxicity for acute and chronic ethanol, *Alcohol. Clin. Exp. Res.,* 14, 28, 1990.

62. Odeleye, O. E. and Watson, R. R., Is the Lieber-DeCarli diet adequate in vitamin E?, *Alcohol Alcohol.,* 25, 433, 1990.

63. Teschke, R., Minzlaff, M., Oldiges, H., and Frenzel, H., Alcohol consumption and tumor incidence due to diamethylnitrosamine administration, *Alcohol Alcohol.,* 18, 129, 1983.

64. Mufti, S. I., Becker, G., and Sipes, I. G., Effect of chronic dietary ethanol consumption on the initiation and promotion of chemically-induced esophageal carcinogenesis in experimental rats, *Carcinogenesis,* 10, 303, 1989.

65. Mufti, S. I., Salvagnini, M., Lieber, C. S., and Garro, A. T., Chronic ethanol consumption inhibit repair of dimethylnitrosamine-induced DNA alkylation, *Biochem. Biophys. Res. Commun.,* 152, 423, 1988.

66. Ohnishi, K., Terabayashi, H., Unuma, T., Takahashi, A., and Okuda, K., Effect of habitual alcohol intake and cigarette smoking on the development of hepatocellular carcinoma, *Alcohol. Clin. Exp. Res.,* 11, 45, 1987.

67. Chance, B., Sies, H., and Boveris, A., Hydroperoxide metabolism in mammalian organ, *Physiol. Rev.*, 59, 527, 1979.
68. Burk, R. F., Protection against free radical injury by seleno enzymes, *Pharmacol. Ther.*, 45, 383, 1990.
69. Marklund, S. L., Caeruloplasm extracellular superoxide dismutase and scavenging, superoxide anion radicals, *J. Free Radicals Biol. Med.*, 2, 255, 1987.
70. McCay, P. B., Gibson, D. D., Fong, K. L., and Hornbrook, K. R., Effect of glutathione peroxidase activity on lipid peroxidation in biological membranes, *Biochim. Biophys. Acta*, 431, 459, 1976.
71. Burk, R. F., Lawrence, R. A., and Lane, J. M., Liver necrosis and lipid peroxidation in the rat as the result of paraquat and diquat administration, *J. Clin. Invest.*, 65, 1024, 1980.
72. Mercurio, S. D. and Combs, G. F., Selenium-dependent glutathione peroxidase inhibitors increase toxicity of pro-oxidant compounds, *J. Nutr.*, 116, 1726, 1986.
73. Takahashi, K., Newberger, P. E., and Cohen, H. J., Glutathione peroxidase protein. Absence of selenium deficiency states and correlation of enzymatic activity, *J. Clin. Invest.*, 77, 1402, 1986.
74. Nordmann, R., Ribiere, C., and Rovach, H., Ethanol-induced peroxidation and oxidative stress in extrahepatic tissues, *Alcohol Alcohol.*, 25, 231, 1990.
75. Strubelt, O., Yones, M., and Pentz, R., Enhancement by glutathione depletion of ethanol-induced acute hepatotoxicity *in vitro* and *in vivo*, *Toxicology*, 45, 213, 1987.
76. Videla, L. A., Ugarte, F. G., and Valenzuela, A., Effect of acute ethanol intoxication on the content of glutathione of the liver in relation to its lipoperoxidative capacity in the rat, *FEBS Lett.*, 111, 6, 1980.
77. Fernandez, V. and Videla, L. A., Effect of acute and chronic ethanol ingestion on the content of reduced glutathione of various tissues of the rat, *Experientia*, 37, 392, 1981.
78. Vendemials, G., Altomase, E., Grattagliano, I., and Albano, O., Increased plasma levels of glutathione and malondialdehyde after acute ethanol ingestion in humans, *J. Hepatol.*, 9, 359, 1989.
79. Pierson, J. L. and Mitchell, M. C., Increased hepatic efflux of glutathione after chronic ethanol feeding, *Biochem. Pharmacol.*, 35, 1533, 1986.
80. Spiesky, H., McDonald, A., Giles, G., Orrego, H., and Isreal, Y., Increased loss and decreased synthesis of hepatic glutathione after acute ethanol administration, *Biochem. J.*, 225, 565, 1985.
81. Vina, J., Estrella, J. M., Guerri, D., and Romero, F. J., Effect of ethanol on glutathione concentration in isolated hepatocyte, *Biochem. J.*, 188, 549, 1980.
82. Videla, L. A. and Valenzuela, A., Alcohol ingestion, liver glutathione and lipoperoxidation. Metabolic interrelationship and pathological implication, *Life Sci.*, 31, 2395, 1982.
83. Lieber, C. S., Metabolic effects of ethanol and its interaction with other drugs, hepatotoxic agents, vitamins and carcinogens: a 1988 update, *Semin. Liver Dis.*, 8, 47, 1988.

84. Nagasawa, H. T., Elberling, J. A., and DeMaster, E. G., Structural requirements for the sequestration of metabolically generated acetaldehyde, *J. Med. Chem.,* 23, 140, 1980.

85. Marklund, S. F., Westman, N. G., Lundgren, E., Roos, G., Copper and zinc containing superoxide dismutase, manganese-containing superoxide dismutase, catalase, and glutathione peroxidase in normal and neoplastic human cell lines and normal human tissues, *Cancer Res.,* 42, 1955, 1982.

86. Nicholls, P. and Schonbaum, G. R., Catalases, in *The Enzymes,* Vol. 8, Boyer, P. D., Hardy, H., and Myrback, H., Eds., Academic Press, New York, 1963, 147.

87. Cedarbaum, A. I. and Dicker, E., Inhibition of microsomal oxidation of alcohols and of hydroxyl radical scavenging agents by the iron-chelating agent desferrioxamine, *Biochem. J.,* 210, 107, 1983.

88. Nordman, R., Ribiere, C., and Rovach, H., Involvement of iron and iron-catalysed free radical production in ethanol metabolism and toxicity, *Enzyme,* 37, 57, 1987.

89. Halliwell, B. and Gutteridge, J. M., *Free Radicals in Biology and Medicine,* Clarendon Press, Oxford, 1989, 189.

90. Brown, J. T. and Charlwood, B. V., The accumulation of essential oils, tissue cultures of *Pelargonium fragrans* (wild), *FEBS Lett.,* 205, 117, 1986.

91. Ingold, I. C. U., Webb, A. C., Willer, D., Burton, G. W., Metcalfe, T. A., and Muller, D. P., Vitamin E remains the major lipid soluble, chain breaking antioxidant in human plasma, even in individuals suffering severe vitamin E deficiency, *Arch. Biochem. Biophys.,* 259, 224, 1987.

92. Gruger, E. H. and Tappel, A. L., Reactions of biological antioxidants. Composition of biological membranes, *Lipids,* 6, 147, 1971.

93. Benedetti, A. and Comporti, M., Formation, reactions and toxicity of aldehydes produced in the course of lipid peroxidation in cellular membranes, *Bioelectrochem. Bioenerg.,* 18, 187, 1987.

94. Odeleye, O. E., Eskelson, C. D., Watson, C. O., Watson, R. R., Mufti, S. I., and Chvapil, M., Vitamin E reduction of lipid peroxidation products in rats fed cod liver oil and ethanol, *Alcohol,* 8, 273, 1990.

95. Machlin, L. J., *Handbook of Vitamins,* Machlin, L. J., Ed., Marcel Dekker, New York, 96, 1987.

96. Niki, E., Saito, T., Kawakani, A., and Kamiya, Y., Inhibition of oxidation of methyl linoleate in solution by vitamin C and vitamin C, *J. Biol. Chem.,* 259, 4177, 1984.

97. Leung, H. W., Vang, M. J., and Mavis, R. D., The cooperative interaction between vitamin E and vitamin C in suppression of peroxidation of membrane phospholipids, *Biochim. Biophys. Acta,* 664, 266, 1981.

98. Packer, J. E., Slater, T. F., and Willson, R. L., Direct observation of a free radical interaction between vitamin A and vitamin C, *Nature,* 278, 737, 1979.

99. Niki, E., Tsuchiya, J., and Tanimura, Y., ESR study of radicals reactions with vitamin C, glutathione and thiophenol, *Chem. Lett.,* 789, 1982.

100. Wafers, H. and Sies, H., The protection by ascorbate and glutathione against lipid peroxidation is dependent on vitamin E, *Eur. J. Biochem.,* 174, 353, 1988.

101. Odeleye, O. E., Eskelson, C. D., Watson, R. R., Mufti, S. I., and Earnest, D., The effects of chronic ethanol and cod liver oil consumption on rat liver lipid composition: modulatory role of vitamin E, submitted to *Alcohol Alcoholism,* 1992.

102. Bendich, A. and Olson, J. A., Biological actions of the carotenoids, *FASEB J.,* 48, 292, 1988.

103. Straub, O., *Key to Carotenoids,* 2nd ed., Pfander, H., Ed., Birkhausen Verlag, Basel, 1987, 1.

104. Burton, G. W., Antioxidant actions of carotenoids, *J. Nutr.,* 119, 109, 1989.

105. Foote, C. S., Photosensitized oxidation and singlet oxygen: consequences in biological membranes, in *Free Radicals in Biology,* Vol. 2, Pryor, W. A., Ed., Academic Press, New York, 1976, 85.

106. Burton, G. W. and Ingold, K. U., B-carotene: an unusual type of lipid antioxidant, *Science,* 224, 569, 1984.

107. Mayne, S. T. and Parker, R. E., Antioxidant activity of dietary canthaxanthin, *Nutr. Cancer,* 12, 225, 1989.

108. Diliberto, E. J., Dean, G., Carter, C., and Allen, P. L., Tissue, subcellular and submitochondrial, distribution of semidehydroascorbate reductase. Possible role of semidehydroascorbate reductase in cofactor regeneration, *J. Neurochem.,* 39, 563, 1982.

109. Forni, L. G. and Willson, R. L., Vitamin C and consecutive hydrogen atom and electron transfer reaction in free radical protection: a novel catalytic role for glutathione, in *Protective Agents in Cancer,* McBrien, D. C. and Slatter, T. F., Eds., Academic Press, London, 1983, 159.

110. Kallitratos, G., Fasske, E., Donos, A., Vadalouka-Kalfaka, A., and Kou, V., The prophylactic and therapeutic effect of vitamin C on experiental malignant tumors, in *Protective Agents in Cancer,* McBrien, D. C. and Slatter, T. F., Eds., Academic Press, London, 1983, 221.

111. Bendich, A., The antioxidant role of vitamin C, *Adv. Free Radicals Biol. Med.,* 2, 419, 1986.

112. Nikki, E., Saito, T., and Kamiya, Y., The role of vitamin C as an antioxidant, *Chem. Lett. (Japan),* 631, 1983.

113. Halliwell, B., Wasil, M., and Grootveld, M., Biologically-significant scavenging of the myeloperoxidase-derived oxidant hypochlorous acid by ascorbic acid, *FEBS Lett.,* 213, 15, 1987.

114. Kunert, K. J. and Tappel, A. L., The effect of vitamin C on *in vivo* lipid peroxidation in guinea pigs as measured by pentane and ethane exhalation, *Lipids,* 18, 271, 1983.

115. Denney, R. C. and Johnson, R., Nutrition, alcohol, and drug abuse, *Proc. Nutr. Soc.,* 43, 265, 1984.

116. Lieber, C. S., The influence of alcohol on nutritional status, *Nutr. Rev.,* 46, 241, 1988.

117. Brenout, D., Peterman, M., Ugarte, G., Barrera, G., and Ituoriaga, H., Nitrogen economy in alcoholic patients without liver disease, *Metabolism,* 36, 651, 1987.

118. Schreiber, S. S., Dratz, M., Rothschild, M. A., Reff, F., and Evans, C., Alcoholic carcinopathy. II. Inhibition of cardiac microsomal protein synthesis by acetaldehyde, *J. Mol. Cell Cardiol.,* 6, 207, 1974.

119. Stamm, D., Hansert, E., and Feurlein, W., Excessive consumption of alcohol in men as biological influence factor in clinical laboratory investigations, *J. Clin. Chem. Clin. Biochem.*, 22, 65, 1984.
120. Lieber, C. S., Alcohol and nutrition: an overview, *Alcohol Health Res. World*, 13, 197, 1989.
121. Tuma, D. J., Casey, C. A., and Sorrell, M. F., Effects of ethanol on hepatic protein trafficking. Impairment of receptor-mediated endocytosis, *Alcohol Alcohol.*, 25, 117, 1990.
122. Cunningham, C. C., Coleman, W. B., and Spach, P., The effect of chronic ethanol consumption hepatic mitochondrial energy metabolism, *Alcohol Alcohol.*, 25, 127, 1990.
123. Tuma, D. J. and Sorrell, M. F., Effects of ethanol on protein trafficking in the liver, *Semin. Liver Dis.*, 8, 69, 1988.
124. Mohs, M. E. and Watson, R. R., Changes in nutrient status and balance associated with alcohol abuse, in *Diagnosis of Alcohol Abuse*, Watson, R. R., Ed., CRC Press, Boca Raton, FL, 1989, 125.
125. Guthrie, G. D., Myers, J. K., Gesar, E. J., White, G. W., and Koehl, J. R., Alcohol as a nutrient: interreaction between ethanol and carbohydrate, *Alcohol. Clin. Exp. Res.*, 14, 17, 1990.
126. Crouse, J. R. and Grundy, S. M., Effect of alcohol on plasma lipoproteins, cholesterol and triglyceride metabolism in man, *J. Lipid Res.*, 25, 486, 1984.
127. Tsutsumi, M., Laskez, J. M., Shiniqu, M., Rosman, A. S., and Lieber, C. S., The intralobular distribution of ethanol-inducible P450IIE1 in rat and human liver, *Hepatology*, 10, 437, 1989.
128. Spait, P. I., Bottenus, R. E., and Cunningham, C. C., Control of adenine mitochondria from rats with ethanol-induced fatty liver, *Biochem. J.*, 202, 445, 1982.
129. Arai, M., Gordon, E. R., and Lieber, C. S., Decreased cytochrome oxidase activity in hepatic mitochondria after chronic ethanol consumption and the possible role of decreased cytochrome aa3 content and changes in phospholipid, *Biochem. Biophys. Acta*, 797, 327, 1984.
130. Lieber, C. S., Baroana, E., Hernandez-Munoz, R., Kubota, S., Sato, N., Kawano, S., Matsumura, T., and Inatomi, N., Impaired oxygen utilization: a new mechanism for the hepatotoxicity of ethanol in sub-human primates, *J. Clin. Invest.*, 83, 1682, 1989.
131. Guthrie, G. D., Myers, K. J., Gesser, E. J., White, G. W., and Koehl, J. R., Alcohol as a nutrient: interactive between ethanol and carbohydrate, *Alcohol. Clin. Exp. Res.*, 14, 17, 1990.
132. Takase, S., Yasuhura, M., Takada, A., and Ueshima, Y., Changes in blood acetaldehyde levels after ethanol administration in alcoholics, *Alcohol*, 7, 37, 1990.
133. Rubin, E., Beattie, D. S., and Lieber, C. S., Effect of ethanol on the biogenesis of mitochondrial functions, *Lab. Invest.*, 23, 620, 1970.
134. SanKaran, H., Nishimura, C. Y., Lin, J. C., Larkin, E. C., and Rao, G. A., Regulation of pancreatic amylase by dietary carbohydrase in chronic alcoholic rats, *Pancreas*, 4, 733, 1989.

135. Sotaniemi, E. A., Keinamen, K., Lahtela, J. T., Costas, R. D., Cruz-Vidal, M., Abbott, R. D., and Havik, R. J., Carbohydrate intolerance associated with reduced hepatic glucose phosphorylating and releasing enzymes activities and peripheral insulin resistance in alcoholics with liver cirrhosis, *J. Hepatol.*, 1, 277, 1985.

136. Arakawa, M., Taketomi, S., Furuno, K., Matsuo, T., Iwatsuka, H., and Suzuoki, S., Metabolic studies on the development of ethanol-induced fatty liver in KK-AY mice, *J. Nutr.*, 105, 1500, 1975.

137. Salaspuro, M. P., Ross, W. A., Jayatilleke, E., Shaw, S., and Lieber, C. S., Attenuation of the ethanol induced hepatic redox change after chronic alcohol consumption in baboons: metabolic consequences *in vivo* and *in vitro*, *Hepatology*, 1, 33, 1981.

138. Nikkila, E. A. and Ojala, K., Role of hepatic L-alpha-glycero phosphate and triglyceride synthesis in production of fatty acid liver by ethanol, *Proc. Soc. Exp. Biol. Med.*, 113, 814, 1963.

139. Brunengraber, H., Boutry, M., Lowenstein, L., and Lowenstein, J. M., The effect of ethanol on lipogenesis by the perfused liver, in *Alcohol and Aldehyde Metabolizing Systems*, Wurman, R. G., Yonetani, T., Williamson, J. R., and Chance, B., Eds., Academic Press, New York, 1974, 329.

140. Savolainen, M. J. and Hassinen, T. E., Effect of ethanol on hepatic phosphotidate phosphohydroxylase. Dose-dependent enzyme induction and its abolition by adrenalectomy and pyrazole treatment, *Arch. Biochem. Biophys.*, 201, 640, 1980.

141. Savolainen, M. J., Stimulation of hepatic phosphotidate phosphohydrolase activity by a single dose of ethanol, *Biochem. Biophys. Res. Commun.*, 75, 511, 1977.

142. Odeleye, O. E., Eskelson, C. D., Watson, R. R., and Mufti, S. I., Composition of hepatic lipids after ethanol, cod liver oil and vitamin E feeding in rats, *Adv. Exp. Biol. Med.*, 283, 785, 1991.

143. Uthus, E. O., Skurdal, D. N., and Cornatzer, W. E., Effect of ethanol ingestion on choline phosphotransferase and phosphatidyl ethanol amine methyltransferase activities in liver microsomes, *Lipids*, 11, 641, 1976.

144. Mezey, E., Potter, J. J., Slusser, R. T., Brandes, D., Romero, J., Tanura, T., and Halsted, C. H., Effect of ethanol feeding on hepatic lysosomes in the monkey, *Lab. Invest.*, 43, 83, 1980.

145. Takeuchi, N., Ito, N., and Yamamura, Y., Esterification of cholesterol and hydrolysis of cholesteryl ester in alcohol induced fatty liver of rats, *Lipids*, 9, 353, 1974.

146. Boyer, J. L., Effect of chronic ethanol feeding on bile formation and secretion of lipids in the rat, *Gastroenterology*, 62, 294, 1972.

147. Lefevre, A. F., DeCarli, L. M., and Lieber, C. S., Effect of ethanol on cholesterol and bile acid metabolism, *J. Lipid Res.*, 13, 48, 1972.

148. Cunnane, S. C., McAdoo, K. R., and Horrobin, D. F., Long-term ethanol consumption in the hamster: effects on tissue lipids, fatty acids and erythrocyte hemolysis, *Ann. Nutr. Metab.*, 31, 265, 1987.

149. Rottenberg, H., Membrane solubility of ethanol in chronic alcoholism: the effect of ethanol feeding and its withdrawal on the protection by alcohol of rat red blood cells from hypotonic hemolysis, *Biochem. Biophys. Acta*, 855, 211, 1986.

150. Benedetti, A., Birabell, A. M., Brunell, E., Curatola, G., Feretti, G., Del-
     Prete, U., Jezequel, A. M., and Orlandi, F., Modification of lipid com-
     position of erythrocyte membranes in chronic alcoholism, *Pharm. Res. Com-
     mun.*, 19, 657, 1987.
151. Harris, R. A., Baxter, D. M., Mitchell, M. A., and Hitzemann, R. J.,
     Physical properties and lipid composition of brain membranes from ethanol
     tolerant dependent mice, *Mol. Pharm.*, 25, 401, 1984.
152. Taraschi, T. F., Ellingson, J. S., Wu, A. G., Zimmerman, R., and Rubin,
     E., Membrane tolerance to ethanol is rapidly lost after withdrawal: a model
     for studies of membrane adaptation, *Proc. Natl. Acad. Sci. U.S.A.*, 83,
     3669, 1986.
153. Aloia, R. C., Paxton, J., Daviau, J. S., Van Gelb, O., Mlekusch, W.,
     Truppe, W., Meyer, J. A., and Bralles, E. S., Effect of chronic ethanol
     consumption on brain microsome lipid composition, membrane fluidity and
     Na+-K+-ATPase activity, *Life Sci.*, 36, 1003, 1985.
154. Alling, C., Gustavsson, L., Kristensson, A. A. S., and Wallersteid, S.,
     Changes in fatty acid composition of major glycerophospholipids in eryth-
     rocyte membranes from chronic alcoholics during withdrawal, *Scand. J.
     Clin. Lab. Invest.*, 44, 283, 1984.
155. Harris, R. A., Baxter, D. M., Mitchell, M. A., and Hitzemann, R. J.,
     Physical properties and lipid composition of brain membranes from ethanol
     tolerant-dependent mice, *Mol. Pharm.*, 25, 401, 1984.
156. Neiman, J., Cursted, T., and Cronholm, T., Composition of platelets phos-
     phatidylinositol and phosphatidycholine after ethanol withdrawal, *Thromb.
     Res.*, 46, 295, 1987.
157. Salem, N., Jr. and Karanian, J. W., Polyunsaturated fatty acids and ethanol,
     Adv. Alcohol Substance Abuse, 7, 183, 1988.
158. La-Droitte, P., Lamboeuf, Y., DeSaint-Blanquat, G., and Bezaury, J. P.,
     Sensitivity of individual erythrocyte membrane phospholipid to changes in
     fatty acid composition in chronic alcoholic patients, *Alcohol. Clin. Exp.
     Res.*, 9, 135, 1985.
159. Horrobin, D. F. and Manku, M. S., Possible role of prostaglandin E_1 in
     affective disorders and in alcoholism, *Br. Med. J.*, 280, 1363, 1980.
160. Glen, E., MacDonnell, L., Glen, I., and Mackenzie, J., Possible phar-
     macological approaches to the prevention and treatment of alcohol related
     CNS impairment: results of a double blind trial of essential fatty acid, in
     Pharmacological Treatments for Alcoholism, Edward, G. and Littleton, J.,
     Eds., Methuen, New York, 1984, 331.
161. Nieman, J., Hillbom, M., Benthin, G., and Anggard, E. E., Urinary ex-
     cretion of 2,3-dinor-6-keto prostaglandin F1 alpha and platelets thromboxane
     formation during ethanol withdrawal in alcoholics, *J. Clin. Pathol.*, 5, 512,
     1987.
162. Engler, M. M., Karanian, J. W., and Salem, N., Jr., The effect of gamma-
     linoleic acid (18:3 w-6) on alcohol-induced changes in fatty acid compo-
     sition, blood pressure and its reactivity, *Fed. Proc.*, 46, 1467, 1987.
163. Reitz, R. C., Helsabeck, E., and Mason, D. P., Effect of chronic alcohol
     ingestion on the fatty acid composition of the heart, *Lipids*, 8, 80, 1973.

164. Littleton, J. M., John, G. R., and Grieve, S. J., Alterations in phospholipid composition in ethanol tolerance and dependence, *Alcohol. Clin. Exp. Res.,* 3, 50, 1979.
165. McIntyre, N., The effects of alcohol on water, electrolyte and minerals, in *Clinical Biochemistry of Alcoholism,* Rosalski, S. E., Ed., Churchill Livingstone, New York, 1984, 117.
166. Morgan, M. Y., Alcohol and the endocrine system, *Med. Bull.,* 38, 35, 1982.
167. Krawitt, E. L., Ethanol inhibits intestinal calcium transport in rats, *Nature,* 243, 88, 1973.
168. Flink, E. B., Magnesium deficiency in alcoholism, *Alcohol. Clin. Exp. Res.,* 10, 590, 1986.
169. Iseri, L. T., Freed, J., and Bures, A. R., Magnesium deficiency and cardiac disorders, *Am. J. Med.,* 58, 837, 1975.
170. Burton, W. N. and Gladstone, L., M.I.L.T., Laboratory clues to the diagnosis of alcoholism, *Int. Med. J.,* 161, 265, 1982.
171. Van der Weyden, M. B., Fong, H., Salem, H. H., Batey, R. G., and Dudley, F. J., Erythrocyte ferritin content in idiopathic haemochromatosis and alcoholic liver disease with iron overload, *Br. Med. J.,* 286, 752, 1983.
172. Savage, D. and Lindenbaum, J., Anemia in alcoholics, *Medicine (Baltimore),* 65, 322, 1986.
173. Feinman, L., Absorption and utilization of nutrients in alcoholism, *Alcohol Health Res. World,* 13, 207, 1989.
174. Wu, C. T., Lee, J. N., and Shen, W. W., Serum zinc, copper, and ceruloplasmin levels in male alcoholics, *Biol. Psychiatry,* 19, 1333, 1984.
175. McClain, C. J. and Su, L. C., Zinc deficiency in the alcoholics: a review, *Alcohol. Clin. Exp. Res.,* 7, 5, 1983.
176. Canalese, J., Sewell, R. B., Poston, L., and Williams, R., Zinc abnormalities in fulminant hepatic failure, *Aust. N.Z. J. Med.,* 15, 7, 1985.
177. McClain, C. J., Antonow, D. R., Cohen, D. A., and Shedlofsky, S. I., Zinc metabolism in alcoholic liver disease, *Alcohol. Clin. Exp. Res.,* 10, 582, 1986.
178. Richard, B., Flint, D. M., and Wahlquist, M. L., Acute effects of food and ethanol on plasma zinc concentration, *Nutr. Rep. Int.,* 23, 939, 1981.
179. Anon., Review. Zinc deficiency impairs ethanol metabolism, *Nutr. Rev.,* 43, 158, 1985.
180. Aturokala, R. M. and Herath, C. A., Zinc and vitamin A status of alcoholics in Sri Lanka, in 13th Int. Congr. Nutr. (Abstract), Brighton, U.K., August 18, 1985, p. 136.
181. Hartoma, T. R., Sotaniemi, E. A., and Maathanen, J., Effects of zinc on some biochemical indices of metabolism, *Nutr. Metab.,* 23, 203, 1979.
182. Chandra, R. R. and Au, B., Single nutrient deficiency and cell mediated immune responses. I. Zinc, *Am. J. Clin. Nutr.,* 33, 736, 1980.
183. Yeh, L. C. and Cerklewski, F. L., Interaction between ethanol and low dietary zinc during gestation and lactation in the rat, *J. Nutr.,* 114, 2027, 1985.

184. Tanner, A. R., Bantock, I., Hinks, L., Lloyd, B., Turner, N. R., and Wright, R., Depressed selenium and vitamin E levels in an alcoholic population: possible relationship to hepatic injury through lipid peroxidation, *Dig. Dis. Sci.,* 31, 1307, 1986.

185. Dutta, S. K., Miller, P. A., Greenberg, L. B., and Levander, O. A., Selenium and acute alcoholism, *Am. J. Clin. Nutr.,* 38, 713, 1983.

186. Dworkin, B., Rosenthal, W. S., Jankowski, R. H., and Haldea, D., Low blood selenium levels in alcoholics with and without advanced liver disease: correlation with clinical and nutritional status, *Dig. Dis. Sci.,* 30, 838, 1985.

187. Korpela, H., Kampulainen, J., and Luoma, P. V., Decreased serum selenium in alcoholics as related to liver structure and function, *Am. J. Clin. Nutr.,* 42, 147, 1985.

188. Valimaki, M. J., Harju, K. J., and Ylikahri, R. H., Decreased serum selenium in alcoholics: a consequence of liver dysfunctions, *Clin. Chem. Acta,* 130, 291, 1983.

189. Shah, H., Smith, A., and Picciano, M. F., Plasma selenium levels in alcoholic liver disease and primary biliary cirrhosis, *Nutr. Res.,* Suppl. I, 385, 1985.

190. Wood, B. and Breen, K. J., Vitamin deficiency in alcoholism with particular reference to thiamine deficiency, *Clin. Exp. Pharm. Physiol.,* 6, 457, 1979.

191. Leevy, C. M., Baker, H., Tenhove, W., Frank, O., and Cherrick, G. R., B-complex vitamins in liver disease of the alcoholic, *Am. J. Clin. Nutr.,* 16, 339, 1965.

192. Neville, J. N., Eagles, J. A., Samson, G., and Olson, R. E., Nutritional status of alcoholics, *Am. J. Clin. Nutr.,* 21, 1329, 1968.

193. Baines, M., Detection and incidence of B and C vitamin deficiency in alcohol related illnesses, *Ann. Clin. Biochem.,* 15, 307, 1978.

194. Truswell, A. S., Konno, T., and Hansen, J. D., Thiamine deficiency in adult hospital patients, *S. Afr. Med. J.,* 46, 2079, 1972.

195. Baker, H. and Frank, O., Absorption, utilization and clinical effectiveness of allithiamines compared to water-soluble thiamines, *J. Nutr. Sci. Vitaminol.,* 22(Suppl.), 63, 1978.

196. Hoyumpa, A. M., Breen, K. J., Schenker, S., and Wilson, F. A., Thiamine transport across the rat intestine. II. Effect of ethanol, *Lab. Clin. Med.,* 86, 803, 1975.

197. Fennelly, J., Frank, O., Baker, H., and Leevy, C. M., Peripheral neuropathy of the alcoholic. I. Aetiological role of aneurin and other B-complex vitamins, *Br. Med. J.,* 2, 1290, 1964.

198. Kershaw, P. W., Blood thiamine and nicotine acid levels in alcoholism and confusional states, *Br. J. Psychiatry,* 113, 387, 1967.

199. Periera, V. G., Masuda, Z., Katz, A., and Tronchini, V., Shonstin beriberi report of two successfully treated patients with hemodynamic documentation, *Am. J. Cardiol.,* 53, 1467, 1984.

200. Whyte, K. F., Dunnigan, M. G., and McIntosh, W. B., Excessive beer consumption and beri-beri, *Scott. Med. J.,* 27, 288, 1982.

201. Baines, M., Detection and incidence of B and C vitamin deficiency in alcohol-related illnesses, *Ann. Clin. Biochem.,* 15, 307, 1978.

202. Shehata, M. and Saad, S., The effects of aliphatic alcohols on certain vitamins of the B-complex group in the liver of the rat, *Pol. J. Pharmacol. Pharm.*, 30, 35, 1978.
203. Thomson, A. D., Baker, H., and Leevy, C. M., Patterns of [31]S-thiamine hydrochloride absorption in the malnourished alcoholic patient, *J. Lab. Clin. Med.*, 76, 34, 1970.
203a. Pekkanen, L. and Rusi, M., The effects of dietary niacin and riboflavin on voluntary intake and metabolism of ethanol in rats, *Pharmacol. Biochem. Behav.*, 11, 575, 1979.
204. Rosenthal, W. S., Adham, N. F., Lopez, R., and Cooperman, J. M., Riboflavin deficiency in complicated chronic alcoholism, *Am. J. Clin. Nutr.*, 26, 858, 1973.
205. Kim, C. I. and Roe, D. A., Development of riboflavin deficiency in alcohol fed hamsters, *Drug Nutr. Int.*, 3, 99, 1985.
206. Baries, M., Detection and incidence of B and C vitamin deficiency in alcohol related illness, *Ann. Clin. Biochem.*, 15, 307, 1978.
207. Walsh, M. P., Howorth, P., and Marks, V., Pyroxidine deficiency and tryptophan metabolism in chronic alcoholics, *Am. J. Clin. Nutr.*, 19, 379, 1966.
208. Sarles, R., An international survey on nutrition and pancreatitis, *Digestion*, 9, 378, 1973.
209. Devgun, M. S., Fiabane, S., Paterson, C. R., and Zarembski, P., Vitamin and mineral nutrition in chronic alcoholics including patients with Korsakoff's psychosis, *Br. J. Nutr.*, 45, 469, 1981.
210. Vanderlinde, R. E., Review of pyridoxal phosphate and the transaminase in liver disease, *Ann. Clin. Lab. Sci.*, 16, 79, 1986.
211. Veitch, R. L., Lumeng, L., and Li, T. K., The effect of ethanol and acetaldehyde on vitamin B_6 metabolism in liver, *Gastroenterology*, 66, 868, 1974.
212. Ryle, P. R. and Thomson, A. D., Nutrition and vitamins in alcoholism, in *Clinical Biochemistry of Alcoholism*, Rosalski, S. B., Ed., Churchill Livingstone, New York, 1984, 188.
213. Fatteb, F., Alcohol is dangerous to your health, *JAMA*, 20, 2959, 1985.
214. Weir, D. G., McGing, P. G., and Scott, J. M., Folate metabolism, the enterohepatic circulation and alcohol, *Biochem. Pharmacol.*, 34, 1, 1985.
215. Herbert, V., Zalusky, R., and Davison, C. S., Correlation of folate deficiency with alcoholism and associated macrocytosis, anemia and liver disease, *Ann. Intern. Med.*, 58, 977, 1968.
216. Davis, R. E., Clinical chemistry of folic acid, *Adv. Clin. Chem.*, 25, 233, 1986.
217. Halsted, C. H., Folate deficiency in alcoholism, *Am. J. Clin. Nutr.*, 33, 2736, 1980.
218. Wu, A., Chanarin, I., Slavin, G., and Levi, A. J., Folate deficiency in the alcoholic — its relationship to clinical and haematological abnormalities, liver disease and folate stress, *Br. J. Hematol.*, 29, 469, 1975.
219. Halsted, C. H., Robles, E. A., and Mezey, E., Intestinal malabsorption in folate-deficient alcoholics, *Gastroenterology*, 64, 526, 1973.

220. Russell, R. M., Rosenberg, I. H., Wilson, P. D., Iber, F. L., Daks, E. B., Biovetti, A. C., Otradovac, C. L., Karowski, P. A., and Press, W. A., Increased urinary excretion and prolonged turnover time of folic acid during ethanol ingestion, *Am. J. Clin. Nutr.,* 38, 64, 1983.

221. Eichner, E. R. and Hillman, R. S., Effect of alcohol on serum folate level, *J. Clin. Invest.,* 52, 584, 1973.

222. Paine, C., Eichner, E. R., and Dickson, V., Concordance of radioimmunoassay and microbiological assay in the study of the ethanol-induced field in serum folate level, *Am. J. Med. Sci.,* 266, 135, 1973.

223. Halsted, C. H., Griggs, R. C., and Harris, J. W., The effect of alcoholism on the absorption of folic acid (H³-PGA) evaluated by plasma levels and urine excretion, *J. Lab. Clin. Chem.,* 69, 116, 1967.

224. Lane, F., Goff, P., McGuffin, R., Eichner, E. R., and Hillman, R. S., Folic acid metabolism in normal, folate deficient and alcoholic man, *Br. J. Haematol.,* 34, 489, 1976.

225. Halsted, C. H., Robles, E. A., and Mezey, E., Decreased jejunal uptake of labeled folic acid (3H-PGA) in alcoholic patients: roles of alcohol and nutrition, *New Engl. J. Med.,* 285, 701, 1971.

226. Bonjour, J. P., Vitamins and alcoholism. II. Folate and B12, *Int. J. Vitam. Nutr. Res.,* 50, 96, 1980.

227. Eichner, E. R., Buchanan, B., Smith, J. W., and Hillman, R. S., Variation in the hematological and medical status of alcoholics, *Am. J. Med. Sci.,* 263, 35, 1972.

228. Kimber, C., Deller, D. J., Ibbotson, R. N., and Lander, H., The mechanism of anemia in chronic liver disease, *Q. J. Med.,* 34, 33, 1965.

229. Lindenbaum, J. and Lieber, C. S., Alcohol induced malabsorption of vitamin B12 in man, *Nature,* 224, 806, 1969.

230. Lindenbaum, J. and Lieber, C. S., Effects of chronic ethanol administration on intestinal absorption in man in the absence of nutritional deficiency, *Ann. N.Y. Acad. Sci.,* 252, 228, 1975.

231. Dastur, D. K., Santhadevi, Q., Quadros, E. V., Avari, F. C., Wadia, N. H., Desai, M. M., and Bharucha, E. P., The B-vitamins in malnutrition with alcoholism, *Br. J. Nutr.,* 36, 143, 1976.

232. Fennelly, J., Frank, O., Baker, H., and Leevy, C. M., Effect of alcohol on excretion of some water soluble vitamins, *Br. Med. J.,* 2, 1290, 1964.

233. Rossouw, J. E., Labadarios, D., Davis, M., and Williams, R., The degradation of tryptophan in severe liver disease, *Int. J. Vitam. Nutr. Res.,* 48, 281, 1978.

234. Barboriak, J. J., Rooney, C. B., Leitshuh, T. H., and Anderson, A. J., Alcohol and nutrient intake of elderly men, *J. Am. Diet. Assoc.,* 72, 493, 1978.

235. Payne, I. R., Lu, G. H., and Meyer, K., Relationship of dietary tryptophan and niacin to tryptophan metabolism in alcoholics and non-alcoholics, *Am. J. Clin. Nutr.,* 27, 572, 1974.

236. Tao, H. G. and Fox, H. M., Measurements of urinary pantothenic acid excretions of alcoholic patients, *J. Nutr. Sci. Vitaminol.,* 23, 333, 1976.

237. Baker, H., Frank, O., Zetterman, R. K., Rajan, K. S., Tenhove, W., and Leevy, C. M., Inability of chronic alcoholics with liver disease to use food as a source of folates thiamin and vitamin B$_6$, *Am. J. Clin. Nutr.*, 28, 1377, 1975.

238. National Academy of Science, Biotin, in *Recommended Dietary Allowance*, NAS, Washington, D.C., 1980, 120.

239. Bonjour, J. P., *Int. J. Vitam. Nutr. Res.*, 47, 107, 1977.

240. Dow, J. and Goldberg, A., Ethanol metabolism in the vitamin C deficient guinea pig, *Biochem. Pharmacol.*, 24, 863, 1975.

241. Shugalei, I. U., Features of vitamin C metabolism and the functional status of the liver in alcoholism and alcoholic delirium in the stage of detoxification therapy, *Zh. Neuropathol. Psychiatry*, 87, 240, 1987.

242. Yunice, A. A., Hsu, J. M., Fahmy, A., and Henry, S., Ethanol-ascorbate interrelationship in acute and chronic alcoholism in the guinea pig, *Proc. Soc. Exp. Biol. Med.*, 177, 262, 1984.

243. Sprince, H., Parker, C. M., Smith, G. G., and Gonzalez, L. J., Protection against acetaldehyde toxicity by ascorbic acid plus reserpine or atropine, *Fed. Proc.*, 2, 34, 1975.

244. Sprince, H., Parker, C. M., Smith, G. G., and Gonzales, L. J., Protection action of ascorbic acid and sulfur compounds against acetaldehyde toxicity: implications in alcoholism and smoking, *Agents Actions*, 5, 164, 1975.

245. Susick, R. L., Jr. and Zannoni, V. G., Ascorbic acid and alcohol oxidation, *Biochem. Pharmacol.*, 33, 3963, 1984.

246. Russell, R. M., Vitamin A and zinc metabolism in alcoholism, *Am. J. Clin. Nutr.*, 33, 2741, 1980.

247. Majundar, S. K., Shaw, G. K., and Thomson, A. D., Blood B-carotene status in chronic alcoholics — a good biochemical marker for malnutrition, *Drug Alcohol Depend.*, 12, 111, 1983.

248. Gruchow, H. W., Sobocinski, K. A., Barboriak, J. J., and Scheller, J. G., Alcohol consumption, nutrient intake and relative body weight among US adults, *Am. J. Clin. Nutr.*, 422, 289, 1985.

249. Hillers, V. N. and Massey, L. K., Interrelationship of moderate and high alcohol consumption with diet and health status, *Am. J. Clin. Nutr.*, 41, 356, 1985.

250. Kvale, G., Bjelke, E., and Gart, J. J., Dietary habits and lung cancer risk, *Int. J. Cancer*, 31, 397, 1983.

251. Mak, K. M., Leo, M. A., and Lieber, C. S., Ethanol potentiates squamous metaplasia of the rat trachea caused by vitamin A deficiency, *Trans. Assoc. Am. Phys.*, 98, 210, 1984.

252. Nettesheim, P. and Williams, M. L., The influence of vitamin A on the susceptibility of the rat lung by 3-methylcholanthrease, *Br. J. Cancer*, 17, 351, 1976.

253. Leo, M. A. and Lieber, C. S., Hepatic vitamin A depletion in alcoholic liver injury, *N. Engl. J. Med.*, 307, 597, 1982.

254. Sato, M. and Lieber, C. S., Hepatic vitamin A depletion after chronic ethanol consumption in the baboons and rats, *J. Nutr.*, 111, 2015, 1981.

255. Leo, M. A., Kim, C., and Lieber, C. S., Increased vitamin A in esophagus and other extrahepatic tissues after chronic ethanol consumption in the rat, *Alcohol. Clin. Exp. Res.*, 10, 487, 1986.

256. Leo, M. A. and Lieber, C. S., Hypervitaminosis A: a liver lovers lament, *Hepatology,* 8, 412, 1988.
257. Sato, M. and Lieber, C. S., Changes in vitamin A status after acute ethanol administration in the rat, *J. Nutr.,* 112, 1188, 1982.
258. Sporn, M. B., Roberts, A. B., and Goodman, D. S., Eds., *The Retinoids,* Academic Press, New York, 1984, 1.
259. Odeleye, O. E., Eskelson, C. D., Alak, J. I., Watson, R. R., Chvapil, M., and Mufti, S. I., The effects of vitamin E supplementation on hepatic levels of vitamin A and E in ethanol and cod liver oil fed rats, *Int. J. Vitam. Nutr. Res.,* 61, 143, 1990.
260. Long, R. K., Skinner, R. K., Willis, M. R., and Sherlock, S., Vitamin D deficiency in alcoholics, *Lancet,* 2, 650, 1978.
261. Posner, D. B., Russell, R. M., Absood, S., Connor, T. B., Davis, C., Martin, L., Williams, J. B., Norris, A. H., and Merchant, C., Effective 25-hydroxylation of vitamin D_2 in alcoholic cirrhosis, *Gastroenterology,* 74, 866, 1978.
262. Dutta, S. K., Costa, B. S., Russell, R. M., and Connor, T. B., Fat soluble vitamin deficiency in treated patients with pancreatic insufficiency, *Gastroenterology,* 76, 1126, 1979.
263. Jung, R. T., Davis, M., Hunter, J. O., Chalmer, T. M., and Lawson, D. E., Abnormal vitamin D metabolism in cirrhosis, *Gut,* 19, 290, 1978.
264. Mezey, E., Metabolic effects of alcohol, *Fed. Proc.,* 44, 134, 1985.
265. Gedik, O. and Akaline, S., Effects of vitamin D deficiency and repletion on insulin and glucagon secretion in man, *Diabetologia,* 29, 142, 1986.
266. Nyomba, B. L., Bouillon, R., and De Moor, P., Influence of vitamin D status on insulin secretion and glucose tolerance in the rabbit, *Endocrinology,* 115, 191, 1984.
267. Clark, S. A., Stumpf, W. E., and Sar, M., Effect of 1,25-dihydroxyvitamin D_3 on insulin secretion, *Diabetes,* 30, 382, 1981.
268. Kadawaki, S. and Norman, A. W., Demonstration that the vitamin D metabolite 1,25$(OH)_2$-vitamin D_3 and not 24,25$(OH)_2$-vitamin D_3 is essential for normal insulin secretion in the perfused rat pancreas, *Diabetes,* 34, 315, 1984.
269. McCay, P. B., Vitamin E. Interaction with free radicals and ascorbate, *Annu. Rev. Nutr.,* 5, 323, 1985.
270. Nikki, E., Interaction of ascorbate and alpha-tocopherol, *Ann. N.Y. Acad. Sci.,* 498, 186, 1987.
271. Bjorneboe, G. E., Bjorneboe, A., Hagen, B. F., Morland, J., and Drevon, C. A., Reduced hepatic alpha-tocopherol content after long-term administration of ethanol to rats, *Biochim. Biophys. Acta,* 918, 236, 1987.
272. Bjorneboe, A., Bjorneboe, G. A., Bodd, E., Hagan, B. F., Kveseth, N., and Drevon, C. A., Transport and distribution of alpha-tocopherol in lymph, serum and liver cells in rats, *Biochim. Biophys. Acta,* 889, 310, 1986.
273. Bjorneboe, G. E., Johnsen, J., Bjorneboe, A., Bache-Wigg, J.-E., Morland, J., and Drevon, G. A., Diminished serum concentrations of vitamin E and selenium in alcoholics, *Ann. Nutr. Metab.,* 32, 56, 1988.

274. Bjorneboe, G. E., Jonsen, J., Bjorneboe, A., Marklund, S. L., Skylv, N., Hoiseth, A., Bache-Wigg, J. E., Morland, J., and Drevon, C. A., Some aspects of antioxidant status in blood from alcoholics, *Alcohol. Clin. Exp. Res.,* 12, 806, 1988.

275. Dworkin, E. M., Rosenthal, W. S., Gordon, G. G., and Jankowski, R. H., Diminished serum concentration of selenium and vitamin E in alcoholics, *Alcohol. Clin. Exp. Res.,* 8, 535, 1984.

276. Bonjour, J. P., Vitamins and alcoholism. X. Vitamin D. XI. Vitamin E. XII. Vitamin K, *Int. J. Vitam. Nutr. Res.,* 51, 307, 1981.

277. Kawase, T., Kato, S., and Lieber, C. S., Lipid peroxidation and antioxidant defense system in rat liver after chronic ethanol feeding, *Hepatology,* 10, 815, 1989.

278. Morgan, A. G., Kelleher, J., Walker, B. E., Losowsky, M. S., Droller, H., and Middleton, R. S., Increased prothrombin time in chronic hepatic disease, *Int. J. Vitam. Nutr. Res.,* 45, 448, 1972.

279. Mohs, M. and Watson, R. R., Alcohol-induced changes in nutrition, in *Focus on Biochemistry and Physiology of Substance Abuse,* Vol. 1, Watson, R. R., Ed., CRC Press, Boca Raton, FL, 1989.

2 Dietary Factors and Alcohol Consumption

INTRODUCTION

It is well known that chronic, excessive use of alcohol often leads to adverse nutritional consequences. Such effects result from decreased food intake or appetite and/or impaired digestion, absorption, and utilization of nutrients. A less studied, but at least equally important issue, however, is whether nutritional interventions can reduce alcohol usage among problem drinkers. Indeed, despite the dearth of well-controlled nutritional research with human subjects, nutritional counseling and nutritional therapy have already become common components of in-patient alcoholism treatment programs.[1]

In this chapter, the authors review research on nutritional interventions to reduce alcohol consumption. Most of the presentation focuses on animal studies dealing with the effects of various nutrients on drinking. Following this is a summary of the results of the small number of human studies dealing with the possible relations between nutritional variables and the decrease in alcohol consumption. The authors then propose a neurochemical model as the stratum in which nutrients might modify drinking behavior. Finally, they suggest promising directions for future research and present what they consider the major clinical issues and concerns for nutritional interventions in alcoholism treatment.

ROLE OF NUTRITIONAL FACTORS IN ALCOHOL CONSUMPTION IN EXPERIMENTAL ANIMALS

PROTEIN, CARBOHYDRATE, AND FAT DIETS

A range of studies have suggested that altering the protein, carbohydrate, and fat intake of animals can modify their levels of drinking. While investigations of protein changes have yielded rather consistent results,

TABLE 1
Effects of Dietary Intervention on Alcohol Intake Using Experimental Animal Models: Carbohydrate, Protein, and Fat Diet

Animal model	Nutritional intervention	Alcohol intake	Study
Albino male rat	Increased carbohydrate 46–63%	Decrease	Lester and Greenberg[8]
Rats	Presence of sucrose solution	Decrease	Mardones et al.[9]
	Changing sucrose from 29–81%	No change	
Male and female mice (black C_{57})	Low-protein, high-carbohydrate diet	No change	Mirone[2]
	High-protein, low-carbohydrate diet	Increase	
	High-fat, low-protein, and low-carbohydrate diet	Increase	
Albino rats	High-fat, low-carbohydrate diet	Decrease	Eriksson[10]
Male and female minipigs (Sinclair)	Decreasing protein from 16–4% diet	Decrease	Brown and Hutcheson[3]
Male albino rats (Sprague-Dawley)	Low-protein, high-carbohydrate diet	Decrease	Pekkanen et al.[4]
	High-carbohydrate, low-fat diet	No change	
	High-fat, low-carbohydrate diet	Increase	
Male rats (Holtzman)	Long-term low-protein, high-carbohydrate diet	Decrease (day 76) No change (days 176 and 276)	Hanig et al.[5]
Female rats (alcohol-preferring)	Low-protein, high-carbohydrate diet	Decrease	Forsander and Sinclair[7]
Female rats (alcohol nonpreferring)	Low-protein, high-carbohydrate diet	No change	Forsander and Sinclair[7]

research on fats and carbohydrates has produced variable findings. Table 1 summarizes these results.

Early studies by Mirone[2] showed that mice maintained on a diet high in protein and low in carbohydrate increased their levels of alcohol consumption. Similarly, Brown and Hutcheson[3] found that minipigs on a 16% protein diet, drank 3 to 4 times more alcohol than those maintained on a 4% protein diet. The low-protein consuming animals obtained only 15% of their calories from alcohol, while the high protein animals derived 37% of their calories from alcohol. In agreement with these findings, Pekkanen et al.[4] demonstrated that rats assigned a low-protein, high-carbohydrate diet drank only half as much as control rats. Since there was no difference in alcohol consumption between the control group and a group of rats maintained on a low-fat, high-carbohydrate diet, protein rather than carbohydrate seemed more important in influencing alcohol intake. Pursuing this line of research, Hanig et al.[5] investigated the long-term sequential effects of protein restriction by imposing a low-protein diet during life stages of gestation, lactation, youth, and adulthood (300 d old). At day 76, rats fed the low-protein diet (8% of diet) consumed 47% less alcohol than rats fed an isocaloric normal protein diet (24% of diet). Interestingly, at subsequent 100-d follow-ups, the differences disappeared, indicating some unknown behavioral or metabolic adaptation to the protein deficiency.

As noted, results from research on dietary fat and carbohydrate and alcohol consumption have been less consistent. Rats fed a high-carbohydrate, low-protein diet have been found to drink significantly less than those on a normal diet.[4-7] Lester and Greenberg[8] found that rats maintained on a 46% carbohydrate diet drank more than those maintained on the same diet, but at 63% carbohydrate. A recent study by Forsander and Sinclair[7] revealed a negative correlation between alcohol and carbohydrate intake in alcohol-preferring rats. Mardones et al.[9] found that when a solution of sucrose or dextrose was given to rats with water and alcohol present, a significant reduction in alcohol intake was observed. Interestingly, the investigators, however, did not find that further changes in sucrose from 29 to 81% were associated with changes in alcohol consumption. Mirone[2] also failed to see a change in voluntary alcohol intake in mice administered a high-carbohydrate diet. These contradictory results may be due, in part, to different methodologies and animal species.

Finally, several animal studies have indicated that changes in the composition of dietary fat can alter alcohol intake. An early study by Mirone[2] found that a high-fat, low-protein, low-carbohydrate diet significantly decreased alcohol consumption by 45% in mice. While Eriksson[10] also demonstrated that a diet consisting of high fat and no carbohydrate lowered alcohol intake in rats, a subsequent study by Pekkanen et al.[4] showed that rats fed a high-fat low-carbohydrate diet markedly increased their intake of alcohol. Pekkanen and co-workers hypothesized that the contradictory results may have been caused by differences in methods of measuring vitamin intake across the three experimental studies. The Mirone and Eriksson studies computed vitamin intake on a weight basis, whereas Pekkanen et al. based their estimate of vitamin intake on total energy content. Since the high-fat, low-carbohydrate diet yielded high energy, Pekkanen et al. postulated that in the Mirone and Eriksson studies, a vitamin deficiency resulted from a dietary imbalance. Perhaps it was this vitamin deficiency that led to diminished alcohol intake (see below).

An important question concerning these and other dietary relationships with alcohol consumption is whether dietary factors differently affect the drinking behavior of alcohol-preferring animals vs. nonalcohol-preferring animals. A recent study involving alcohol-preferring and alcohol-avoiding rat lines suggests that such differences do exist. Forsander and Sinclair[7] found that rats of the alcohol-preferring line drank fully nine times more alcohol when maintained on a 40% (by energy) protein diet than on a 5% protein diet. By contrast, rats of the alcohol-avoiding line were unaffected by the changes in their protein diet. However, it is unknown if the difference is due to the nature of the alcohol-preferring line or the nature of the alcohol-avoiding line or both. Rats not selectively bred are also influenced by protein diet (Table 1). Nevertheless, these findings suggest that dietary influence on alcohol intake may be somehow related to a genetic predisposition to alcohol preference, thus perhaps accounting for some of the mixed results cited above.

The mechanisms ultimately responsible for the effect of dietary protein, carbohydrate, and fat on alcohol intake remain largely unknown. Changes in rates of metabolism and clearance of alcohol have been postulated. Several investigators,[4,7,11] for example, have shown that rats maintained on a low-protein, high-carbohydrate diet have both lower rates of alcohol elimination and alcohol intake. Conversely, rats maintained on a diet of excess protein eliminate alcohol more rapidly and increase their alcohol intake. Interestingly, the rates of alcohol elimination and alcohol intake are strongly influenced by changes in the protein/carbohydrate ratio in the alcohol-preferring line of rats, while alcohol elimination rates are not affected by changes in this ratio in alcohol-avoiding rats (with the exception that with an excess protein diet alcohol elimination rate is increased).[7] It is unlikely, however, that a change in the rate of alcohol elimination is the sole regulator of alcohol intake or vice versa. Forsander and Sinclair[7] plotted alcohol intake against rate of alcohol elimination. The relationship deviated substantially from linearity and the regression line did not intersect the y-axis at the origin. Also, Pekkanen et al.[4] reported a dissociation in the relationship between alcohol intake and rate of alcohol elimination. They observed decreases in both alcohol intake and rate of alcohol elimination in rats fed a high-carbohydrate, low-protein diet, in contrast to an increase in alcohol intake and a decrease in alcohol elimination rate in rats fed a high-fat, low-carbohydrate diet.

The physiological agency underlying these relationships may well involve acetaldehyde, the first metabolic product of ethanol oxidation. Changes in acetaldehyde may also mediate the effects of dietary factors on alcohol consumption. When accumulated in sufficient quantities, acetaldehyde produces toxic effects and causes a reduction in drinking. Several studies have reported increases in blood levels of acetaldehyde, along with diminished alcohol intake in rats maintained on a low-protein diet.[4,12] Higher levels of acetaldehyde have also been reported in the alcohol-avoiding line of rats, but not in alcohol-preferring rats.[13] The enzyme responsible for the catabolism of acetaldehyde, aldehyde dehydrogenase, is also depressed in rats on a low-protein diet.[11] In addition, a high association ($r = 0.83$) has been observed between the brain activity of aldehyde dehydrogenase and alcohol consumption in rats.[14] Alcohol dehydrogenase, the enzyme responsible for converting ethanol into acetaldehyde, is also depressed under conditions of the low-protein diet, although not to the extent of aldehyde dehydrogenase.[11,15]

Several questions concerning the acetaldehyde theory remain. Lindros et al.[12] showed that acetaldehyde levels in rat blood and liver increase as the protein diet is reduced from 50 to 12%; however, acetaldehyde levels begin to decrease as the amount of protein in the diet is reduced below 12%. Also, Pekkanen et al.[4] reported a decrease in drinking and an increase in the blood acetaldehyde level for rats maintained on a low-protein, high-carbohydrate diet, in contrast to an increase in drinking and no change in blood acetaldehyde levels with rats kept on a high-fat, low-carbohydrate diet. Hence, dietary protein and fat may evoke different mechanisms for influencing drinking or perhaps a low level of acetaldehyde is only one basis for increased drinking. For example, prevention of acetaldehyde accumulation in Long-Evans or alcohol-nonpreferring rats does not appear to alter their alcohol intake.[14] Finally, methodological problems in measuring acetaldehyde levels have been reported.[16] Thus, some caution must be observed in interpreting the changes reported above.

VITAMINS

Variations in vitamin content of diet may also influence voluntary alcohol intake (Table 2). An early study by Brady and Westerfeld[17] revealed that rats fed a diet deficient in vitamin B complex increased voluntary alcohol consumption. Similarly, Williams et al.[18] found an increase in

TABLE 2
Effects of Dietary Intervention on Alcohol Intake Using Experimental Animal Models: Vitamins

Animal model	Nutritional intervention	Alcohol intake	Study
Rats	Deficient vitamin B complex diet	Increase	Brady and Westerfeld[17]
Female rats (Wistar)	Deficient thiamin diet	No change	Westerfeld and Lawrow[20]
Male and female rats (Wistar)	Deficient multivitamin diet	Increase	Williams et al.[18]
Male and female mice (black C_{57})	Deficient vitamin B complex diet	Increase	Mirone[2]
	Deficient thiamin diet	Increase	
	Deficient pyridoxine diet	Increase	
	Deficient pantothenic acid diet	No change	
Male and female albino rats	Deficient thiamin diet	No change	Purdy and Lee[21]
	Deficient riboflavin diet	No change	
Male and female mice (DBA/2; 129/ J; BALB/c; and A/J)	Deficient niacin diet	Increase	Brown[19]
	Deficient pantothenic acid diet	No change	
	Deficient thiamin diet (female only)	Increase	
	Deficient pyridoxine diet (male only)	Increase	

alcohol intake in rats given a multivitamin-deficient diet. In a third study, Mirone[2] discovered that a diet deficient in either thiamin (B_1) or pyridoxine (B_6) was associated with an increase in voluntary alcohol consumption in mice, while a diet deficient in pantothenic acid (part of the B_2 complex) resulted in no change in alcohol intake. Brown[19] also showed that mice fed a niacin-deficient diet increased their alcohol intake, but that those fed with pantothenic acid deficiency experienced no change in voluntary alcohol consumption. (Interestingly, female mice deficient in thiamin and pyridoxine consumed more alcohol than did male mice on the same diet, who did not differ from controls.)

Not all of the early studies showed vitamin-induced changes in alcohol intake. Westerfeld and Lawrow[20] found that rats deficient in thiamin did not alter their voluntary alcohol consumption. Purdy and Lee[21] also reported that rats fed a diet deficient in thiamin or deficient in riboflavin failed to significantly increase their voluntary alcohol intake. (In the latter study, changes in alcohol consumption were more closely associated with food intake.)

While several early studies indicated that deficiencies in certain B vitamins may alter voluntary alcohol consumption, unfortunately, little recent work has been performed to substantiate or refute these results. Also, no projects seem to have been undertaken to investigate the physiological mechanisms underlying these changes.

AMINO ACIDS

Amino acids have also been reported to influence alcohol consumption (see Table 3). In one study, oral doses of glutamine in rats resulted in a decrease in voluntary alcohol consumption.[22] Surprisingly, however, glutamine injected intraperitoneally (i.p.) did not alter alcohol consumption. Also, while glutamine reduced drinking, asparagine, glutamic acid, sodium glutamate, and glycine failed to produce demonstrable effects on alcohol consumption.[23] In a recent report by Blum et al.,[24] however, a reduction in alcohol consumption was observed in alcohol-preferring mice when injected i.p. with D-phenylalanine.

Several investigations have also shown that tryptophan and 5-hydroxy-tryptophan influence alcohol intake. Sprince et al.[25] reported a meaningful increase in voluntary alcohol consumption in rats fed a 1% D,L-tryptophan diet, while only a slight effect was observed with D,L-tyrosine and D,L-leucine. In the same vein, Myers and Melchior[26] found an increase in alcohol intake with a 1 to 3% L-tryptophan diet using female rats of the Royal Victoria strain. However, this effect appeared to be strain dependent since only a slight effect occurred in the male Long-Evans strain and no effect at all was experienced in the male Sprague-Dawley rats. In contrast to the effects of tryptophan, Geller[27] found that D,L-5-hydroxytryptophan (hydroxylated form of tryptophan), administered i.p. in Sprague-Dawley rats, reduced alcohol intake. Walters[28] reported a similar finding with D,L-5-hydroxytryptophan in addition to a peripheral decarboxylase inhibitor in male Holtzman albino rats. Zabik et al.[29] also found that at a range of doses of i.p. injected D,L-5-hydroxytryptophan, alcohol intake was reduced in rats, while water intake was unaltered. Later, Zabik et al.[30] showed that i.p. administration of L-tryptophan or L-5-hydroxytryptophan resulted in a significant decrease in the amount of alcohol consumed. Since D-5-hydroxytryptophan failed to reduce alcohol consumption, it appears that the L-isomer is the physiologically active form. Finally, McBride et al.[31] reported a 68% reduction in alcohol consumption with i.p. administration of D,L-5-hydroxytryptophan in alcohol-preferring rats.

TABLE 3
Effect of Dietary Intervention on Alcohol Intake Using Experimental Animal Models: Amino Acids

Animal model	Nutritional intervention	Alcohol intake	Study
Male and female rats (Wistar)	Glutamine (diet)	Decrease	Rogers et al.[22]
	Glutamine (i.p.)	No change	
	Glutamine (diet)	Decrease	Rogers et al.[23]
	Asparagine (diet)	No change	
	Glutamic acid (diet)	No change	
	Sodium glutamate (diet)	No change	
	Glycine (diet)	No change	
Male albino rats	D,L-Tryptophan (diet)	Increase	Sprince et al.[25]
	D,L-Tyrosine (diet)	No change	
	D,L-Leucine (diet)	No change	
Male rats (Sprague-Dawley)	D,L-5-Hydroxytryptophan diet	Decrease	Geller[27]
Rats (Royal Victoria, Long-Evans, and Sprague-Dawley)	L-Tryptophan diet, female Royal Victoria strain	Increase	Myers and Melchior[26]
	L-Tryptophan diet, male Long-Evans strain	Slight increase	
	L-Tryptophan diet, male Sprague-Dawley strain	No change	
Male albino rats (Holtzman)	D,L-5-Hydroxytryptophan (i.p.) plus MK-486 (decarboxylase inhibitor)	Decrease	Walters[28]
Male rats (Sprague-Dawley)	D,L-5-Hydroxytryptophan (i.p.)	Decrease	Zabik et al.[29]
	L-Tryptophan (i.p.)	Decrease	Zabik et al.[30]
	L-5-Hydroxytryptophan (i.p.)	Decrease	
	D-5-Hydroxytryptophan (i.p.)	No change	
Alcohol-preferring mice (C57BL/6J)	D-Phenylalanine (i.p.)	Decrease	Blum et al.[24]
Alcohol-preferring line of rats	D,L-5-Hydroxytryptophan (i.p.)	Decrease	McBride et al.[31]

It has been hypothesized that amino acids increase neurotransmitter levels. Tryptophan and 5-hydroxytryptophan are serotonin precursors, while glutamine has been shown to increase the brain content of γ-aminobutyric acid (GABA).[32] Changes in each of these neurotransmitters have been postulated to alter the craving response for drinking.[33]

TABLE 4
Effects of Dietary Intervention on Alcohol Intake Using Experimental Animal Models: Minerals

Animal model	Nutritional intervention	Alcohol intake	Study
Male and female mice (black C$_{57}$)	Deficient Na diet	No change	Mirone[2]
	Deficient K diet	No change	
	Deficient I diet	Increase	
Male albino rats (Wistar)	Deficient I diet	Decrease (first 4 d, followed by increase)	Maenpaa and Forsander[34]
Male rats (Sprague-Dawley)	Deficient Z diet	Increase	Collipp et al.[35]
Male and female rats (Wistar)	Low Na diet plus furosemide (salt-losing diuretic)	Decrease	Grupp et al.[38,39]
Male rats (Wistar)	Na-supplemented diet	Increase	Grupp et al.[40]

MINERALS

Minerals may also play a role in drinking (see Table 4). Mirone[2] fed mice diets variously deficient in sodium (Na), potassium (K), and iodine (I). While Na and K deficiency did not alter the alcohol intake, I deficiency increased voluntary alcohol consumption. Later, Maenpaa and Forsander[34] observed that rats fed an I-deficient diet reduced their drinking over the first 4 d, but subsequently increased their consumption of alcohol. Reintroduction of I to the diet reduced the drinking to the low levels initially found.

Recently, Collipp et al.[35] observed an increase in voluntary consumption by rats of different ages when fed a zinc (Zn)-deficient diet. When the rats were returned to a normal diet, alcohol consumption declined. Ahmed and Russell[36] also showed that if rats were fed a Zn-deficient diet and given alcohol, they went into a negative Zn balance and had decreased amounts of Zn in most of their tissues when contrasted with pair-fed Zn-deficient (no alcohol) rats. (A related and curious human finding is that children of alcoholics have lower Zn concentrations in their hair than do other children,[37] suggesting a possible link between Zn and the predisposition of alcoholism.)

In two similar experiments, Grupp et al.[38,39] showed that a low-Na diet in combination with a salt-depleting diuretic, furosemide, significantly reduced voluntary alcohol drinking in rats. This reduction was not accompanied by a change in water intake. Conversely, a dietary Na supplement (up to 6%) produced an increase in alcohol consumption.[40] The mechanism of action may involve the renin-angiotensin system. When Na levels are decreased, a compensatory increase occurs in plasma renin and angiotensin I and II. Grupp et al.[41] found that alcohol intake is inversely related to plasma renin activity in both the alcohol-preferring and -nonpreferring lines of rats. The alcohol-preferring line drank significantly more alcohol and had significantly lower renin activity than did the alcohol-nonpreferring line of rats. Grupp et al.[42] also observed a greater consumption of alcohol by salt-sensitive rats, which have a lower renin-angiotensin activity than the salt-resistant rats.[43,44] The β-adrenergic agonist, isoproterenol, a potent releaser of renin, also suppressed voluntary intake of alcohol.[45] Finally, subcutaneous (s.c.) injections of angiotensin II reduced voluntary alcohol intake in rats. Conversely, the angiotensin II antagonist, Sar-1 Thr-8 angiotensin II, restored the level of voluntary intake of alcohol.[46,47] Angiotensin II appears to act directly on the central nervous system (CNS) since a lesion in the subfornical organ attenuated its effect on intake.[48]

SUMMARY

Over the past 4 decades, many studies have been conducted on the influence of dietary factors on alcohol intake. A wide range of animal models have been used with varying levels of sophistication in their experimental design. The overall results of the studies indicate that through some unknown mechanisms, alteration in the diet can cause a change in alcohol consumption. Interestingly, these changes appear to be greater with the alcohol-preferring rats compared to the alcohol-nonpreferring rats.

Many questions remain to be answered. Additional studies should focus on the differences between alcohol-preferring and alcohol-nonpreferring lines of rats. Also, further animal studies are needed to understand the mechanisms responsible for changes in alcohol consumption. This will demand well-designed experiments conceived to answer specific questions. Finally, any significant animal findings need to be confirmed in humans.

NUTRITIONAL INTERVENTIONS IN REDUCING ALCOHOL CONSUMPTION IN HUMANS

Only a small number of studies have examined nutritional aids to reduce drinking behavior in alcoholics. An early study by Rogers and Pelton[49] reported that glutamine supplements diminished the desire to drink, decreased ''nervousness'', and improved the ability to sleep in subjects with extensive histories of excessive drinking. More recently, Yung et al.[50] evaluated the possible relationship between drinking and diet in recently detoxified alcoholics. Those who maintained sobriety longer consumed significantly more carbohydrates, including twice as much sugar. It is unknown whether sobriety caused the increase in sugar intake, or if the heightened sugar intake facilitated sobriety, or indeed, if some underlying mechanism was responsible for both. In addition, patients who supplemented their diet with multivitamins and/or vitamin B complex were also more effective in maintaining sobriety. Despite the correlational nature of this project, the results are intriguing and compellingly argue the need for additional causal research in the topic.

In a recent double-blind, placebo-controlled study, Blum et al.[51] investigated the effects of an amino acid and vitamin mixture (called ''SAAVE'') on alcohol and polydrug abusers in an inpatient treatment program. The compound consisted of D- and L-phenylalanine, L-tryptophan, L-glutamine, and pyridoxal 5'-phosphate (activated form of vitamin B_6). Patients receiving SAAVE for 21 d revealed lower skin conductance and improvement in several physical responses (e.g., flushing response, muscular coordination, seizure activity, sweating, and tremors) as well as improvement in behavioral, emotional, social, and spiritual (''BESS'') indices than did their peers receiving placebo.

Blum and colleagues[33,51] postulated that the effectiveness of SAAVE was due to an alteration in the levels of neurotransmitters either by acting as a precursor or as a cofactor. For instance, D-phenylalanine seemed to inhibit enkephalinase, thereby increasing brain levels of enkephalin, an endogenous opioid. Earlier, Blum et al.[24] showed that i.p. injections of D-phenylalanine significantly reduced alcohol intake in alcohol-preferring (C57BL/6J) mice, apparently by increasing the availability of enkephalin. Amino acids were used as neurotransmitter precursors: phenylalanine, to increase levels of the catecholamine dopamine and norepinephrine; L-tryptophan, for serotonin; and L-glutamine, to elevate brain GABA. Pyridoxal 5'-phosphate was used as a cofactor to increase the aminergic neurotransmitters (serotonin, dopamine, GABA, and norepinephrine) and to enhance the gastrointestinal absorption of amino acids.[51]

While thought provoking, Blum and co-workers' research is not definitive as to whether the substances directly caused the changes in neurotransmitters or whether they altered other functional mechanisms within the body. Also, the study did not examine the role of the individual amino acids. Since the physical measures and BESS scores are subjective, it is also possible that the patients were able to discriminate between the inert placebo and the SAAVE capsule, thus accounting for at least part of the observed difference. It is also difficult to generalize from their research, since the investigators did not fully describe the samples, nor did they specify how diagnosis were given, how severely patients were dependent on alcohol, or whether subjects suffered colateral psychopathology. Nevertheless, the Blum group's research should stimulate future investigations using nutritional supplements as an adjunct in treatment of alcoholism.

ROLE OF NEUROTRANSMITTERS IN AFFECTING ALCOHOL CRAVING AND DRINKING BEHAVIOR

Several of the studies mentioned above suggest that nutritional therapy may ultimately modify drinking behavior by altering levels of neurotransmitters in the brain. Candidate neurotransmitters include serotonin, norepinephrine, dopamine, GABA, and endogenous opiates.

Recent research has associated serotonin with behavioral patterns of drinking. Rats selectively bred to prefer alcohol have lower serotonin levels in several regions of the brain than do alcohol-nonpreferring rats.[31,52] These areas, such as the nucleus accumbens, hypothalamus, hippocampus, and frontal cortex, correspond to behavioral reward activity. In addition, i.p. administration of agents, which increases levels of serotonin (e.g., fluoxetine, a serotonin uptake inhibitor, and fenfluramine, a releaser of serotonin) or which mimic the action of serotonin (e.g., serotonin agonists), have been shown to decrease the alcohol intake of alcohol-seeking rats.[31] In several randomized, double-blind, placebo-controlled studies with humans, the serotinin uptake inhibitors, fluoxetine, citalopram, viqualine, and zimelidine, reduced alcohol intake in social drinkers, early problem drinkers, and chronic alcoholics.[53-58] The operative mechanism responsible for this remains unspecified.

Dopamine is also believed to be involved with proclivity to drinking. McBride et al.[31] found significantly lower levels of dopamine in the nucleus accumbens in the alcohol-preferring and the high alcohol-drinking lines of rats than in rats of the alcohol-nonpreferring and low alcohol-drinking lines. The i.p. administration of GBR 12909 (a dopamine uptake inhibitor), amphetamine (a dopamine releaser), or bromocriptine (a dopamine agonist) resulted in a significant decrease in alcohol intake of high alcohol-seeking rats.[31] Similarly, Koob and Weiss[59] reported a decrease in alcohol intake and an increase in water intake in alcohol-preferring rats treated with bromocriptine. In a double-blind, placebo-controlled study, Borg[60] found that bromocriptine reduced craving in alcoholics over a 6-month period.

GABA, another neurotransmitter, has been proposed to be involved in mediating drinking behavior. Hwang et al.[61] reported more GABAergic terminals in the nucleus accumbens region of the brain in both alcohol-preferring and high alcohol-drinking lines of rats as contrasted with alcohol-nonpreferring and low alcohol-drinking lines. When the benzodiazepine inverse agonist Ro 15-4513 was administered to rats, alcohol intake decreased significantly.[31,62] (Ro 15-4513 binds to the GABA receptor, a part of a macromolecular complex receptor containing GABA, barbiturate, picrotoxin, and benzodiazepine binding sites.)

Mechanisms for the reinforcement properties of alcohol may be related to norepinephrine action. In several animal studies, turnover of brain norepinephrine is increased following the administration of alcohol.[63] During acute intoxication and acute alcohol withdrawal, heightened levels of norepinephrine have been found in the CNS of alcoholics as well as in healthy human controls.[64-66] A significant correlation has been observed between alcohol consumption and level of cerebrospinal fluid (CSF) 3-methoxy-4-hydroxy-phenylethyleneglycol (MHPG), a metabolite of norepinephrine.[65] Moreover, a lower MHPG level has been observed among subjects with first-degree relatives with alcohol problems, suggesting that a hypoadrenergic system may be associated with increased alcohol craving.[65]

During the 1980s, a great deal of research implicated opiates in the regulation of alcohol consumption. For instance, the narcotic antagonists naltrexone and naloxone were shown to reduce alcohol consumption in rats and monkeys.[67-69] A recent report by Volpicelli et al.[70] noted that naltrexone also reduced alcohol consumption and craving in alcohol-dependent patients following treatment. In addition, a difference has been demonstrated in the brain met-enkephalin levels between the alcohol-preferring line and alcohol-nonpreferring line of rats, particularly in the hypothalamus, anterior striatum, and posterior striatum.[71] Also, Gianoulakis et al.[72] has shown that high-risk human subjects (strong positive history of alcoholism) have a lower plasma level of β-endorphin than that measured in low-risk individuals (negative history of alcoholism). In the presence of alcohol, the percent increase in plasma β-endorphin is greater in the high-risk individuals than that observed in the low-risk individuals. Finally, a class of compounds, known as the tetrahydroisoquinoline (TIQ) alkaloids (formed from the condensation of acetaldehyde and dopamine), are believed to bind to opiate receptors in the brain.[73] Several investigators[74-76] have reported that the TIQ alkaloids cause an increase in alcohol intake, which is blocked by the opiate antagonists, naloxone and naltrexone.

Research is currently underway to identify the neuroanatomical circuitry involved in regulating alcohol drinking behavior and to determine more specifically the alterations that occur in alcoholism. Such research is difficult since the network is exceptionally complex and probably involves several areas within the limbic system, resulting in a range of intricate interactions.[31,73,77] In searching for differences between the alcohol-drinking (alcohol-preferring line and high alcohol-drinking line) rats and the nonalcohol-drinking (alcohol-nonpreferring line and low alcohol-drinking line) rats, McBride et al.[31] concluded that abnormalities exist in the serotonergic system of the nucleus accumbens and medial prefrontal cortex, the dopaminergic system of the nucleus accumbens, and the GABA system also within the nucleus accumbens.

CONSIDERATIONS FOR FUTURE RESEARCH

In light of the positive studies on nutritional interventions on drinking in animals and an intuitively appealing scientific rationale for such effects, several types of research are now needed. These projects could profitably focus in the nutritional pathophysiology of alcoholism, operative components of nutritional interventions, neurochemical bases of alcoholism, and neurobiological relationships between alcoholism and other addictive disorders.

At the most basic level, research should be directed toward determining if alcoholics and problem drinkers are actually deficient in nutrients for which a role in alcohol consumption has been imputed. Most impressive would be longitudinal studies demonstrating exacerbation of such nutritional deficiencies or excesses with development on alcoholism.

Another yet to be undertaken research task would involve measuring neurotransmitter levels *in vivo* and relating these levels to changes in drinking and alcoholism recovery status. Sophisticated imaging techniques are rapidly becoming available and may be employed to better quantify neurotransmitter levels.

Efforts to clearly specify the underlying physiological and psychological bases of drinking behavior and alcohol craving should accompany applied nutritional research. If one were to adopt a purely pragmatic approach to the development of nutritional interventions (i.e., looking for effective interventions without attempting to understand the mechanism for their effectiveness), it would be unclear whether the nutritional approach worked indirectly (''psychologically''), for example, by making patients feel better or healthier or less in need of the effects of alcohol, or whether the nutritional adjunct directly affected mechanisms related to drinking, craving, or satiety.

The need to conduct nutritional studies, with alcohol-dependent human subjects cannot be too greatly emphasized. Several of the studies noted above suggest species-specific differences in alcohol-nutrition relationships, and others have found differences between alcohol-dependent and alcohol-nondependent organisms. Beyond this, alcohol consumption in humans, especially problematic drinking, likely involves significant learned as well as genetic components. (To date, it seems no nutritional research has been conducted on animals conditioned, as opposed to bred, to drink excessively.) Only one controlled study has been performed on humans in which a significant improvement in the treatment of alcoholism was reported,[51] and, as noted, this study both failed to evaluate the effects of nutrition on actual drinking or to specify the level of dependency in the subjects. Alcohol consumption among humans differs in fundamental ways from drinking by animals. For example, social stimuli, expectancy for alcohol effects, and personality characteristics, such as impulsiveness, have been associated with problematic drinking in humans. Indeed, the psychosocial correlates of drinking seem to differ even between alcoholics and social drinkers.

As with certain types of drug abuse, alcoholism is believed to involve dysfunction in the neurotransmitter serotonin. Several other types of psychiatric disorders, including depression, compulsive eating, and seasonal affective disorder (SAD) also seem to be influenced by serotonin. All have been treated with pharmacologic agents that increase levels of serotonin (e.g., fluoxetine and D-fenfluramine).[56,78-80] In addition, alcoholism, depression, compulsive eating, and SAD have been associated with the increased intake of high-carbohydrate, low-protein meals.[50,80,81] The ingestion of a high-carbohydrate meal results in an increase in insulin which, in turn, augments transport of tryptophan across the blood-brain barrier, apparently leading to increased levels of brain serotonin.[80,81] More studies are needed to understand the relationships among drinking behavior, depression, neurotransmitters, and diet.

Finally, investigations involving other types of addictions are needed. Many researchers believe that alcoholism and drug addiction may derive from some common neurobiological mechanism.[82] Recent reports have suggested that dietary therapy may assist in the treatment of cocaine addiction.[83,84] Blum et al.[83] developed an amino acid, vitamin, and mineral mixture called Tropamine as a neurochemical support to treat cocaine abusers. In a double-blind clinical trial, they found that patients receiving Tropamine were less agitated, more cooperative and "focused", reported less drug craving, and had a lower treatment dropout rate. It would be interesting to repeat this study with individuals simultaneously dependent on both alcohol and cocaine as well as alcohol-only patients.

CLINICAL ISSUES AND CONCERNS

Should alcoholism be found to respond to nutritional interventions, several clinical issues must be resolved. The first issue deals with the nature and dosage of the nutritional adjunct. This will likely vary among alcoholics as a function of their other nutritional requirements. A wide range of factors can, of course, alter dietary needs. Most importantly, other health conditions must be considered. For example, phenylketonuria, liver disease, renal disease, and pregnancy can impede phenylalanine metabolism, thus increasing the blood levels of phenylalanine after taking aspartame or phenylalanine.[85] Stage and severity of alcoholism in the individual will probably also make a difference. Beneficial dietary adjuncts for an alcoholic may differ during acute alcohol withdrawal vs. long-term abstinence. Also, the age of the alcoholic and level of activity (exercise) may influence the amount of the nutritional agent needed. Carbohydrate metabolism declines with age, a condition that may be further exacerbated by alcohol abuse.[86] Thus, it will probably be important to carefully match the composition and dosage of the nutritional intervention with the physiological status of the patient.

As with any treatment intervention, patient compliance will be critical in nutritional therapy. To enhance prospects for compliance, effective programs in nutritional education, counseling, aftercare, and monitoring must be developed. Psychosocial aids to augment compliance will probably prove necessary. Experience with disulfiram may provide some guidance in this regard. Compliance with disulfiram has been facilitated through reinforcement paradigms, contracts with the patient, and involvement of family members.[87-91] Similar strategies might well increase compliance with nutritional adjuncts. Finally, aftercare plans should include frequent consultations to monitor compliance with the dietary intervention and to assess eating patterns, physical condition, and status of abstinence from alcohol.

As nutritional therapies are developed for alcoholism, consideration must be given to comorbid psychiatric disorders and/or associated drug abuse. As noted earlier, several types of psychiatric disorders (eating disorders, SAD, and depression) and drug dependencies have been associated with diet-induced changes in neurotransmitters. Various types of drug abuse may require specific nutrient regimes. For example, as noted earlier, Blum et al.[83] reported that Tropamine was more effective in treating cocaine abusers than the multinutrient SAAVE used to treat alcoholics.

Consideration of possible short- and long-range side effects of nutritional agents is also essential for appropriate therapy. Today, most vitamins, minerals, and amino acids are available without prescription and are being marketed to the public as beneficial for numerous problems. Unfortunately, many agents risk significant toxicities when taken in large amounts.[85] Clinically effective amounts of nutrients are often a function of patient characteristics and accompanying diet. For instance, L-tryptophan is accumulated in the brain when taken with a high-carbohydrate, low-protein snack.[80,81] Therefore, "individualizing" dietary supplements would be necessary. Finally, the way in which the nutrients are prepared, processed, and manufactured may itself produce differing side effects. For example, L-tryptophan is currently banned in the U.S. because of a contaminant resulting from the manufacturing process, causing eosinophilia-myalgia syndrome, a serious blood disorder. Nutritional regimens that cause side effects uncomfortable to the patient, even if helpful in alcoholism treatment, are, of course, less likely to be voluntarily followed.

Finally, if a successful dietary intervention is ultimately developed for alcoholism, this intervention must be effectively integrated with other psychosocial and pharmacological interventions. Short- and long-term goals of these interventions should be specified. After their identification, it should be possible to develop an optimal temporal phasing or integration of the psychosocial, dietary, and pharmacological interventions to maximize treatment outcome. For instance, an initial treatment protocol might consist of treatment for acute alcohol withdrawal, cognitive impairment, and medical stabilization, followed by a broad-based behaviorally oriented rehabilitation program.[93]

SUMMARY

Over the past 40 years, researchers have studied the role of nutrition in alcohol consumption. Recent research on diet and on basic mechanisms of alcohol drinking behavior has provided evidence of a possible association between nutrition and alcohol consumption. Changes in protein diet appear to alter alcohol consumption, while mixed results have been reported with diets varying in carbohydrate and fat content. The mode of action of these changes is unknown, though alterations in metabolism, clearance, acetaldehyde levels, and neurotransmitters have been postulated. Deficiencies in vitamin B complex have also produced changes in alcohol intake. However, more research is needed before strong conclusions can be drawn. L-glutamine, L-tryptophan, L-5-hydroxytryptophan, and L-phenylalanine act as precursors for several neurotransmitters that have been implicated in altering alcohol consumption, and are thus potentially effective agents to curb drinking. In addition to the amino acids, I, Zn, and Na seem to modify alcohol seeking in several experimental animal models.

Only a few studies have examined the effectiveness of nutritional interventions in humans with alcohol problems. The recent work of Blum et al.,[51] using the amino acid and vitamin mixture, SAAVE, has had optimistic results, although more research is clearly needed to confirm the results and then to determine if SAAVE results in a long-term decrease of alcohol consumption.

The neurotransmitters, serotonin, norepinephrine, dopamine, GABA, and the opioids, seem related to alcohol consumption. Modifications in the levels of these neurotransmitters by nutrient therapy may prove an important adjunct to treatment for regulating drinking behavior.

New areas of research include determination of the biological basis of alcohol drinking behavior, performance of more double-blind, placebo-controlled studies with humans, and exploration of a possible common neurobiological mechanism of chemical dependency and several types of psychiatric disorders that seem to share common neurotransmitter dysfunctions with alcoholism.

Finally, the research on nutritional therapy for alcoholism is currently in a preliminary phase. If effective nutritional interventions derive from research, several clinical issues and concerns will require resolution. These include matching precise compositions and dosages of the nutritional intervention with physiological and psychological status variables in the individual; insuring patient compliance through nutritional education, counseling, and aftercare; determining the short- and long-term effects of nutritional therapy; and successfully integrating nutritional interventions into alcoholism treatment programs.

REFERENCES

1. ADA Reports, Position of the American Diabetic Association: nutrition intervention in treatment and recovery from chemical dependency, *J. Am. Diet. Assoc.*, 90, 1274, 1990.
2. Mirone, L., Dietary deficiency in mice in relation to voluntary alcohol consumption, *Q. J. Stud. Alcohol*, 18, 552, 1957.
3. Brown, R. V. and Hutcheson, D. P., Nutrition and alcohol consumption in the Sinclair miniature pig, *Q. J. Stud. Alcohol*, 34, 758, 1973.
4. Pekkanen, L., Eriksson, K., and Sihvonen, M. L., Dietary-induced changes in voluntary ethanol consumption and ethanol metabolism in the rat, *Br. J. Nutr.*, 40, 103, 1978.
5. Hanig, J. P., Yoder, P., Kropp, S., and Lao, C., Effect of long-term restriction of protein intake, from gestation onward, on free-choice consumption of ethanol by rats, *Life Sci.*, 23, 1881, 1978.
6. Norton, V. P., Interrelationships of nutrition and voluntary alcohol consumption in experimental animals, *Br. J. Addict.*, 72, 205, 1977.
7. Forsander, O. A. and Sinclair, J. D., Protein, carbohydrate, and ethanol consumption: interactions in AA and ANA rats, *Alcohol*, 5, 233, 1988.

8. Lester, D. and Greenberg, L. A., Nutrition and the etiology of alcoholism, *Q. J. Stud. Alcohol,* 13, 553, 1952.
9. Mardones, J., Segovia-Riquelme, N., Hederra, A., and Alcaino, F., Effect of some self-selection conditions on the voluntary alcohol intake of rats, *Q. J. Stud. Alcohol,* 16, 425, 1955.
10. Eriksson, K., Factors affecting voluntary alcohol consumption in the albino rat, *Ann. Zool. Fenn,* 6, 227, 1969.
11. Lindros, K. O., Pekkanen, L., and Koivula, T., Enzymatic and metabolic modification of hepatic ethanol and acetaldehyde oxidation by the dietary protein level, *Biochem. Pharmacol.,* 28, 2313, 1979.
12. Lindros, K. O., Pekkanen, L., and Kiovula, T., Biphasic influence of dietary protein levels on ethanol-derived acetaldehyde concentrations, *Acta Pharmacol. Toxicol.,* 43, 409, 1978.
13. Eriksson, C. J. P., Ethanol and acetaldehyde metabolism in rat strains genetically selected for their ethanol preference, *Biochem. Pharmacol.,* 22, 2283, 1973.
14. Sinclair, J. D. and Lindros, K. O., Suppression of alcohol drinking with brain aldehyde dehydrogenase inhibition, *Pharmacol. Biochem. Behav.,* 14, 377, 1981.
15. Preston, A. M., Tumbleson, M. E., and Hutcheson, D. P., Ethanol consumption and enzyme activities in Sinclair miniature pigs, *Q. J. Stud. Alcohol,* 34, 1293, 1973.
16. Eriksson, C. J. P., Problems and pitfalls in acetaldehyde determinations, *Alcohol. Clin. Exp. Res.,* 4, 22, 1980.
17. Brady, R. A. and Westerfeld, W. W., The effect of B-complex vitamins on the voluntary consumption of alcohol by rats, *Q. J. Stud. Alcohol,* 7, 499, 1947.
18. Williams, R. J., Pelton, R. B., and Rogers, L. L., Dietary deficiencies in animals in relation to voluntary alcohol and sugar consumption, *Q. J. Stud. Alcohol,* 16, 234, 1955.
19. Brown, R. V., Vitamin deficiency and voluntary alcohol consumption in mice, *Q. J. Stud. Alcohol,* 30, 592, 1969.
20. Westerfeld, W. W. and Lawrow, J., The effects of caloric restriction and thiamin deficiency on the voluntary consumption of alcohol by rats, *Q. J. Stud. Alcohol,* 14, 378, 1953.
21. Purdy, M. B. and Lee, J. G., The effect of restricted food intake, thiamine deficiency and riboflavin deficiency on the voluntary consumption of ethanol by the albino rat, *Q. J. Stud. Alcohol,* 23, 549, 1962.
22. Rogers, L. L., Pelton, R. B., and Williams, R. J., Voluntary alcohol consumption by rats following administration of glutamine, *J. Biol. Chem.,* 214, 503, 1955.
23. Rogers, L. L., Pelton, R. B., and Williams, R. J., Amino acid supplementation and voluntary alcohol consumption by rats, *J. Biol. Chem.,* 220, 321, 1956.
24. Blum, K., Briggs, A. H., Trachtenberg, M. C., Delallo, L., and Wallace, J. E., Enkephalinase inhibition: regulation of ethanol intake in genetically predisposed mice, *Alcohol,* 4, 449, 1987.

25. Sprince, H., Parker, C. M., Smith, G. G., and Gonzales, L. J., Alcoholism: biochemical and nutritional aspects of brain amines, aldehydes, and amino acids, *Nutr. Rep. Int.,* 5, 185, 1972.

26. Myers, R. D. and Melchior, C. L., Dietary tryptophan and the selection of ethyl alcohol in different strains of rats, *Psychopharmacologia,* 42, 109, 1975.

27. Geller, I., Effects of parachlorophenylalanine and 5-hydroxytryptophan on alcohol intake in the rat, *Pharmacol. Biochem. Behav.,* 1, 361, 1973.

28. Walters, J. K., Effects of PCPA on the consumption of alcohol, water, and other solutions, *Pharmacol. Biochem. Behav.,* 6, 377, 1977.

29. Zabik, J. E., Liao, S. S., Jeffreys, M., and Maickel, R. P., The effects of DL-5-hydroxytryptophan on ethanol consumption by rats, *Res. Commun. Chem. Pathol. Pharmacol.,* 20, 69, 1978.

30. Zabik, J. E., Binkerd, K., and Roache, J. D., Serotonin and ethanol aversion in the rat, in *Research Advances in New Psychopharmacological Treatments for Alcoholism,* Naranjo, C. A. and Sellers, E. M., Eds., Elsevier, New York, 1985, 87.

31. McBride, W. J., Murphy, J. M., Lumeng, L., and Li, T.-K., Serotonin, dopamine and GABA involvement in alcohol drinking of selectively bred rats, *Alcohol,* 7, 199, 1990.

32. Ostrovsky, S. Y., Glutamine-induced alterations in the content of brain amino acid neurotransmitters in rats with different alcohol motivation, *Subst. Alcohol Actions/Misuse,* 5, 247, 1985.

33. Blum, K. and Trachtenberg, M. C., Neurogenetic deficits caused by alcoholism: restoration by SAAVE, a neuronutrient intervention adjunct, *J. Psychoactive Drugs,* 20, 297, 1988.

34. Maenpaa, P. H. and Forsander, O. A., Influence of iodine deficiency on free choice between alcohol and water in rats, *Q. J. Stud. Alcohol,* 27, 596, 1966.

35. Collipp, P. J., Kris, V. K., Castro-Magana, M., Shih, A., Chen, S. Y., Antoszyk, N., Baltzell, J., Noll, J., and Trusty, C., The effects of dietary zinc deficiency on voluntary alcohol drinking in rats, *Alcohol. Clin. Exp. Res.,* 8, 556, 1984.

36. Ahmed, S. B. and Russell, R. M., The effect of ethanol feeding on zinc balance and tissue zinc levels in rats maintained on zinc-deficient diets, *J. Lab. Clin. Med.,* 100, 211, 1982.

37. Kern, J. C., Hassett, C. A., Collipp, P., Bridges, C., Solomon, M., and Condren, R. J., Children of alcoholics: locus of control mental age, and zinc level, *J. Psychiatric Treat. Eval.,* 3, 169, 1981.

38. Grupp, L. A., Stewart, R. B., and Perlanski, E., Salt restriction and the voluntary intake of ethanol in rats, *Physiol. Psychol.,* 12, 242, 1984.

39. Grupp, L. A., Perlanski, E., and Stewart, R. B., Diet and diuretics in the reduction of voluntary alcohol drinking in rats, *Alcohol Alcohol.,* 21, 75, 1986.

40. Grupp, L. A., Perlanski, E., and Stewart, R. B., Dietary salt and DOCA-salt treatments modify self-selection in rats, *Behav. Neural Biol.,* 40, 239, 1984.

41. Grupp, L. A., Kalant, H., and Leenen, F. H. H., Alcohol intake is inversely related to plasma renin activity in the genetically selected alcohol-preferring and -nonpreferring lines of rats, *Pharmacol. Biochem. Behav.*, 32, 1061, 1989.

42. Grupp, L. A., Perlanski, E., Wanless, I. R., and Stewart, R. B., Voluntary alcohol intake in the hypertension prone Dahl rat, *Pharmacol. Biochem. Behav.*, 24, 1167, 1986.

43. Iwai, J., Dahl, L. K., and Knudsen, K. D., Genetic influences on the renin-angiotensin system. Four renin activities in hypertension-prone rats, *Circ. Res.*, 32, 678, 1973.

44. Rapp, J. P., Tan, S. Y., and Margolius, H. S., Plasma mineralocorticoids, plasma renin, and urinary kallikrein in salt-sensitive and salt-resistant rats, *Endocrinol. Res. Commun.*, 5, 35, 1978.

45. Grupp, L. A., Sneddon, B., Solway, E., Perlanski, E., and Stewart, R. B., The beta adrenergic agonist isoproterenol suppresses voluntary alcohol intake in rats, *Pharmacol. Biochem. Behav.*, 33, 493, 1989.

46. Grupp, L. A., Killian, M., Perlanski, E., and Stewart, R. B., Angiotension II reduces voluntary alcohol intake in the rat, *Pharmacol. Biochem. Behav.*, 29, 479, 1988.

47. Grupp, L. A., Perlanski, E., and Stewart, R. B., Angiotensin II-induced suppression of alcohol intake and its reversal by the angiotensin antagonist Sar-1 Thr-8 angiotensin II, *Pharmacol. Biochem. Behav.*, 31, 813, 1989.

48. Grupp, L. A., Perlanski, E., and Stewart, R. B., Systemic angiotensin II acts at the subfornical organ to suppress voluntary alcohol consumption, *Pharmacol. Biochem. Behav.*, 34, 201, 1989.

49. Rogers, L. L. and Pelton, R. B., Glutamine in the treatment of alcoholism, *Q. J. Stud. Alcohol*, 18, 581, 1957.

50. Yung, L., Gordis, E., and Holt, J., Dietary choices and likelihood of abstinence among alcoholic patients in an outpatient clinic, *Drug Alcohol Depend.*, 12, 355, 1983.

51. Blum, K., Trachtenberg, M. C., Elliott, C. E., Dingler, M. L., Sexton, R. L., Samuels, A. I., and Cataldie, L., Enkephalinase inhibition and precursor amino acid loading improves inpatient treatment of alcohol and polydrug treatment of alcohol and polydrug abusers: double-blind placebo-controlled study of the nutritional adjunct SAAVE, *Alcohol*, 5, 481, 1989.

52. McBride, W. J., Murphy, J. M., Lumeng, L., and Li, T.-K., Serotonin and ethanol preference, in *Recent Developments in Alcoholism Treatment Research*, Vol. 7, Galanter, M., Ed., Plenum Press, New York, 1989, 187.

53. Naranjo, C. A., Sellers, E. M., Roach, C. A., Woodley, D. V., Sanchez-Craig, M., and Sykora, K., Zimelidine-induced variations in alcohol intake by nondepressed heavy drinkers, *Clin. Pharmacol. Ther.*, 35, 374, 1984.

54. Naranjo, C. A., Sellers, E. M., Jullivan, J. T., Woodley, D. V., Kadlec, K., and Sykora, K., The serotonin uptake inhibitor citalopram attenuates ethanol intake, *Clin. Pharmacol. Ther.*, 41, 266, 1987.

55. Amit, Z., Brown, Z., Sutherland, A., Rockman, G., Gill, K., and Selvaggi, N., Reduction in alcohol intake in humans as a function of treatment with zimelidine: implications for treatment, in *Research Advances in New Psychopharmacological Treatments for Alcoholism*, Naranjo, C. A. and Sellers, E. M., Eds., Excerpta Medica, Amsterdam, 1985, 189.

56. Gorelick, D. A., Serotonin uptake blockers and the treatment of alcoholism, in *Recent Developments in Alcoholism Treatment Research,* Vol. 7, Galanter, M., Ed., Plenum Press, New York, 1989, 267.
57. Naranjo, C., Sullivan, J. T., Kadlec, K. E., Woodley-Remus, D. V., Kennedy, G., and Sellers, E. M., Differential effects of viqualine on alcohol intake and other consummatory behaviors, *Clin. Pharmacol. Ther.,* 46, 301, 1989.
58. Naranjo, C. A., Kadlec, K. E., Sanhueza, P., Woodley-Remus, D., and Sellers, E. M., Flouxetine differentially alters alcohol intake and other consummatory behaviors in problem drinkers, *Clin. Pharmacol. Ther.,* 47, 490, 1990.
59. Koob, G. F. and Weiss, F., Pharmacology of drug self-administration, *Alcohol,* 7, 193, 1990.
60. Borg, V., Bromocriptine in the prevention of alcohol abuse, *Acta Psychiatr. Scand.,* 68, 100, 1983.
61. Hwang, B., Lumeng, L., Wu, J.-Y., and Li, T.-K., Increased number of GABAergic terminals in the nucleus accumbens is associated with alcohol preference in rats, *Alcohol. Clin. Exp. Res.,* 14, 503, 1990.
62. Samson, H. H., Tolliver, G. A., Pfeffer, A. O., Sadeghi, K. G., and Mills, F. G., Oral ethanol reinforcement in the rat: effect of the partial inverse benzodiazepine agonist RO 15-4513, *Pharmacol. Biochem. Behav.,* 27, 517, 1987.
63. Blum, K., Briggs, A. H., and Trachtenberg, M. C., Ethanol ingestive behavior as a function of central neurotransmission, *Experientia,* 45, 444, 1989.
64. Sjoquist, B., Borg, S., and Kvande, H., Catecholamine derived compounds in urine and cerebrospinal fluid from alcoholics during and after long-standing intoxication, *Subst. Alcohol Actions/Misuse,* 2, 63, 1981.
65. Borg, S., Liljeberg, R., and Mossberg, D., Clinical studies on central noradrenergic activity in alcohol abusing patients, *Acta Psychiatr. Scand.,* 73(Suppl.), 43, 1986.
66. Linnoila, M., Alcohol withdrawal syndrome and sympathetic nervous system, *Alcohol Health Res. World,* 13, 355, 1989.
67. Hubbell, C. L., Czirr, S. A., Hunter, G. A., Beaman, C. M., LeCann, N. C., and Reid, L. D., Consumption of ethanol solution is potentiated by morphine and attenuated by naloxone persistently across repeated daily administrations, *Alcohol,* 3, 39, 1986.
68. Myers, R. D., Borg, S., and Mossberg, R., Antagonism by naltrexone of voluntary alcohol selection in the chronically drinking macaque monkey, *Alcohol,* 3, 383, 1986.
69. Volpicelli, J. R., Davis, M. A., and Olgin, J. E., Naltrexone blocks the post-shock increase of ethanol consumption, *Life Sci.,* 38, 841, 1986.
70. Volpicelli, J. R., O'Brien, C. P., Alterman, A. I., and Hayashida, M., Naltrexone and the treatment of alcohol-dependence: initial observations, in *Opioids, Bulimia, and Alcohol Abuse and Alcoholism,* Reid, L. D., Ed., Springer-Verlag, New York, 1990, 195.
71. Froehlich, J. C. and Li, T.-K., Enkephalinergic involvement in voluntary drinking of alcohol, in *Opioids, Bulimia, and Alcohol Abuse and Alcoholism,* Reid, L. D., Ed., Springer-Verlag, New York, 1990, 217.

72. Gianoulakis, C., Angelogianni, P., Meaney, M., Thavundayil, J., and Tawar, V., Endorphins in individuals with high and low risk for development of alcoholism, in *Opioids, Bulimia and Alcohol Abuse and Alcoholism*, Reid, L. D., Ed., Springer-Verlag, New York, 1990, 229.
73. Myers, R. D., Anatomical "circuitry" in the brain mediating alcohol drinking revealed by THP-reactive sites in the limbic system, *Alcohol*, 7, 449, 1990.
74. Myers, R. D. and Melchior, C. L., Alcohol drinking: abnormal intake caused by tetrahydropapaveroline in brain, *Science*, 196, 554, 1977.
75. Myers, R. D. and Critcher, E. C., Naloxone alters alcohol drinking induced in the rat by tetrahydropapaveroline (THP) infused ICV, *Pharmacol. Biochem. Behav.*, 16, 827, 1982.
76. Critcher, E. C., Lin, C. I., Patel, J., and Myers, R. D., Attenuation of alcohol drinking in tetrahydroisoquinoline-treated rats by morphine and naltrexone, *Pharmacol. Biochem. Behav.*, 18, 225, 1983.
77. Koob, G. F. and Bloom, F. E., Cellular and molecular mechanisms of drug dependence, *Science*, 242, 715, 1988.
78. Wurtman, J., Wurtman, R., Mark, S., Tsay, R., Gilbert, W., and Growdon, J., d-Fenfluramine selectively suppresses carbohydrate snacking by obese subjects, *Int. J. Eating Disorders*, 4, 89, 1985.
79. Schatzberg, A., Dessain, E., O'Neil, P., Katz, D. L., and Cole, J. O., Recent studies on selective serotonergic antidepressants: trazodone, fluoxetine, and fluvoxamine, *J. Clin. Psychopharmacol.*, 7, 44s, 1987.
80. Wurtman, R. J. and Wurtman, J. J., Carbohydrates and depression, *Sci. Am.*, 260, 68, 1989.
81. Wurtman, R. J., Behavioral effects of nutrients, *Lancet*, 1, 1145, 1983.
82. Miller, N. S. and Mirin, S. M., Multiple drug use in alcoholics: practical and theoretical implications, *Psychiatr. Ann.*, 19, 248, 1989.
83. Blum, K., Allison, D., Trachtenberg, M. C., Williams, R. W., and Loeblich, L. A., Reduction of both drug hunger and withdrawal against advice rate of cocaine abusers in a 30-day inpatient treatment program by the neuronutrient tropamine, *Curr. Ther. Res.*, 43, 1204, 1988.
84. Trachtenberg, M. C. and Blum, K., Improvement of cocaine-induced neuromodulator deficits by the neuronutrient tropamine, *J. Psychoactive Drugs*, 20, 315, 1988.
85. Clark, H. W., Sees, K. L., and Nathan, J. A., Clinical and legal aspects of nonphysician prescription of vitamins, amino acids, and other nutritional supplements, *J. Psychoactive Drugs*, 20, 355, 1988.
86. Patel, D. G., Effects of ethanol on carbohydrate metabolism and implications for the aging alcoholic, *Alcohol Health Res. World*, 13, 240, 1989.
87. Azrin, N. H., Sisson, R. W., Meyer, R., and Godley, M., Alcoholism treatment by disulfiram and community reinforcement therapy, *J. Behav. Ther. Exp. Psychiatry*, 13, 105, 1982.
88. Brewer, C. and Smith, J., Probation linked supervised disulfiram in the treatment of habitual drunken offenders: results of a pilot study, *Br. Med. J.*, 287, 1282, 1983.

89. Keane, T. M., Foy, D. W., Nunn, B., and Rychtarik, R. G., Spouse contracting to increase Antabuse compliance in alcoholic veterans, *J. Clin. Psychol.*, 40, 340, 1984.

90. O'Farrell, T. J. and Bayog, R. D., Antabuse contracts for married alcoholics and their spouses: a method to maintain Antabuse ingestion and decrease conflict about drinking, *J. Subst. Abuse Treat.*, 3, 1, 1986.

91. Sereny, G., Sharma, V., Holt, J., and Gordis, E., Mandatory supervised Antabuse therapy in an outpatient alcoholism program: a pilot study, *Alcohol. Clin. Exp. Res.*, 10, 290, 1986.

92. Meyer, R. E., Prospects for a rational pharmacotherapy of alcoholism, *J. Clin. Psychiatry*, 50, 403, 1989.

3 Nutritional Status of Alcoholics from Different Social Groups

INTRODUCTION

The incidence of malnutrition in alcoholics can be related to the severity and duration of alcohol abuse as well as to several somatic complications caused by or related to excessive chronic heavy drinking.[1-15] With regards to the pathogenesis of alcohol-related diseases the relative contribution of nutritional deficiencies on the one hand, and the direct toxicity of ethanol and its metabolites on the other hand, have thus far been an intensive topic of contradictory opinions. Modern techniques in formulating reliable nutritional surveys and in assessing the nutritional status of alcoholic individuals have greatly improved the possibility of understanding the discrepancies in earlier findings.

SECONDARY NATURE OF MALNUTRITION IN ALCOHOLICS

Most of the early nutritional studies on alcoholics concentrated either on indigent, ''skid row'' alcoholics or on alcoholic patients with significant somatic complications.[16-19] Based on patient materials from a derelict population with severe alcoholic liver injury it was concluded in the 1940s that the relationship between nutritional deficiency and cirrhosis is significant and that the clinical course of the disease can be improved by a diet high in protein and vitamins.[20] This study included 304 alcoholic patients, who were admitted to the hospital because of medical complications, and about 60% of those had cirrhosis of the liver. The protein intake of these alcoholics constituted only 6% of the total calories; i.e., 30 to 50% of the recommended amount. Similar conclusions have been reached in many

ISBN 0-8493-7933-4
© 1992 by CRC Press, Inc.

TABLE 1
Possible Causes of Malnutrition Among Chronic Alcoholics

Poor dietary intake
Lack of effective caloric value of alcohol
Enhanced metabolic rate
Maldigestion and malabsorption:
   Delayed gastric emptying
   Accelerated small intestinal transit
   Intestinal villous injury produced by ethanol or vitamin deficiency
   Pancreatic exocrine insufficiency
   Decreased biliary secretion
Impaired metabolism of nutrients
Decreased hepatic storage of nutrients
Increased requirements of nutrients
Increased urinary and fecal losses

other studies dealing with alcoholics hospitalized because of alcoholic liver injury.[6,7,12,21-23] However, due to many confounding factors, the conclusions on the primary cause of malnutrition — liver injury or poor nutrition — in patients with liver cirrhosis should be drawn extremely carefully.[19]

It is generally agreed that the primary cause of malnutrition among alcoholics can be multifactorial (Table 1). Malnutrition may be caused by the lack of effective caloric value of alcohol associated with the enhanced metabolism of ethanol.[24] High ethanol concentrations may delay gastric emptying and cause maldigestion.[25] Ethanol may cause villous injury in intestinal epithelial cells[26] and malabsorption may be further potentiated by associated folate deficiency.[27] Steatorrhea is a frequent finding in patients with alcoholic cirrhosis,[28] most often caused by decreased biliary secretion of bile acids,[29] but malabsorption of fats may also be secondary to pancreatic exocrine insufficiency. Finally, alcoholic liver cirrhosis may lead to impaired metabolism of (at least) thiamin, folate, and pyridoxine and may interfere with the hepatic storage of these and many other vitamins.[5]

The laboratory tests used to diagnose protein calorie malnutrition are often abnormal in patients with alcoholic liver disease (ALD).[30-33] These abnormalities are multifactorial and therefore may considerably hamper both the assessment of the hepatic function of the patient as well as the evaluation of their nutritional status. Reduced levels of serum albumin, prealbumin, and transferrin are frequently found in patients with alcoholic cirrhosis, hepatitis, or fatty liver.[33-36] Furthermore, a negative correlation is apparent between the serum levels of these secretory proteins and the degree of alcoholic liver injury.[33] In the assessment of the nutritional status of a patient with mild alcoholic liver injury only serum transferrin appears to have some nutritional significance.[33]

NUTRITIONAL STATUS OF ALCOHOLICS WITHOUT LIVER DISEASE

GENERAL NUTRITION

The assessment of the nutritional status of an alcoholic may be hampered by the unreliability of the information concerning individual alcohol consumption. In a study of 28 alcoholic patients, Eagles and Longman[37] reported no significant difference when dietary histories were obtained either from the patients or from the spouse or another family member. However, individual patient history of alcohol intake at times may be much more unreliable. The frequency and quantity of alcohol intake reported by an alcoholic upon entry for treatment may still be valid.[38] However, 10 to 15% of alcoholics who have recently imbibed underreport to such an extent that they may be incorrectly classified as nonalcoholics.[38]

Neville et al.[18] were the first to assess the nutritional status of chronic alcoholics who were not admitted to hospitals due to medical problems. Their study group consisted of 34 alcoholics (26 men, 8 women) with sufficient annual incomes. The average nutrient intake (food, alcoholic beverages, and vitamin supplements) were determined by dietary history for 1 month prior to the hospitalization and vitamin excretion tests. In alcoholics the intake of calories was higher and the intakes of protein and fat somewhat lower than in controls. The results did not generally support the view that the nutritional status of alcoholics without medical complications is markedly inferior to that of nonalcoholics, particularly among those with similar economic and health histories.

Confirmatory results were obtained in two later studies.[39,40] The study group of Hurt et al.[39] consisted of 43 men and 15 women. They were consecutively admitted for the treatment of alcoholism to the Alcoholism and Drug Dependence Unit of Rochester Methodist Hospital, Rochester, MN, which is the major chemical dependency treatment facility for patients of the Mayo Clinic. The patients represented a broad cross-section of middle-class people; most of the men were blue- or white-collar non-professional workers, and most of the women chose to remain at home. Only three of the patients were unemployed. A thorough dietary history was taken by the same clinical dietician within 72 h of admission. A standardized method of obtaining and recording the dietary history was used: typical daily nutrient intake, including food habits, meal and snack pattern, restaurant eating, food frequency data, and beverage intake. The pretreatment dietary histories of the 58 alcoholics were compared with their actual intake while the patients were hospitalized for the treatment of alcoholism. It was concluded that the mean calorie, protein, fat, and carbohydrate intake of the patients was adequate and was well within the U.S. Recommended Dietary Allowances (RDA) ranges. After the patients stopped drinking, they increased their intake of all major nutrients, especially carbohydrates.

The study[39] also included a subgroup of 11 patients whose recent dietary intake by history was corroborated by their urinary nitrogen excretion. Among these patients no change in total caloric intake after cessation of drinking could be observed. The authors concluded that although several patients had selected nutritional intake deficiencies, the nutrient intake of most middle-class alcoholic patients is adequate.

Goldsmith et al.[40] compared the nutritional status of 50 middle-class alcoholics to 50 lower-class alcoholics. Standard measurements included height, weight, triceps skinfold, midarm circumference, hematocrit, and hair-pulling strength. The study indicated that the differences in socioeconomic class can make a significant difference in nutritional status between the middle-income alcoholic and the lower-income alcoholic. Lower-income alcoholics had significantly lower weight-to-height indices, lower triceps skinfold, lower arm muscle circumference, lower microhematocrit, and lower epilation force (force required to pull hairs from the head). Nevertheless, neither group was revealed to be greatly malnourished.

SELECTIVE MALNUTRITION

Hillers and Massey[41] studied the relationships between habitual alcohol consumption and diet and nutritional status in 179 middle-income males with a wide range of alcohol consumption. The study group included 51 undergraduate students, 46 nonfaculty university employees, 35 men arrested for driving while intoxicated (DWI), and 47 alcoholics admitted to in-patient treatment. The Dietary Intake Form based on assessing intakes of the four basic food groups was used to assess each subject's long-term food intake. In addition a 24-h dietary recall was collected from each subject. Blood samples were analyzed for 33 clinical laboratory tests. In linear regression a trend toward increased energy intake occurred as alcohol consumption increased. When the population was divided into tertiles based on alcohol consumption, however, energy intake was not significantly different between the tertile groupings. As alcohol intake increased, there was a decrease in percentage of energy derived from protein, fat, and carbohydrate and the nutritional quality of the diet declined. Changes in health status, as measured by blood chemistries, were associated with both moderate and high alcohol consumption. However, only three abnormal mean values were found in the tertile with the highest alcohol consumption. These were vitamin A, vitamin C, and thiamin with 75, 73, and 79%, respectively, of the RDA.

Salaspuro and co-authors[42] have assessed the impact of heavy alcohol consumption on the diet and nutritional status of employed Finnish men with special reference to vitamins and trace elements with anitoxidative properties. They studied 26 male problem drinkers fulfilling the American Psychiatric Association's *Diagnostic and Statistical Manual of Mental Disorders* (DSM-III) criteria of alcoholism and 49 controls (male). Dietary interviews and anthropometric measurements were performed by a trained nutritionist using standardized techniques and protocols. The dietary history covered the average diet of the previous month and included a set of questions that focused on drinking and meal patterns.

Because of their greater alcohol consumption, the daily energy intake for the alcoholic significantly exceeded that of the control males.[42] Other dietary deficiencies, however, were negligible. As compared to controls, alcoholics had thicker fat folds but reduced body mass and arm muscle circumference. Mean circulating levels of vitamin C and α-tocopherol were normal and equal in alcoholics and controls, but serum retinol was elevated and β-carotene reduced in alcoholics. Serum concentration and 24-h urinary excretion of selenium were significantly lower in alcoholics than in the controls. Serum levels of magnesium (Mg) and zinc (Zn) were similar in both groups, but urinary excretion was higher in alcoholics. It was concluded that heavy drinking does not result in florid nutritional deficiencies in socially intact men, but its role in subtle nutritional alterations deserves further study.[42]

NUTRITIONAL STATUS OF LOWER
SOCIAL CLASSES

The data on the nutritional indices and dietary adequacy of lower social classes, including urban homeless adults and "skid row" alcoholics, are rather limited. However, homeless persons frequently suffer several health disorders such as mental illness, alcoholism, tuberculosis, coronary artery disease, hypertension, and diabetes mellitus.[43-45] The early studies on indigent and malnourished lower-class alcoholics revealed low levels of circulating vitamins in 40 to 95% of the patients.[46-48] In 1975 and 1976 13.1% of lower-class alcoholics and 9.5% of middle-class alcoholics at the Addiction Research Foundation of Ontario could be considered to be malnourished.[49]

Laven and Brown[50] assessed the nutritional status and socioeconomic characteristics of 49 men attending a soup kitchen in a residential neighborhood of Birmingham, AL. Laboratory or anthropometric evidence of nutrient deficiency was present in 94% of the subjects. The incidence of alcohol problems among the men was not mentioned. The incidences of ascorbate (63%), folate (35%), and thiamin (29%) deficiencies were significantly higher among these men than in either other patients or presumably healthy adults.

Luder et al.[51] surveyed the nutritional adequacy of dietary intake, quality of shelter meals, and objective clinical parameters of nutritional status in a heterogenous group of urban homeless persons. The group was comprised of mentally ill persons, alcohol and illicit drug users, and temporarily unemployed persons. Although 90% of the subjects (n = 96) reported that they obtained adequate amounts of food, the quality of their diets was inadequate. Shelter meals and diet records showed a high level of saturated fat and cholesterol. Serum cholesterol levels were frequently elevated and a high incidence of hypertension and obesity was discovered. Luder et al. concluded that persons who obtain meals at shelters are getting enough to eat; however, the shelter meals should be modified to meet the nutritional needs and dietary prescriptions of the large number of clients who suffer from various health disorders.[51]

The thiamin status of 107 homeless men was analyzed in Sydney by Darnton-Hill and Truswell.[52] Via 24-h recall methods, the mean dietary thiamin intake of the men was significantly less than the recommended dietary intake of the vitamin. This finding was associated with a rather high prevalence of signs that were consistent with thiamin deficiency. For instance, 24% of the subjects showed three or more symptoms of Wernicke-Korsakoff syndrome: ophthalmoplegia, nystagmus, ataxia, peripheral neuropathy, and global confusion.

CONCLUSIONS

Modern techniques in formulating reliable nutritional surveys and in assessing the nutritional status of alcoholic individuals have greatly improved knowledge of the nutritional status of alcoholics from different social groups. In earlier studies the rather high incidence of malnutrition could be related to the patient materials of indigent, "skid row" alcoholics or patients with severe somatic complications, liver cirrhosis, pancreatic insufficiency, etc. Later studies revealed that the differences in the general nutrition of alcoholics from different social classes and without significant somatic complications are minimal. Nevertheless, some subtle nutritional deficiencies may occur and the incidence of selective malnutrition may be higher among those from lower-income and homeless populations.

REFERENCES

1. Blackburn, G. L., Bistrain, B. R., Maini, B. S., Schlamm, B. A., and Smith, M. F., Nutritional and metabolic assessment of the hospitalized patient, *J. Parent. Nutr.*, 1, 11, 1977.
2. Baines, M., Detection and incidence of B and C vitamin deficiency in alcohol-related illness, *Ann. Clin. Biochem.*, 15, 307, 1978.
3. Thomson, A. D., Alcohol and nutrition, *Clin. Endocrinol. Metab.*, 7, 405, 1978.
4. Devgun, M. S., Fiabane, A., Paterson, C. R., and Zarembski, P., Vitamin and mineral nutrition in chronic alcoholics including patients with Korsakoff's psychosis, *Br. J. Nutr.*, 45, 469, 1981.
5. Morgan, M. Y., Alcohol and nutrition, *Br. Med. Bull.*, 38, 21, 1982.
6. Simko, V., Connell, A. M., and Banks, B., Nutritional status in alcoholics with and without liver disease, *Am. J. Clin. Nutr.*, 35, 197, 1982.
7. Bunout, D., Gattas, V., Iturriaga, H., Perez, C., Pereda, T., and Ugarte, G., Nutritional status of alcoholic patients. Its possible relationship to alcoholic liver damage, *Am. J. Clin. Nutr.*, 38, 469, 1983.
8. World, M. J., Ryle, P. R., Pratt, O. E., and Thomson, A. D., Alcohol and body weight, *Alcohol Alcohol.*, 19, 1, 1984.

9. Ryle, P. R. and Thomson, A. D., Nutrition and vitamins in alcoholism, *Contemp. Issues Clin. Biochem.,* 1, 188, 1984.

10. World, M. J., Ryle, P. R., and Thomson, A. D., Alcoholic malnutrition and the small intestine, *Alcohol Alcohol.,* 20, 89, 1985.

11. Gruchow, H. W., Sobocinski, K. A., Barboriak, J. J., and Scheller, J. G., Alcohol consumption, nutrient intake and relative body weight among US adults, *Am. J. Clin. Nutr.,* 42, 289, 1985.

12. Mendenhall, C. L., Tosch, T., Weesner, R. E., Garcia-Pont, P., Goldberg, S. J., Kiernan, T., Seeff, L. B., Sorell, M., Tamburro, C., Zetterman, R. et al., VA cooperative study on alcoholic hepatitis. II. Prognostic significance of protein-calorie malnutrition, *Am. J. Clin. Nutr.,* 43, 213, 1986.

13. Morgan, M. Y. and Levine, J. A., Alcohol and nutrition, *Proc. Nutr. Soc.,* 47, 85, 1988.

14. Mezey, E., Kolman, C. J., Diehl, A. M., Mitchell, M. C., and Herlong, H. F., Alcohol and dietary intake in chronic pancreatitis and liver disease in alcoholism, *Am. J. Clin. Nutr.,* 48, 148, 1988.

15. Watanabe, J., Shiota, T., Okita, M., and Nagashima, H., Lasting nutritional imbalance following abstinence in patients with alcoholic cirrhosis, *J. Med.,* 20, 331, 1989.

16. Joske, K. A. and Turner, C. N., Studies in chronic alcoholism. I. The clinical findings in seventy-eight cases of chronic alcoholism, *Med. J. Aust.,* 1, 729, 1952.

17. Olsen, A. Y., A study of dietary factors, alcoholic consumption, and laboratory findings in one hundred patients with hepatic cirrhosis and two hundred non-cirrhotic controls, *Am. J. Med. Sci.,* 220, 477, 1950.

18. Neville, J. N., Eagles, J. A., Samson, G., and Olson, R. A., Nutritional status of alcoholics, *Am. J. Clin. Nutr.,* 21, 1329, 1968.

19. Patek, A. J., Jr., Toth, I. G., Saunders, J. G., Castro, G. A. M., and Engel, J. J., Alcohol and dietary factors in cirrhosis: an epidemiological study of 304 alcoholic patients, *Arch. Intern. Med.,* 135, 1053, 1975.

20. Patek, A. J., Jr. and Post, J., Treatment of cirrhosis of the liver by a nutritious diet and supplements rich in vitamin B complex, *J. Clin. Invest.,* 20, 481, 1941.

21. Bollet, A. J. and Owens, S., Evaluation of nutritional status of selected hospitalized patients, *Am. J. Clin. Nutr.,* 26, 931, 1973.

22. Morgan, M. Y., Enteral nutrition in chronic liver disease, *Acta Chir. Scand., Suppl.,* No. 507, 81, 1981.

23. Achord, J. L., Malnutrition and the role of nutritional support in alcoholic liver disease, *Am. J. Gastroenterol.,* 82, 1, 1987.

24. Lieber, C. S., Interactions of alcohol and nutrition, *Alcohol. Clin. Exp. Res.,* 7, 2, 1983.

25. Barboriak, J. J. and Meade, R. C., Effect of alcohol on gastric emptying in man, *Am. J. Clin. Nutr.,* 23, 1151, 1970.

26. Persson, J., Alcohol and the small intestine, *Scand. J. Gastroenterol.,* 26, 3, 1991.

27. Halsted, C. H., Robles, E. A., and Mezey, E., Intestinal malabsorption in folate-deficient alcoholics, *Gastroenterology,* 64, 526, 1973.

28. Losowsky, M. S. and Walker, B. E., Liver disease and malabsorption, *Gastroenterology*, 56, 589, 1969.
29. Vlahcevic, Z. R., Juttijudata, P., Bell, C. C., Jr., and Swell, L., Bile acid metabolism in patients with cirrhosis. II. Cholic and chenodeoxycholic acid metabolism, *Gastroenterology*, 62, 1174, 1972.
30. Skrede, S., Blomhoff, J. P., Elgjo, K., and Gjone, E., Serum proteins in diseases of the liver, *Scand. J. Clin. Lab. Invest.*, 35, 399, 1975.
31. Shenkin, A., Assessment of nutritional status: the biochemical approach and its problems in liver disease, *J. Human Nutr.*, 33, 341, 1979.
32. O'Keefe, S. J. D., Abraham, R., Elzayadi, A., Marshall, W., Davis, M., and Williams, R., Increased plasma tyrosine concentrations in patients with cirrhosis and fulminant hepatic failure associated with increased plasma tyrosine flux and reduced hepatic oxygen capacity, *Gastroenterology*, 81, 1017, 1981.
33. Naveau, S., Molla-Hosseini, C., Poynard, T., Agostini, H., Abella, A., and Chaput, J.-C., Nutritional status in alcoholics with and without liver disease: are serum albumin, transferrin, prealbumin liver function tests or nutritional parameters useful?, *Eur. J. Gastroenterol. Hepatol.*, 3, 143, 1991.
34. Hallen, J. and Laurel, L., Plasma protein patterns in cirrhosis of the liver, *Scand. J. Clin. Lab. Invest.*, 29(Suppl.), 97, 1972.
35. Marisini, B., Agostino, A., Stabilini, R., and Dioguardi, N., Serum proteins of hepatic and extrahepatic origin in alcoholic cirrhosis, *Clin. Chim. Acta*, 40, 501, 1972.
36. Mills, P. R., Shenkin, A., and Anthony, R. S., Assessment of nutritional status and *in vivo* immune responses in alcoholic liver disease, *Am. J. Clin. Nutr.*, 38, 849, 1983.
37. Eagles, J. A. and Longman, D., Reliability of alcoholics' reports of food intake, *J. Am. Diet. Assoc.*, 42, 136, 1963.
38. Armor, D. J., Polich, J. M., and Stambul, H. B., *Alcoholism and Treatment*, Rand Corporation, Santa Monica, CA, 1976, 165.
39. Hurt, R. D., Higgins, J. A., Nelson, R. A., Morse, R. M., and Dickson, R. E., Nutritional status of a group of alcoholics before and after admission to an alcoholism treatment unit, *Am. J. Clin. Nutr.*, 34, 386, 1981.
40. Goldsmith, R. H., Iber, F. L., and Miller, P. A., Nutritional status of alcoholics of different socioeconomic class, *J. Am. Coll. Nutr.*, 2, 215, 1983.
41. Hillers, V. N. and Massey, L. K., Interrelationships of moderate and high alcohol consumption with diet and health status, *Am. J. Clin. Nutr.*, 41, 356, 1985.
42. Rissanen, A., Sarlio-Lähteenkorva, S., Alfthan, G., Keso, L., and Salaspuro, M., Employed problem drinkers: a nutritional risk group?, *Am. J. Clin. Nutr.*, 45, 456, 1987.
43. Robertson, M. J. and Cousineau, M. R., Health status and access to health services among the urban homeless, *Am. J. Public Health*, 76, 561, 1986.
44. Cellberg, L. and Linn, L. S., Assessing the physical health of homeless adults, *JAMA*, 262, 1973, 1989.

45. Breakey, W. R., Fischer, P. J., Kramer, M., Nestadt, G., Romanoski, A. J., Ross, A., Royall, R. M., and Stine, O. C., Health and mental health problems of homless men and women in Baltimore, *JAMA*, 262, 1352, 1989.
46. Leevy, C. M., Cardi, L., Frank, O., Gellene, R., and Baker, H., Incidence and significance of hypovitaminemia in a randomly selected municipal hospital population, *Am. J. Clin. Nutr.*, 17, 259, 1965.
47. Herbert, V., Zalusky, R., and Davidson, C. S., Correlation of folate deficiency with alcoholism and associated macrocytosis, anemia and liver disease, *Ann. Intern. Med.*, 58, 977, 1963.
48. Leevy, C. M., Baker, H., Ten Hove, W., Frank, O., and Cherrick, G. R., B-complex vitamins in liver disease of the alcoholic, *Am. J. Clin. Nutr.*, 16, 339, 1965.
49. Ashley, M. J., Olin, J. S., LeRiche, W. H., Kornaczewski, A., Schmidt, W., and Rankin, J. G., Social class and morbidity in clinically treated alcoholics, *Drug-Alcohol Depend.*, 1, 263, 1976.
50. Laven, G. T. and Brown, K. C., Nutritional status of men attending a soup kitchen: a pilot study, *Am. J. Public Health*, 75, 875, 1985.
51. Luder, E., Ceysens-Okada, E., Koren-Roth, A., and Martinez-Weber, C., Health and nutrition survey in a group of urban homeless adults, *J. Am. Diet. Assoc.*, 90, 1387, 1990.
52. Darnton-Hill, I. and Truswell, A. S., Thiamin status of a sample of homeless clinic attenders in Sydney, *Med. J. Aust.*, 152, 5, 1990.

4 Interaction of Nutrients and Alcohol: Absorption, Transport, Utilization, and Metabolism

INTRODUCTION

The relationship between vitamin deficiency, alcohol metabolism, and tissue injury is complex and has given rise to a number of areas of confusion. Nutrients of importance include a dozen vitamins, at least eight minerals, a similar number of essential amino acids, and various unsaturated fatty acids. The roles of these in tissue metabolism are highly complex. Almost any organ of the body may be affected by one or more deficiencies and many interactions occur between nutrients. For example, lack of one of the B-group vitamins, niacin, is of little consequence if an adequate supply exists of the essential amino acid, tryptophan, since the latter can be converted to niacin, although only rather slowly. The classic vitamin deficiency syndromes are well described, related to clinical signs that are obvious, but occur late in response to a usually prolonged inadequate vitamin supply to the tissues. The effects of less severe deficiencies may also be important, although this has been the subject of debate, in part because the deficiencies have been clinically and morphologically more difficult to characterize. The early work from Baker's group[1,2] included surveys that demonstrated that reduced circulating levels of vitamins frequently occur in alcoholic patients and are usually multiple. Since then, many other surveys have been conducted that have found varying degrees of depletion, depending upon the particular populations studied and on the methodology used. The interpretation of these data has been made more

ISBN 0-8493-7933-4

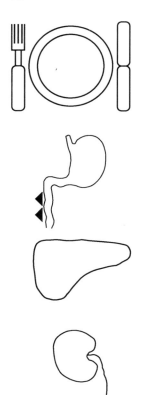

Factors reducing nutrient intake

- "Empty" calories of high ethanol intake
- Loss of appetite
- Alcoholic beverage costs reduce food expenditure
- Addiction reduces intake of nutrients
- Loss of social integration, from behavior changes and brain damage

Impaired absorption

- Impaired digestion
- Impaired transport accross intestinal wall

Impaired Utilization of Nutrients

- Tissue damage interferes with nutrient utilization
- Deficiency of one nutrient may impede utilization of other nutrients
- Individual variations in susceptibility
- Deficiency of one nutrient maqy aggravate lack of another

Increased Nutrient Losses

- Hepatic storage of nutrients reduced
- Other tissue damage increases losses

FIGURE 1. The main reasons that nutritional deficiencies develop in alcoholism.

difficult because no clear functional "cut-off" point has been in evidence that would allow a precise definition of deficiency.[3]

THE EVOLUTION OF MALNUTRITION

Malnutrition is a disease process in evolution that differs in its reactions at each stage of the process. Starting with a well-nourished individual who begins to drink heavily, the first disorder is likely to arise from the toxic effects of metabolizing large quantities of ethanol. For a variety of reasons (Figure 1) deficiencies develop, especially of B-group vitamins. Even though the dietary intake of nutrients may still be within recommended requirements, the toxic effects of alcohol metabolism begin to damage

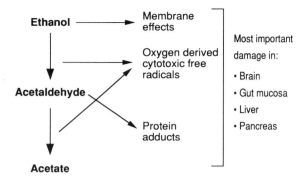

FIGURE 2.   The main mechanisms by which tissues may be damaged in alcoholism.

many organs or tissues (Figure 2). The consequences of such damage are wide ranging: injury to the gastrointestinal (GI) tract interfering with nutrient absorption, that to the pancreas interfering with the digestion of fats and proteins, liver damage reducing vitamin storage and increasing losses by excretion, and damage to membranes inhibiting the transport of various nutrients. The nutrient quality of the diet itself is likely to fall at this stage for various reasons (Figure 1). As nutrition deteriorates due to any of the factors or a combination of them, tissue damage will be increased for a variety of reasons (Figure 3).

The disturbance in the function of certain organs is important in exacerbating nutritional deficiencies and accelerating the evolution of a generalized toxic-deficiency syndrome. Thus, damage to the GI tract or the pancreas impairs nutrient absorption and digestion at the same time as liver injury increases the toxic effects of ethanol metabolism. The resulting brain impairment impedes rehabilitation and further aggravates social factors, leading to more malnutrition. Also, the evolution of the toxic-deficiency state may be accelerated by interaction between nutrients since a deficiency of one may impair the storage or utilization of another. Further deterioration will occur if toxic damage, for example, from acetaldehyde, fails to be repaired properly due to malnutrition.

This evolutionary process constitutes a discrete entity and describes in general terms the pattern of development of the pathology associated with long-term abuse of alcohol. An appropriate name for it would seem to be the toxic alcoholic malnutrition syndrome (TAMS).

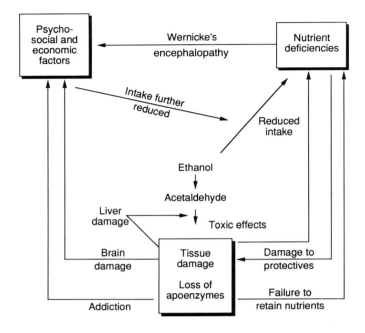

FIGURE 3.   Some ways in which TAMS may evolve over a period of years.

PRIMARY FACTORS

It is often not appreciated that malnutrition as well as ethanol abuse can separately, or in combination, reduce absorption of actively transported molecules (Figure 3). Some aspects of thiamin absorption and metabolism are discussed to illustrate the more general principles that may also operate with other nutrients.

DAMAGE TO GUT MUCOSA

This area has been studied in more detail for thiamin, but problems have been reported also for B_{12}, folates, riboflavin, the fat-soluble vitamins, and proteins.

The contribution made by thiamin malabsorption to depletion is complex and our knowledge is still incomplete. Early on, Thomson[4] developed a test using radioactive thiamin hydrochloride together with adequately demonstrated flushing doses of the nonradioactive vitamin as a test for absorption in man. Much of the detailed investigations substantiating the test and answering possible criticisms has not been published and thus readers are referred to the original work. Briefly, it was possible to show that thiamin was not broken down prior to absorption from the intestine and malabsorption was already reflected by low concentrations in the human portal vein, indicating a block at the mucosal level. Virtually all of the radioactivity absorbed was recovered in the urine, which allowed quantitation of absorption; no evidence was found of any significant entero-hepatic circulation. Thiamin is absorbed by a rate-limiting process that showed that, on average, the maximum amount of thiamin that can be absorbed from a single oral dose by man is approximately 4.5 mg in healthy subjects. The size of the oral dose required to produce half-maximum absorption was 8 mg; when oral doses greater than twice this dose were given, the amount excreted did not exceed the maximum predicted value. A marked decrease in the V_{max} occurred in malnourished alcoholics (V_{max} = 1.55), interpreted as evidence that receptor sites were damaged by prolonged receipt of ethanol or nutritional deficiency, or a combination of both of these factors. The block in absorption was demonstrated to be at the intestinal level and only returned to normal following receipt of a high-protein, vitamin-supplemented diet for 6 to 8 weeks. It is important to point out that these observations were made on a limited number of patients. Some of these patients appeared to absorb extremely small amounts of thiamin, confirmed by the fact that repeated flushing doses were given and the pattern of absorption was not altered when this was done, indicating that the luminal concentration of thiamin was not changed. Questions remain unanswered as to how long the patients had been in this condition; perhaps those with the greatest impairment were at greater risk of developing neurological damage in the long run.

Investigations in other patients showed that ethanol (1.5 g/kg), given either parenterally or orally, caused a 50% reduction in thiamin absorption in 4 of 12 healthy subjects, providing an explanation for the occurrence of thiamin deficiency syndromes, despite the ingestion of food containing minimum requirements of this vitamin. How frequently this occurs in different human populations and the extent to which it is dependent upon the dose of ethanol taken remains uncertain. In many alcoholic subjects prior to admission to the hospital one can assume malabsorption secondary to malnutrition will be further increased by the high level of ethanol consumed. Whereas 50 mg of thiamin hydrochloride in patients with Wernicke encephalopathy was minimally absorbed, an equivalent dose of thiamin propyldisulfide (the lipid-soluble form) which is absorbed by diffusion consistently produced high blood and cerebrospinal fluid (CSF) levels and was shown to be metabolically effective by relieving the symptoms of encephalopathy.

As found elsewhere in this volume, a number of studies both in animals and humans followed which initially gave confusing results. However, much of the results were clarified when it was realized that whereas lower levels of ethanol, e.g., 0.4 g/l, did not inhibit thiamin absorption, higher levels, i.e., >0.7 g/l reduced transport; similar observations were made of human chronic alcoholics.

PANCREATITIS

Acute alcoholism is a common cause of chronic pancreatitis, especially in young males. Painful episodes caused by acute attacks lead to pancreatic insufficiency,[5,6] often with calcified pancreatic calculi. Such patients will have impaired absorption of vitamin B_{12} and of amino acids from protein. Feeding pancreatic enzymes orally can improve their nutritional status.[7] Failure of fat digestion from pancreatic insufficiency or alcoholic liver damage can lead to deficiencies of fat-soluble vitamins. Although only a minority of alcoholics develop this sort of tissue damage a linear relation exists between the log of the risk and the mean daily ethanol intake, with no threshold.[8]

DAMAGE TO THE LIVER

Alcohol is directly toxic to the liver, even in the absence of any nutritional deficiency, in contrast to the situation in the brain, and here this issue is still unclear. Metabolism of the major part of ingested ethanol within the liver through the alcohol dehydrogenase pathway produces a redox shift that disrupts the metabolism of lipids, sugars, proteins, and purines. Evidence of the metabolic disturbance is provided by the increase in liver fat within days of initiating heavy drinking. Even at the fatty liver stage dramatic reductions occur in the liver stores of nutrients.[2,9] A very important further finding is that ethanol can be oxidized in microsomes with the induction of cytochrome P-450 IIE1, which affects the response of the alcoholic to various potential toxins. Substances that may be activated by this induced enzyme include not only analgesics and other drugs, solvents, and environmental carcinogens, but also a nutrient, vitamin A.[10] Induction of this microsomal enzyme also leads to an increased production of acetaldehyde, even to the point at which this toxic first metabolite of ethanol escapes into the circulation. Acetaldehyde combines with amino group side chains of proteins to form Schiff bases which can be reduced to stable adducts. This damage to proteins results in antibody production, loss of enzyme activity, and impeded repair of DNA. In the liver the ability to use oxygen is sharply reduced. Additionally, cytotoxic free radicals derived from the metabolism of acetaldehyde (and sometimes also of ethanol itself) not only damage tissue, but may also deplete various micronutrients and react with unsaturated fatty acids in cell membrane lipids forming lipid peroxides. The nutrients depleted by oxygen-derived free radicals are the antioxidants and those forming part of the protective mechanisms. These include the enzymes, superoxide dismutase (SOD) and catalase, which remove the cytotoxic free radicals, and the antioxidants, vitamins E and C, and glutathione. These interactions involve in various ways the metals, iron (Fe), manganese (Mn), selenium (Se), copper (Cu), and zinc (Zn).

EFFECT ON THE BRAIN
Shrinkage

The brains of heavy drinkers are smaller at post-mortem than those of nondrinkers, a difference confirmed by brain scans.[11,12] Much of this shrinkage is due to loss of fibers and synapses and is reversible, at least in the early stages. The picture shown by brain scans — enlarged ventricular spaces and widened sulci — has been confirmed by post-mortem measurements. The increase in the proportion of the space within skull surrounding the brain has been used as a post-mortem measure of brain tissue loss (not all necessarily permanent). This fluid-filled space is increased from 7.3% in controls to 9.8% in moderately heavy drinkers. A statistically significant increase also occurs for all groups of alcoholics to between 11 and 16%, the higher values being shown by patients who had cirrhosis or Wernicke's encephalopathy.[13]

Wernicke-Korsakoff Syndrome

Wernicke's encephalopathy has long been known to be caused by thiamin deficiency and is characterized by clouding of consciousness, eye muscle disorders, and ataxia. If thiamin is not given brain damage becomes irreversible, with lesions in the mamillary bodies, the brainstem, and the thalamic nuclei. This produces the chronic form of the syndrome, Korsakoff's psychosis, showing a short-term memory deficit, but with relative preservation of other intellectual functions.[14] This seems to be a relatively rare disease, but only apparently because various surveys suggest

TABLE 1
Incidence of Wernicke's Encephalopathy
Calculated from Serial Post-Mortem Examinations
in Various Parts of the World

Post-mortems	Wernicke's encephalopathy	Incidence (%)	No. of alcoholics	Ref.
1600	28	1.7	27	72
1539	29	1.9		73
2891	51	1.7	45	74
8735	70	0.8	65	75
4677	131	2.8	119	47
285	6	2.1		76
6964	52	0.75	604	77

Note: Around 2% of brains show the morphological lesions of the Wernicke-Korsakoff syndrome in and near the mamillary bodies. In contrast, clinical detection of the Wernicke-Korsakoff syndrome is uncommon; incidence is around 0.1% of hospital admissions[73] and even less in the general population.

(Table 1) it is relatively common, although the proportion of cases diagnosed clinically is very low, around 1 or 2%. Many cases show only mild memory defects with a wide spectrum of disability, often corresponding to other types of organic brain disorder.[15]

These findings are consistent with the Wernicke-Korsakoff syndrome being a subset of TAMS. If so, Wernicke's encephalopathy is diagnosed when the predominant effect upon the brain is that caused by acute thiamin deficiency, and the damage affects mainly the brainstem structures concerned with memory and eye muscle coordination. A diagnosis of Korsakoff psychosis is likely at any stage in the evolution of TAMS when the chronic effects of the Wernicke episode(s) predominate over damage to other structures or general toxic effects, such as loss of cells from the frontal cortex. In many cases of TAMS, a Wernicke-Korsakoff diagnosis will only be made at post-mortem and not while the patient is alive, either because memory deficit symptoms did not predominate or were not appreciated at any stage or because the patient did not seek treatment at the relevant time.

EFFECT UPON NUTRIENT TRANSPORT

Only thiamin is considered in detail since enough work has been carried out on this vitamin for a general pattern to emerge. Thiamin is transported across membranes, either of the intestine or the brain capillary endothelium, by two processes. It is phosphorylated within cells to the functional diphosphate, with some 10% being the mono- or triphosphates.[16,17] At low physiological concentrations (up to 2 mM) the main mechanism is carrier mediated, being active and sodium dependent in the gut and in brain cells, but it is only facilitated diffusion at the blood-brain barrier (BBB). Although the vitamin is phosphorylated in the mucosal cells, it is dephosphorylated again before entering the portal blood. Thiamin is phosphorylated in the brain and liver cells; at the latter site 35% is found in the mitochondria and 55% in the cytosol.[18] Although the liver is the main site of thiamin phosphorylation,[19] it must be dephosphorylated again since transport into other tissues is mainly of the free form.

Role of Intestinal Transport

Experimental work in rats using either intact intestinal loops or inverted jejunal segments showed that thiamin uptake was maximal in the upper small intestine and that the active (low concentration) absorption alone was susceptible to ethanol inhibition. Like the Na/K ATPase inhibitor, ouabain, this blocked the exit of thiamin from the mucosal cell.[20] This conclusion has been confirmed by the finding that the reduction of Na/K ATPase activity of the basolateral enterocyte membrane, produced by ethanol, was correlated with a reduction in serosal thiamin appearance.[21]

These animal experiments are not necessarily incompatible with clinical observations for the maximum dose given to healthy human subjects, 50 mg (0.15 mmol). This easily could be diluted to very low concentrations by the time it reached the small intestine, as suggested by the data of Sklan and Trostler.[22] However, since the thiamin intake of alcoholics is extremely low, the critical process is the active absorption of the vitamin. This absorption process may be independently affected by ethanol and by malnutrition in man.[3] Folic acid administration may marginally improve the latter situation, and the patient returns to normal after a 6 to 8 week course of a high-protein, vitamin-supplemented diet.

The conclusion from animal experiments that the impairment of thiamin transport depends upon the concentration of ethanol bathing the enterocyte membranes receives some support from a clinical survey that also points to malabsorption as the most important cause of thiamin deficiency in some alcoholic patients.[23] In such a case, binge drinking is the possible factor that precipitates a Wernicke crisis. Further work is required to define the role of thiamin malabsorption in the alcoholic, but it seems likely that impaired absorption in the face of poor intake is a critical factor determining which patients suffer from the Wernicke-Korsakoff syndrome. Further work is particularly required to quantify the net loss that may occur with the passage of nutrients from the blood into the lumen of the intestine, secondary to the effects of ethanol, when the diffusion gradient is appropriate.

Role of the Blood-Brain Barrier

Evidence for a possible effect of ethanol upon transport across the BBB remains controversial. It was long ago suggested that ethanol may adversely affect the rate of transport of various metabolites across the BBB,[24] although later workers failed to find such an effect.[25,26] No change apparently occurs in the kinetic parameters of influx at the BBB of the rat during a chronic ethanol regime, although a decrease in flux was seen after an acute dose, which produces transient but much higher blood concentrations of ethanol and its metabolites.[28] A similar effect has been demonstrated for thiamin transport across the wall of the intestine of the rat,[20] comparing the effects of chronic and acute ethanol administration. It seems likely that the peak concentration of the ethanol rather than the duration of exposure determines whether thiamin transport systems are affected by alcohol.

Findings contrary to this hypothesis were reported by other workers,[25] who, after an acute dose of ethanol, found no change in the entry of thiamin into the central nervous system (CNS). In these experiments, however, the plasma ethanol concentrations achieved were not reported and from the dose given were probably not much higher than those found in chronically intoxicated rats.

In chronic alcoholism, adaptation may occur via a change in cellular membranes caused by the incorporation of larger amounts of lipids such as cholesterol that "stiffen" the membrane and counteract the increase in its fluidity caused by ethanol. Such changes are likely to alter the properties of transport carriers located in the cell membranes and may account for the acute effects of ethanol upon transport. If the alcoholic insult is removed, the membranes lose the fluidizing agent and hence become overcompensated. The occurrence of such an effect on the surfaces of brain cells, it has been suggested, may be a causative factor in the withdrawal syndrome.[28] During this period of readjustment it is conceivable that the function of carrier molecules situated within the membrane will be affected. However, animals during alcohol withdrawal showed no difference in thiamin influx from controls,[27] suggesting that at least insofar as thiamin is concerned the membrane perturbations caused by chronic (unlike acute) ethanol administration do not affect the carrier.

INTERFERENCE WITH NUTRIENT UTILIZATION

The B-group vitamin, pyridoxine, is converted in the body to pyridoxal phosphate. Acetaldehyde, the first metabolite of ethanol, interferes with the binding of this form to protein[29,30] and may explain inhibition of hepatic pyridoxal phosphate accumulation after alcohol ingestion. Both pyridoxal phosphate and acetaldehyde are aldehydes and have in common the ability to form complexes, known as Schiff bases, by reversible reactions with amino groups. Much of the vitamin is held in this form on the lysine side chains of proteins. Acetaldehyde competes with the pyridoxal phosphate for these sites.[31]

SOCIOECONOMIC FACTORS REDUCE NUTRIENT INTAKE

The nutrient intake of a heavy drinker tends to be reduced not only because alcoholic beverages lack other nutrients but also because of expense. Thus, to buy equal energy content, the cost of gin is some five times that of milk at current U.K. prices.

CHEMICAL ADDICTION

After a prolonged period of heavy drinking many patients become chemically dependent upon ethanol for reasons which are still controversial, but must involve changes in the tissues and/or in their metabolism of ethanol. The physical effects of addiction are highly likely to aggravate one or more of the socioeconomic factors that tend to cause malnutrition (Figure 3).

SECONDARY FACTORS

ADDICTION REDUCES NUTRIENT INTAKE

The chemically addicted alcoholic consumes commonly some 50% of his/her calories in the form of ethanol in beverages containing either no other nutrients (in spirits) or negligible amounts (other beverages). The nonalcohol components of the diet are likely to be of low nutritional quality. The intake of many nutrients is likely to be dangerously low compared to recommended values.

Although a number of attempts have been made to estimate the micronutrient intake of different populations of alcoholic patients, it is understandably difficult to get accurate information, although very few people would disagree that patients with severe problems often eat very little. However, little information is available concerning what happens earlier in the development of alcoholism, the eating patterns of heavy drinkers, also those who remain at home and especially women. Researchers would find it helpful to have more information on the levels of intake that precede hepatic and pancreatic damage and to observe which micronutrients might be displaced in the diet. Supplementation may possibly prevent organ damage, which would subsequently affect absorption storage and utilization. It should be said, however, that although information is limited, much of the supposition has been validated by the use of animal models. Care must be taken not to extrapolate these findings to patients uncritically.

TISSUE DAMAGE INCREASES NUTRIENT LOSSES

In vitro perfusion of rat liver with ethanol causes the release of all vitamins from liver stores except biotin, vitamins C and E, and β-carotene, which are subsequently unable to rebind while ethanol is circulating.[32] Thus, induction of a hepatic microsomal enzyme increases the catabolism and loss of vitamin A. Generally, losses are also increased as a result of liver damage, as exemplified by vitamin B_6, folates, and vitamin B_{12}. Vitamin B_{12} deficiency is rare because normal stores suffice for many years without dietary intake but the rise in plasma B_{12} in alcoholics provides a sensitive index of the severity of liver damage.[33]

Vitamin B_6 is active in the form of pyridoxal phosphate as a cofactor for many enzymes of amino acid metabolism. Liver damage interferes with the formation of pyridoxal phosphate, increasing its deficiency, which may also be made worse by accelerated destruction of the vitamin.[34]

Lack of folate is one of the most common deficiencies in alcoholics, the majority of binge drinkers having low serum levels and about one third having megaloblastic bone marrow.[35] Storage of the vitamin depends upon efficient biliary recycling and uptake by the liver or peripheral tissues.

This process may become inefficient in alcoholism due to liver damage or to decreased transport across enterocyte or hepatocyte membranes, which increases urinary losses of the vitamin.[36] The minimum daily requirement of folate is 50 µg, which is high relative to the body stores of 7 to 10 mg, so that lack of dietary folate results in a serious deficiency in about 140 d. Alcoholics, however, develop deficiency more rapidly because of lower body folate stores.[37] The reduced body folate storage is due either to a catabolic effect of ethanol on folate metabolism or to impaired enterocyte or hepatocyte membrane transport leading to defective conservation.[38] Alcohol intake in folate-deficient patients decreased jejunal uptake of fluid, electrolytes, glucose, and folic acid, suggesting a mechanism for diarrhea (increased loss) and malabsorption.[39]

Alcoholic cirrhosis greatly increases the losses from the liver of Zn,[40] Cu, and Mn,[41,42] and these changes are paralleled by reductions in the hepatic activity of the important free radical defense enzyme, Cu-Zn SOD. Chronic alcohol ingestion without dietary deficiency of Se causes loss from the liver and reduced activity of another free radical protective enzyme, glutathione peroxidase (GSH-peroxidase), for which Se is a cofactor.[43]

EXAMPLES OF DEFICIENCIES THAT IMPEDE THE UTILIZATION OF OTHER NUTRIENTS

Vitamin B_6, or pyridoxine, is a cofactor in its phosphorylated form for many of the enzymes of amino acid metabolism, including many amino acid decarboxylases and glutamate-oxaloacetate or glutamate-pyruvate transaminases, as well as enzymes of heme synthesis. Its role in the decarboxylation of tryptophan or of tyrosine make it essential for the synthesis of the neurotransmitters, serotonin and catecholamines, respectively. The dietary requirement for pyridoxin or other forms of vitamin B_6 is therefore roughly proportional to the protein content of the diet. It is needed for the synthesis of nicotinamide from the amino acid tryptophan.

INDIVIDUAL VARIATIONS ALTERING THE EVOLUTION OF THE DISEASE PROCESS

Genetically determined differences exist in the distribution of the isoenzymes of alcohol dehydrogenase and of aldehyde dehydrogenase, which must affect the severity of the toxic effects of chronic alcoholism, although the mechanisms are not yet fully understood.

Evidence is available that individual factors may alter the requirements for some B-group vitamins.[44] Thus, inborn errors of metabolism may impair the function of one of the pyridoxal phosphate-dependent enzymes of amino acid metabolism. If the loss of activity is not complete, feeding large amounts of vitamin B_6 may increase the activity to adequate levels to prevent metabolic damage. The effect of oral contraceptives upon tryptophan metabolism temporarily increases the need for vitamin B_6.

TERTIARY FACTORS IN THE EVOLUTION OF THE SYNDROME

SEVERE LIVER DAMAGE INCREASES TOXIC EFFECTS

Over a period liver damage tends to become more severe. As a result, therefore, acetaldehyde escapes more frequently into the circulation to damage the brain and other organs. Formation of cytotoxic oxygen-derived free radicals is also likely to be increased and the resulting damage more widespread.

LOSS OF PROTECTION AGAINST FREE RADICAL CYTOTOXICITY

Some acute alcoholic patients show evidence of loss of SOD, one of the enzymes that inactivates oxygen-derived free radicals.[45] Acetaldehyde can damage the enzyme, GSH-reductase, which normally recycles GSH.[46] Such damage will cause a deficiency of the reduced form of this important antioxidant. Supplies of vitamins C and E may also be low due to reduced intake. Such loss of protective mechanisms will tend to make the tissue damage from activated oxygen species more severe.

ACUTE CEREBRAL CRISIS

This is Wernicke's encephalopathy, due to acute thiamin deficiency superimposed upon a chronic deficiency, or perhaps occasionally due to niacin deficiency. It is of great importance since further irreversible brain damage is likely if the condition is not treated promptly by vitamin repletion. Since the proportion of the population, some 2%, showing such irreversible damage in the brain greatly exceeds the apparent prevalence of the Wernicke-Korsakoff syndrome[47] (Table 1), most of the cases remain undetected in life. This apparent contradiction is explicable if Wernicke's encephalopathy is not an isolated disease but an intermittent episode in a fairly common condition, TAMS.

DEFICIENCY OF ONE NUTRIENT MAY
AGGRAVATE LACK OF ANOTHER

The effects of certain deficiencies are largely additive. Thus, a low niacin diet is more likely to have serious effects upon metabolism if tryptophan depletion or pyridoxal lack also occurs, since either of these conditions will prevent the synthesis of niacin from tryptophan. This synthesis depends not only upon a supply of tryptophan, but also upon an enzyme containing pyridoxal phosphate as its cofactor. Acute niacin deficiency occasionally causes a syndrome resembling Wernicke's encephalopathy, normally due to lack of thiamin.

In thiamin deficiency one thiamin-dependent enzyme, transketolase, is partially converted to the apoenzyme without the thiamin-containing cofactor. In this form it becomes unstable.[48,49] Some patients with reduced activity of this enzyme fail to respond to vitamin therapy alone because they are also protein deficient and cannot replace the damaged apoenzyme.

PSYCHOSOCIAL EFFECTS OF BRAIN DAMAGE

The cognitive deficit, memory difficulties, and dementia caused by structural damage, especially cerebral atrophy or Korsakoff's psychosis, are associated with long periods of intoxication. Social effects include loss of employment, rejection by family and friends, violent behavior, and criminal convictions. Other problems include loss of income and habitation. All this tends to reduce the intake of nutrients and worsen malnutrition.

CLINICAL IMPLICATIONS OF NUTRIENT-ALCOHOL INTERACTIONS

MAJOR SITES OF DAMAGE

The manifold effects of chronic alcoholism differ widely in their dependence upon nutritional deficiencies. In this respect, two major areas of injury can be contrasted.[46] Thus, nutritional deficiency seems to play only a minor role in the frequently fatal hepatotoxic effects of alcoholism, whereas the debilitating damage to the CNS is commonly secondary to nutritional deficiency, especially of thiamin. It is tempting to assume that the occurrence of severe liver or brain damage, affecting only a minority of alcoholic patients, is determined by the severity of secondary nutritional deficiencies. However, this assumption is much more likely to be valid for brain than liver damage. Little is known about the prevalence of nutritional factors in other types of alcohol-related damage, for example, to muscles or gonads. However, some evidence has been uncovered that maternal Zn deficiency contributes to fetal alcohol syndrome,[50,51] although such prenatal damage to the brain does not seem to be related to B-group vitamin deficiency, but rather to the timing of a high alcohol intake in relation to rapid cell proliferation in the developing neural plate.

PREVALENCE OF THE EVOLVING NUTRIENT-ALCOHOL INTERACTION SYNDROME

Only a minority of heavy drinkers develop serious liver damage, but the partially reversible loss of brain tissue universally found in heavy drinkers probably provides a good indication of patients beginning to develop TAMS. Irreversible brain lesions of the Wernicke Korsakoff type are found in some 2% of serial post-mortems,[47] a proportion corresponding to the prevalence of heavy drinking in the U.K. population.[52] In support of this hypothesis is the evidence that thiamin deficiency is common among acute alcoholics,[52,53] and the view of Victor and Adams[54] that thiamin deficiency is involved in all alcohol-related brain damage.

WHEN MICRONUTRIENT SUPPLEMENTATION IS EFFECTIVE

Whether nutrient supplementation of normal populations significantly improves cognitive performance remains highly controversial.[55,56] In contrast, considerable evidence is mounting for the occurrence of deficiencies in the chronic alcoholic population; vitamin supplementation is a justifiable part of the standard treatment of this condition.

Researchers have found that the timing of supplementation is critical. Once the tissues are replete with any of the B-group vitamins, little is stored; i.e., incipient deficiency states need to be detected and treated promptly. This is especially true of the prevention of brain damage by avoiding thiamin deficiency in the CNS. The high incidence of the morphological damage of the Wernicke-Korsakoff syndrome in the midbrain and associated structures in serial post-mortems in different parts of the world indicates that much of the acute phase of this disorder, the encephalopathy, escapes medical recognition and treatment. It cannot be emphasized too strongly that thiamin administration will have no value for treating established morphological damage in the brain caused by acute deficiency episodes, perhaps years earlier. On the other hand, the reported high incidence of thiamin deficiency in such patients would seem to justify thiamin supplementation on a continuing basis to prevent future acute deficiency episodes that include further morphological damage.

EFFECTS OF MICRONUTRIENT REPLETION

The effect of repleting the malnourished patients with micronutrients varies according to the stage reached in the evolution of the syndrome. In the early stages, since vitamins and minerals are so intimately involved in cell metabolism, it is to be expected that the effects of depletion would be more clearly apparent as a generalized functional inefficiency and the effects of repletion difficult to demonstrate, for example, by cognitive tests. There may well be no obvious gain but, despite this repletion will restore the reserves and possibly prevent a nutritional crisis which otherwise would have eventually occurred. Surveys show that many alcoholics without liver disease and lacking any physical signs of nutritional deficiency have reduced tissue supplies of vitamins.[48,49] On the basis of vitamin-mineral supplementation, not only of children, but also of adults, Yudkin[57] postulates a group with less than optimal vitamin supplies for mental functions, such as intelligence, and perhaps even social behavior. It is likely that many alcoholics developing TAMS are included within this category, although the surveys did not look for alcoholism.

Alcoholism is a problem often extending over a considerable period, and as the disease process evolves, different multiple deficiencies are likely to appaer at varying times. Their combined effect on a tissue will also be dependent upon how much damage already has been caused to that organ. Damage to particular organs, especially the liver and GI tract, may well interfere with absorption, utilization, transport, and excretion, aggravating one or more of the deficiencies (Figure 3). Treatment of nutritional deficiencies must occur parenterally to bypass the problems of malabsorption, especially for B-group vitamins, the lack of which risks irreversible brain damage. Variations also exist in the amount that different patients drink and in the amount the same person drinks at different times. There is little doubt that malnutrition will increase as patients deteriorate and the importance of the interplay between undernutrition and alcohol metabolism will vary depending upon the patient's genetic predisposition. Therefore, the combined contribution to tissue injury made by alcohol and malnutrition will not only vary from one patient to another, but from one time to another within the same patient's life. The damage of the past is often cumulative, especially in the brain.

In view of this complex relation between alcoholism and nutritional deficiencies evolving over a prolonged period, it is not surprising that alcoholism is the most common cause of malnutrition in the developed world. The many reasons are summarized in Figure 1 and fall into two major categories: (1) reduced intake, whether due to the high alcohol content or to social factors leading to a poor diet; and (2) the inefficiency of nutrient use, from various problems of transport, metabolism, or excretion.

IMPLICATIONS FOR DIAGNOSIS AND TREATMENT OF ACUTE DEFICIENCIES

Research has uncovered two reasons that the timing of micronutrient repletion is of considerable importance: (1) micronutrient storage may be severely reduced due to liver damage, especially in the tertiary stage of the syndrome; and (2) correct timing is an absolute necessity for the prevention of brain damage due to an acute lack of thiamin or other B-group vitamins. The brain-damaged patient in the tertiary stage of the syndrome may well not have any current deficiency of B-group vitamins. The memory problems and other cognitive handicaps in such a case are due to irreversible morphological changes in the brain, and repletion with B-group vitamins will have no effect. The damage to the brain is likely to have been the result of one or more episodes of unrecognized and untreated acute thiamin deficiency, occurring perhaps many years earlier. Had such episodes been recognized and B-group vitamin repletion given in time, irreversible brain damage would have been prevented. The following includes two methods for remedying this situation, making use of improved procedures for diagnosis of tissue thiamin lack.[58,59]

First, alcoholic patients should be screened regularly for B-group vitamin deficiencies, especially of thiamin. When they are screened,[48,49] around 25% are found to show early signs of thiamin deficiency. These patients are at risk for further episodes of a Wernicke-type acute deficiency with aggravation of morphological brain damage. Ongoing supplementation with B-group vitamins should be considered to prevent such a recurrence.

Second, it should be realized that the classical signs of Wernicke's encephalopathy may be difficult to detect in practice in alcoholics. Any alcoholic patients suspected to lack thiamin (as defined below) should be treated as follows. A blood sample should be taken to test for possible deficiency and assess the risks of future Wernicke-type eposides. Meanwhile, in view of the possible urgency of the need for treatment, if they are in fact deficient, they should be repleted immediately with parenteral B-group vitamins. Patients to be treated in such a manner thus should include:

- Acute alcoholics requiring detoxification
- Alcoholics with evidence of any type of ophthalmoplegia
- Alcoholics showing acute ataxia not due to current intoxication
- Alcoholics showing acute confusion not due to current intoxication
- Alcoholics in whom ophthalmoplegia, ataxia, and confusion would not be detectable because they are comatose or unconscious
- Alcoholics showing an acute peripheral neuropathy
- Alcoholics with other evidence of malnutrition

CLINICAL IMPLICATIONS OF BLOOD-BRAIN BARRIER THIAMIN TRANSPORT

Cerebral thiamin economy is of considerable importance since deficiency so rapidly causes irreversible brain damage. The value of 0.52 μM for the Michaelis constant for the transport of thiamin across the BBB is close to the normal free plasma thiamin concentration of 0.268 μM, thus allowing for good control of influx over the physiological range and ensuring that the tissue levels will remain reasonably constant despite any wide fluctuations in the plasma concentration.

Because of the essential nature of thiamin for the CNS, the carrier mechanism is of utmost importance to normal brain function. As has been demonstrated, the rate of influx of thiamin by the nonsaturable component of flux within the normal thiamin plasma range is not sufficient to meet the needs of the brain. Moreover, the rate of total thiamin influx at normal plasma concentrations is within the same order of magnitude as turnover, which implies that during thiamin deficiency, with low circulating thiamin levels, insufficient influx occurs. Because of this, harmful effects are more likely to occur when the blood thiamin level is below normal, a condition that is possible because of the small reserves of thiamin present in tissue and because of the irreducible losses of thiamin. Loss of thiamin occurs mainly via the continuous excretion in urine and perspiration,[60] there being apparently no tubular reabsorption of thiamin in the kidney.[61] Such a condition is particularly likely to occur, for example, in the malnourished chronic alcoholic patient in whom interference commonly occurs with alimentary absorption of the vitamin,[62] in conjunction with a poor diet and liver damage. By increasing the blood concentration of thiamin one can raise its flux into the brain by increasing the rate of entry by both the carrier-mediated and nonsaturable components of transport. This may have a bearing upon the nutritional treatment of various conditions, including chronic alcoholism[63] and Leigh's disease.[64] Moreover, lipid-soluble derivatives of thiamin may be used which are not restricted from entering the CNS. Having crossed the BBB and entered the cells of the brain the lipid-soluble moiety is enzymatically split off, releasing free thiamin into the metabolic pool.[63]

Carrier molecules resemble enzymes in many respects. Therefore, like enzymes, the values within any population of V_{max} and K_t for the transport of thiamin into the brain can be expected to vary due to chemical individuality.[65-67] Because of this variability certain individuals may, under normal conditions, possess sufficient carrier activity to provide an adequate supply of thiamin to the brain. During alcoholism with secondary malnutrition, however, the supply of the vitamin to the brain will fall more easily to a critically low level, resulting in a deficiency of the vitamin within the CNS. Thus, Garrod's[65] concept of inborn predispositions, first proposed in relation to enzymes, seems just as likely to be applicable to transport processes.

Although defects of carrier processes within animals are difficult to demonstrate, a mutant strain of *Escherichia coli* that possesses a defective thiamin transport mechanism has been isolated.[66] It was found that this mutant strain required a thiamin concentration in the growth medium 150-fold higher than the parent strain. It remains to be seen, however, whether a condition in mammals exists in which the thiamin carrier is defective. Although should such a defect occur, it is likely that it will either be fatal shortly after conception or be subclinical under normal conditions, according to the severity of the defect.

The importance of the BBB for thiamin homeostasis of the CNS is in the maintenance of relatively constant levels of thiamin within the brain during a state of deficiency. This occurs as a result of the binding of thiamin more tightly in the CNS to its dependent enzymes than in other tissues with a subsequent reduction in turnover. Experimental evidence suggests that the turnover of thiamin within the CNS in rats is from 2 to 10% of the total thiamin content per hour, which is similar in order of magnitude to the turnover in other tissues.[67,68] Furthermore, the affinity of thiamin for the dependent enzymes in the brain seems to be similar to that in other tissues.[69] Therefore, apparently both influx and efflux are strictly controlled, and loss of thiamin from the CNS is due mainly to the net efflux of free thiamin. If such efflux of thiamin occurs by carrier-facilitated diffusion at the capillary endothelium, transport becomes critical only when blood and subsequently brain capillary levels drop sufficiently for a concentration gradient to exist that would be conducive to efflux.

Because thiamin, amino acids, and probably most other nutrients cross the BBB by passive carrier-facilitated diffusion, they cannot move against a concentration gradient. Adequate supplies of the vitamin to the brain can therefore only be achieved when the concentration of free thiamin in the blood plasma is sufficiently greater than that of the extracellular space in the brain. The efflux of free thiamin from the brain to the blood also appears to be limited. This phenomenon protects the CNS during adverse conditions by maintaining near-normal levels of thiamin within the brain for periods longer than would otherwise be possible, thus prolonging the period of survival of the deficient animal.

CONCLUSIONS

In the evolution of what should be called TAMS a continuous and widespread interaction occurs between the various toxic and metabolic effects of ethanol metabolism and the deficiencies of many micronutrients that commonly develop. Much of this interaction is mediated through tissue damage, especially to the liver, brain, GI tract, and pancreas, but other interactions are mediated by psychosocial or economic factors. Thus, the primary disorder, excessive alcohol intake, evolves into a secondary stage with tissue damage (reversible, at least in part) that interacts with chronic malnutrition to become episodically acute. Further evolution leads to a tertiary stage with much irreversible tissue damage, further malnutrition, and probably an increased vulnerability to micronutrient lack with a loss of social integration.

This evolution usually occurs over many years, and individual variations lead to diverse patterns of irreversible tissue and organ damage, with a variety of diagnostic labels. Despite this, TAMS is believed to include the majority of alcoholic patients, with a prevalence of the order of 2% in the general population.

REFERENCES

1. Baker, H. and Frank, O., *Clinical Vitaminology*, John Wiley & Sons, New York, 1969.
2. Leevy, C. M., Baker, H., Ten Hove, W., Frank, O., and Cherrick, G., B-complex vitamins in liver disease of the alcoholic, *Am. J. Clin. Nutr.*, 16, 339, 1965.
3. Thomson, A. D., Vitamin deficiency and its role in alcoholic tissue damage, *Eur. J. Gastroenterol. Hematol.*, 2, 411, 1990.
4. Thomson, A. D., Thiamine Absorption in Man, Ph.D. thesis, University of Edinburgh, Edinburgh, Scotland, 1969.
5. Bernades, P., Belghiti, J., Althouel, M., Mallardo, N., Breil, P., and Fekete, F., Histoire naturelle de la pancreatite chronique: etude de 120 cas, *Gastroenterol. Clin. Biol.*, 7, 8, 1983.
6. Shaw, G. K., Pratt, O. E., and Thomson, A. D., unpublished data, 1991.
7. Sarles, H., Bernard, J. P., and Johnson, C., Pathogenesis and epistemiology of chronic pancreatitis, *Annu. Rev. Med.*, 40, 453, 1989.
8. Baker, H., Frank, O., Ziffer, H., Goldfarb, S., Leevy, C. M., and Sobotka, H., Effect of hepatic disease on liver B-complex vitamin titres, *Am. J. Clin. Nutr.*, 14, 1, 1964.
9. Frank, O., Luisada-Opper, A., Sorrell, M. F., Thomson, A. D., and Baker, H., Vitamin deficits in severe alcoholic fatty liver of man calculated from multiple reference units, *Exp. Mol. Pathol.*, 15, 191, 1971.
10. Lieber, C. S., Biochemical mechanisms of alcohol-induced hepatic injury, *Alcohol Alcohol.*, 26(Suppl. 1), 283, 1991.
11. Ron, M. A., Acker, W., Shaw, G. K., and Lishman, W. A., Computerised tomography of the brain in chronic alcoholics: a survey and follow-up study, *Brain*, 105, 498, 1982.
12. Phillips, S. C., Harper, C., and Kril, J., A quantitative histological study of the cerebellar vermis in alcoholic patients, *Brain*, 110, 301, 1987.
13. Harper, C. and Kril, J., If you drink your brain will shrink: neuropathological considerations, *Alcohol Alcohol.*, 26(Suppl. 1), 375, 1991.
14. Victor, M., Adams, R. D., and Collins, G. H., The Wernicke-Korsakoff syndrome, 1989.
15. Torvik, A., Wernicke's encephalopathy — prevalence and clinical spectrum, *Alcohol Alcohol.*, 26(Suppl. 1), 381, 1991.
16. Moran, J. R. and Greene, H. L., The B-vitamins and vitamin C in human nutrition, *Am. J. Dis. Child.*, 133, 192, 1979.
17. Tanphaichitr, V. and Wood, B., Thiamin, in *Present Knowledge in Nutrition*, Olsen, R. E. et al., Eds., The Nutrition Foundation, Washington, D.C., 1984, 273.
18. Dianzani, M. U. and Dianzani, M. A., Displacement of thiamine pyrophosphate from swollen mitochondria, *Biochim. Biophys. Acta*, 24, 564, 1957.
19. Westenbrink, H. G., Biochemical features of thiamine metabolism, in *Proc. 4th Int. Congr. Biochemistry, Vienna*, Vol. 11, 1958, 73.
20. Hoyumpa, A. M., Breen, K. J., Schenker, S., and Wilson, F. A., Thiamine transport across the rat intestine; the effect of ethanol, *J. Lab. Clin. Med.*, 86, 803, 1975.

21. Hoyumpa, A. M., Nicholls, S., Wilson, F. A., and Schenker, S., Effect of ethanol on intestinal (Na,K)-ATPase and intestinal thiamine transport in rats, *J. Lab. Clin. Med.*, 90, 1086, 1977.
22. Sklan, D. and Trostler, N., Site and extent of thiamine absorption in the rat, *J. Nutr.*, 107, 353, 1977.
23. Camilo, M. E., Morgan, M. Y., and Sherlock, S., Erythrocyte transketolase activity in alcoholic liver disease, *Scand. J. Gastroenterol.*, 16, 273, 1981.
24. Lee, J. C., Effect of alcohol injections on the blood-brain barrier, *Q. J. Stud. Alcohol.*, 23, 4, 1962.
25. Leslie, C. A., Gottesfeld, Z., and Elliott, K. A. C., Effect of ethanol on entry of some substances into the brain of rats, *Can. J. Physiol. Pharmacol.*, 49, 833, 1971.
26. Shaw, S., Gorkin, B. D., and Lieber, C. S., Effects of chronic alcohol feeding on thiamine status: biochemical and neurological correlates, *Am. J. Clin. Nutr.*, 34, 856, 1981.
27. Greenwood, J. and Pratt, O. E., The effect of ethanol upon thiamine transport across the blood-brain barrier in the rat, *J. Physiol.*, 348, 61p, 1984.
28. Littleton, J., Alcohol tolerance and dependence at the cellular level, *Br. J. Addict.*, 73, 347, 1978.
29. Vietch, R. L., Lumeng, L., and Li, T. K., Vitamin B6 metabolism in chronic alcohol abuse, *J. Clin. Invest.*, 55, 1026, 1975.
30. Lumeng, L. and Li, T. K., Characterisation of the pyridoxal 5'-phosphate and pyridoxamine 5'-phosphate hydrolase activity in the rat liver, *J. Biol. Chem.*, 250, 8126, 1975.
31. Lumeng, L., The role of acetaldehyde in mediating the deleterious effect of ethanol on pyridoxal 5'-phosphate metabolism, *J. Clin. Invest.*, 62, 286, 1978.
32. Sorrell, M. F., Baker, H., Barak, A. J., and Frank, O., Release by ethanol of vitamins into rat liver perfusates, *Am. J. Clin. Nutr.*, 27, 743, 1974.
33. Baker, H., Frank, O., and DeAngelis, B., Plasma vitamin B12 titres as indicators of disease severity and mortality of patients with alcoholic hepatitis, *Alcohol Alcohol.*, 22, 1, 1987.
34. Lumeng, L. and Li, T.-K., Vitamin B6 metabolism in chronic alcohol abuse, *J. Clin. Invest.*, 53, 693, 1974.
35. Savage, D. and Lindenbaum, J., Anemia in alcoholics, *Medicine*, 65, 322, 1986.
36. McMartin, K. E., Increased urinary folate excretion and decreased plasma folate levels in the rat after acute alcohol treatment, *Alcohol. Clin. Exp. Res.*, 8, 172, 1984.
37. Eichner, E. R. and Hillman, R. S., Effect of alcohol on serum folate level, *J. Clin. Invest.*, 52, 584, 1973.
38. Halsted, C. H. and Keen, C. L., Alcoholism and micronutrient metabolism and deficiencies, *Eur. J. Gastroenterol. Hepatol.*, 2, 399, 1990.
39. Halsted, C. H., Robles, E. A., and Mezey, E., Intestinal malabsorption in folate-deficient alcoholics, *Gastroenterology*, 64, 526, 1973.
40. Sullivan, J. F. and Burch, R. E., Potential role of zinc in liver disease, in *Trace Elements in Human Health and Disease*, Vol. 1, Prasad, A., Ed., Academic Press, New York, 1976, 67.

41. Keen, C. L., Tamura, T., Lonnerdal, B., Hurley, L. S., and Halsted, C. H., Changes in hepatic superoxide dismutase activity in alcoholic monkeys, *Am. J. Clin. Nutr.,* 41, 929, 1985.

42. Zidenberg-Cherr, S., Halsted, C. H., Olin, K. L., Reisenaur, A. M., and Keen, C. L., The effect of chronic alcohol ingestion on free radical defense in the miniature pig, *J. Nutr.,* 120, 213, 1990.

43. Schisler, N. J. and Singh, S. M., Modulation of selenium-dependent glutathione peroxidase activity in mice, *Free Radical Biol. Med.,* 4, 147, 1985.

44. Bartlett, K., Vitamin responsive inborn errors, *Adv. Clin. Chem.,* 23, 141, 1983.

45. Rooprai, H. K., Pratt, O. E., Shaw, G. K., and Thomson, A. D., Superoxide dismutase in the erythrocytes of acute alcoholics during detoxification, *Alcohol Alcohol.,* 24, 503, 1989.

46. Pratt, O. E., Rooprai, H. K., Shaw, G. K., and Thomson, A. D., The genesis of alcoholic brain tissue injury, *Alcohol Alcohol.,* 25, 217, 1990.

47. Harper, C., The incidence of Wernicke's encephalopathy in Australia — a neuropathological study of 131 cases, *J. Neurol. Neurosurg. Psychiatry,* 46, 593, 1983.

48. Jeyasingham, M. D., Pratt, O. E., Shaw, G. K., and Thomson, A. D., Reduced stability of rat brain transketolase after conversion to the apo form, *J. Neurochem.,* 47, 278, 1986.

49. Jeyasingham, M. D. and Pratt, O. E., Rat brain apotransketolase: activation and inactivation, *J. Neurochem.,* 50, 1537, 1988.

50. Halmesmaki, E., Ylikorkala, O., and Alfthan, G., Concentrations of zinc and copper in pregnant problem drinkers and their newborn infants, *Br. Med. J.,* 291, 1470, 1985.

51. Keen, C. L. and Hurley, I. S., Zinc and reproduction: effect on fetal and postnatal development, in *Zinc in Human Biology,* Mills, C. F., Ed., Springer-Verlag, New York, 1989, 184.

52. Jeyasingham, M. D., Pratt, O. E., Burns, A., Shaw, G. K., Thomson, A. D., and Marsh, A., The activation of red blood cell transketolase in groups of patients especially at risk from thiamin deficiency, *Psychol. Med.,* 17, 311, 1987.

53. Jeyasingham, M. D., Pratt, O. E., Shaw, G. K., and Thomson, A. D., Changes in the activation of red blood cell transketolase of alcoholic patients during treatment, *Alcohol Alcohol.,* 22, 359, 1987.

54. Victor, M. and Adams, R. D., The alcoholic dementias, in *Handbook of Clinical Neurology,* Frederiks, J. A. M., Ed., Elsevier, Amsterdam, 1985, 335.

55. Schoenthaler, S. J., Amos, S. P., Eysenck, H. J., Peritz, E., and Yudkin, J., Controlled trial of vitamin-mineral supplementation: effects on intelligence and performance, *Personal Individual Differences,* 12, 351, 1991.

56. Peto, R., Vitamins and IQ, *Br. Med. J.,* 302, 906, 1991.

57. Yudkin, J., Intelligence of children and vitamin-mineral supplements: the DRF study discussion, conclusions and consequences, *Personal Individual Differences,* 12, 363, 1991.

58. Jeyasingham, M. D., Pratt, O. E., and Rooprai, H. K., Interaction between pyridine nucleotide coenzymes and heme protein as a possible source of error in assay of activities of coenzyme-linked enzymes, *Clin. Chem.*, 35, 2129, 1989.

59. Rooprai, H. K., Pratt, O. E., Shaw, G. K., and Thomson, A. D., The age dependence of the activity and activation of human red blood cell transketolase, *Alcohol Alcohol.*, 25, 435, 1990.

60. Pearson, W. N., Blood and urinary vitamin levels as potential indices of body stores, *Am. J. Clin. Nutr.*, 20, 514, 1967.

61. Carleen, M. H., Weissman, N., and Ferrebee, J. W., Subclinical vitamin deficiencies. IV. Plasma thiamin, *J. Clin. Invest.*, 23, 297, 1944.

62. Thomson, A. D., Baker, H., and Leevy, C. M., Patterns of 35S-thiamine hydrochloride absorption in the malnourished alcoholic patient, *J. Lab. Clin. Med.*, 76, 34, 1970.

63. Thomson, A. D., Alcohol-related structural brain changes, *Br. Med. Bull.*, 38, 87, 1982.

64. Pincus, J. H., Solitaire, G. B., and Cooper, J. R., Thiamine triphosphate levels and histopathology: correlation in Leigh's disease, *Arch. Neurol.*, 33, 759, 1976.

65. Garrod, A., *Inborn Factors in Disease*, Oxford University Press, New York, 1931.

66. Childs, B. and Der Kaloustian, V. M., Genetic heterogeneity, *N. Engl. J. Med.*, 249, 1205, 1968.

67. Childs, B., Sir Archibald Garrod's conception of chemical individuality: a modern appreciation, *N. Engl. J. Med.*, 282, 71, 1970.

68. Kawasaki, T., Miyata, I., Esaki, K., and Nose, Y., Thiamine uptake in *Escherichia coli*, *Arch. Biochem. Biophys.*, 131, 231, 1969.

69. Rindi, G., Patrini, C., Comincioli, V., and Reggiani, C., Thiamine content and turnover rates of some rat nervous regions, using labelled thiamine as a tracer, *Brain Res.*, 181, 369, 1980.

70. Sen, I. and Cooper, J. R., The turnover of thiamine and its phosphate esters in rat organs, *Neurochem. Res.*, 1, 65, 1976.

71. Blass, J. P., Piacentini, S., Bolzsar, E., and Baker, A., Kinetic studies of mouse brain transketolase, *J. Neurochem.*, 39, 729, 1982.

72. Cravioto, H., Korein, J., and Silberman, J., Wernicke's encephalopathy, *Arch. Neurol.*, 4, 510, 1961.

73. Victor, M., Adams, R. D., and Collins, G. H., *The Wernicke-Korsakoff Syndrome*, Blackwell Scientific, Oxford, 1971.

74. Harper, C., Wernicke's encephalopathy: a more common disease than realised, *J. Neurol. Neurosurg. Psychiatry*, 42, 226, 1979.

75. Torvik, A., Lindboe, Ch. F., and Rogde, S., Brain lesions in alcoholics: a neuropathological study with clinical correlations, *J. Neurol. Sci.*, 56, 233, 1982.

76. Harper, C., The incidence of Wernicke's encephalopathy in Australia — a neuropathological study of 131 cases, *J. Neurol. Neurosurg. Psychiatry*, 46, 593, 1989.

77. Lindboe, Ch. F. and Lobert, E. M., "Wernicke's" encephalopathy in non-alcoholics: an autopsy study, *J. Neurol. Sci.*, 90, 125, 1989.

5 Alcohol and Glucose Homeostasis

INTRODUCTION

Ethanol (alcohol), the most common and oldest addictive substance used by man, has profound effects on energy metabolism. Chronic alcohol abuse is recognized to be a primary cause of malnutrition in developed countries.[1-4] The origins of this malnutrition are complex and multifactorial. One factor relates to the nutritional quality of the diet and it is well established that the percent of energy derived from carbohydrate, fat, and protein declines as alcohol intake increases.[5] A second facet of alcohol-related malnutrition is impaired energy metabolism: alcohol abuse has deleterious effects on carbohydrate, lipid and protein metabolism. Although the focus of this chapter concerns the interaction between alcohol abuse and glucose homeostasis, it is important to recognize that carbohydrate, lipid, and protein metabolism are interdependently regulated and that disorders in glucose homeostasis are invariably accompanied by disturbances in lipid and protein metabolism.

GLUCOSE HOMEOSTASIS

The maintenance of plasma glucose concentrations within relatively narrow limits is a primary homeostatic function in man. This is presumably because both hypo- and hyperglycemia are associated with severe metabolic and functional abnormalities. Episodes of hyperglycemia may cumulatively lead to the onset of chronic complications in susceptible tissues, at least in diabetic patients,[6] whereas hypoglycemia is associated with brain damage and mental retardation. A major factor in the evolution of homeostatic mechanisms to maintain circulating glucose concentrations is commonly recognized to be the obligate requirement by the central nervous system (CNS) and other specialized tissues for glucose as a substrate. Why the brain has this obligate requirement for glucose remains a mystery.

ISBN 0-8493-7933-4
© 1992 by CRC Press, Inc.

The steady-state plasma glucose concentration is determined by the balance between the rate of glucose production by the liver and, to a lesser extent, the kidney, and the rate of glucose utilization. Both gluconeogenesis and glycogenolysis contribute to hepatic and renal glucose production, whereas many tissues make important contributions to the rate of glucose utilization and oxidation. Whereas approximately one third of an oral glucose load is taken up by the splanchnic bed,[7] studies of glucose exchange across the leg in normal man during a euglycemic insulin clamp indicate that muscle may account for up to 85% of the disposal of an infused glucose load.[8] Other tissues, particularly the brain and splanchnic bed, account for the remaining glucose. The balance between the rates of glucose production and utilization is determined to a significant extent by the balance between insulin and its counterregulatory hormones, including glucagon, cortisol, growth hormine, and the catecholamines. Insulin, which is the body's primary anabolic hormone, stimulates glucose uptake and disposal by oxidative and nonoxidative pathways in peripheral tissues, particularly skeletal muscle. This stimulation is complex and multifaceted and is mediated by effects on glucose transport, glycolytic flux, glycogen synthesis, and the pyruvate dehydrogenase (PDH) complex. In the liver insulin reduces glucose production via the inhibition of gluconeogenic flux and stimulates net glucose disposal. The maintenance of normal glucose homeostasis is dependent upon the coordinate regulation of three inter-dependent processes: (1) insulin secretion by the pancreatic β cells, (2) the suppression by insulin of hepatic glucose output, and (3) the stimulation by insulin, in association with hyperglycemia, of peripheral and splanchnic glucose uptake. Counterregulatory hormones oppose the action of insulin by a variety of mechanisms, including effects on insulin secretion, hepatic glucose production, and splanchnic and peripheral glucose utilization, and by the modulation of plasma levels of fatty acids (the glucose/fatty acid cycle).

The Glucose/Fatty Acid Cycle

To understand the interdependent nature of the relationship between glucose homeostasis and lipid and protein metabolism, it is first necessary to examine the mechanisms that govern fuel metabolism under normal circumstances. The body uses two primary fuels in energy generation, glucose and the lipid-derived fuels (viz., fatty acids, ketone bodies), and a well-established reciprocal relationship exists between the use of these fuels as substrates.[9,10] This relationship, commonly termed the glucose/ fatty acid or Randle cycle, serves to promote the preferential oxidation of lipid-derived fuels by muscle in response to starvation or diets low in available carbohydrate. This preferential oxidation leads to the suppression of glucose uptake and oxidation and to diminished whole-body glucose utilization. Glucose metabolism by the brain is oxidative, with the production of CO_2, and leads to diminution of the body's glucose pool. Under conditions of dietary carbohydrate restriction ("carbohydrate stress"), there is a mandatory requirement for *de novo* glucose synthesis to occur to compensate for the glucose carbon irrevocably "lost" from the body by oxidative metabolism, particularly by the brain. It is important to recognize in this context that gluconeogenesis is not synonymous with *de novo* glucose synthesis. Gluconeogenesis from the products of incomplete glucose metabolism (*viz.*, lactate, pyruvate, alanine) recycles existing carbohydrate carbon via the Cori and glucose/alanine cycles, and therefore has no capacity to increase the whole body glucose pool. By contrast, gluconeogenesis from precursors of noncarbohydrate origin, particularly amino acids and glycerol, provides a route of *de novo* glucose synthesis and compensates for net glucose loss via oxidation to CO_2.[11] The functional link between carbohydrate and protein metabolism under conditions of dietary carbohydrate restriction is that enhanced proteolysis, particularly by skeletal muscle, is a prerequisite to the sustained provision of precursors for hepatic gluconeogenesis.

An important facet of the operation of the glucose/fatty acid cycle is that dietary carbohydrate restriction results in the activation of triacylglycerol lipolysis in adipose tissue and the release of free fatty acids (FFA) into the bloodstream. The first and flux-generating reaction in FFA release by adipose tissue is catalyzed by triacylglycerol lipase. This enzyme exists in two forms, an active phosphorylated form and an inactive dephosphorylated form. Activation and phosphorylation of the enzyme is via cyclic adenosine monophosphate (cAMP)-dependent protein kinase and is promoted by a number of hormones ("lipolytic hormones"), including the catecholamines. This activation is opposed by insulin. FFA release is, therefore, determined by the balance between the antilipolytic action of insulin and the counterregulatory lipolytic hormones. The FFA and ketone bodies produced by their partial oxidation in the liver are preferentially oxidized in muscle, their oxidation generating metabolites that inhibit glucose utilization and oxidation. The mechanism underlying this inhibition is multifactorial and is mediated via the coordinate inhibition of hexokinase, phosphofructo-1-kinase, and PDH complex.[9,10,12,13] Although the basic features of the glucose/fatty acid cycle were recognized over 25 years ago, it has only been recently that direct evidence has been obtained of its operation in normal man.[14]

ACUTE ALCOHOL ABUSE AND GLUCOSE HOMEOSTASIS

Alcohol (ethanol) is metabolized predominantly in the liver via a pathway comprising the enzymes alcohol dehydrogenase (EC 1.1.1.1.) and aldehyde dehydrogenase (EC 1.2.1.3.).[15] This pathway oxidizes ethanol to acetate via the intermediate acetaldehyde with the concomitant production of excess reducing equivalents, mainly as the reduced form of cytosolic nicotinamide adenine dinucleotide (NADH). The products of this pathway, particularly excess NADH and acetate, are recognized to be the primary mediators of the acute effects of ethanol on fuel metabolism.[15-17] Although ethanol oxidation via the alcohol dehydrogenase pathway is primarily hepatic, up to 80% of the ethanol oxidized appears as free acetate in the hepatic vein and its further oxidation to CO_2 occurs at extrahepatic sites, particularly skeletal muscle.[18-20]

ETHANOL AND FASTING HYPOGLYCEMIA

In individuals whose hepatic glycogen stores have been depleted by poor nutrition and fasting, ethanol may acutely provoke severe and often life-threatening hypoglycemia.[21,22] Infants and children are especially vulnerable to ethanol-induced fasting hypoglycemia, which is commonly associated with plasma glucose concentrations of <2.2 mM. This hypoglycemic response is attributed primarily to the specific inhibition by ethanol of hepatic gluconeogenic flux, although other factors, particularly adrenocortical insufficiency, may influence individual susceptibility.[23] The extrahepatic effects of ethanol may contribute to the reduction in gluconeogenic flux; ethanol via the inhibition of triacylglycerol lipolysis in adipose tissue reduces plasma glycerol concentration.[24] In the absence of adequate glycogen stores in the liver, the inhibition of gluconeogenesis leads inexorably to the suppression of hepatic glucose production. The inhibition of gluconeogenesis occurs secondary to ethanol oxidation by the liver and is abolished by 4-methylpyrazole, an inhibitor of alcohol dehydrogenase.[25] Excess NADH is acknowledged to be the primary factor that mediates the inhibition of gluconeogenic flux. The mechanism of this inhibition has been reviewed extensively elsewhere[16,21,26] and is not discussed in depth here. It is important, however, to emphasize that the inhibition of gluconeogenic flux is one of a series of related derangements in hepatic metabolism provoked by acute alcohol abuse. These derangements include decreased flux via the tricarboxylic acid (TCA) cycle, decreased fatty acid oxidation, enhanced lipogenesis and triacylglycerol esterification, and impaired hepatic lactate and alanine utilization.

In fasted human volunteers ethanol administration reduces rates of glucose synthesis from lactate[27] and rates of glucose appearance in both the postabsorptive state and during euglycemic hyperinsulinemia.[28-30] Starvation is, therefore, not a prerequisite for the inhibition by ethanol of hepatic gluconeogenesis, but is necessary for the development of hypoglycemia. In individuals with adequate hepatic glycogen reserves, the inhibition of gluconeogenesis is presumably compensated for by increased rates of glycogenolysis.

ETHANOL AND IMPAIRED HEPATIC GLYCOGEN STORAGE

Recent research[12,31] has put into question the textbook view that hepatic glycogen synthesis during the starved-to-fed transition is predominantly from glucose via its direct phosphorylation to glucose 6-phosphate and conversion via glucose 1-phosphate and UDP-glucose to glycogen. It is now recognized that a substantial proportion (up to 70%) of the liver glycogen deposited in response to carbohydrate refeeding is synthesized from glucose following its conversion to lactate and related 3-carbon metabolites. Sustained gluconeogenic flux is, therefore, a prerequisite to active glycogen deposition following carbohydrate refeeding. The inhibition of hepatic gluconeogenic flux secondary to ethanol oxidation may, therefore, not only lead to fasting hypoglycemia, but it also severely comprises the capacity of the liver to store glycogen, at least in the rat.[32] This finding has important nutritional implications since it implies that acute alcohol abuse may diminish the capacity of the liver to produce glucose via parallel derangements in gluconeogenesis and hepatic glycogen storage.[33]

ACUTE EFFECTS OF ETHANOL ON INSULIN
SECRETION

Whereas glucose tolerance may be impaired by the simultaneous administration of ethanol,[34,35] the consensus view is that ethanol pretreatment leads to the potentiation of the insulin secretory response on subsequent oral or intravenous (i.v.) glucose challenge.[36-40] Plasma insulin levels are elevated if ethanol and glucose are given concurrently,[34,41] implying that pretreatment is not an absolute prerequisite to ethanol stimulation of glucose-mediated insulin secretion.

Insulin release from the pancreatic β cells in response to secretagogues is biphasic, the initial burst of release within the first few minutes being followed by a sustained phase of gradual release of the hormone over several hours.[42] Ethanol pretreatment increases both first- and second-phase insulin secretory responses to glucose loading in normal subjects, but the stimulation of the first-phase response may be attenuated in obese and diabetic subjects.[37,39] Ethanol pretreatment not only increases the insulin secretory response to glucose but also to other β cell secretagogues, including arginine[43] and tolbutamide,[44] but not cAMP[45] or glucagon.[37] This may imply that the priming effect of ethanol is mediated via a cAMP-dependent pathway, a conclusion supported by the observation that ethanol may increase adenylcyclase activity in islet tissue homogenates.[46] Other indirect mechanisms may be involved in ethanol-mediated potentiation, including reduction in the rate of hepatic insulin extraction (but see Reference 47) and potentiation by release of gastrointestinal (GI) hormones. Acetate, a product of hepatic ethanol oxidation, potentiates glucose-induced insulin secretion in the rat,[48] but not in man,[29] which may indicate that the priming of insulin secretion is not mediated by ethanol per se. This occurs not by ethanol per se, but is dependent on its hepatic oxidation to acetate, at least in the rat.

There are indications of important interspecies differences in the responsiveness of the pancreatic β cells to ethanol. In contrast to the situation in man, in fasted rats ethanol administered prior to or in conjunction with glucose or tolbutamide results in glucose intolerance, inhibition of glucose- or tolbutamide-induced insulin response, and impaired glucose disappearance rate.[48,49] This derangement may involve the inhibition by ethanol of insulin secretion mediated via hypocalcemia[48] or its effects on the integrity of the β cell microtubular system.[50-52] In the pig an inverse relationship exists between serum ethanol concentration and glucose-induced insulin secretion, implying that low doses of ethanol are a prerequisite to the priming response, at least in this species.[47]

Evidence exists that the early phases of both insulin-dependent and noninsulin-dependent diabetes mellitus are associated with diminished first-phase insulin secretion in response to i.v. glucose,[53,54] and that this deficiency may precede and be an important factor in the pathogenesis of glucose intolerance in diabetes.[55] This deficiency in the first-phase response may lead to the delayed inhibition of hepatic glucose production in response to postprandial hyperglycemia.[56]

ETHANOL AND REACTIVE HYPOGLYCEMIA

The potentiation by ethanol of glucose-induced insulin secretion may provoke a profound, often symptomatic, reactive hypoglycemia following the ingestion of carbohydrate-rich foods.[21] Reactive hypoglycemia associated with increased plasma insulin levels, for example, may be induced in normal volunteers several hours after the consumption of gin and tonic, which contains sucrose (60 g) and ethanol (50 g).[41] The hypoglycemia is absent if the gin and tonic is substituted by either sucrose or ethanol alone, consistent with its mediation via ethanol priming of glucose-induced insulin secretion. The potentiation of glucose-induced insulin secretion by ethanol may also cause severe hypoglycemia in sulfonylurea-treated diabetic patients,[57] in athletes following severe exercise in cold weather,[58] and may also lead to nocturnal hyperinsulinemia in healthy individuals who drink alcoholic beverages with their evening meal.[39]

ACUTE ALCOHOL ABUSE, GLUCOSE DISPOSAL, AND INSULIN RESISTANCE

Controversy surrounds the acute effects of ethanol on glucose tolerance in normal man with contradictory reports of unchanged,[39,59] impaired,[34,60] and improved glucose tolerance.[40] It is well established that ethanol, in addition to decreasing hepatic glucose production, impairs peripheral glucose utilization and causes acute insulin resistance. In overnight-fasted individuals ethanol decreases glucose utilization in the basal state and during euglycemic hyperinsulinemia,[29,30,61] reduces the conversion of glucose to lactate,[27] inhibits glucose uptake by leg muscles in overnight-fasted volunteers,[62] and reduces the stimulatory effects of prolonged exercise on glucose uptake by the exercising leg.[28] Ethanol also decreases peripheral glucose utilization in 2- to 3-d fasted dogs[63] and impairs glucose uptake by the isolated rat diaphragm.[64] It is important to recognize that acute ethanol-induced insulin resistance may be compensated for to varying degrees by the hypersecretion of insulin. The extent to which this compensation is achieved, which depends to a significant extent on the dose of ethanol and its route of administration, will determine whether ethanol administration is associated with glucose intolerance. Small doses of ethanol, for example, are sufficient to inhibit basal rates of glucose appearance and disappearance[29] and potentiate glucose-induced insulin secretion,[47] whereas inhibition of insulin-stimulated glucose disposal requires a moderate ethanol dose.[29]

The mechanism of acute ethanol-induced insulin resistance remains a puzzle. Indirect calorimetric studies indicate that in normal man ethanol decreases total body fat oxidation (by 79%) and protein oxidation (by 39%), and attenuates the rise in carbohydrate oxidation after glucose infusion.[30] The implication is that ethanol acts as a preferred oxidative fuel, largely replacing fat and protein as the substrate for oxidation in the postabsorptive state and suppressing glucose oxidation following glucose administration. One cause of this preferential oxidation is the depression of TCA cycle activity in the liver secondary to ethanol oxidation and the inhibition of hepatic oxidation of fatty and amino acids.[16] In man up to 80% of the ethanol oxidized by the liver appears as free acetate in the hepatic vein. The blood concentration of acetate rapidly increases following ethanol consumption and soon reaches a steady-state level of approximately 0.8 mM. This acetate is rapidly oxidized at extrahepatic sites, particularly skeletal muscle.[18-20] Muscle, by contrast, has a negligible capacity to oxidize ethanol. The oxidation of acetate by skeletal muscle consequently serves to redistribute ethanol carbon from the liver to extrahepatic sites. Acetate oxidation in skeletal muscle, like that of long-chain fatty acids, is inhibitory to glucose utilization and oxidation in both the perfused rat heart and the perfused rat hindquarter,[65,66] and uptake of glucose by the leg in human volunteers is reduced to the same magnitude as acetate is taken up.[61] Therefore, the question posed is whether, by analogy to the glucose/fatty acid cycle, ethanol exerts a glucose-sparing action via its oxidation to acetate in the liver, the preferential oxidation of which in peripheral tissues suppresses peripheral glucose utilization and oxidation. Recent research[29] indicates that acetate infusion has no effect on rates of glucose production and utilization in normal man either in the basal state or during a euglycemic hyperinsulinemic clamp. It would appear likely, therefore, that acetate is not the mediator of ethanol-induced insulin resistance. The possibility remains, however, that acetate oxidation in muscle and other peripheral tissues may selectively impair glucose oxidation as opposed to nonoxidative routes of glucose disposal. In the perfused rat heart, acetate is reported to abolish glucose oxidation but to have little effect on rates of glucose uptake.[65] Another dimension exists to the interrelationship between ethanol and fatty acid oxidation, since it is well established that acetate inhibits triacylglycerol lipolysis in adipose tissue in normal man, and as a consequence reduces circulating FFA concentrations via the suppression of peripheral fatty acid release.[67,68]

The conclusion that acetate is unlikely to mediate this acute insulin resistance raises the question of the role of other ethanol metabolites, notably excess NADH. Hepatic ethanol oxidation, in addition to producing acetate, generates excess reducing equivalents as NADH. This alteration in hepatic redox balance abolishes the normal uptake of lactate by the liver and leads to net splanchnic release of lactate and hyperlactacidemia.[62] Excess NADH, mediated by the decrease in the mitochondrial $NAD^+/NADH$ ratio, has the capacity to inhibit pyruvate dehydrogenase kinase and lead to the net dephosphorylation and inactivation of the PDH complex in muscle. In theory, therefore, the acute hyperlactacidemia associated with ethanol consumption may impair peripheral glucose oxidation via the inhibition of the PDH complex in muscle. Whether ethanol-induced hyperlactacidemia, particularly in combination with increased circulating acetate concentrations, inhibits glucose oxidation in skeletal muscle remains to be established.

Ethanol has pronounced acute effects on the plasma concentrations of a number of counterregulatory hormones, but it is questionable whether these changes contribute to the genesis of ethanol-induced insulin resistance. Ethanol activates adrenal glucocorticoid secretion by a central hypothalamic-pituitary effect that leads to acute increases in plasma corticosterone levels,[16] and moderate doses of ethanol have been shown to produce a rise in both plasma and urinary catecholamines in normal subjects.[69] Ethanol also acutely increases fasting plasma glucagon levels in man,[40,70] as well as in the pig[71] and rat.[72] No consistent changes, however, in the plasma levels of corticosol, catecholamines, glucagon, or growth hormone accompany the onset of acute ethanol-induced insulin resistance in normal man.[29,30,61]

SELECTIVE EFFECTS OF ETHANOL ON
GLUCOSE DISPOSAL IN OXIDATIVE MUSCLES

Skeletal muscle is heterogeneous in structure and function. One important facet of this heterogeneity relates to differences between individual muscles in their capacity for glucose utilization. The diaphragm, heart, and postural skeletal muscles, which are constantly working and contain a high proportion of oxidative fibers, have far higher rates of glucose uptake and phosphorylation than nonoxidative muscles in the fed state, and unlike the nonoxidative muscles, respond to starvation by the pronounced suppression of glucose uptake.[73,74] Starvation,[73] like anesthesia,[75] is associated with a pronounced (40%) reduction in glucose utilization which can be largely accounted for by the selective suppression of glucose utilization by cardiothoracic and postural muscles. Differences also occur between individual muscles in their capacity for pyruvate oxidation in response to progressive starvation[74,76] and refeeding after starvation.[77] The flux-generating step in pyruvate oxidation is that catalyzed by the PDH complex, the activity of which is regulated by phosphorylation and dephosphorylation. Starvation is associated with the net dephosphorylation and inactivation of the PDH complex. The reduction in glucose utilization and pyruvate oxidation after starvation is commonly attributed to the operation of the glucose/fatty acid cycle.[72] It is important to recognize, however, that activity of the PDH complex is more rapidly suppressed than glucose utilization (measured as 2-deoxyglucose uptake and phosphorylation) in response to starvation or acute elevation in fatty acid concentrations.[77]

Starvation leads to the mobilization of glycogen reserves in both oxidative and nonoxidative muscles. Carbohydrate refeeding after starvation in the rat is associated with rapid increases in rates of glucose utilization by oxidative and nonoxidative muscles[77] and the repletion of glycogen reserves, the rate of glycogen deposition being influenced either by muscle fiber composition[33] or the extent of glycogen depletion elicited by starvation.[76,78] Glycogen synthesis accounts for most of the glucose phosphorylated in the first few hours of refeeding, implying that the oxidative disposal of glucose in skeletal muscle continues to be suppressed, possibly via sustained *in situ* fatty acid oxidation.[33,79] An important question is the extent to which ethanol acutely influences glycogen repletion in different muscles following carbohydrate refeeding after starvation. Recent research in this laboratory indicates that ethanol may selectively suppress glycogen deposition in oxidative as opposed to nonoxidative muscles during the starved-to-fed transition. Glucose refeeding of rats starved for 40 h is normally associated with rapid rates of glycogen deposition in skeletal muscles, particularly in oxidative muscles. Our results indicate that ethanol pretreatment in the rat inhibits glycogen deposition in response to glucose refeeding in oxidative muscles (*viz.*, diaphragm, soleus) but not in non-oxidative muscles (*viz.*, extensor digitorum longus, tibialis anterior, plantaris, gastrocnemius) (Figure 1). This inhibition, which is accompanied by impaired glucose uptake and phosphorylation (measured by the tracer 2-deoxyglucose[80]), resulted in the total abolition of glycogen deposition in diaphragm and soleus muscles, but had no effect on rates of glycogen deposition in nonoxidative muscles.

In contrast to its effects on glucose utilization in skeletal muscles during the starved-to-fed transition, ethanol administration in the postabsorptive state produces no major impairment in glucose utilization in individual muscles in the rat, except for the gastrocnemius.[81] Ethanol does, however, have a potent effect on endotoxin-enhanced glucose utilization in the postabsorptive state.[81] Endotoxemia is associated with enhanced glucose production resulting in a transient hyperglycemia[82,83] and increased rates of glucose utilization, particularly by macrophage-rich tissues, including the liver, spleen, lungs, skin, GI tract and skeletal muscle.[84] These changes in glucose metabolism may be an integral element of the body's response to sepsis. Ethanol is recognized to cause changes in glucose production and utilization that are the opposite of those provoked by endotoxin. The question posed, therefore, is whether ethanol opposes the effects of endotoxin on glucose turnover and whether this contributes to the increased susceptibility to infection that is a feature of alcoholism. Spitzer's laboratory established that ethanol infusion attenuates the endotoxin-induced increases in both glucose production and glucose utilization,[84,85] including those seen in individual oxidative and nonoxidative skeletal muscles,[81] and suppresses endotoxin-mediated increases in circulating levels of tumor necrosis factor (TNF).[86]

ACUTE ALCOHOL ABUSE AND GLUCOSE HOMEOSTASIS: AN OVERVIEW

The preceding discussion focused on the acute effects of alcohol abuse on glucose metabolism. This acute interaction of ethanol with glucose homeostasis is multifaceted and is mediated by inhibitory effects of ethanol

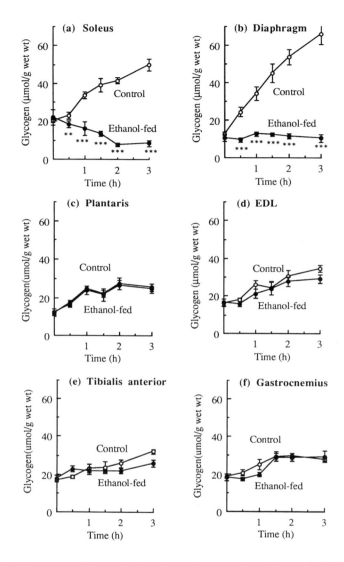

FIGURE 1. The acute effects of ethanol on glycogen deposition in individual skeletal muscles in response to glucose refeeding of 40-h starved rats. Rats starved for 40 h were administered ethanol (50% aqueous solution, 75 mmol/kg body weight) or an equivalent volume of water 1 h before refeeding with glucose (2 *M* solution, 20 mmol/kg body weight) and animals were sampled at time intervals thereafter (see Reference 32 for experimental details). The values for muscle glycogen content are shown for (a) soleus, (b) diaphragm, (c) plantaris, (d) extensor digitorum longus, (e) tibialis anterior, and (f) gastrocnemius, and results (expressed as μmol glucose equivalents per g wet weight) are the means ± S.E.M. of six animals. Statistically significant effects of ethanol as opposed to water pretreatment are denoted as *** $p < 0.001$.

TABLE 1
Acute Alcohol Abuse and Glucose Homeostasis: An Overview

Target organ	Effect	Consequence
Liver	Inhibition of hepatic gluconeogenic flux	Fasting hypoglycemia and diminished hepatic glycogen storage
Muscle	Inhibition of glucose utilization	Glucose intolerance and acute insulin resistance
Pancreas	Potentiation of glucose-induced insulin secretion	Hyperinsulinemia
Adipose tissue	Inhibition of triacylglycerol lipolysis	Reduced plasma fatty acid concentrations

on rates of glucose production (*viz.*, hepatic gluconeogenesis, diminished hepatic glycogen storage) and disposal (acute insulin resistance) coupled with the potentiation by ethanol of glucose-induced insulin secretion (Table 1). An outstanding question concerns the mechanism of acute ethanol-induced insulin resistance and its relationship, if any, to the insulin resistance associated with alcoholic liver disease (ALD), particularly cirrhosis.

GLUCOSE HOMEOSTASIS AND CHRONIC ALCOHOL ABUSE

The term "chronic alcoholic" is notoriously imprecise. It encompasses individuals with one or more of a complex and heterogeneous group of related disabilities, the only common feature of which is that they develop as a consequence of alcohol abuse. These reviewers have chosen to restrict discussion to abnormalities in glucose homeostasis associated with two specific sequelae of chronic alcohol abuse. For a broader view of alcohol-related pathology, readers are referred to Lieber, 1982.[16]

GLUCOSE INTOLERANCE IN ALCOHOLIC LIVER DISEASE

The majority of cases of cirrhosis of the liver are related to alcohol abuse and a close correlation exists between per capita alcohol consumption and mortality due to cirrhosis. It has been recognized for many years that glucose intolerance and overt diabetes mellitus are features associated with cirrhosis,[87] with almost three fourths of all cirrhotic patients being intolerant to oral glucose. The question posed concerns the relationship between alcohol abuse, glucose intolerance, and overt diabetes. Early studies, including that by Allen,[88] reported beneficial effects of moderate ethanol intake in diabetic patients, which may relate to the potentiation by ethanol of insulin secretion. There are, however, reports that in rare instances abstinence from excessive ethanol intake may alleviate diabetic symptoms in insulin-dependent diabetic patients.[89] A common feature of those patients who showed remission was a strong family history of diabetes, which may imply predisposition to the diabetogenic effects of ethanol abuse. There are also reports that ethanol consumption over a period of a few days may induce clinically significant diabetes associated with hyperinsulinemia in apparently healthy volunteers.[38] The basis for these diabetogenic effects remains obscure. Since the abnormalities in glucose homeostasis associated with cirrhosis have been recently reviewed in some detail,[90] the focus here is on the pathogenesis of these disorders.

The primary defect of glucose homeostasis in cirrhosis is insulin resistance. Rates of insulin-mediated glucose disappearance are consistently reduced by up to one half during euglycemic hyperinsulinemia in cirrhotic patients.[91-96] The cause of this insulin resistance is now recognized as primarily a reduction in glucose utilization by peripheral tissues, a conclusion based on isotope studies,[97] and indirect calorimetry to quantify glucose oxidation during the euglycemic insulin clamp.[90] These studies indicate a reduction by up to 50% in nonoxidative glucose disposal, consistent with a lesion in glycogen synthesis. Studies of forearm glucose uptake indicate that skeletal muscle is an important site of insulin resistance in cirrhosis[98] and measurement of glycogen concentrations in the vastus lateralis muscle during the euglycemic insulin clamp[96] confirms that muscle glycogen storage is compromised. This reduction in glycogen synthesis may be specifically related to a decrease in the active (dephosphorylated) form of glycogen synthase in muscle.[96]

The insulin resistance associated with cirrhosis provokes a compensatory increase in insulin secretion by the pancreatic β cells. Both basal and glucose-stimulated levels of plasma insulin are elevated in cirrhotic patients[91,99] and similar elevations occur in plasma C-peptide levels, at least following oral glucose challenge.[92,100] The primary cause of the hyperinsulinemia is increased insulin secretion as opposed to its impaired hepatic extraction or portosystemic shunting.[99-101] The liver is the main site of insulin degradation in the body; up to 60% of the insulin secreted by the pancreas is extracted by the liver during a single transhepatic passage. The fractional hepatic extraction of insulin is diminished in cirrhotic patients by up to 75%.[102] The increase in insulin secretion is insufficient in magnitude to offset the insulin resistance and glucose intolerance ensues.

The mechanism underlying the insulin resistance in cirrhosis remains a puzzle. Studies of insulin binding to adipocytes or peripheral blood monocytes and erythrocytes yield contradictory results, although many indicate depressed insulin binding in cirrhotic patients.[90] The functional significance of the defects is questionable, particularly in view of the poor correlation between insulin binding and rates of lipogenesis by isolated adipocytes.[95] Cirrhosis is associated with elevations in plasma levels of fatty acids, glucagon, and growth hormone, and with abnormalities in lipoprotein metabolism. It is tempting to implicate fatty acids, via operation of the glucose/fatty acid cycle, as the factor that precipitates the insulin resistance, but this is discounted by studies of palmitate oxidation during the euglycemic insulin clamp.[90] Although hyperglucagonemia may be a contributory factor,[103] hyperinsulinemia, which in the first instance may develop in cirrhotic patients because of defective hepatic insulin degradation secondary to hepatic dysfunction, may be the agent that initiates the insulin resistance via a receptor-mediated defect or, more probably, a postreceptor defect in insulin signaling.

The temporal sequence of events involved in the initiation and progression of liver injury is still only poorly understood. The spectrum of ALD encompasses alcoholic fatty liver (steatosis), early fibrosis (perivenular fibrosis), alcoholic hepatitis, and cirrhosis.[16] An important question is the relationship between the progressive stages of liver injury and the onset of abnormalities in glucose homeostasis. Many studies indicate that chronic alcoholism per se is associated with glucose intolerance and that alcohol abuse exerts a diabetogenic effect in susceptible individuals (see, for example, References 38, and 104 to 106). Asymptomatic liver damage, poor diet,[107] and exocrine pancreatic damage[108] may be contributory factors to this glucose intolerance. The glucose intolerance seen in alcoholic patients without liver disease may be related to lowered plasma insulin levels and is reversible by ethanol infusion.[109] Peripheral insulin resistance is not detectable by the insulin clamp technique in these early abstinent alcoholic patients, although evidence has been found of an increased glucose production rate in the postabsorptive state in these patients.[110]

CHRONIC ALCOHOLIC SKELETAL MYOPATHY

A second important disorder related to chronic alcohol abuse occurs that warrants special mention in relation to glucose homeostasis. Chronic alcohol abuse is commonly associated with functional changes involving the skeletal muscles, typified by weakness, pain, and abnormal gait.[111,112] Chronic alcoholic skeletal myopathy afflicts approximately one half to two thirds of alcohol abusers[113,114] and may lead to the loss of up to one fourth of the body's muscle mass. Most patients with chronic myopathy have a history of alcohol abuse of at least 10 years and have muscle wasting and weakness of the proximal muscle groups, particularly those of the lower extremities. The pathogenesis of the myopathy involves muscle fiber atrophy mediated via a defect in protein synthesis which is selective for type II (fast twitch, glycolytic) fibers.[115,116] Type I (slow twitch, oxidative) fibers are relatively unaffected. The myopathy is associated with abnormal lipid deposition[117] and derangements in carbohydrate metabolism, including decreased activities of glycolytic enzymes[118] and a reduced lactic acid response to ischemic exercise[119] (see Reference 120).

Chronic alcoholic skeletal myopathy may have a major impact on glucose homeostasis, particularly since skeletal muscle accounts for such a large proportion (approximately 40%) of body weight. This conclusion poses the question of the specific effects of severe alcoholic skeletal myopathy on total body fuel metabolism and glucose homeostasis. Studies using the euglycemic insulin clamp technique[121] to evaluate insulin sensitivity in patients with chronic alcoholic myopathy are long overdue. The alcoholic myopathy may be mimicked by chronic alcohol feeding in the rat.[112] During the active phase of the pathogenesis of this disorder in the rat, studies on isolated soleus and extensor digitorum longus muscles have identified a defect in glycogen synthesis, which may indicate a peripheral abnormality in nonoxidative glucose disposal.[33,122]

Chronic Alcohol Abuse and Glucose Homeostasis: An Overview

A number of outstanding questions have been posed relating to the impact of chronic alcohol abuse on glucose homeostasis. ALD, particularly cirrhosis, is commonly associated with impaired glucose metabolism typified by insulin resistance, glucose intolerance, and overt diabetes. We need to identify the site of the primary lesion(s) in cirrhosis that leads to this impairment. Present evidence indicates that the defect may be in the glycogen synthetic pathway[90,96] in skeletal muscle. What is more problematic is the relationship, if any, between peripheral insulin resistance in cirrhosis and abnormalities in muscle metabolism and function. An important question concerns the role of chronic skeletal myopathy or related asymptomatic abnormalities in the genesis of peripheral abnormalities in glucose disposal in alcoholism.

REFERENCES

1. World, M. J., Ryle, P. R., and Thomson, A. D., Alcoholic malnutrition and the small intestine, *Alcohol Alcohol.*, 20, 89, 1985.
2. Morgan, M. Y. and Levine, J. A., Alcohol and nutrition, *Proc. Nutr. Soc.*, 47, 85, 1988.
3. Halsted, C. H. and Keen, C. L., Alcoholism and micronutrient metabolism and deficiencies, *Eur. J. Gastroenterol. Hepatol.*, 2, 399, 1990.
4. Halsted, C. H., Chronic alcoholism, malnutrition, and folate deficiency, in *Alcoholism: A Molecular Perspective*, Palmer, T. N., Ed., Plenum Press, New York, 1991, 237.
5. Hillers, V. N. and Massey, L. K., Interrelationships of moderate and high alcohol consumption with diet and health status, *Am. J. Clin. Nutr.*, 41, 356, 1985.
6. Raskin, P. and Rosenstock, J., Blood glucose control and diabetic complications, *Ann. Intern. Med.*, 105, 254, 1986.
7. Ferrannini, E., Bjorkman, O., Reichard, G. A., Jr., Pilo, A., Olsson, M., Wahren, J., and DeFronzo, R. A., The disposal of an oral glucose load in healthy subjects, *Diabetes*, 34, 580, 1985.
8. DeFronzo, R. A., Jacot, E., Jéquier, E., Maeder, E., and Felber, J. P., The effect of insulin on the disposal of intravenous glucose: results from indirect calorimetry and hepatic and femoral venous catheterization, *Diabetes*, 30, 1000, 1981.
9. Randle, P. J., Molecular mechanisms regulating fuel selection in muscle, in *Biochemistry of Exercise*, Vol. IV-A, Poortmans, J. and Nisbet, G., Eds., University Park Press, Baltimore, 1981, 13.
10. Randle, P. J. and Tubbs, P. K., Carbohydrate and fatty acid metabolism, in *Handbook of Physiology: The Cardiovascular System*, Vol. 1, Berne, R. M., Ed., American Physiological Society, Bethesda, MD, 1979, 805.
11. Palmer, T. N., Caldecourt, M. A., Snell, K., and Sugden, M. C., Alanine and inter-organ relationships in branched-chain amino acid and 2-oxo acid metabolism, *Biosci. Rep.*, 5, 1015, 1985.
12. Sugden, M. C., Holness, M. J., and Palmer, T. N., Fuel selection and carbon flux during the starved-to-fed transition, *Biochem. J.*, 263, 313, 1989.
13. Newsholme, E. A. and Leech, A. R., *Biochemistry for the Medical Sciences*, John Wiley & Sons, Chichester, U.K., 1983.
14. Thiebaud, D., DeFronzo, R. A., Jacot, E., Golay, A., Acheson, K., Maeder, E., Jéquier, E., and Felber, J. P., Effect of long chain triglyceride infusion on glucose metabolism in man, *Metabolism*, 31, 1128, 1982.

15. Lieber, C. S., Pathways of ethanol metabolism and related pathology, in *Alcoholism: A Molecular Perspective*, Palmer, T. N., Ed., Plenum Press, New York, 1991, 1.
16. Lieber, C. S., *Medical Disorders of Alcoholism. Pathogenesis and Treatment*, W. B. Saunders, Philadelphia, 1982.
17. Lieber, C. S., Alcohol and the liver, in *The Molecular Pathology of Alcoholism*, Palmer, T. N., Ed., Oxford University Press, Oxford, 1991, 60.
18. Lundquist, F., Production and utilization of free acetate in man, *Nature*, 193, 579, 1962.
19. Lundquist, F., Tugstrup, N., Winkler, K., Mellemgaard, K., and Munck-Petersen, S., Ethanol metabolism and production of free acetate in the human liver, *J. Clin. Invest.*, 41, 955, 1962.
20. Lundquist, F., Sestoft, L., Damgaard, S. E., Clausen, J. P., and Trap-Jensen, J., Utilization of acetate in the human forearm during exercise after ethanol ingestion, *J. Clin. Invest.*, 52, 3231, 1973.
21. Marks, V., Alcohol and carbohydrate metabolism, *Clin. Endocrinol. Metab.*, 7, 333, 1978.
22. Hoffman, R. S. and Goldfrank, L. R., Ethanol-associated metabolic disorders, *Emerg. Med. Clin. North Am.*, 7, 943, 1986.
23. Arky, R. A. and Freinkel, N., The response of plasma human growth hormone to insulin and ethanol-induced hypoglycemia in two patients with "isolated adrenocorticotropic defect", *Metabolism*, 13, 547, 1964.
24. Feinman, L. and Lieber, C. S., Effect of ethanol on plasma glycerol in man, *Am. J. Clin. Nutr.*, 20, 400, 1967.
25. Salaspuro, M. P., Pikkarainen, P., and Lindros, K., Ethanol-induced hypoglycaemia in normal man: its suppression by the alcohol dehydrogenase inhibitor 4-methylpyrazole, *Eur. J. Clin. Invest.*, 7, 487, 1977.
26. Hawkins, R. D. and Kalant, H., The metabolism of ethanol and its metabolic effects, *Pharmacol. Rev.*, 24, 67, 1972.
27. Kreisberg, R. L., Siegel, A. M., and Owen, W. C., Glucose-lactate interrelationships: effect of ethanol, *J. Clin. Invest.*, 50, 175, 1971.
28. Juhlin-Dannfelt, A., Ahlborg, G., Hagenfeldt, L., Jorfeldt, L., and Felig, P., Influence of ethanol on splanchnic and skeletal muscle substrate turnover during prolonged exercise in man, *Am. J. Physiol.*, 233, E195, 1977.
29. Yki-Järvinen, H., Koivisto, V. A., Ylikahri, R., and Taskinen, M.-R., Acute effects of ethanol and acetate on glucose kinetics in normal subjects, *Am. J. Physiol.*, 254, E175, 1988.
30. Shelmet, J. J., Reichard, G. A., Skutches, C. L., Hoeldke, R. D., Owen, O. E., and Boden, G., Ethanol causes acute inhibition of carbohydrate, fat, and protein oxidation and insulin resistance, *J. Clin. Invest.*, 81, 1137, 1988.
31. McGarry, J. D., Kuwajima, M., Newgard, C. B., and Foster, D. W., From dietary glucose to liver glycogen: the full circle round, *Annu. Rev. Nutr.*, 7, 51, 1987.
32. Cook, E. B., Preece, J. A., Tobin, S. D. M., Sugden, M. C., Cox, D. J., and Palmer, T. N., Acute inhibition by ethanol of intestinal absorption of glucose and hepatic glycogen synthesis on glucose refeeding after starvation in the rat, *Biochem. J.*, 254, 59, 1988.

33. Palmer, T. N., Cook, E. B., and Drake, P. G., Alcohol abuse and fuel homeostasis, in *Alcoholism: A Molecular Perspective*, Palmer, T. N., Ed., Plenum Press, New York, 1991, 213.

34. Dornhorst, A. and Ouyang, A., Effect of alcohol on glucose tolerance, *Lancet*, 2, 957, 1971.

35. Shanley, B. C., Robertson, E. J., Joubert, S. M., and North-Coombes, J. D., Effect of alcohol on glucose tolerance, *Lancet*, 1, 1232, 1972.

36. Metz, R., Berger, S., and Mako, M., Potentiation of the plasma insulin response to glucose by prior administration of alcohol. An apparent islet-priming effect, *Diabetes*, 18, 517, 1969.

37. Friedenberg, R., Metz, R., Mako, M., and Surmaczynska, B., Differential plasma insulin response to glucose and glucagon stimulation following ethanol priming, *Diabetes*, 20, 397, 1971.

38. Phillips, G. B. and Safrit, H. F., Alcoholic diabetes. Induction of glucose intolerance with alcohol, *JAMA*, 217, 1513, 1971.

39. Nikkilä, E. A. and Taskinen, M.-R., Ethanol-induced alterations of glucose tolerance, postglucose hypoglycemia, and insulin secretion in normal, obese, and diabetic subjects, *Diabetes*, 24, 933, 1975.

40. McMonagle, J. and Felig, P., Effect of ethanol ingestion on glucose tolerance and insulin secretion in normal and diabetic subjects, *Metab. Clin. Exp.*, 24, 625, 1975.

41. O'Keefe, O. J. D. and Marks, V., Lunchtime gin and tonic a cause of reactive hypoglycemia, *Lancet*, 1, 1286, 1977.

42. O'Connor, S. P., Nugent, Z., Rudenski, A. S., Hooker, J. P., Burnett, M. A., Darling, P., and Turner, R. C., Comparison of storage- and signal-limited models of pancreatic insulin secretion, *Am. J. Physiol.*, 7, R378, 1980.

43. Andreani, D., Tamburrano, G., and Javicoli, M., Alcoholic hypoglycemia: hormonal changes, in *Hypoglycemia*, Hormone and Metabolism Research Supplement Series, Andreani, D., LeFebvre, P., and Marks, V., Eds., Georg Thieme Verlag, Stuttgart, 1974, 99.

44. Kühl, C. and Anderson, O., Glucose- and tolbutamide-mediated insulin response after preinfusion with ethanol, *Diabetes*, 23, 821, 1974.

45. Colwell, A. R., Jr., Feinzimer, M., Cooper, D. and Zuckerman, L., Alcohol inhibition of cyclic AMP-induced insulin release, *Diabetes*, 22, 854, 1973.

46. Kuo, W. N., Hodgkins, D. S., and Kuo, J. F., Adenylate cyclase in islets of Langerhans. Isolation of islets and regulation of adenylate cyclase activity by various hormones and agents, *J. Biol. Chem.*, 248, 2705, 1973.

47. Kühl, C., Anderson, O., Lindkaer, S., and Van Nielson, O., Effect of ethanol on the glucose-mediated insulin release in triply catheterized anesthetized pigs, *Diabetes*, 25, 752, 1976.

48. Shah, J. H., Wongsurawat, N., and Aran, P. P., Effect of ethanol on stimulus-induced insulin secretion and glucose tolerance. A study of mechanisms, *Diabetes*, 26, 271, 1977.

49. Singh, S. P. and Patel, D. G., Effects of ethanol on carbohydrate metabolism. I. influence on oral glucose tolerance test, *Metabolism*, 25, 239, 1976.

50. Mallaisse, W. J., Malaisse-Lagae, F., and Lacy, P. E., Participation of a microtubular-microfilamentous system in insulin secretion, *Diabetologia*, 6, 638, 1970.
51. Mallaisse, W. J., Malaisse-Lagae, F., Walker, W. O., and Lacy, P. E., The stimulus-secretion coupling of glucose-induced insulin release. V. The participation of a microtubular-microfilamentous system, *Diabetes*, 20, 257, 1971.
52. Bivens, C. H. and Feldman, J. M., Effect of ethanol and its metabolites on insulin secretion, *Q. J. Stud. Alcohol*, 35, 635, 1974.
53. Ganda, O. P., Srikanta, S., Brink, S. J., Morris, M. A., Gleason, R. E., Soeldner, J. S., and Eisenbarth, G. S., Differential sensitivity of β-cell secretatogues in "early" type I diabetes mellitus, *Diabetes*, 33, 516, 1984.
54. Garvey, W. T., Revers, R. R., Koltermann, O. G., Rubenstein, A. H., and Olefsky, J., Modulation of insulin secretion by insulin and glucose in type II diabetes mellitus, *J. Clin. Endocrinol. Metab.*, 60, 559, 1985.
55. Bruce, D. G., Chisholm, D. J., Storlien, L. H., and Kraegen, E. W., Physiological importance of deficiency in early prandial insulin secretion in non-insulin dependent diabetes, *Diabetes*, 37, 736, 1988.
56. Luzi, L. and DeFronzo, R. A., Effect of loss of first-phase insulin secretion on hepatic glucose production and tissue glucose disposal in humans, *Am. J. Physiol.*, 257, E241, 1989.
57. Seltzer, H. S., Drug-induced hypoglycemia: a review based on 473 cases, *Diabetes*, 21, 955, 1972.
58. Haight, J. S. and Keatinge, W. R., Failure of thermoregulation in the cold during hypoglycaemia induced by exercise and alcohol, *J. Physiol. (London)*, 229, 87, 1973.
59. Singh, S. P., Kumar, Y., Snyder, A. K., Ellyin, F. E., and Gilden, J. L., Effect of alcohol on glucose tolerance in normal and non-insulin-dependent diabetic subjects, *Alcoholism*, 12, 727, 1988.
60. Wapnick, S. and Jones, J. J., Alcohol and glucose intolerance, *Lancet*, 2, 180, 1972.
61. Yki-Järvinen, H. and Nikkilä, E. A., Ethanol decreases glucose utilization in healthy man, *J. Clin. Endocrinol. Metab.*, 61, 941, 1985.
62. Jorfeldt, L. and Juhlin-Dannfelt, A., The influence of ethanol on splanchnic and skeletal muscle metabolism in man, *Metabolism*, 27, 97, 1978.
63. Lochner, A., Wulff, J., and Madison, L. L., Ethanol-induced hypoglycemia. I. The acute effects of ethanol on hepatic glucose output and peripheral glucose utilization in fasted dogs, *Metabolism*, 16, 1, 1967.
64. Clarke, D. W. and Evans, R. L., The influence of alcohol upon carbohydrate metabolism in the liver and in isolated diaphragms, *Q. J. Stud. Alcohol*, 21, 13, 1960.
65. Williamson, J. R., Glycolytic control mechanisms. I. Inhibition of glycolysis by acetate and pyruvate in the isolated perfused rat heart, *J. Biol. Chem.*, 240, 2308, 1965.
66. Karsson, N., Fellenius, E., and Kiessling, K.-H., The metabolism of acetate in the perfused hind-quarter of the rat, *Acta Physiol. Scand.*, 93, 391, 1975.
67. Jones, D. P., Perman, E., and Lieber, C. S., Free fatty acid turnover and triglyceride metabolism after ethanol ingestion in man, *J. Lab. Clin. Med.*, 66, 804, 1965.

68. Crouse, J. R., Gerson, C. D., DeCarli, L. M., and Lieber, C. S., Role of acetate in the reduction of plasma free fatty acids produced by ethanol in man, *J. Lipid Res.*, 9, 509, 1968.

69. Anton, H., Ethanol and urinary catecholamines in man, *Clin. Pharmacol. Ther.*, 6, 462, 1965.

70. Palmer, J. P. and Ensinck, J. W., Stimulation of glucagon secretion by ethanol-induced hypoglycemia in man, *Diabetes*, 24, 295, 1975.

71. Tiengo, A., Fedele, D., Frasson, P., Muggeo, M., and Crepaldi, G., Ethanol effect on glucagon secretion in the pig, *Horm. Metab. Res.*, 6, 245, 1974.

72. Jauhonen, V. P., Effect of acute ethanol load on plasma immunoreactive insulin and glucagon, *Horm. Metab. Res.*, 10, 214, 1978.

73. Issad, T., Pénicaud, L., Ferré, P., Kandé, J., Baudon, M.-A., and Girard, J., Effects of fasting on tissue glucose utilization in conscious resting rats. Major glucose-sparing effect on working muscles, *Biochem. J.*, 246, 241, 1987.

74. Holness, M. J. and Sugden, M. C., Glucose utilization in heart, diaphragm and skeletal muscle during the fed-to-starved transition, *Biochem. J.*, 270, 245, 1990.

75. Pénicaud, L., Ferré, P., Kande, J., Leturque, A., Issad, T., and Girard, J., Effect of anesthesia on glucose production and utilization in rats, *Am. J. Physiol.*, 252, E365, 1987.

76. Sugden, M. C. and Holness, M. J., Effects of re-feeding after prolonged starvation on pyruvate dehydrogenase activities in heart, diaphragm and selected skeletal muscles of the rat, *Biochem. J.*, 262, 669, 1989.

77. Sugden, M. C., Liu, Y.-L., and Holness, M. J., Glucose utilization and disposal in cardiothoracic and skeletal muscles during the starved-to-fed transition in the rat, *Biochem. J.*, 272, 133, 1990.

78. Holness, M. J., Schuster-Bruce, M. J. L., and Sugden, M. C., Skeletal-muscle glycogen synthesis during the starved-to-fed transition in the rat, *Biochem. J.*, 254, 855, 1988.

79. Oscai, L. B., Gorski, J., Miller, W. C., and Palmer, W. K., Role of the alkaline TG lipase in regulating intramuscular TG content, *Med. Sci. Sports Exercise*, 20, 539, 1988.

80. Ferré, P., Leturque, A., Burnol, A.-F., Pénicaud, L., and Girard, J., A method to quantify glucose utilization *in vivo* in skeletal muscle and white adipose tissue of the anaesthetized rat, *Biochem. J.*, 228, 103, 1985.

81. Molina, P. E., Lang, C. H., Bagby, G. J., and Spitzer, J. J., Ethanol attenuates endotoxin-enhanced glucose utilization, *Am. J. Physiol.*, 258, R987, 1990.

82. Lang, C. H., Bagby, G. J. and Spitzer, J. J., Glucose kinetics and body temperature after lethal and nonlethal doses of endotoxin, *Am. J. Physiol.*, 248, R471, 1985.

83. Wolfe, R. R., Elahi, D., and Spitzer, J. J., Glucose and lactate kinetics after endotoxin administration in dogs, *Am. J. Physiol.*, 232, E180, 1977.

84. Mészàros, K., Lang, C. H., Bagby, G. J., and Spitzer, J. J., Contribution of different organs to increased glucose consumption after endotoxin administration, *J. Biol. Chem.*, 262, 10965, 1987.

85. Molina, P. E., Lang, C. H., Bagby, G. J., D'Souza, N. B., and Spitzer, J. J., Ethanol administration diminishes the endotoxin-induced increase in glucose metabolism, *Alcohol. Clin. Exp. Res.,* 13, 407, 1989.
86. D'Souza, N. B., Bagby, G. J., Nelson, S., Lang, C. H., and Spitzer, J. J., Acute alcohol infusion suppresses endotoxin-induced serum tumor necrosis factor, *Alcohol. Clin. Exp. Res.,* 13, 295, 1989.
87. Creutzfeldt, W., Frerichs, H., and Sickinger, K., Liver diseases and diabetes mellitus, in *Progress in Liver Diseases,* Vol. 3, Popper, H. and Schaffner, F., Eds., Grune & Stratton, New York, 1970, 371.
88. Allen, F. M., Studies concerning diabetes, *JAMA,* 63, 791, 1914.
89. Feingold, K. R. and Siperstein, M. D., Normalization of fasting blood glucose levels in insulin-requiring diabetes: the role of ethanol abstention, *Diabetes Care,* 6, 186, 1983.
90. Petrides, A. S. and DeFronzo, R. A., Glucose and insulin metabolism in cirrhosis, *J. Hepatol.,* 8, 107, 1989.
91. Proietto, J., Nankervis, A., Aitken, P., Dudley, F. J., Caruso, G., and Alford, F. P., Insulin resistance in cirrhosis: evidence for a postreceptor defect, 21, 677, 1984.
92. Cavallo-Perin, P., Cassader, M., Bozzo, C., Bruno, A., Nuccio, P., Dall'Omo, A. M., Marucci, M., and Pagano, G., Mechanism of insulin resistance in human liver cirrhosis. Evidence for a combined receptor and postreceptor defect, *J. Clin. Invest.,* 75, 1659, 1985.
93. Iversen, J., Vilstrup, H., and Tygstrup, N., Kinetics of glucose metabolism in relation to insulin concentrations in patients with alcoholic cirrhosis and in healthy persons, *Gastroenterology,* 87, 1138, 1984.
94. Vannini, P., Forlani, G., Marchesini, G., Ciavarella, A., Zoli, M., and Pisi, E., The euglycemic clamp technique in patients with liver cirrhosis, *Horm. Metab. Res.,* 16, 341, 1984.
95. Taylor, R., Heine, R. J., Collins, J., James, O. F. W., and Alberti, K. G. M. M., Insulin action in cirrhosis, *Hepatology,* 5, 64, 1985.
96. Kruszynska, Y. T., Williams, N., Perry, M., and Home, P. D., The relationship between insulin sensitivity and skeletal muscle enzyme activities in hepatic cirrhosis, *Hepatology,* 8, 1615, 1988.
97. Proietto, J., Alford, F. P., and Dudley, F. J., The mechanism of carbohydrate intolerance of cirrhosis, *J. Clin. Endocrinol. Metab.,* 51, 1030, 1980.
98. Leatherdale, B. A., Chase, J., Rogers, J., Alberti, K. G. M. M., Davies, P., and Record, C. O., Forearm glucose uptake in cirrhosis and its relationship to glucose tolerance, *Clin. Sci.,* 59, 191, 1980.
99. Johnston, D. G., Alberti, K. G. M. M., Faber, O. K., Binder, C., and Wright, R., Hyperinsulinism of hepatic cirrhosis: diminished degradation of hypersecretion, *Lancet,* 1, 10, 1977.
100. Proietto, J., Dudley, F. J., Aitken, P., and Alford, F. P., Hyperinsulinemia and insulin resistance of cirrhosis: the importance of insulin hypersecretion, *Clin. Endocrinol.,* 21, 657, 1984.
101. Iwasaki, Y., Ohkubo, A., Kajinuma, H., Akanuma, Y., and Kosaka, K., Degradation and secretion of insulin in hepatic cirrhosis, *J. Clin. Endocrinol. Metab.,* 47, 774, 1978.

102. Nygren, A., Adner, N., Sundblad, L., and Wiechel, K.-L., Insulin uptake by the human cirrhotic liver, *Metabolism*, 34, 48, 1985.

103. Keller, U., Sonnenberg, G. E., Burckhardt, D., and Perruchoud, A., Evidence for an augmented glucagon dependence of hepatic glucose production in cirrhosis of the liver, *J. Clin. Endocrinol. Metab.*, 54, 961, 1982.

104. Rehfeld, J. F., Juhl, E., and Hilden, M., Carbohydrate metabolism in alcohol-induced fatty liver. Evidence for an abnormal insulin response to glucagon in alcoholic liver disease, *Gastroenterology*, 64, 445, 1973.

105. Sereny, G. and Endrenyi, L., Mechanism and significance of carbohydrate intolerance in chronic alcoholism, *Metabolism*, 27, 1041, 1978.

106. Nicolson, G. and Paton, A., Glucose intolerance in alcoholics, *J. Stud. Alcohol.*, 40, 997, 1979.

107. Pezzarossa, A., Cervigni, C., Ghinelli, F., Molina, E., and Gnudi, A., Glucose tolerance in chronic alcoholics after alcohol withdrawal: effect of accompanying diet, *Metabolism*, 35, 984, 1986.

108. Nyboe Andersen, B., Hagen, C., Faber, O. K., Lindhol, J., Boisen, P., and Worning, H., Glucose intolerance and B cell function in chronic alcoholism: its relation to hepatic histology and exocrine pancreatic function, *Metabolism*, 32, 1029, 1983.

109. Iturriaga, H., Kelly, M., Bunout, D., Pino, M. E., Pereda, T., Barrera, R., Petermann, M., and Ugarte, G., Glucose intolerance and insulin response in recently drinking alcoholic patients: possible effects of withdrawal, *Metabolism*, 35, 238, 1986.

110. Bunout, D., Petermann, M., Bravo, M., Kelly, M., Hirsch, S., Ugarte, G., and Iturriaga, H., Glucose turnover rate and peripheral insulin sensitivity in alcoholic patients without liver disease, *Ann. Nutr. Metab.*, 33, 31, 1989.

111. Preedy, V. R. and Peters, T. J., Alcohol, nutrition and muscle disease, *Eur. J. Gastroenterol. Hepatol.*, 6, 426, 1990.

112. Peters, T. J. and Preedy, V. R., Chronic alcoholic skeletal myopathy: an overview, in *Alcoholism: A Molecular Perspective*, Palmer, T. N., Ed., Plenum Press, New York, 1991, 301.

113. Peters, T. J., Martin, F., and Ward, K., Chronic alcoholic skeletal myopathy — common and reversible, *Alcohol*, 2, 485, 1985.

114. Urbano-Marquez, A., Estruch, R., Navarro-Lopez, F., Grau, J. M., Mont, L., and Rubin, E., The effects of alcoholism on skeletal and cardiac muscle, *N. Engl. J. Med.*, 320, 409, 1989.

115. Slavin, G., Martin, F., Ward, P., Levi, A. J., and Peters, T. J., Chronic alcohol excess is associated with selective but reversible injury to type 2B muscle fibres, *J. Clin. Pathol.*, 36, 772, 1983.

116. Preedy, V. R. and Peters, T. J., The effect of chronic ethanol ingestion on protein metabolism in Type-I- and Type-II-fibre rich skeletal muscles of the rat, *Biochem. J.*, 254, 631, 1988.

117. Sunnasy, D., Cairns, S. R., Martin, F., Slavin, G., and Peters, T. J., Chronic alcoholic skeletal myopathy: a clinical, histological and biochemical assessment of muscle lipid, *J. Clin. Pathol.*, 36, 778, 1983.

118. Martin, F. C., Levi, A. J., Slavin, G., and Peters, T. J., Glycogen content and activities of key glycolytic enzymes in muscle biopsies from control subjects and patients with chronic alcoholic skeletal myopathy, *Clin. Sci.*, 66, 69, 1984.

119. Perkoff, G. T., Hardy, P., and Vélez-Garcia, E., Reversible acute muscular syndrome in chronic alcoholism, *N. Engl. J. Med.,* 274, 1277, 1966.
120. Ward, K. and Peters, T. J., Ischaemic lactate response in alcoholism — a reappraisal, *Clin. Sci.,* 65, 21P, 1983.
121. DeFronzo, R. A., Tobin, J. D,. and Andres, R., Glucose clamp technique: a method for quantifying insulin secretion and resistance, *Am. J. Physiol.,* 237, E214, 1979.
122. Palmer, T. N., Fuel homeostasis and alcohol abuse, *Eur. J. Gastroenterol. Hepatol.,* 2, 406, 1990.

6 Role of Carbohydrate in Alcohol Metabolism

INTRODUCTION

Recent reviews have included carbohydrate effects in alcohol (ethanol) metabolism.[1-4] By their scope, these reviews demonstrate the ubiquitous effects of ethanol on metabolism, but also illustrate the scant direct evaluation of the influence of carbohydrate on these ethanol effects. Many reports consider carbohydrate as a substrate in metabolism on a par with ethanol and do not consider the direct influence of glucose or other carbohydrates on the total metabolic state of the cell. Consequently, conflicting effects of ethanol are reported which may reflect differences in carbohydrate influence rather than direct effects of ethanol.

This chapter focuses on the overall role of carbohydrate in ethanol metabolism, with special attention to its role in determining the metabolic state of the system. Metabolism in the liver is emphasized since it is the major site of ethanol oxidation, but other tissues or conditions are mentioned where applicable.

ETHANOL AS A NUTRIENT

Ethanol is consumed in nutritional quantities, 25% or more of total calories in many instances, for example, a hot dog and a beer or a beef sandwich and a glass of wine. Most experimental studies include 25 to 50% of calories as ethanol.[5] In rats, 35% of calories as ethanol is necessary in order to maintain adequate blood alcohol levels.[6] As a nutrient, each ethanol molecule provides one equivalent of acetate and two of reduced nicotinamide adenine dinucleotide (NADH) to the general pool of metabolic intermediates. In this initial metabolism, no evidence exists of either control of uptake or regulation of the two oxidizing enzymes, alcohol dehydrogenase (ADH) and aldehyde dehydrogenase, except by substrate or product concentrations.

ISBN 0-8493-7933-4
© 1992 by CRC Press, Inc.

In the liver, where most ethanol metabolism occurs, the activity of a second system, the microsomal ethanol oxidizing system (MEOS),[7] can catalyze the first oxidation reaction in the place of ADH. The activity of MEOS is increased by prolonged alcohol ingestion, but its K_m is 10 to 15 mM vs. 0.2 to 2 mM for ADH so that it competes effectively only at higher ethanol concentrations. Since it is a mixed function oxidase (MFO) system, one reduced coenzyme is reoxidized with each ethanol molecule in a coupled reaction that utilizes molecular oxygen. Thus, in the MEOS pathway there is no net production of reducing equivalents for the conversion of ethanol to acetate.

The end result of this unregulated ethanol oxidation either by the ADH pathway alone or in combination with MEOS is an abnormal increase in reduced coenzymes and acetate. Therefore, because of a lack of metabolic controls, the excessive accumulation of C-2 units (acetate) and reduced coenzymes (NADH) from ethanol oxidation must be further metabolized in other pathways. It is in these subsequent steps that the role of carbohydrate in ethanol metabolism becomes significant, and carbohydrate is thereby linked directly to the degree of toxicity of ethanol that occurs when the system is unable to handle these excesses.

In contrast, the metabolism of other macronutrients (proteins, carbohydrates, and fats) is subjected to regulation at various levels from the beginning. That is, while ethanol is only regulated at the most immediate level of substrate and product in its initial metabolic pathway, all other nutrients and all general metabolic pathways are further regulated at higher levels, including allosteric control, covalent activation, and gene induction of key enzymes. These regulatory mechanisms respond to different levels of dietary nutrients, balance nutrient input against the needs of the system, and thereby create an appropriate metabolic state.

ROLES OF CARBOHYDRATE IN METABOLISM

Carbohydrate, primarily glucose, has four functions in normal metabolism:

1. It is a nutrient (bulk fuel) in several pathways, including glycolysis and gluconeogenesis (pyruvate, lactate, and glucogenic amino acids are the input in the latter pathway), glycogenesis and glycogenolysis, the hexose monophosphate (pentose) shunt, and endogenous fatty acid synthesis.

2.   Associated with its function as a fuel molecule, carbohydrate supplies and maintains the intermediate pools for these and other metabolic pathways, e.g., the tricarboxylic acid (TCA) cycle. In this role, when it is present in adequate amounts, glucose can spare the utilization of glucogenic amino acids to maintain these pools.

3.   It is a short-term metabolic signal, as glucose concentration, in the covalent activation/inactivation control of enzymes primarily through its influence on the insulin/glucagon hormone signal balance.

4.   In the longer term, carbohydrate is a metabolic signal at the gene level,[8] through insulin and perhaps other metabolites,[9,10] for induction or suppression of many enzymes located in the pathways listed above.

Therefore, carbohydrate plays several primary roles in establishing a metabolic state.

METABOLISM OF ETHANOL

Since ethanol is a ketogenic rather than a glucogenic metabolite and does not exert controls on metabolic pathways above the substrate/product level, it is instead subject to the controls exerted on the system by the other nutrients. Specifically, carbohydrate continues to play all four of its metabolic roles during ethanol metabolism. The only carbohydrate function ethanol can fulfill is as a substrate in fatty acid synthesis. All the rest of the roles of carbohydrate must be filled by the carbohydrate present in the diet or by glucogenic amino acids. If ethanol is substituted for carbohydrate, as it often is in experimental alcohol diets, the remaining reduced carbohydrate will not have the same effect as it does in the control diet. Therefore, in any study of the metabolic effects of ethanol it is essential to determine the specific roles of carbohyrate and ethanol. Similar determinations for protein are usually not necessary when protein calories are kept the same for experimental and control diets. However, if carbohydrate is low enough, protein may be affected due to role (2) of carbohydrate, outlined above.

ROLES OF CARBOHYDRATE IN ETHANOL METABOLISM

GLYCOLYSIS AND GLUCONEOGENESIS

The decrease in the cytosol $NAD^+/NADH$ ratio during ethanol oxidation should inhibit glycolysis, promote gluconeogenesis, and permit blood glucose levels to be maintained. However, hypoglycemia is a common symptom of alcohol ingestion and hyperglycemia has also been observed.[1] Consequently, the effect of ethanol oxidation on gluconeogenesis has been extensively investigated. Early studies of acute ethanol effects with liver slices and perfused liver suggested that ethanol was inhibitory to gluconeogenesis in spite of the increased supply of NADH. The inhibition could be relieved by pyruvate or certain other glucogenic intermediates.[11,12] Subsequently, ethanol was also found to stimulate gluconeogenesis.[13,14] It is now accepted that gluconeogenesis is promoted in liver in the fed state and inhibited in the fasted state, and each of these conditions may contribute to the observed abnormal blood glucose levels, although hormonal control may also be involved.[15] In any event, the metabolic state of the liver and the relative availability of glucose and glucogenic substrates is now recognized as a significant factor in gluconeogenic activity and the maintenance of blood glucose during ethanol oxidation.[1]

Short-term (hormonal) regulation was examined by Topping et al.[13] using livers from fed rats perfused with recirculating whole blood. Ethanol stimulated gluconeogenic flux from lactate in this system and produced a rise in circulating glucose concentration. Insulin alone caused a drop in the perfusing blood glucose concentration, presumably through its normal stimulation of glycolysis in the liver. With ethanol and insulin together, circulating glucose was the same as in control liver preparations, suggesting that the substrate level effect of ethanol (high NADH) that promoted gluconeogenesis was being counterbalanced by the hormone level, covalent activation/inactivation, and signal of insulin on key regulatory glycolytic and gluconeogenic enzymes to promoted glycolysis. Thus, an ethanol control and an independent carbohydrate control were being expressed together in this metabolic state to control glycolysis/gluconeogenesis. In a different hormonal study, stimulation of gluconeogenesis by alanine in isolated livers from T_4-treated (thyrotoxic) rats was measured.[16] Livers from thyroxine-treated rats and ethanol-treated livers from control rats both exhibited alanine stimulation of gluconeogenesis; however, ethanol added to the thyroxine-treated livers did not show any added effect. Thus, in this case, where both signals stimulated gluconeogenesis, either signal alone appeared to have caused maximum stimulation of the system and no apparent interaction occurred.

Mascord et al.[17] examined the effect of diet on oxidation of an acute ethanol dose in humans. After 5 d of receiving a high (65%) or low (20%)

carbohydrate diet, the [lactate]/[pyruvate] ratio (L/P) generated by constant perfusion of an (acute) ethanol load was determined. While no difference was found in the initial (prealcohol) L/P ratios or subsequent ethanol clearance rate, the subjects who received the high carbohydrate diet conditioning maintained a smaller steady-state L/P ratio during ethanol metabolism. Furthermore, the smaller L/P ratio was a combination of both higher pyruvate and lower lactate concentrations in the equilibrium ratio. The L/P ratio is most closely associated with glycolysis/gluconeogenesis, but the difference could be related to activity changes of any number of enzymes that might contribute to reducing equivalents' clearance and cause a shift in the L/P ratio because the conditioning period was long enough for many diet-induced enzyme changes to be nearly complete. The study is of further interest because it was carried out in humans, and it suggests that if the L/P ratio is a measure of the metabolic stress on the liver during alcohol oxidation, then it is relatively easy to lessen this stress by dietary manipulation of carbohydrate.

GLYCOGENESIS AND GLYCOGENOLYSIS

Precursors for glycogen synthesis in the liver can come from free glucose or from gluconeogenic synthesis in the fed state. In the fasted state the latter is the more important pathway because of the fall in plasma insulin and the related loss of glucokinase due to its decay in the absence of dietary glucose (half-life approximately 12 h).

Rifkin et al.[18] examined glycogen synthesis in hepatocytes from rats after chronic administration (3 to 4 weeks) of ethanol or control (isocaloric carbohydrate) liquid diets or lab chow. They observed significant reductions in glycogen synthesis in ethanol and pair-fed rats compared to the chow controls. They concluded that this was the result of caloric deprivation, because of ethanol-decreased diet consumption by experimental and pair-fed animals. However, they proposed that a further reduction of glycogen synthesis and an additional plasma hypoinsulinemia in the experimental animals was caused by ethanol. There was no recognition of the additional reduction of carbohydrate in the alcohol diets due to its isocaloric substitution with ethanol and the probable effect of this on circulating insulin levels or glycogen-synthesizing capacity of these animals. This points to a common flaw in many studies using the isocaloric liquid diet technique which is that, too often, carbohydrate is considered a "neutral" caloric source and potential effects of its removal, such as a reduction of plasma insulin and a loss of glycogen-synthesizing capacity in this instance, are ignored. Instead, data are evaluated so that changes are attributed to the addition of ethanol and not the removal of carbohydrate.

Cook et al.[19] demonstrated the coupling between liver glycogen synthesis and gluconeogenesis in hepatocytes from 24-h starved rats. Neither basal level glycogen synthesis from glucose (10 mM) nor the approximately 20-fold increase caused by added dihydroxyacetone (20 mM), a glucogenic substrate, was inhibited by ethanol. However, the 12-fold increase caused by lactate (18 mM) + pyrivate (2 mM) in control cells was inhibited 23% by ethanol. The stimulation by added glucogenic substrates and the selective inhibition by ethanol indicated that the majority of glycogen synthesis in hepatocytes from starved rats was being synthesized from C-3 units by the gluconeogenic pathway and the center of the pathway, between pyruvate and dihydroxyacetone phosphate, was inhibited by ethanol oxidation. These data are consistent with those for glucose synthesis in liver tissue from starved rats, as referenced above.

It therefore appears that the role of carbohydrate in glycogen metabolism is closely linked to the metabolism of glucogenic intermediates in the gluconeogenic pathway and that the primary mechanism connecting carbohydrate and ethanol here is the NAD^+/NADH status of the cytosol. If sufficient nonreduced glucogenic precursors are available, as they presumably are in the fed state, ethanol can increase gluconeogenic flux, but if the dominant glucogenic precursor its lactate, which is already reduced, then ethanol reduces the flux.

In chronic studies, the use of a low concentration of dietary carbohydrate by replacing most if it with ethanol shifts the burden of maintaining blood glucose almost entirely to gluconeogenesis. Even when glycogen stores are used for blood glucose, the gluconeogenic pathway appears to be the one used to maintain glycogen stores because low glucose reduces circulating insulin, which in turn lowers the concentration of glucokinase and favors glycogen synthesis from C-3 over C-6 precursors.

PRODUCT REMOVAL IN ETHANOL OXIDATION

For ethanol oxidation via ADH, a 2:1 relationship exists between reducing equivalents and C-2 units (NADH:acetate); for the MEOS pathway the relationship is 0:1. Three options are available for clearance of these products:

1. Oxidation to produce energy using NADH directly in the electron transport system and acetate in the TCA cycle coupled to electron transport.

2. Transport from liver to other tissues by increased lactate circulation to transport excess reducing equivalents, increased acetate circulation for excess C-2, or by ketone body synthesis for export of both reducing equivalents and acetate in a ratio of <1:2, depending on the hydroxybutyrate/acetoacetate ratio.

3. Recombination of reducing equivalents and C-2 substrates into fatty acids for export and storage with a ratio of 2:1.

These options are not mutually exclusive and are presumably used in proportion to the relevant pathway activities of a particular metabolic state.

Direct Reoxidation of NADH

Increased oxygen uptake by hepatocytes is observed in ethanol metabolism. Factors that promote reoxidation of NADH can further increase oxygen uptake. These factors include increased shuttle activity to move reducing equivalents from the cytosol into mitochondria, increased adenosine triphosphate (ATP) hydrolysis to accelerate oxidative phosphorylation and hence reoxidation of NADH, and perhaps other energy-consuming reactions that increase the tightly coupled reoxidation reactions of NADH to NAD^+.

While the acceleration of ethanol oxidation by fructose, including its demonstration in humans,[20] has been well documented,[21] some reports concluded that fructose acts in the same way as lactate, pyruvate, and other glucogenic intermediates to replenish intermediate pools[22] (role 2 in carbohydrate metabolism, above). Subsequently, it was shown with rat hepatocytes that during ethanol oxidation fructose increases glucose synthesis above that caused by lactate or pyruvate alone, and a concomitant decrease occurs in ATP. Thus, the hydrolysis of ATP provides the conditions for accelerated oxidative phosphorylation, increased reoxidation of NADH, and an increased rate of ethanol oxidation, as outlined above. However, the rate of ethanol oxidation is not increased beyond that observed with added lactate or pyruvate alone.[23] The paradox of whether a fructose effect exists may have been resolved by the work of Crownover et al.,[21] which demonstrated that whether the increase in oxidation rate is observed depends on experimental conditions. In humans, if fructose is given with ethanol, the peak ethanol concentration is reduced due to a "first pass" effect of fructose on ethanol entering the liver together through the portal system, and this effect obscures the general increase in oxidation. If ethanol is first allowed to equilibrate, the increase in oxidation rate upon the addition of fructose is clearly evident. Therefore, the proposed mechanism for an increased ethanol oxidation rate with fructose incorporates the depletion of ATP by the unregulated fructokinase reaction, its regeneration by the electron transport system, and the coupled acceleration of NADH reoxidation. Whatever the actual mechanism, it is clear that with fructose carbohydrate directly intervenes to accelerate ethanol oxidation. It is worth noting, however, that fructose metabolism itself causes an increase in blood lactate which will oppose the lowering of lactate resulting from the increased clearance rate of ethanol.

Direct Metabolism of Acetate

Acetate appears to leave the liver freely and circulate throughout the peripheral tissues. Experiments designed to relate glucose turnover to acetate metabolism in humans[24] led to the conclusion that both production and utilization of glucose are reduced by ethanol which results in no net change in blood glucose. However, no involvement of acetate could be demonstrated as part of the mechanism for maintaining this glucose balance even though a substantial rise in circulating acetate was found. One difficulty with the technique used was that splanchnic and peripheral changes could not be assessed separately.

In another study in humans,[25] it was possible to measure the metabolic responses of both forearm and adipose to acute ethanol ingestion. These experiments measured the same increase in circulating acetate reported by others, and oxidation of acetate could be measured in muscle but not in adipose. Further, it was possible to calculate that in spite of significant circulation, only about 3% of the total acetate produced by liver ethanol oxidation was metabolized by muscle. This suggests that even though acetate circulates to a significant amount, most of it is still metabolized in the liver during repeated passes. There are a number of earlier reports of significant acetate oxidation in muscle suggesting that further investigation may be needed; however, the experimental design of the transmuscle and transadipose measurements summarized here appears to be sound.

Synthesis and Transport of Ketones

Some of the earliest work on the effects of ethanol involved studies of ketone metabolism.[26] These studies also represent the effective use of diet manipulation for studying ethanol effects. In this work, four metabolic states were established: a lipolytic state using high dietary fat (82% fat, 5% carbohydrate calories); a lipogenic state using high carbohydrate (51% carbohydrate, 36% fat), a lipolytic/alcohol state (36% fat, 46% ethanol, and 5% carbohydrate), and a lipogenic/alcohol state (5% fat, 46% ethanol, and 36% carbohydrate). Compared to initial values, ketones rose 30-fold with the lipolytic/alcohol diet, 8- to 10-fold with the lipolytic diet, and no increase in ketogenesis occurred with either the lipogenic or the lipogenic/alcohol diets. Many subsequent investigations have essentially supported this relationship between the lipolytic state and alcohol in the biogenesis of ketones. Thus, the export of ethanol metabolites as ketones has a negative correlation with dietary carbohydrates.

Production of Fatty Acids from Ethanol

Based on the relative proportions of the substrates, conversion of ethanol metabolites directly to fatty acids seems the most logical answer to the problem of ethanol oxidation in the liver. The ratio of reducing equivalents to C-2 is right (2:1), the liver is the right location for fatty acid synthesis, and fatty liver is a common result of alcohol ingestion both acutely and chronically. Doubts about this logical solution arose very early from both human and rat studies,[27,28] when it was recognized that transient liver lipid accumulation following an acute ethanol load resembled adipose fatty acids in composition, while the composition of accumulated fatty acids following chronic intake resembled either exogenous (dietary) fatty acids or endogenous (synthesized) fatty acids *depending on the proportion of triglyceride to carbohydrate in the diet.*

The results of fatty acid accumulation following ethanol ingestion were clearly not being substrate determined by ethanol oxidation products or even by a single mechanism. While fatty acid collection in the liver occurred in each case, acute ingestion leading to mobilization of adipose lipids implied an impairment of insulin action which caused the mobilization of depot fat, chronic ethanol ingestion with a diet high in lipid implied impairment of peripheral lipid uptake or retention plus continuous inadequate lipoprotein formation to clear the liver, and finally, from chronic ethanol ingestion with high carbohydrate there was the added effect of excessive endogenous synthesis. These findings suggested the involvement of at least two types of carbohydrate metabolism, one related to a failure of lipid retention in adipose similar to that observed in insulin-dependent diabetes mellitus and a second related to excessive lipogenesis reflecting the result of carbohydrate-stimulated lipogenic enzyme induction. The failure of adequate lipoprotein synthesis would not be related to carbohydrate metabolism unless glucogenic amino acids were being removed from amino acid pools by a shortage of carbohydrate, preventing adequate synthesis of apolipoproteins.

Unfortunately for the role of carbohydrate in ethanol metabolism, the liquid pair-fed diet technique was introduced because of these early studies.[29] The standard diet, commonly referred to as the Lieber-DeCarli diet, included carbohydrate as 48% of calories and fat as 35%, with carbohydrate reduced to 12% when ethanol was substituted for 36% of the total calories. These diets became part of the standard paradigm for studying chronic alcohol effects in rats.[5] Research on the role of carbohydrate was not promoted because the initial description of the diet included the assertion, supported with data, that the control diet was "nutritionally adequate" and the further implication that therefore the isocaloric ethanol diet was also nutritionally adequate. Acceptance of this interpretation led to two unfortunate results: (1) there was little impetus to investigate correlations between ethanol and carbohydrate, and (2) lipogenesis data derived from studies comparing the effects of a low carbohydrate ethanol diet to a high carbohydrate control diet were interpreted as being the total result of the added ethanol, with the removal of carbohydrate being insignificant. This unfortunate approach has persisted in spite of other early work that recognized the importance of employing both high carbohydrate and high fat controls in alcohol studies to determine if ethanol is the sole cause of the effect.[30]

Recently, the importance of using both a glucogenic (isocaloric carbohydrate) and ketogenic (isocaloric triglyceride) control has been demonstrated, and the report includes data illustrating that the kind of carbohydrate used in the ethanol diet may also have a bearing on its effects on ethanol metabolism.[31] The study shows that the activities of lipogenic enzymes are primarily determined by the carbohydrate content of the diet, even though ethanol provides the bulk of the reducing equivalents and C-2 substrates for fatty acid synthesis. The levels of lipogenic enzymes in the ethanol-fed rats are essentially the same as those in the isocaloric fat controls; i.e., there is no difference between animals receiving the same carbohydrate in the diet, even when the dietary fat content is as high as 70%. In these studies, the ethanol-fed animals were in a lipolytic state with the standard Lieber-DeCarli proportion of carbohydrate (12% in the

ethanol diet). The morphology of the livers showed the expected fat infiltration, even though the feeding period was only 18 d. However, using
an ethanol diet with 35% carbohydrate, enzyme activities were increased
to a lipogenic level and only minimal lipid accumulated in the liver. These
studies illustrate the importance of using different supporting carbohydrate
concentrations in ethanol diets and using both glucogenic and ketogenic
isocaloric substitutes in control diets in order to distinguish ethanol effects
from carbohydrate effects.

In a study by Savolainen et al.,[32] the effect of dietary carbohydrate
content on the utilization of substrates produced from ethanol oxidation
for fatty acid synthesis was directly demonstrated by measuring triglyceride
content in livers from rats on low-fat/high-carbohydrate base diets containing an additional 36% ethanol as calories (experimental) or 36% carbohydrate (control). In one comparison, in which the control contained
77% carbohydrate and the experimental 41% plus 36% ethanol, the triglyceride content of the ethanol rat livers was nearly twice that of the
control. In another, in which the fat was doubled but the carbohydrate still
high enough to maintain a lipogenic state, the same approximately twofold
increase in triglycerides was found. Thus, with sufficient lipogenic enzymes, a substantial amount of the ethanol oxidation products can be
converted to fatty acids.

In a study limited to the pentose phosphate portion of the inducible
lipogenic enzymes a similar reduction of glucose-6-phosphate dehydrogenase activity was observed when carbohydrate was replaced by ethanol.[33]
In this study, an associated increase occurred in the activity of a microsomal
MFO (for the oxidation of 7-ethoxycoumarin) which was used to measure
dehydrogenase activity *in situ*. The increase of MFO activity by carbohydrate removal is discussed later with carbohydrate effects on MEOS.

Finally, diet-induced reductions of lipogenic enzyme activities similar
to those found in liver have been reported for adipose.[34] Unfortunately,
only the high carbohydrate pair-fed control diet was used in this study and
the reduction was interpreted as being a direct effect of ethanol addition
rather than of carbohydrate removal, even though carbohydrate is known
as the lipogenic signal in adipose just as it is in liver. However, a subsequent
study from the same laboratory did show that the changes in lipogenic
enzyme activity were also reflected in an *in vitro* assay system for fatty
acid synthesis from various precursors including acetate.[35] These studies,
in conjunction with those summarized above concerning transadipic

measurement of acetate concentrations in humans[25] and those using induction of different metabolic states with high and low carbohydrate diets in humans,[17] might provide a new paradigm for comparing the rat and human models while exploring the roles of carbohydrate in ethanol metabolism.

OTHER CARBOHYDRATE AND ETHANOL INTERACTIONS

Two other aspects of the role of carbohydrate in ethanol metabolism are worth noting. One is the effect of limited carbohydrate on induction of a variety of MFOs of the endoplasmic reticulum. The other is the implication of a carbohydrate influence on alcohol consumption in a genetically determined alcohol-preferring strain of rat.

MICROSOMAL ETHANOL OXIDIZING SYSTEM

The function and importance of the microsomal cytochrome P-450 system and associated MFOs has been recently reviewed.[4] In addition to its potential importance in ethanol metabolism, changes in the metabolism of a variety of drugs and other organic compounds have been associated with the proliferation of MEOS brought on by chronic ethanol ingestion. However, substantial evidence exists that carbohydrate plays a significant although differential role in the activities of the MFOs of the cytochrome P-450 system.

The relationship between rat liver activities of MFOs and diet was investigated.[36] It was demonstrated that chronic (3-week) feeding of various combinations of carbohydrate in diets with or without ethanol produces activities of MFOs that are a function of both carbohydrate content and ethanol in the diets with a negative correlation to carbohydrate. The greatest increase in activity was always with the diet having combined ethanol and lower carbohydrate. That combination led both to increased activities of the MFOs tested and to an increase in the actual amount of the cytochrome P-450 system in the liver. The study concluded that a significant effect in MEOS proliferation in chronic alcohol studies with the Lieber-DeCarli diet is due to the low-carbohydrate content of the ethanol diet.

In a second, more complete report[37] two aspects of the effects of carbohydrate on the cytochrome P-450 system were described. The result of chronic low carbohydrate exposure, described above, was coupled to an immediate effect of carbohydrate deprivation. This immediate effect could be elicited simply by a single day of feeding the low-carbohydrate diet. Thus, it was separate from any microsomal proliferation that would have required the extended feeding regimen used in the chronic alcohol studies. With respect to the longer term induction, it was found that the combined effect of chronic carbohydrate deprivation and ethanol ingestion was an inverse function of the amount of carbohydrate in the diet. In further studies with partially purified rat liver extracts, Sato et al.[38] determined a spectrum of effects of carbohydrate and ethanol on MFO activity for a variety of organic compounds oxidized by specific parts of the cytochrome P-450 system. As with their previous studies, both carbohydrate deprivation and ethanol were factors in developing the increased activity. For the activities reported, linkage apparently occurred between the carbohydrate and ethanol effects because the oxidation of a particular compound was either affected by both or neither of the dietary manipulations.

It is worth noting that the ethanol-inducible cytochrome P-450 fraction (P-450 IIE1) is also susceptible to dietary manipulation.[39] It is induced by fasting and by diabetes. It can also be induced in rats using an ''obesity-producing energy-dense diet'' that contains 60% fat and 3.55% sucrose. Thus, the role of carbohydrate in modifying the proliferation of the MEOS system is broadened to include other pathologic metabolic states such as increased effects of toxins.

CARBOHYDRATE METABOLISM IN
ALCOHOL-PREFERRING RATS

In a series of studies, Forsander et al.[40-42] examined dietary influences on intermediary metabolism in alko alcohol (AA) and alko nonalcohol (ANA) strains of rats. The first series of experiments, acute studies, showed that while both strains produce glucose via gluconeogenesis at the same rate under control conditions, AA rats have higher gluconeogenic rates in the presence of ethanol and the ANA rats do not. Further calculations showed that in the presence of ethanol all glucose produced by AA rats was through gluconeogenesis whereas half had to come from glycogenolysis in the ANA rats. In the second series, AA rats were given access to three macronutrients, carbohydrate, protein, and fat. During the first phase of the experiment, the rats selected an appropriate balance between the three nutrients. In the second phase, when alcohol was added as a fourth nutrient choice, they maintained about the same caloric intake by increasing the proportion of calories from alcohol and selectively reducing the calories obtained from carbohydrate. There was individual variation to the adaptation to ethanol consumption, which suggested a more complex set of determinants than a simple trade off between ethanol and carbohydrate. A relationship was established between ethanol consumption and the proportion of protein to carbohydrate calories (P/C ratio) such that selection of ethanol increased but with a diminishing rate as the P/C ratio changed from 5/85 to 40/50. In a second set of experiments, both AA and ANA rats were pretreated, with the diets differing in P/C ratio. They were then challenged with an acute dose of ethanol. The rate of ethanol elimination increased with increasing P/C for the AA rats. The rate of ethanol elimination by the ANA rats was much lower and was only slightly and non-significantly increased by increasing the P/C ratio in the diets. Finally, in the third series of experiments, the high-protein diet and a methylene blue diet, used to relieve the high $NADH/NAD^+$ caused by ethanol oxidation, were compared to a normal rat chow diet. Under these conditions, it was demonstrated that not only can the AA rats carry out effective gluconeogenesis, but with the high-protein diet they are able to maintain a higher blood glucose concentration than the ANA rats. It was suggested that this ability to maintain blood glucose through the gluconeogenic pathway is important in promoting the increased consumption of ethanol. Thus, again, and now at the genetic level, carbohydrate, and especially the metabolism of glucogenic intermediates, appears to be significant in ethanol metabolism.

SUMMARY AND CONCLUSION

The metabolic effects of ethanol are those of an uncontrolled nutrient taken to excess. The research reviewed shows that each role of normal carbohydrate metabolism adapts and provides some measure of added stability to the system while ethanol is being metabolized. The brunt of the work falls to gluconeogenesis because even glycogen metabolism is dependent on it during ethanol metabolism. Gluconeogenesis is also the connection between carbohydrate and glucogenic substrates in the protein and amino acid pools. That is what makes the AA strain of rat and the connection between gluconeogenesis and ethanol preference so interesting.

Fatty acid synthesis holds great potential for a permanent solution to excess ethanol oxidation products. However, it is only partially successful even when a lipogenic state is created with sufficient carbohydrate in the diet.

Finally, it was interesting to find that the effect of removal of carbohydrate went beyond its own pathways and helped ethanol promote the proliferation of the endoplasmic reticulum. Thus, there is a significant role of carbohydrate in the one effect ethanol seemed to cause by itself.

The roles of carbohydrate encompass the width and depth of intermediary metabolism. In a like manner, nearly complete permeation of this same metabolic network has been achieved by ethanol.[4] It is neither surprising that carbohydrate plays many roles in ethanol metabolism, nor that these carbohydrate roles are often not emphasized and are too often ignored. Ethanol naturally dominates the thinking in ethanol research. It should be kept in mind, therefore, that presentation of this subject has required the review of published reports whose purpose was to describe the effects of ethanol, not carbohydrate. This necessity forced a substantial degree of selection in the papers cited as well as a redirection of some of the emphasis placed on data within a report. As a total picture, the studies reviewed provide convincing evidence of the intimate and important role of carbohydrate in ethanol metabolism.

REFERENCES

1. Sneyd, J. G. T., Interactions of ethanol and carbohydrate metabolism, in *Human Metabolism of Alcohol*, Vol. 3, Crow, K. E. and Batt, R. D., Eds., CRC Press, Boca Raton, FL, 1989, chap. 8.
2. Kondrup, J., Grunnet, N., and Dich, J., Interactions of ethanol and lipid metabolism, in *Human Metabolism of Alcohol*, Vol. 3, Crow, K. E. and Batt, R. D., Eds., CRC Press, Boca Raton, FL, 1989, chap. 7.
3. Lieber, C. S., Mechanism of ethanol induced hepatic injury, *Pharmacol. Ther.*, 46, 1, 1990.
4. Lieber, C. S., Hepatic, metabolic and toxic effects of ethanol: 1991 update, *Alcohol. Clin. Exp. Res.*, 15, 573, 1991.
5. Lieber, C. S., DeCarli, L. M., and Sorrell, M. F., Experimental methods of ethanol administration, *Hepatology*, 10, 437, 1989.
6. Lieber, C. S. and DeCarli, L. M., The feeding of alcohol in liquid diets: two decades of applications and 1982 update, *Alcohol. Clin. Exp. Res.*, 6, 523, 1982.
7. Lieber, C. S. and DeCarli, L. M., Hepatic microsomal ethanol-oxidizing system: *in vitro* characteristics and adaptive properties *in vivo*, *J. Biol. Chem.*, 245, 2505, 1970.
8. Gibson, D. M., Lyons, R. T., and Scott, D. F., Synthesis and degradation of the lipogenic enzymes of rat liver, *Adv. Enzyme Regul.*, 10, 187, 1972.

9. Gimenez, M. S. and Johnson, B. C., Pair-feeding in the dietary control of glucose 6-phosphate dehydrogenase, *J. Nutr.*, 111, 260, 1981.

10. Mariash, C. N. and Oppenheimer, J. H., Stimulation of malic enzyme formation in hepatocyte culture by metabolites: evidence favoring a non-glycolytic metabolite as the proximate induction signal, *Metabolism*, 33, 545, 1983.

11. Freinkel, N., Cohen, A. K., Arky, R. A., and Foster, A. E., Ethanol hypoglycemia. II. A postulated mechanism of action based on experiments with rat liver slices, *J. Clin. Endocrinol.*, 25, 76, 1965.

12. Krebs, H. A., Freedland, R. A., Hems, R., and Stubbs, M., Inhibition of hepatic gluconeogenesis by ethanol, *Biochem. J.*, 112, 117, 1969.

13. Topping, D. L., Clark, D. G., Illman, R. J., and Trimble, R. P., Inhibition by insulin of ethanol-induced hyperglycaemia in perfused livers from fed rats, *Horm. Metab. Res.*, 14, 361, 1982.

14. Topping, D. L., Clark, D. G., Storer, G. B., Trimble, R. P., and Illman, R. J., Acute effects of ethanol on the perfused rat liver, *Biochem. J.*, 184, 97, 1979.

15. Erwin, G. V. and Towell, J. F., Ethanol-induced hyperglycaemia mediated by the central nervous system, *Pharmacol. Biochem. Behav.*, 18, 559, 1983.

16. Singh, S. P. and Snyder, A. K., Interrelation between the effects of ethanol and thyroid hormones on gluconeogenesis from alanine in perfused rat liver, *J. Lab. Clin. Med.*, 99, 746, 1982.

17. Mascord, D., Rogers, J., Smith, J., Starmer, G. A., and Whitfield, J. B., Effect of diet on [lactate/cb/[pyruvate] ratios during alcohol metabolism in man, *Alcohol Alcohol.*, 24, 189, 1989.

18. Rifkin, R. M., Todd, W. W., Toothaker, D. R., Sussman, A., Trowbridge, M., and Draznin, B., Effects of *in vivo* and *in vitro* alcohol administration on insulin binding and glycogenesis in isolated rat hepatocytes, *Ann. Nutr. Metab.*, 27, 313, 1983.

19. Cook, E. B., Preece, J. A., Tobin, S. D. M., Sugden, M. C., Cox, D. J., and Palmer, T. N., Acute inhibition by ethanol of intestinal absorption of glucose and hepatic glycogen synthesis on glucose refeeding after starvation in the rat, *Biochem. J.*, 254, 59, 1988.

20. Sprandel, U., Troger, H.-D., Liebhardt, E. W., and Zollner, N., Acceleration of ethanol elimination with fructose in man, *Nutr. Metab.*, 24, 324, 1980.

21. Crownover, B. P., La Dine, J., Bradford, B., Glassman, E., Forman, D., Schneider, H., and Thruman, R. G., Activation of ethanol metabolism in humans by fructose: importance of experimental design, *J. Pharm. Exp. Ther.*, 236, 574, 1986.

22. Cornell, N. W. and Veech, R. L., Effect of fructose on ethanol metabolism by isolated hepatocytes, *Biochem. Soc. Trans.*, 8, 525, 1980.

23. Crow, K. E., Newland, K. M., and Batt, R. D., Factors influencing rates of ethanol oxidation in isolated rat hepatocytes, *Pharmacol. Biochem. Behav.*, 18, 237, 1983.

24. Yki-Järvinen, H., Koivisto, V. A., Ylikahri, R., and Taskinen, M., Acute effects of ethanol and acetate on glucose kinetics in normal subjects, *Am. Physiol. Soc.*, E175, 1988.

25. Frayn, K. N., Coppack, S. W., Walsh, P. E., Butterworth, H. C., Humphreys, S. M., and Pedrosa, H. C., Metabolic responses of forearm and adipose tissues to acute ethanol ingestion, *Metabolism,* 39, 958, 1990.

26. Lefevre, A., Adler, H., and Lieber, C. S., Effect of ethanol on ketone metabolism, *J. Clin. Invest.,* 49, 1775, 1970.

27. Lieber, C. S. and Spritz, N., Effects of prolonged ethanol intake in man: role of dietary, adipose, and endogenously synthesized fatty acids in the pathogenesis of the alcoholic fatty liver, *J. Clin. Invest.,* 45, 1400, 1966.

28. Lieber, C. S., Spritz, N., and DeCarli, L. M., Role of dietary, adipose, and endogenously synthesized fatty acids in the pathogenesis of the alcoholic fatty liver, *J. Clin. Invest.,* 45, 51, 1966.

29. DeCarli, L. M. and Lieber, C. S., Fatty liver in the rat after prolonged intake of ethanol with a nutritionally adequate new liquid diet, *J. Nutr.,* 91, 331, 1967.

30. Lieber, C. S., Jones, D. P., and DeCarli, L. M., Effects of prolonged ethanol uptake: production of fatty liver despite adequate diets, *J. Clin. Invest.,* 44, 1009, 1965.

31. Guthrie, G. D., Myers, K. J., Gesser, E. J., White, G. W., and Koehl, J. R., Alcohol as a nutrient: interactions between ethanol and carbohydrate, *Alcohol. Clin. Exp. Res.,* 14, 17, 1990.

32. Savolainen, M. J., Hiltunen, J. K., and Hassinen, I. E., Effect of prolonged ethanol ingestion on hepatic lipogenesis and related enzyme activities, *Biochem. J.,* 164, 169, 1977.

33. Reinke, L. A., Tupper, J. S., Smith, P. R., and Sweeny, D. J., Diminished pentose cycle flux in perfused livers of ethanol-fed rats, *Mol. Pharmacol.,* 31, 631, 1987.

34. Wilson, J. S., Korsten, M. A., Colley, P. W., and Pirola, R. C., Decrease in lipogenesis and glucose oxidation of rat adipose tissue after chronic ethanol feeding, *Biochem. Pharmacol.,* 35, 2025, 1986.

35. Wilson, J. S., Korsten, M. A., Donnelly, L. P., Colley, P. W. et al., Chronic ethanol administration depresses fatty acid synthesis in rat adipose tissue, *Biochem. J.,* 251, 547, 1988.

36. Sato, A., Nakajima, T., and Koyama, Y., Interaction between ethanol and carbohydrate on the metabolism in rat liver of aromatic and chlorinated hydrocarbons, *Toxicol. Appl. Pharmacol.,* 68, 242, 1983.

37. Sato, A. and Nakajima, T., Dietary carbohydrate- and ethanol-induced alteration of the metabolism and toxicity of chemical substances, *Nutr. Cancer,* 6, 121, 1984.

38. Sato, A., Yonekura, I., Asakawa, M., Nakahara, H., Nakajima, T., Ohta, S., and Ito, N., Augmentation of ethanol-induced enhancement of dimethylnitrosamine and diethylnitrosamine metabolism by lowered carbohydrate intake, *Jpn. J. Cancer Res.,* 77, 125, 1986.

39. Raucy, J. L., Lasker, J. M., Kraner, J. C., Salazar, D. E., Lieber, C. S., and Corcoran, G. B., Induction of cytochrome P450IIE1 in the obese overfed rat, *Mol. Pharmacol.,* 39, 275, 1990.

40. Forsander, O. A. and Poso, A. R., Hepatic carbohydrate metabolism in rats bred for alcohol preference, *Biochem. Pharmacol.,* 37, 2209, 1988.

41. Forsander, O. A. and Sinclair, J. D., Protein, carbohydrate, and ethanol consumption: interactions in AA and ANA rats, *Alcohol,* 5, 233, 1988.
42. Poso, A. R. and Forsander, O. A., Dietary regulation of voluntary alcohol consumption in rats. Influence of a high protein diet and a methylene blue diet, *Biochem. Pharmacol.,* 40, 1295, 1990.

7 Protein Metabolism in Alcoholism

INTRODUCTION

This chapter is primarily concerned with the ways in which protein synthesis and protein degradation in the different types of muscle (skeletal, cardiac, and intestinal smooth) and bone are affected by alcohol. Musculoskeletal tissues have been especially selected for examination because comparatively very little attention has been paid to the ways in which they respond to ethanol toxicity, even though alcoholic muscle and bone disease are far more common than cirrhosis. The reason for this is probably self-explanatory; although cirrhosis frequently leads to death, skeletal and intestinal myopathies and osteopathies are not acutely life threatening. Nevertheless, it is important to note that a large percentage of alcoholics die because of cardiovascular disease and myocardial damage may represent one end of the spectrum of a disease process in which all types of muscle are affected. Persistent skeletal muscle weakness and osteopathy may also contribute to the impaired life qualities of alcoholics. Furthermore, the tissues we have chosen to examine in this chapter may be used to illustrate how basic processes, inherent in the regulation of organ protein content, are measured and controlled. In addition, the gastrointestinal (GI) tract, muscle, and bone are major contributors to whole-body protein synthesis and together account for at least half of the whole-body value. Changes in any one of these tissues may, therefore, have important physiological implications. This chapter recognizes the central role of the liver in nutritional metabolism. Ethanol-induced changes in hepatic protein synthesis are therefore described, although briefly. Attention is drawn to changes in liver protein turnover relative to the effects of ethanol on other tissues.

It is difficult to define precisely what ''protein metabolism'' encompasses: on the one hand, it is the supply and compartmentalizing of amino acids for subsequent assembly into polypeptides. On the other, protein

ISBN 0-8493-7933-4

metabolism may include the oxidation of amino acids proceeding from the degradation of endogenous tissue proteins. Each of these processes are themselves specialist areas of protein metabolism that have their own homeostatic control mechanisms; they may merit in-depth coverage, but space precludes this option. We have resolved this dilemma by embracing a chapter that is principally concerned with "protein turnover". Its core centers on protein synthesis and protein degradation. At the periphery are the ways in which these processes might be controlled (i.e., by the amount of tissue RNA) or measured (i.e., by incorporation of labeled amino acids, or release of suitable markers of protein degradation). For the sake of brevity the sections pertaining to methodology are exemplified by those techniques that have been used in alcohol toxicity studies.

Most of the work cited is derived from laboratory animal studies, largely because very little reliable information has been obtained from man. This is primarily because a principal determinant of protein turnover is nutritional intake[1,2] and in many situations this has not been adequately controlled or accounted for. Additionally, technical problems exist in routinely measuring protein turnover in man. Animal studies are much more conducive for controlling nutritional variables and protein synthesis can be accurately determined in a large number of animals (especially with the flooding dose technique, described below). Nevertheless, clinical studies have been cited where applicable.

PROTEIN TURNOVER

Protein metabolism can be divided into two components, protein synthesis and protein breakdown. Both are integrally combined in protein turnover, which is defined as the process whereby proteins are continually being synthesized and degraded. The amount of tissue protein at a particular point in time is dependent upon the balance between their respective rates. It follows, therefore, that the rate of protein synthesis will equal the rate of protein degradation only in the steady state, i.e., when the tissue protein content is unaltered. An example of this steady state would be the adult individual or animal in which the tissue protein content is generally considered to be constant.[1] In anabolic phases, such as during growth or cardiac hypertrophy, the synthesis rate will exceed the rate of protein degradation.[3,4] In catabolic phases, in contrast, the degradation rate will exceed the rate of protein synthesis. The latter situation can occur in metabolic stresses, such as those imposed by acute injury and infection[2,5] or chronic metabolic disturbances, such as those occurring in malnutrition and cancer cachexia.[6] More pertinent disease states characterized by reductions in tissue protein content occur in response to alcoholism. This includes alcoholic myopathy,[7] osteopathy,[8] and intestinal atrophy.[9]

It is a common misunderstanding that reductions in tissue protein content occur solely via a fall in the rate of protein synthesis. Reductions in protein content may also arise as a consequence of:

1. Increases in both protein synthesis and protein breakdown, in which the increase in protein breakdown is greater than the increase in protein synthesis.
2. An increase in the rate of protein breakdown, without alterations in protein synthesis.
3. A decrease in the rate of protein synthesis, without alterations in protein breakdown.
4. A decrease in both protein synthesis and breakdown, but the decrease in protein synthesis is disproportionately greater than the decrease in protein breakdown.

From the above, it is evident that both synthetic and degradative processes should be measured in any investigative study into the regulatory mechanisms responsible for changes in tissue protein mass. However, the *in vivo* estimation of rates of protein degradation is not always reliable, as illustrated below.

PROTEIN METABOLISM *IN VIVO* AND *IN VITRO*

A variety of studies investigating the alterations in protein metabolism by alcohol have been carried out in isolated systems *in vitro*. These include the use of perfused organs such as the heart,[10] tissue slices,[11] or isolated cells such as hepatocytes[12] or HeLa cells.[13] While these *in vitro* studies are useful for dissecting biochemical events or metabolic pathways, it is important to emphasize that the results derived from these experiments must eventually be translated into events and mechanisms that occur *in vivo*, i.e., in the intact animal or the whole person. Protein synthetic rates in tissue preparation *in vitro* may be considerably lower than *in vivo* rates. These low protein synthesis rates may arise because of impaired nutrient supply, disruption of membranes and subcellular organelles, or even due to the absence of humoral factors that may be essential for overall signal processing. During the 1980s, considerable awareness has grown of the need to consider the metabolic viability or state of isolated preparations *in vitro*. Perturbed integrity may be reflected by alterations in the rate of protein synthesis.[14] Nevertheless, recent studies have shown that perfused skeletal and cardiac muscle *in vitro* are able to synthesize protein at a rate similar to that occurring *in vivo*.[15-18] These systems, therefore, offer potentially useful methods for investigating the metabolic regulation of protein metabolism in acute and chronic states of alcohol myotoxicity. However, a major cautionary note is required, as the composition of the extracellular medium may determine the qualitative results.[16] For these reasons the authors have decided to focus their attention toward *in vivo* observations. Unfortunately, the measurement of protein synthesis in the intact organism is technically more demanding than studies *in vitro*. This is illustrated by the fact that labeled phenylalanine can be used to measure protein synthesis in isolated muscles, as this amino acid is not metabolized by this tissue (other than its incorporation into protein). All the radioactivity in the muscle protein at the completion of the study occurs exclusively in phenylalanine.[19] *In vivo*, however, a substantial proportion of the phenylalanine is converted to tyrosine, largely in the liver, and the radioactivity in the muscle protein is derived from both phenylalanine and tyrosine.[20] Therefore, techniques must be applied to the extraction and subsequent isolation of phenylalanine in muscle hydrolysates. Similar problems occur *in vivo* with other amino acids.[1]

MEASUREMENT OF PROTEIN SYNTHESIS

Reliable rates of protein synthesis can be obtained providing the time course changes of the precursor and the product are accurately characterized and defined.[1] In practical terms, this entails measuring the specific radioactivity of the labeled amino at the site of protein synthesis, namely the aminoacyl tRNA (i.e., the precursor) and the labeled amino acid in the tissue protein (i.e., the product). In general, measurements of protein synthesis in man are usually undertaken with stable isotopes, while in laboratory animals radiolabeled compounds are used.[1,2]

One must consider that the routine measurements of aminoacyl tRNA-specific radioactivities are encumbered with numerous practical difficulties. These relate to the fact that tissue tRNA comprises only a small proportion of total RNA species and the aminoacyl tRNA is extremely labile and may even be compartmentalized.[21,22] To resolve this the specific radioactivity of the free amino acid in the intra- or extracellular compartments are usually measured and taken to represent the aminoacyl tRNA.[1] These are usually determined by appropriate assays on acid-soluble phases of tissue homogenates and plasma, respectively.[1] In human studies using stable isotopic infusions of ^{13}C-labeled leucine, the enrichment of [13]C α-ketoisocaproic acid is considered to be representative of the precursor pool.[23] The specific radioactivity of the amino acid in the tissue protein also needs to be isolated and assayed. Many protein turnover studies have measured the amount of radioactivity per unit protein at the end of the experiment, however, as mentioned above, the *in vivo* administration of labeled amino acids is complicated because the label may be transferred to other compounds and amino acids, for example, glycine to serine.[20,24] Another added complication is the fact that in catabolic states, individual or groups of tissue proteins, each with their own amino acid profiles, may be preferentially affected, i.e., a selective loss of nonstromal proteins.[25] Thus, the amount of radioactivity per unit protein will represent not only the transfer of isotope from one amino acid to another, but also changes in the amino acid profile of the tissue protein. To resolve this, it is essential that tissue proteins are hydrolyzed to their constituent amino acids, and the labeled amino acid extracted by suitable procedures. In the case of stable isotopes this may include application of gas chromatography (GC) and isotopic mass spectroscopy (MS).[26] For radiolabeled isotopes a variety of methods have been employed, including column chromatography, split-stream splitting, and scintillation spectroscopy,[27] or by enzymatic isolation followed by fluorimetry and scintillation spectroscopy.[28]

ADMINISTRATION OF THE LABELED AMINO ACID

Methods for administering the labeled amino acid to determine the rate of tissue protein synthesis *in vivo* have been extensively reviewed by Waterlow et al.[1] and Garlick.[29] In some alcohol studies, rates of protein synthesis have been measured after the administration of a single injection of a tracer amount of labeled amino acid, but the reservations inherent in these methods were described previously.[1,29] More suitable methods are by (1) the constant infusion of a tracer amount of isotope and (2) by the pulse injection of a large flooding dose of isotope.[1,29,30] The utilization of both these methods provides relatively accurate rates of protein synthesis;[1,29,30] however, quite recently controversy has arisen over which is the more suitable of the two. The constant infusion method involves administration of the isotope over a protracted period of time, i.e., about 3 to 6 h in laboratory rats.[1,29,30] Concomitant immobilization, cessation of food intake (to achieve a "steady state"), or withdrawal of alcohol feeding and surgical manipulations, including cannulation, may also occur. Some of these factors themselves may modify tissue protein synthesis.[31,32] In contrast, the measurement of protein synthesis by the flooding dose technique does not require any of these procedures, as measurements are made over acute periods, i.e., in as little as 10 min.[28] Rats are intravenously (i.v.) injected with 150 mmol/l of either L-[4-^{3}H]- or L-[U-^{14}C]phenylalanine at a dose of 1 ml/100 g body weight. Immediately following the administration of the isotope, animals are returned to their cages and have continued (albeit for an acute period) access to food or ethanol.[28] Some adaptations have been devised for the administration of the isotope via the intraperitoneal (i.p.) route.[33,34] However, the authors showed that for the GI tract, ethanol represses the transfer of [^{3}H]phenylalanine from the extracellular to the intracellular compartments, although the errors involved in calculating k_s were small.[35] In the flooding dose technique, fractional rates of protein synthesis, i.e., the percentage of tissue protein renewed each day (k_s, %/day) are calculated from the formula:[28]

$$k_s = \frac{S_B \times 100}{(S_i \text{ or } S_p) \times t} \%/d \tag{1}$$

where S_i is tissue-free phenylalanine-specific radioactivity, S_p is plasma-free phenylalanine-specific radioactivity, S_B is protein-bound phenylalanine-specific radioactivity (after hydrolysis), and t is the radiolabeling period (the time between injection of the isotope and immersion of the tissue in iced water or liquid nitrogen, in days).[28] For hepatic protein turnover measurements the protein-bound phenylalanine-specific radioactivities reflect labeling of both structural and cytoplasmic proteins as well as those proteins that are destined for subsequent secretion, i.e., albumin. Most of the labeled export proteins are secreted after 15 to 30 min.[36] In constant infusion studies the values of k_s largely reflect the structural and nonexportable proteins.[1,29,30] A flooding dose method has been devised for human studies,[37] but this has not yet been applied to the investigation of alcohol toxicity.

Three criticisms have been made of the flooding dose technique that necessitate close scrutiny. The first pertains to the possibility that the amino acid used to measure protein synthesis may alter protein synthesis per se. Originally, studies used a flooding dose of leucine,[27] which has been implicated as having an important regulatory role in muscle protein synthesis.[38] However, the amino acid currently used to measure protein synthesis, i.e., phenylalanine, does not appear to be of primary importance in altering tissue protein synthesis *in vivo*.[28] Nonetheless, rates of protein synthesis using the flooding dose technique are apparently higher than those obtained by the constant infusion technique in comparable animals.[30] This may partly be due to the fact that the immobilization procedure may perturb protein synthesis,[39] or that during immobilization animals do not have access to food, which may possibly elicit a starvation-induced reduction in protein synthesis.[40] It is also possible that during acute labeling periods proteins with short half-lives are preferentially labeled.[30,41]

The second point relates to the recent argument by Samarel,[42] who suggested that in cardiac tissue at least, a brief delay may occur in aminoacyl tRNA equilibration after a flooding dose of amino acid (leucine and proline). Theoretically, this deficiency in aminoacyl labeling will produce a lag in the incorporation of the isotope into the tissue protein. More importantly, this may seriously underestimate the rate of tissue protein synthesis if the lag period is a significant proportion of the total labeling period. However, this can be tentatively refuted as we now have evidence that in glycolytic muscle *in vivo* no such delay occurs with phenylalanine. For example, in young rats muscle protein-bound phenylalanine-specific radioactivities (i.e., S_B) at t = 2.7 min, were 0.044 ± 0.002 dpm/nmol. At t = 10.7 min, S_B was 0.184 ± 0.010, which indicates almost linear incorporation after injection of the isotope.[43] Similar results with a flooding dose of labeled phenylalanine have been obtained for oxidative skeletal muscles[44] and virtually all the regions of the GI tract.[45]

The third point of contention pertains to the possibility that the high concentration of phenylalanine may alter other aspects of tissue or whole-body metabolism. In this regard, a comprehensive evaluation has recently been made into the outcome of injecting a large dose of phenylalanine i.v.[46] Plasma sodium (Na) and calcium (Ca) were slightly reduced (by 2 to 7%) 10 min after the i.v. injection, but no effects were observed on plasma potassium (K) or phosphate concentrations.[46] Creatine kinase activities were, however, significantly increased by phenylalanine injection (by 39%), but the activities of alkaline phosphatase and alanine amino-transferase were unaltered.[46] The plasma concentrations of triglycerides, urea, creatinine, total protein, albumin, cholesterol, and glucose were also unchanged.[46] This implies that some metabolic perturbations may have occurred in membrane structure or function, as reflected by enhanced creatine kinase release, but the significance of these observations is not known, largely because we do not unequivocally know the origins of the increased creatine kinase activities (though it probably reflects skeletal muscle) nor whether it was due to the injection process rather than the phenylalanine per se.[46] Nevertheless, the prevalent experimental evidence favors the contention that after 10 min the high concentration of phenyl-alanine (150 μmol/100 g body weight) does not overtly alter plasma an-alytes or hormones such as insulin and glucagon,[47] which alter protein synthesis.[40,47-49] Thus, the flooding dose technique with phenylalanine appears to be eminently suitable for investigating the effects of ethanol on protein synthesis.

MEASUREMENT OF PROTEIN DEGRADATION

No reliable methods are available for directly measuring the rate of protein breakdown *in vivo* in the absence of invasive procedures. Methods based on monitoring the rate of decay of prelabeled protein are invariably subject to problems due to the reincorporation of the label and complex kinetics of decay.[1,29,30] The application of these methods is also limited; for example, acute changes are usually difficult to measure. This subject is reviewed in greater depth by Waterlow et al.[1] Nevertheless, indirect methods exist for estimating degradation rates. Three relatively accurate methods have been used for estimating rates of protein degradation *in vivo* in many clinical and experimental situations. These have also been applied to alcohol studies, and are exemplified in the following.

Excretion of Urinary Markers

This includes the excretion of 3-methylhistidine, which is formed by post-translational modification of histidine,[50] and is found in the acto-myosin fraction of skeletal muscle.[51,52] In man and laboratory rats it is neither reincorporated into tissue protein nor metabolized, but is quanti-tatively excreted in the urine.[50-53] As skeletal muscle contains substantial amounts of 3-methylhistidine, urinary concentrations have been used as an index of muscle protein degradation.[53,54] The validity of these mea-surements has been disputed by Millward and colleagues[55] because protein-

TABLE 1
Protein Synthesis in Different Tissues of the
Rat[28,32,56,57]

	k_s (%/d)	
	Young male rats (100 g)	Mature female rats (220 g)
Skeletal muscle	17	5
Brain	ND	12
Heart	20	9
Lung	33	22
Spleen	68	38
Liver	86	81
Small intestine	119	76
Skin	64	ND
Bone	90	21
Uterus	ND	34
Kidney	ND	35

Note: Fractional rates of protein synthesis (k_s) were measured in fed rats with a large flooding dose of [^{3}H]phenylalanine. Data compiled from References 28, 32, 56, and 57. ND, not determined. Skeletal muscle and bone are represented by the gastrocnemius muscle and tibia, respectively. The small intestine pertains to whole segments (mucosa and seromuscular layers combined) of duodenum plus jejunum (young rats) or the entire small bowel (mature rats). Skin protein synthesis was measured in the protein fraction that was soluble in 0.3 mol/l Na hydroxide.

bound 3-methylhistidine is also found in other organs, such as the GI tract, skin, and heart. Even though the amounts of 3-methylhistidine in these tissues are low, methodological problems arise because the fractional rates of protein turnover in skin and the GI tract are high[32,56-58] (also see Table 1). Despite these reservations the measurement of urinary 3-methylhistidine still provides useful data on whole-body metabolism. Theoretically, if the amount of urinary 3-methylhistidine and creatinine from nonskeletal muscle sources is known, then changes attributable to skeletal muscle per se can also be computed. This is the basis of the "Afting correction" and is derived from the known concentrations of 3-methylhistidine and creatinine in the urine of a patient with neither micro- nor macroscopically detectable skeletal muscle tissue.[59]

Urinary hydroxyproline has also been used to monitor collagen breakdown and has traditionally been used to investigate bone protein metabolism. Collagen is perhaps the most common protein in the mammalian body, and therefore the criticisms applied to the measurement of urinary 3-methylhistidine may similarly be applied to hydroxyproline excretion. Although hydroxyproline comprises approximately one tenth of total collagen residues it is also found in elastin and complement and, in addition, urinary concentrations may reflect changes in skin, liver, and muscle collagens.[1,60] Furthermore, a relatively large proportion of hydroxyproline is oxidized before its urinary excretion.[1,60] Other suitable urinary markers for assessing collagen breakdown exist, namely the pyridinium cross-links deoxypyridinoline (hydroxylysyl pyridinoline) and pyridinoline (lysyl pyridinoline).[60] These markers are thought to be specific for types I, II, and IX collagens of cartilage and bone[60] and can be routinely assayed by high performance liquid chromatography (HPLC).[61]

Indirect Methods as Applied to the Whole-Body and Individual Tissues

One method is based on the fact that the fractional rate of growth is dependent upon the difference between the fractional rate of protein synthesis and the fractional rate of protein degradation:

$$k_g = k_s - k_d \qquad (2)$$

where k_g, k_s, and k_d are the fractional rates of growth, synthesis, and degradation, respectively.[1,3] By measuring the rates of protein synthesis and growth, the rate of protein degradation is easily calculated. The reliability of the method is largely dependent upon the accuracy of the protein synthetic data, but other complicating factors have been reviewed by Preedy and Peters.[62] An alternative method for measuring rates of whole-body breakdown is based on constant infusion methodology, using the formula:

$$Q = I + B = E + Z \qquad (3)$$

where Q is the flux, I is the intake of the amino acid from food, B is the amino acid derived from protein breakdown, E is the amount of oxidized and excreted amino acid, and Z is the amino acid synthesized to protein.[1,2] Fasting patients overnight reduces I to zero, so Q = B. If flux is accurately known from the dilution of the tracer, then B can be calculated.

Tissue Protease Activities

As tissue proteins are broken down by proteases (lysosomal and non-lysosomal) it follows that the activities of these enzymes may be convenient for assessing the impact of pathogenic treatments on degradative pathways.[63] In practice, they only provide an index of the potential or capacity for protein degradation. Nevertheless, studies by Goldspink and Lewis[63] showed a very good correlation between the *in vitro* release of tyrosine and the activities of muscle cathepsin D and B.

CONTRIBUTION OF TISSUES TO THE OVERALL RATE OF PROTEIN TURNOVER

In most mammalian species, including man and the laboratory rat, skeletal muscle contributes to approximately 40% of body mass.[1] This does not imply that skeletal muscle contributes to a large proportion of whole-body protein turnover, as the rate of skeletal muscle protein synthesis is low compared to almost all other tissues. This is illustrated by Table 1, which contains data on protein synthetic rates in almost all visceral and nonvisceral tissues of immature and mature rats.[28,32,56,57] As the mature animals exhibited negligible or very low growth rates (approximately 1%/d) it may be inferred that fractional synthesis rates are similar to the fractional degradation rates. Although there are scattered reports on synthesis rates in different tissues of man, the most comprehensive studies relate to those in laboratory animals.

In mature female rats the rates of protein synthesis in skeletal muscles, such as the plantaris and gastrocnemius, are approximately 4 to 5%/d.[32] In other more oxidative muscles, such as the diaphragm, soleus, and heart, the synthesis rates are slightly higher, i.e., 6 to 8%/d.[32] Rates of protein synthesis in hepatogastrointestinal tissues are even higher still (approximately 50 to 80%/d).[32] Similar relationships between the k_s values in different tissues occur in rapidly growing young immature rats, in which synthesis rates are generally much higher than in slowly growing mature rats.[28,56,57] In addition, rates of protein synthesis in skeletal tissue (as represented by the tibia) are extraordinarily high (i.e., 90%/d).[56] The estimated contributions of individual tissues to protein synthesis in the whole-body can be calculated from the product of the protein content and the synthesis rate. Skeletal muscle thus contributes to approximately 20% of whole-body rates of protein synthesis, and similar contributions are ascribed to the liver, GI tract, and combined skin and bone. However, it is important to note that within each tissue considerable heterogeneity exists in synthesis rates (see Tables 4 to 6, which contain data on GI tissues).

EXPERIMENTAL ETHANOL STUDIES AND NUTRITIONAL CONSIDERATIONS

A clear distinction must be made between acute and chronic ethanol studies, because in the latter adaptive changes may occur. In the authors' acute studies, animals are injected i.p. with a bolus of ethanol (1 ml/100 g body weight) at a dose of 75 mmol/kg body weight. The i.p. route of injection is preferred as we are also interested in the responses of the tissues in the proximal digestive tract: esophagus, stomach, and duodenum. We, therefore, needed to distinguish between the tissue necrosis caused by localized chemical effects and those attributable to pathophysiological levels of ethanol. Administration of i.p. dosages achieves high plasma levels of ethanol that are sustained for up to 4 h.[64] Although adequate, administration of acute intragastric doses of ethanol undoubtedly induces gross lower esophageal and gastric lesions and the plasma ethanol concentrations may decline more rapidly.[65] Animal studies have also been undertaken using the i.v. infusions of ethanol, but the technique may also cause hemolysis.[66]

For chronic ethanol studies in laboratory animals the best technique is clearly that based on the Lieber-DeCarli regime.[67] Very simply, this involves feeding a nutritionally adequate liquid diet, containing either ethanol or isocaloric glucose *ad libitum*. The ethanol content comprises approximately one third of total calories. It is possible that the stringency of the liquid diet might cause some localized effects (for example, to the esophagus and stomach), but the ethanol concentration is only approximately 5 to 6% (v/v).[68] Thus, in chronic studies, effects are due to the actions of ethanol, rather than nutritional limitation.[67,68]

In man we find considerable problems relating to the investigation of protein metabolism, as alcoholics may have impaired nutritional status.[69-71] This may occur as a result of socioeconomic lifestyles, anorexia induced by ethanol, the caloric displacement of foods containing important micronutrients, malabsorption due to a variety of causes, and by the altered metabolic utilization and retention of macro- or micronutrients.[69-72] In situations in which impaired nutritional status and anorexia causes tissue wasting, protein turnover is undoubtedly affected. Thus, it is essential that due consideration is given to these possible differences and when possible, carry out studies on protein metabolism in situations in which controls and alcoholic subjects have identical nutritional parameters.

The aim of achieving identical nutritional status leads to an important facet of experimental feeding studies; it is possible for control and ethanol-treated animals to be in contrasting nutritional states, i.e., either fed or starved. This is because ethanol-fed rats are incapable of consuming any more diet than the amount they drink *ad libitum*.[68] The glucose-fed control rats are potentially able to consume more diet, but the principles of the pair-feeding technique precludes them from doing so, i.e., they are partially malnourished and consume their daily food allowance in a few hours. Thus, after episodic engorgement of the diet, controls may be postabsorptive or starved for a significant part of the time.[73] Preedy and Peters have attempted to resolve this by carrying out protein synthesis measurements in alcohol studies when both controls and treated rats are in the fed state. This problem was discussed in greater depth previously.[73] Another way of resolving this difficulty is by investigating protein metabolism via 24-h urinary analysis.[74]

EFFECTS OF ETHANOL

SKELETAL MUSCLE

A common feature of chronic and excessive ethanol consumption is skeletal muscle myopathy, which is characterized by a selective reduction in the area of type II skeletal muscle fibers (anaerobic, glycolytic fast-twitch), while type I (aerobic, oxidative slow-twitch) fibers are only marginally affected, if at all.[75-77] This myopathy occurs in between one half to two thirds of all alcoholics,[77-80] and constitutes one of the most common, but least studied, of muscle diseases. For example, comprehensive textbooks on muscle diseases usually devote $<1\%$ of the text to alcohol muscle disease, and mainly to the acute form (rhabdomyolysis). In contrast, considerable attention is devoted to rarer muscle diseases, such as Duchenne muscle dystrophy.

Skeletal muscle biopsies from patients with alcoholic myopathy exhibit reduced protein contents,[7,76,77] implying they have a defect in protein synthesis and/or protein breakdown. Although much attention has focused on the proximal muscles, there are scattered reports implicating involvement of other muscle groups,[7] and data from urinary creatinine excretion suggest that affected patients may lose 20% or more of their entire muscle mass.[81]

TABLE 2
Whole-Body Leucine and Protein Metabolism in Chronic Alcoholics[82]

Skeletal Muscle Protein Synthesis

	Control	Alcoholic	% Change	p
Fractional rate (%/d)	1.10 ± 0.12	0.66 ± 0.09	−40	<0.001
Percent of whole-body synthesis	27 (range 23–36)	15 ± 2	−44	<0.001

Whole-Body Leucine Kinetics

	Control	Alcoholic	% Change	p
Breakdown (mmol/kg/d)	2.64 ± 0.19	2.32 ± 0.10	−12	NS
Oxidation (mmol/kg/d)	0.43 ± 0.02	0.34 ± 0.04	−21	<0.05
Synthesis (mmol/kg/d)	2.21 ± 0.17	1.98 ± 0.09	−10	NS
Plasma α-KIC (μmol/l)	34 ± 2	30 ± 4	−12	NS

Whole-Body Protein Kinetics

	Control	Alcoholic	% Change	p
Breakdown (g/d)	273 ± 28	255 ± 15	−7	NS
Synthesis (g/d)	226 ± 24	218 ± 12	−4	NS

Note: Whole-body and skeletal muscle protein metabolism was investigated in 6 fully ambulant alcoholics (4 males, 2 females; mean 45 years), and who had a daily alcoholic intake of 100 g or more for over 10 years. Comparisons were made with age- and sex-matched controls. α-KIC denotes α-ketoisocaproic acid. All data are mean ± SEM (n = 6). NS, $p > 0.05$, not significant.

Muscle protein synthesis measurements have been carried out in chronic alcoholics, with a primed constant infusion of L-[1-^{13}C]-leucine and NaH^{13}CO$_3$.[82] In these studies, protein synthesis was measured in the post-absorptive state (i.e., after overnight fasting) and after administration of the isotopic bolus, L[1-^{13}C]-leucine was infused for 8 h. Skeletal muscle biopsies were taken at 2 and 8 h postinjection of the priming dose.[82] The results of these studies (Table 2) showed that chronic alcoholics (>100 g/d, >10 years) had impaired rates of skeletal muscle protein synthesis; k_s was reduced by approximately 40%. The contribution of muscle protein synthesis to whole-body protein synthesis also fell from approximately 27 to 15%.[82]

The activities of neutral protease in skeletal muscle biopsies of control and myopathic alcoholics have been measured and found to be similar in both groups.[83] Whether neutral protease activity confers a relatively minor or major importance to the overall rate of muscle protein degradation is not known. Nevertheless, these observations were seemingly supported by data that showed that urinary 3-methylhistidine excretion was relatively unaltered in chronic alcoholics with skeletal muscle myopathy.[83] However, when nonskeletal muscle sources of 3-methylhistidine and creatinine were taken into consideration using the Afting correction, myofibrillar protein breakdown was significantly reduced in alcoholics with histologically proven myopathy, as compared to those without myopathy.[83] The latter conclusions are more plausible. This is because if rates of muscle protein synthesis were reduced by 40% without adjustments in the rate of protein breakdown, then the entire muscle protein mass would be considerably reduced ($>75\%$) in a few years.

In laboratory rat studies we found that chronic ethanol feeding for 6 weeks reduced the weight and protein content of the entire skeletal musculature.[62,68,73,84-87] In young rats the reductions in muscle protein content were rapid, and occurred as early as 14 d of alcohol feeding.[86] The reductions thereafter were less marked, suggesting an adaptive response.[86] However, skeletal muscle is a composite mixture of fiber types and consideration must be given to the fact that in man the myopathy largely affects type II fibers.[75-77] Individual muscles have also been taken to represent type I (i.e., soleus) and type II (i.e., plantaris) skeletal muscle fibers in a spectrum of metabolic studies on protein turnover in laboratory animals, and we have similarly adopted this convention to the investigation of alcoholic muscle disease. In chronic ethanol-fed rats the type II fiber-predominant plantaris muscle was more susceptible to the deleterious effects of ethanol than the type I fiber-predominant soleus.[84] There were also indications that the diameter of type II fibers in the soleus were reduced by ethanol, confirming fiber-type specificity of the disease process, rather than its effects on anatomically distinct skeletal muscles.[87] Thus, the preferential effect of ethanol on type II fibers of rat muscle is similar to the selective effect of ethanol in type II fibers of human. This confirms the suitability of our model for investigative studies into chronic alcoholic myopathy.

The authors examined the effect of both acute and chronic ethanol toxicity on fractional rates of muscle protein synthesis using a flooding dose of [^{3}H]phenylalanine (Table 3). Acute ethanol dosage profoundly reduced the fractional synthetic rates of proteins in the gastrocnemius muscle (containing a mixture of type I and II fibers and therefore considered to be representative of the entire muscle mass).[88,89] It was also evident that the principal fractions of skeletal muscle, i.e., the cytoplasmic, myofibrillar, and stromal fractions, were affected equally by ethanol.[88] In the type II fiber-predominant plantaris, k_s fell by 30%. The type I fiber-predominant soleus was also responsive to acute ethanol dosage, but marginally less sensitive, i.e., k_s was reduced by 22% (Table 3).[88]

In chronic studies, i.e., at 6 weeks, the effects on muscle protein synthesis are far from clear.[84] In young rats, fractional rates of protein synthesis in soleus and plantaris were reduced by 12 and 6%, but these changes did not achieve statistical significance (Table 3).[84] This seems to imply that an adaptation to the ethanol occurred. In mature rats, significant reductions in k_s were observed, though reductions in muscle protein contents were not marked.[84] It is possible that reductions in protein synthesis represent precipitating or transitional events prior to actual reductions in protein content. Thus, although no loss was seen in muscle protein content of mature rats at 6 weeks, the myopathy is apparent at 12 weeks.[90] Alternatively, it is possible that protein degradation plays an important role in the pathogenesis of the myopathy.

We indirectly measured the rates of degradation of cytoplasmic, myofibrillar, and stromal fractions as the difference between fractional rates of protein synthesis and growth.[62] In both young and mature rats, the fractional rate of cytoplasmic, myofibrillar, and stromal protein degradation decreased by approximately 10 to 20%.[62] These directional changes in protein degradation are contrary to the observations obtained by Tiernan and Ward,[91] who indicated that in chronically fed rats the urinary excretion of 3-methylhistidine was increased. However, as mentioned previously, urinary 3-methylhistidine excretion also reflects protein degradative pathways in skin and GI tissues, as well as skeletal muscle. Furthermore, as the study of Tiernan and Ward[91] unfortunately did not employ a pair-feeding regime, it is difficult to ascertain whether their results were due to ethanol-induced anorexia or the ethanol per se.

In the chronic rat model, neutral protease activity in gastrocnemius muscle homogenates was marginally reduced, i.e., by 15%, but did not achieve statistical significance.[92] Different results were obtained upon analysis of skeletal muscle cathepsin B activities, which were increased

TABLE 3
Skeletal Muscle Protein Synthesis in Acute and Chronic Ethanol Toxicity Studies[62,84,88]

Acute Effects: Immature Rats

	k_s (%/d)			
	Control	Ethanol	% Change	*p*
Gastrocnemius				
Sarcoplasmic	18.2 ± 0.6	13.4 ± 1.3	− 26	<0.01
Myofibrillar	13.8 ± 0.6	10.3 ± 1.0	− 26	<0.01
Stromal	14.6 ± 0.4	10.3 ± 1.1	− 29	<0.01
Soleus	22.5 ± 0.7	17.6 ± 1.1	− 22	<0.01
Plantaris	16.9 ± 0.5	11.9 ± 0.6	− 30	<0.001

Chronic Effects: Immature Rats

	k_s (%/d)			
	Control	Ethanol	% Change	*p*
Gastrocnemius				
Sarcoplasmic	8.1 ± 0.2	7.2 ± 0.3	− 12	NS
Myofibrillar	5.7 ± 0.2	5.1 ± 0.3	− 11	NS
Stromal	7.2 ± 0.3	6.4 ± 0.3	− 11	<0.05
Soleus	11.2 ± 0.5	9.9 ± 0.4	− 12	NS
Plantaris	6.9 ± 0.2	6.6 ± 0.2	− 6	NS

Chronic Effects: Mature Rats

	k_s (%/d)			
	Control	Ethanol	% Change	*p*
Gastrocnemius				
Sarcoplasmic	6.2 ± 0.2	5.2 ± 0.2	− 16	<0.001
Myofibrillar	4.1 ± 0.3	3.2 ± 0.1	− 22	<0.05
Stromal	5.4 ± 0.2	4.5 ± 0.3	− 16	NS
Soleus	9.3 ± 0.8	7.5 ± 0.3	− 19	NS
Plantaris	5.2 ± 0.2	4.1 ± 0.3	− 21	<0.025

Note: Young (initial body weight = 0.1 kg) or mature (initial body weight = 0.3 kg) male rats were acutely treated with either saline (controls) or ethanol (75 mmol/kg, i.p., 2.5 h) or chronically treated with nutritionally complete liquid diets containing 35% of total calories as glucose (controls) or ethanol. At the end of the studies fractional rates of protein synthesis (k_s) were measured with a large flooding dose of [^{3}H]phenylalanine. All data are mean ± SEM (n = 6 to 9). NS, $p > 0.05$, not significant.

by 25% (p <0.01), though cathepsin D activities were unaltered. It appears, however, that ethanol itself alters the activities of muscle protease. Addition of ethanol to the muscle homogenates of glucose-fed control animals caused a decrease (20% reductions, p <0.01) in the activities of neutral protease.[92] In contrast cathepsin B activities were increased approximately 10% (p <0.05) by the addition of ethanol to homogenates of control muscle.[92]

The information based on the analysis of protease activity must be treated with caution, primarily because it provides indices on the potential or capacity to degrade proteins *in vivo*. Nevertheless, the information does suggest that degradative pathways are perturbed by ethanol. Tentatively, the data derived from the analysis of the different proteases appear to be contradictory. However, consideration must be given to the fact that the relative contractile and noncontractile protein composition of the skeletal muscles were maintained,[62] and the synthesis rate of contractile and noncontractile proteins were apparently equally affected by both acute and chronic ethanol feeding (Table 3).[62,88] This suggests that there must have been some sort of differential effect on individual protein degradative pathways to maintain the relative composition of the muscle.

GASTROINTESTINAL TRACT

Acute and chronic ethanol studies on the small intestine are usually directed toward mucosal function (such as impairment of nutrient absorption) and morphology (such as villus shortening). In contrast, the effects on the seromuscular layer have been relatively neglected. Various reports have shown that GI motility is markedly perturbed by alcohol which may have important physiological implications.[93-95] This is because intestinal contractility is an integral part of nutritional metabolism, but the concept that a reduction in the amount of smooth muscle contractile protein may not be conducive for optimum motility patterns has not been adequately addressed. Moreover, no clinical studies exist on the effects of ethanol on GI protein metabolism. However, recently our group has been comprehensively investigating the relationship between ethanol and GI protein turnover in the laboratory rat.[96-98]

In response to ethanol feeding the contents of mixed proteins in the entire small intestine was reduced by approximately 20%.[96] More detailed investigations showed that the composition of the myofibrillar proteins was also reduced.[97] Paradoxically, the fractional synthesis rates of the myofi-

TABLE 4
Protein Synthesis in the Seromuscular Layers of the Rat GI Tract[99]

Region	k_s (%/d)			ADH activity (μmol/mg protein/h)
	Control	Ethanol	% Change	
Liver	86 ± 2	78 ± 4	−10[NS]	0.82 ± 0.26
Esophagus	30 ± 1	24 ± 1	−19[a]	
Stomach	77 ± 6	59 ± 4	−23[b]	0.20 ± 0.04
Duodenum	61 ± 4	56 ± 7	−9[NS]	0.16 ± 0.07
Jejunum	70 ± 5	55 ± 2	−22[b]	0.11 ± 0.06
Ileum	63 ± 3	54 ± 5	−15[NS]	0.03 ± 0.03
Colon	44 ± 1	40 ± 3	−8[NS]	
Rectum	47 ± 1	41 ± 2	−13[b]	

Note: Young male rats were injected with ethanol at a dosage of 75 mmol/kg body weight, i.p., and rates of protein synthesis measured after 2.5 h. All data are mean ± SEM (n = 5 to 9). Esophagus pertains to the mixed seromuscular layer plus mucosa, while the remaining regions of the GI tract pertain to the isolated seromuscular layer. ADH activities were derived from Bode.[102] NS, not significant, $p > 0.05$.

[a] $p < 0.001$.
[b] $p < 0.05$.

brillar protein were unaffected in chronic ethanol feeding.[97] The refractory response of protein synthesis in the small intestine may reflect adaptive responses and/or that protein degradation had increased.

Acute ethanol dosage (75 mmol/kg body weight) profoundly reduced the fractional rate of myofibrillary protein synthesis in the combined duodenum and proximal jejunum by approximately 40% after 2.5 h.[98] Mixed tissue protein synthesis rates were reduced by approximately 15%.[98] We have now extended these acute ethanol studies to include all regions of the rat GI tract.[99] Table 4 shows that there is considerable variability in the synthesis rates of mixed tissue proteins (from 30%/d in the esophagus to approximately 80%/d in the stomach) and ethanol appears to exert selective effects on individual regions. The pattern of response is complex.[99] This is perhaps more evident when the myofibrillary fractions are purified from each anatomical location; the rate of myofibrillary protein synthesis falls in the jejunum but is unaltered in the duodenum (Table

TABLE 5
Contractile Protein Synthesis in GI Tissues and Their Response to Acute Ethanol Toxicity[100]

| Contractile proteins | k_s (%/d) | | % Change | p |
	Control	Ethanol		
Stomach	29.9 ± 2.2	24.8 ± 0.9	−14	NS
Duodenum	33.2 ± 1.2	33.1 ± 2.8	0	NS
Jejunum	49.1 ± 2.7	34.1 ± 0.7	−30	<0.001
Ileum	38.3 ± 2.8	26.6 ± 2.5	−31	<0.025
Cecum	51.9 ± 2.1	43.2 ± 3.0	−17	<0.05
Colon	33.3 ± 3.3	28.0 ± 1.6	−16	NS
Rectum	36.2 ± 2.3	32.6 ± 2.2	−10	NS

Note: Rats were injected with ethanol (75 mmol/kg body weight, i.p.) and fractional rates of myofibrillary (contractile) protein synthesis (k_s) measured after 2.5 h. Contractile proteins were isolated from the seromuscular layers by combined differential solubility and high-speed centrifugation procedures. All data are mean ± SEM (n = 6 to 9). NS, not significant, $p > 0.05$.

5).[100] There is also selectivity in the way the mucosa responds to ethanol (Table 6); k_s is virtually unaltered in the colon and rectum but reduced (by approximately 20%) in the mucosa of the stomach, duodenum, and jejunum.[101] The reasons for this variability are not yet known, but regional sensitivity to ethanol-induced reductions in k_s may be related to the fact that susceptible regions have higher alcohol dehydrogenase activity.[102] In other words, endogenously derived acetaldehyde may inhibit protein synthesis. The hypothesis, although very simple, is flawed by the observation that the liver has very high alcohol dehydrogenase levels (Table 4), yet the overall rate of protein synthesis in this tissue is not overtly affected by acute ethanol dosage.[89] However, one has to consider not only the potential rate of acetaldehyde formation but its subsequent oxidation to acetate by acetaldehyde dehydrogenases. In addition, a distinction should be made between acetaldehyde concentrations in the seromuscular and mucosal layers: most studies on acetaldehyde dehydrogenase activities have either analyzed whole intestinal segments or the mucosa itself. Various isoforms of ethanol-oxidizing enzymes also exist that have their own physiobiochemical properties and kinetics. For example, Pares et al.[103] have

TABLE 6
Muscosal Protein Synthesis in the GI Tract[101]

Mucosa	k_s (%/d)		% Change	p
	Control	Ethanol		
Stomach	106 ± 3	85 ± 3	− 20	<0.001
Duodenum	109 ± 3	95 ± 5	− 13	<0.025
Jejunum	111 ± 4	91 ± 6	− 18	<0.025
Ileum	91 ± 4	81 ± 5	− 11	NS
Colon	59 ± 2	56 ± 4	− 5	NS
Rectum	68 ± 5	65 ± 4	− 5	NS

Note: Young rats were injected with an i.p. dose of ethanol (75 mmol/kg body weight) and after 2.5 h fractional rates of protein synthesis (k_s) were measured in the mucosal layer. All data are mean ± SEM (n = 5 to 7). NS, not significant, $p > 0.05$.

demonstrated that rat stomach contains a fourth class of mammalian alcohol dehydrogenase (ADH), distinct from hepatic alcohol dehydrogenase. Nevertheless, the concept that acetaldehyde is a potent inhibitor of protein synthesis is interesting. Unfortunately, the testing of this hypothesis via the administration of acetaldehyde *in vivo* poses numerous practical problems because acetaldehyde is extremely toxic. Nonetheless, there are potential advantages in using suitable inhibitors of ADH and acetaldehyde dehydrogenase to investigate the complexity of acetaldehyde involvement in mediating changes in tissue protein turnover. Although this has not yet been described for the small intestine, their usage in investigating cardiac protein turnover is described below.

HEART

Clinical studies have shown that chronic alcoholism causes a disturbance of myofibrillary structure and function. ADP (adenosine diphosphate)-mediated actin-myosin interaction is inhibited by alcohol and concomitant myofibril derangement has been found.[104,105] Urbano-Marquez et al.[78] also recently reported that electron microscopic examinations of biopsies from alcoholics revealed loss of myofibrils. This implies an ethanol-induced defect in ventricular contractile protein turnover, but as with intestinal studies, no appropriate turnover studies have been carried out in man. We have shown small reductions in the contractile apparatus, by direct assay of myocardial myofibrillary proteins in rats chronically fed ethanol for 6 weeks.[106] These changes were accompanied by a significant increase in protein synthetic rates, thereby implying that protein degradation increased.[106] However, the heart has an adaptive response, as the acute and chronic effects of ethanol are quite different.

In response to acute ethanol toxicity, the synthetic rates of cardiac proteins were reduced by approximately 20%.[107] Subsequently, we addressed the question of whether this was due to alcohol or acetaldehyde. The ADH activity in the heart is exceedingly low, which tentatively suggests that endogenous acetaldehyde production may not mediate these reductions in k_s. Alternatively, the heart tissue may be especially sensitive to low concentrations of endogenously derived acetaldehyde or hepatic-derived acetaldehyde in the plasma which may be possibly mediating changes in k_s. To investigate the role of acetaldehyde, we used the inhibitors, cyanamide and 4-methylpyrazole, which inhibit acetaldehyde dehydrogenase and ADH, respectively.[108,109] Thus, the concomitant administration of ethanol in the presence of either cyanamide or 4-methylpyrazole increases or decreases acetaldehyde levels, respectively. These results are summarized in Table 7, which clearly shows that myocardial protein synthesis was markedly sensitive to acetaldehyde; i.e., k_s was reduced by approximately 80% when ethanol-dosed rats were pretreated with cyanamide.[110] Pretreatment with 4-methylpyrazole produced a very similar response to ethanol alone. Very low levels of acetaldehyde were also injected (Table 7, study 2) but the reductions in k_s (approximately 15%) did not achieve statistical significance.[111] Thus, it is likely that both alcohol and acetaldehyde are protein synthetic perturbatives in the myocardium *in vivo*.

BONE

One of the original studies in this field was conducted by Saville,[112] who nearly 30 years ago demonstrated that the bodies of alcoholics at autopsy have reduced bone mass. Subsequent studies have shown that chronic ethanol consumption induces a variety of pathogenic changes in skeletal tissue, including osteoporosis and osteopenia.[113-115] A composite analysis of these and other recent studies encompassing a total of 308 subjects has shown that approximately half of all alcoholics have bone damage, predominantly osteoporosis.[116] The suggested loss of bone mass indicates an imbalance between the synthetic rates of the organic and inorganic matrix and its resorption.

TABLE 7
Acute Effects of Ethanol With and Without Acetaldehyde Dehydrogenase and ADH Inhibitors on Fractional Rates of Ventricular Protein Synthesis in the Rat[110,111]

Study 1

Pretreatment (30 min)	Treatment (150 min)	k_s (%/d)	% Change (from saline + saline)	p (vs. saline + saline)
Saline	Saline	24.0 ± 0.9		
Saline	Ethanol	18.8 ± 1.2	-22	<0.01
CYN	Saline	24.6 ± 1.5	$+3$	NS
CYN	Ethanol	4.8 ± 0.8	-80	<0.001
4MP	Saline	23.8 ± 1.7	-1	NS
4MP	Ethanol	18.9 ± 1.5	-21	<0.01

Study 2

Pretreatment (30 min)	Treatment (150 min)	k_s (%/d)	% Change (from saline + saline)	p (vs. saline + saline)
Saline	Saline	17.4 ± 1.3		
4MP	Saline	18.1 ± 2.0	$+14$	NS
Saline	Acetaldehyde	15.1 ± 0.4	-13	NS
4MP	Acetaldehyde	14.6 ± 0.9	-16	NS

Note: Male Wistar rats were given i.p. injections of either saline, cyanamide (CYN), or 4-methylpyrazole (4MP) 30 min before i.p. injections of either saline, ethanol, or acetaldehyde. Rates of protein synthesis (k_s) were measured in mixed ventricular homogenates 150 min after the latter treatments. All data are mean $\pm$ SEM (n = 4 to 9). NS, $p > 0.05$ not significant.

Diamond et al.[113] and Crilly et al.[114] have suggested that bone resorption is increased in alcoholism, as inferred from an increase in urinary hydroxyproline excretion. However, it is difficult to ascribe these changes to the effects of ethanol per se, as Crilly et al.[114] demonstrated that dietary calcium intake in alcoholics with a high incidence of bone disease was lower than in abstaining controls. Feitelberg et al.[115] concluded that alcoholic bone disease may be contributed by vitamin D-deficient diets. This raises the question of whether ethanol-induced changes in bone protein metabolism can occur independently of overt nutritional deficits. The issue has been addressed by using suitable animal models, in which both controls and alcoholics received identically matched diets.

TABLE 8

Collagen Degradation in Chronic Alcoholic Rats as Determined by Hydroxyproline, Pyridinoline, and Deoxypyridinoline[117,118]

Urinary excretion (nmol/d/rat)	Control	Ethanol	% Change	p
Hydroxyproline	4370 ± 460	6130 ± 690	+40	<0.01
Pyridinoline	7.03 ± 0.33	6.06 ± 0.48	−14	<0.05
Deoxypyridinoline	7.88 ± 0.45	4.21 ± 0.26	−47	<0.001
Tibia composition (mg/bone)				
Hydroxyproline	3.27 ± 0.16	2.73 ± 0.10	−17	<0.05
Ca	43.1 ± 0.9	38.5 ± 1.0	−11	<0.05
Mg	0.84 ± 0.04	0.73 ± 0.03	−13	$p = 0.06^a$
Phosphate	14.58 ± 1.96	9.57 ± 3.20	−34	$p = 0.06^a$
K	0.31 ± 0.04	0.29 ± 0.02	−6	NS
Na	1.29 ± 0.17	1.07 ± 0.06	−17	NS

Note: Data are from chronic ethanol-feeding studies in which young rats were fed a nutritionally complete liquid diet containing either glucose (controls) or ethanol as 35% of total calories.

[a] Although all pairs demonstrated unidirectional changes, $p = 0.06$.

The protein-bound hydroxyproline content of tibia was reduced by approximately 20% at 4 weeks, although no effect was observed at either 1 or 2 weeks (Table 8).[117] These changes in bone collagen content were relatively slow compared to the protein loss in skeletal muscle. The bone changes were supported by the observation that urinary hydroxyproline excretion increased by approximately 40% in chronic (i.e., 6-week fed) alcohol-fed rats,[117] which was similar to the clinical results of Crilly et al.[114] and Diamond et al.[113] Decreases also occurred in total mineral content in the tibia of the rat, i.e., Ca, phosphate, and magnesium (Mg). Trace element composition (Zn, Cu, and Fe) was also measured, partially as complementary indices of nutritional status, but these were either unaltered or increased slightly.[117]

As mentioned earlier, urinary hydroxyproline cannot be reliably ascribed exclusively to bone, and may well reflect alterations in nonskeletal

TABLE 9
Effects of Chronic Ethanol Feeding on Body Composition

Immature Rats

	Control	Ethanol	% Change	p
Body weight (g)	225 ± 3	197 ± 4	−12	<0.001
Carcass (g)	125 ± 2	102 ± 4	−19	<0.001
Bone, tibia (mg)	367 ± 9	340 ± 7	−7	<0.05
Skeletal muscle mass (g)	114 ± 2	92 ± 4	−20	<0.001
Gastrocnemius (mg)	2520 ± 40	1980 ± 50	−21	<0.001
Lung (mg)	1210 ± 110	1040 ± 70	−14	NS
Skin (g)	36 ± 1	29 ± 2	−19	<0.01
Kidney (mg)	872 ± 16	827 ± 19	−5	NS
Liver (g)	9 ± 1	7 ± 1	−17	<0.001

Mature Rats

	Control	Ethanol	% Change	p
Body weight (g)	390 ± 8	361 ± 9	−7	<0.001
Carcass (g)	217 ± 6	194 ± 7	−10	<0.001
Bone, tibia (mg)	608 ± 6	594 ± 12	−2	NS
Skeletal muscle mass (g)	198 ± 5	177 ± 7	−11	<0.01
Gastrocnemius (mg)	4160 ± 80	3940 ± 110	−5	NS
Lung (mg)	1610 ± 130	1500 ± 100	−7	NS
Skin (g)	63 ± 3	55 ± 3	−13	<0.01
Kidney (mg)	1300 ± 40	1210 ± 50	−7	NS
Liver (g)	14 ± 1	13 ± 1	−6	NS

Note: Male Wistar rats of either 0.1 (young or immature) or 0.3 kg (mature) body weight were chronically fed with nutritionally complete liquid diets containing 35% of total calories as glucose (controls) or ethanol. All data are mean ± SEM (n = 6 to 9). NS, $p > 0.05$, not significant.

tissues.[1,60] For example, Table 9 shows that in response to chronic ethanol feeding the weight of the skin in immature and mature rats were reduced by 19 and 13%, respectively.[85] The weight of other tissues that also contain appreciable concentrations of collagen, i.e., the lung, was also reduced (Table 9).[85] Measurement of the urinary pyridinium cross-links revealed contrasting results to the hydroxyproline data. Pyridinoline is found in types II and IX collagens of cartilage and to a lesser extent in type I

TABLE 10
Urinary Excretion of Free and Conjugated Forms of Pyridinoline and Deoxypyridinoline in Chronic Ethanol-Fed Rats

Pyridinoline	Excretion (nmol/rat/d)			
	Control	Ethanol	% Change	p
Free	2.99 ± 0.20	2.90 ± 0.22	−3	NS
Conjugated	4.04 ± 0.25	3.16 ± 0.48	−22	NS
Free/conjugated ratio	0.426 ± 0.023	0.490 ± 0.046	+15	NS
Deoxypyridinoline				
Free	1.58 ± 0.13	1.18 ± 0.08	−25	<0.05
Conjugated	6.30 ± 0.38	2.86 ± 0.35	−55	<0.001
Free/conjugated ratio	0.201 ± 0.013	0.281 ± 0.013	+40	<0.01

Note: Urine was collected from rats chronically fed liquid diets containing either glucose (controls) or ethanol as 35% of total dietary energy, as described in the legend to Table 8.[118]

collagen of bone.[60,61] Deoxypyridinoline is found predominantly in type I collagen of bone, although trace amounts are contained in dentine.[60,61] Although skin substantially contributes to the whole-body collagen pool, neither pyridinoline nor deoxypyridinoline are found in this tissue.[60]

Chronic alcohol feeding caused the total 24-h urinary pyridinoline excretion to fall only slightly, i.e., by 15%, and no statistically significant effects occurred to either the free or conjugated forms (Tables 8 and 10).[118] The urinary excretion of total, free, and conjugated deoxypyridinoline was significantly reduced.[118] Table 10 shows that differential effects also occurred on the individual cross-link species and the decline in the conjugated form (i.e., 55%) was significantly greater than the decline in free deoxypyridinoline (i.e., 25%).[118] The significance of these differential effects on conjugated and free forms is not entirely clear at present. The formation of free and conjugated moieties may represent the end products of different degradative pathways. The data also indicate that chronic ethanol consumption reduces the absolute rate of bone collagen degradation, and perhaps the involvement of more than one route of type I collagen breakdown is perturbed. Very little is known about the relative distribution of these pyridinium cross-links in cortical and trabecular bone of the ethanol-fed rat, or whether the skeletal collagen contents in individual bones are differentially altered. Nevertheless, the important message arising from these studies is primarily that the absolute rate of bone collagen degradation decreases in experimental alcoholism and contrasting conclusions are obtained when two different markers of protein breakdown are employed. Thus, one must remain aware of the potential limitations in interpreting data derived from urinary markers of protein turnover. Our data also suggest that perturbations in collagen turnover can occur in alcoholism in the absence of deficiencies in nutritional intake. The caveat to this is that ethanol may disturb or interfere with the metabolic handling of nutrients essential for normal skeletal maturation (i.e., calcium, vitamin D) via defects in absorption, excretion, or interhepatic conversions. By the same token it is possible that clinical and experimental chronic alcoholic myopathy may also be mediated by liver dysfunction.

LIVER

Studies have been carried out in which rates of protein turnover have been measured in alcoholic subjects with cirrhosis, including the excretion of 3-methylhistidine and estimation of whole-body turnover rates with stable isotopes. However, it is necessary to distinguish between the effects of liver dysfunction on whole-body metabolism and the effects of ethanol on the liver per se. The important relationship between impaired hepatic function and the extrahepatic metabolism of protein is beyond the scope of this chapter.

The pathological effects of ethanol on the liver and its relationship to nutrition have formed the basis of various reviews, and the reader is referred to these articles.[119-121] Some specifically mention aspects of protein metabolism, but none point out the comparative effects on the liver relative to other tissues. As mentioned earlier, the contribution of the liver to whole-body protein synthesis is comparable to combined skin and bone, skeletal muscle, or the GI tract. The evaluation of the contribution of hepatic tissue as it relates to these organs is complicated by the fact that one of the major functions of the liver is the synthesis and subsequent export of the plasma proteins, with the exception of the immunoglobulins. Severe liver disease is often associated with a fall in the concentrations of plasma albumin,[122] which might be expected to be the result of perturbed synthesis or possibly defects in albumin degradation. However, hepatomegaly is also a common feature of alcoholism, which may be due to defects in the export

TABLE 11

Acute Effects of Ethanol: A Comparative Study of Liver, Small Intestine, Skin, Bone, and Skeletal Muscle[57,58,89,98,148]

Tissue	Contribution to whole-body synthesis (%)	k_s (%/d) Control	Ethanol	% Change	p
Skeletal muscle	20–25	15 ± 1	10 ± 1	− 29	<0.001
Small intestine	15–20	119 ± 3	101 ± 8	− 18	<0.001
Liver	20–25	86 ± 2	78 ± 4	− 10	NS
Skin	15–20	62 ± 2	47 ± 4	− 24	<0.001
Bone	5–10	63 ± 2	45 ± 4	− 29	<0.001

Note: The effects of an acute dose of ethanol (75 mmol/kg body weight: 2 to 5 h) was examined in 100 g rats.

processes.[123] Moreover, cirrhosis is an added complication, which eventually develops in 15 to 20% of all chronic alcoholics.[124] Thus, collagen metabolism becomes an increasingly important component of hepatic protein turnover.

Unfortunately, the manner in which liver protein turnover is modified by ethanol has not been fully elucidated in man. Some indirect estimates of liver protein turnover have been measured in alcoholic subjects, i.e., collagen mRNA levels[125] and circulating serum collagen peptides,[125-127] but reservations are attached to indirect indices. Nevertheless, appropriate studies have been carried out in laboratory animal models *in vivo* in which protein synthesis has been directly measured.[128-130] In general, the results derived from acute (i.e., up to 2 weeks of ethanol treatment) studies arrive at the same conclusion, namely that ethanol has no overt effect on hepatic protein synthesis.[128-130] Chronic ethanol feeding for longer than 2 weeks reduces liver protein synthesis.[129,130] Preedy and associates[89,131] have investigated the effects of both acute and chronic ethanol toxicity on liver protein synthesis using ethanol treatment regimes that have been shown to induce pathogenic changes in nonhepatic tissues. In response to acute dosage we showed that only a small reduction in liver k_s occurs, which does not achieve statistical significance when k_s is calculated from S_i (Table 11).[89] Concomitant analysis of the skeletal muscle shows a more marked reduction in k_s, and indeed fractional synthesis rates in bone and skin are also reduced by 20 to 30% (see Table 11).

In chronic ethanol-feeding studies the authors[131] could find no evidence of the previously reported increase in hepatic protein mass, and by contrast, we found that protein content was either reduced in immature rats by 13% or unaltered in slowly growing mature rats after 6 weeks. Rates of mixed hepatic protein synthesis were reduced by approximately 20 to 25% in both immature and mature rats, confirming the observations of Smith-Kielland et al.[129] and Donohue et al.[130] The paradoxical decrease in k_s in large rats without reductions in protein content may represent a transitional phase or may reflect that protein breakdown was also reduced.[131] It was not possible to provide an accurate value for k_d because the export and/or the retention of plasma proteins complicates such measurements.[36,131]

WHOLE-BODY

A comprehensive clinical study into the relationship between alcohol ingestion and metabolic nitrogen balance was undertaken by McDonald and Margen,[132] who showed that subjects on alcohol-feeding regimes lose weight when compared to those on isocaloric control regimes. There were also significant increases in urinary excretion of total nitrogen, uric acid, and urea.[132] Fecal nitrogen output was not overtly altered, but patients on alcohol-feeding regimes were generally in negative nitrogen balance, largely due to urinary nitrogen losses.[132] Urinary creatinine levels were not generally altered, although one patient in the study who showed a fall in this variable (ascribed to reductions in muscle mass) also displayed the greatest weight loss.[132] Other studies have also shown that ethanol enhances urinary nitrogen losses.[133,134]

Overall, these data imply that ethanolic calories are inadequately employed. This energetically inefficient utilization of ethanol is supported by epidemiological studies, showing, for example, that within the general population male drinkers (i.e., those consuming 56 g of ethanol per day) consumed 16% more calories than nondrinkers, largely due to the intake of alcoholic calories.[135] Abstainers, however, have almost identical body mass indices (kg/m² or Quetelet's Indices), i.e., 26.0, and identical physical activity levels, i.e., mean 3.2 (arbitrary units) as persons consuming ethanol (Quetelet's Index of 26.2 and activity scores of 3.2). Similar conclusions were drawn from an analysis of data derived from female subjects (consuming 40 g of ethanol per day), who, in addition, exhibited significant reductions in Quetelet's Index.[135,136] Other studies have shown weight reductions with alcohol consumption or lack of an increase in body weight when extra calories are consumed as ethanol.[137-139] Thus, one can conclude that despite the higher caloric intake as ethanol, nondrinkers are no more obese than abstainers. The moderate levels of consumption described by Gruchow et al.,[135] for example, should be compared to the groups studied by Peters and colleagues,[76,77,81] whose patients consumed at least 100 g of ethanol per day or more and exhibited an actual deficit in weight.

These metabolic disturbances are probably due to the induction of the hepatic microsomal ethanol oxidizing system (MEOS) of ethanol oxidation, which is energetically wasteful.[140] Also, it has been postulated that besides the futile utilization of calories by the inadequate coupling of adenosine triphosphate (ATP) production, additional metabolic inefficiency may arise as a consequence of elevated ATP hydrolysis of the sodium pump ATPase.[141,142] However, it is apparently clear from the sections on protein turnover that a major contributing factor may be that circulating levels of ethanol (and possibly derived metabolites such as acetaldehyde) inhibit the deposition of tissue protein. Reductions in tissue protein content (which is approximately 20% of tissue weight) are generally associated with the concomitant loss of cytoplasmic contents that is predominantly water (approximately 70% of tissue weight). Thus, reductions in tissue protein will cause disproportionate decrements in tissue weight.

These issues were also raised by Reinus et al.,[143] who applied both indirect and direct calorimetric techniques to ascertain the mechanisms involved. This entailed the employment of nasogastric infusions of either control (glucose) or alcohol-containing enteral diets, comprising either 30, 40, or 60% of total calories. The rationale of using these levels of ethanol infusion was based on the aim of saturating the hepatic capacity for oxidizing ethanol.[143] There were weight losses and elevations in urinary urea nitrogen excretion. Thermal energy losses, as determined by both indirect and direct calorimetry, were unchanged. It was concluded that the weight loss during ethanol infusion is unrelated to negative energy balance and may be due to protein, mineral, fluid loss.[143] Some of the weight loss may have been contributed by the loss of myofibrillary proteins, as urinary 3-methylhistidine excretion was increased.[143] (The apparent contradiction between the studies of Reinus et al.[143] and Martin and Peters[83] may be explained by the subjects in the latter study being abstinent at the time of measurement.) Nevertheless, the conclusions by Reinus et al.[143] are also in accordance with our clinical and experimental findings that the largest mass of tissue, i.e., skeletal muscle that comprises 40% of mammalian body weight, is reduced in chronic alcoholism. This is partly due to a reduction in muscle k_s. Is whole-body protein synthesis also affected?

Rates of whole-body protein turnover have been measured with 8-h infusions L[1-^{13}C]-leucine.[82] Whole-body data were based on the formula: Flux (Q) = I + B = E + Z.[1] Because leucine oxidation was accurately known, whole-body synthesis rates were equated from Z = Q − E. The results of these studies showed that although chronic alcoholics (>100 g/d, >10 years) had reduced rates of skeletal muscle protein synthesis, rates of whole-body protein synthesis and breakdown were only slightly reduced, and these changes did not achieve statistical significance (Table 2).[82] This may have reflected limitations in the analytical techniques as comparisons were made with historical controls and subjects were investigated in the postabsorptive state (which raises the question of whether the responses to food withdrawal were being examined).[82] Despite these reservations, an important finding of our studies was that whole-body amino acid oxidation was significantly reduced (Table 2). The significance of these results relate to the known pathways of leucine catabolism which is predominantly oxidized in skeletal muscle. Subsequently, the labeled carbon (i.e., $^{13}CO_2$) enters into the biocarbonate pool.[144] Thus, production of labeled CO_2 during expiration represents the component of flux that is oxidation of leucine. Since no other pathways of leucine metabolism exist, the remaining part of the flux must be synthesized into protein. The reduction in leucine oxidation in alcoholism evidently represents a paradoxical observation. This is because if both controls and alcoholics are receiving identical nutritional, and by implication leucine, intakes, then excess leucine must be oxidized if synthesis is unaltered or reduced. Nevertheless, it is possible that as chronic alcoholics have reduced muscle mass and muscle is the principal site of leucine oxidation, then the reductions in leucine oxidation may reflect the myopathy. The alternative explanation, that rates of whole-body protein synthesis may increase, is precluded as the results in Table 2 show a small reduction in this component of protein metabolism.[82] The interpretation of these whole-body data is complicated by the fact that turnover measurements were made in alcoholics who were not intoxicated with ethanol during the isotopic infusions. It is possible that more marked perturbations in whole-body protein metabolism would have been apparent if blood ethanol levels were high.

TABLE 12
Urinary Excretion in the Chronically Treated Alcohol-Fed Rat[74]

Excretion	Control	Ethanol	% Change	p
Total nitrogen (mg/d)	137 ± 11	169 ± 12	$+23$	<0.05
Uric acid (μmol/d)	5.3 ± 0.9	12.1 ± 1.4	$+128$	<0.01
Urea (mmol/d)	2.1 ± 0.2	3.4 ± 0.2	$+62$	<0.005
Creatinine (μmol/d)	50 ± 3	46 ± 4	-8	NS
Ethanol (μmol/d)	106 ± 23	1320 ± 100	$+92$	<0.001
Alanine (μmol/d)	9 ± 1	13 ± 3	$+44$	<0.025

Note: Data are derived from chronic ethanol-feeding studies in which young rats were fed a nutritionally complete liquid diet containing either glucose (controls) or ethanol as 35% of total calories. Urine was collected after 6 weeks of treatment.

Similar changes in whole-body protein metabolism have been obtained in rat models of chronic alcohol toxicity.[74,145,146] In our studies there were marked perturbations in whole-body nitrogen economy in response to ethanol, including increases in the excretion of urinary nitrogen, urea, and uric acid (Table 12).[74] Tentatively, some of these changes can be ascribed to altered urea generation, including flux of ammonia to hepatocytes, regulation of carbonyl-phosphate synthetase or ornithine transcarbamoylase, aspartate availability, or blood flow.[147] Increases in either hepatic uptake of amino acids or peripheral production of ureagenic substrates may be other factors. The latter is supported by the observation that alcohol (either acutely or chronically) decreases protein synthesis in a variety of organ systems, including skin, bone, skeletal muscle, and hepatogastrointestinal tissues (Table 12).[148] Disturbances in blood flow as a mediating factor can be excluded as this appears to be unaltered in muscle and GI tissues,[149] and we have recently shown that it is also unaltered in livers of chronically fed rats.[150] In this regard, we showed that excretion of other urinary nitrogenous compounds, i.e., alanine, also increased.[74] Although the contribution of alanine to the total urinary nitrogen pool was small, it may have reflected enhanced alanine release by skeletal muscles. For example, after 6 weeks of treatment, the *in vitro* alanine production from type II muscles of ethanol-fed rats and glucose-fed controls was 5.8 ± 0.5 and 3.6 ± 0.5 μmol/g/h, respectively; $p < 0.01$.[151] Similar elevations in alanine production were observed in type I fiber-rich muscles, i.e., 61% increase, $p < 0.05$.[151] As protein degradation falls these changes may reflect increased alanine production via pyruvate.

Whole-body leucine oxidation has also been measured in the rat *in vivo*. The rate of leucine oxidation was apparently unaltered after 28 d of chronic ethanol feeding.[152] However, in acute ethanol dosage studies, ethanol depressed leucine oxidation *in vivo,* which may possibly induce an expansion in the whole-body pool size of free leucine. Paradoxically, however, the free plasma leucine concentration decreased.[152]

It is possible that the inefficient utilization of calories in the form of ethanol may be due to the excretion of significant amounts of unutilized ethanol. This would perhaps cause an energy deficit in the calculation of the dietary intake, which is presumed to be identical in both control and treated groups. Theoretically, this deficit may induce mobilization of gluconeogenic precursors from tissue protein stores, i.e., a semi-starvation effect is induced. This could account for the reductions in muscle mass, which is particularly sensitive to starvation and is also characterized by type II fiber atrophy. However, in the ethanol-fed rat the excretion of urinary ethanol was only approximately 2% of total ethanol intake and therefore <1% of total caloric intake (Table 12).[74] An alternative hypothesis is that the diminished muscle mass may exacerbate inefficient loss of ethanol-derived calories in the form of acetate, as skeletal muscle is an important site of whole-body acetate metabolism.[153-155] We also showed that the energy generation steps in the conversion of acetate to CO_2 and H_2O via the citric acid cycle were probably unimpaired: 24-h urinary acetate concentrations in glucose-fed controls and ethanol-fed rats were identical and only 0.3% of dietary ethanol (Table 12).[74] Thus, the defects in tissue and whole-body protein metabolism do not appear to be due to calorie starvation.

MECHANISMS FOR ALTERATIONS IN PROTEIN TURNOVER IN ALCOHOLISM

Taking the above into account, a fundamental question arises: what exactly are the mechanisms involved in mediating the ethanol-induced changes in protein metabolism? Unfortunately, it is difficult to propose a grand unifying theory that can be attributable to all the different tissues because there are a spectrum of ways in which they are affected. For example, the fractional rate of cardiac myofibillary protein synthesis of young rats is increased at the end of the 6 weeks of treatment,[106] yet in contrast, skeletal muscle protein synthesis is decreased.[62] Furthermore, fractional breakdown rates of cardiac myofibillary proteins are increased, though skeletal muscle myofibillary protein breakdown as a whole is decreased.[62,106] Within the latter tissue, there even appears to be differential regulation of individual proteases.[92] Also, within separate systems, particular tissues may respond with remarkable variability. An example of this concerns the GI tract, in which the rectum and colon are less susceptible than the esophagus and stomach to acute ethanol.[99-101] This is analogous to the differential effects of ethanol on type I and II muscles.[84,87] We do not know the extent of the heterogeneity of other tissues. For example, is protein metabolism in the atria as sensitive as the ventricles or are these responses exacerbated in concomitant disease processes such as hypertension? In addition we do not know if the tibia is more responsive than other components of the skeletal system. Even within the tibia itself the lower weight-bearing regions lose cortical bone mass but proximal regions are unaffected by chronic ethanol toxicity.[117] We believe that the regulation of tissue protein content is complex and pathological responses to ethanol depend not only on causal agents such as free radicals,[156] but also on endogenous protective mediators, for example, antioxidant levels.[157]

To resolve incorporating the above complexities into the ensuing paragraphs, we have decided to exemplify the discussion with reference to the regulation of protein synthesis in striated muscle. This can be approached from various levels. The first level involves the relatively complex cellular and molecular mechanisms, as elegantly reviewed by Sugden and Fuller.[158] These can be simply designated as transcriptional and translational mechanisms. We have a substantial body of evidence that allows us to surmise that in skeletal muscle (and also for some regions of the GI tract) deranged transcription may be an important pathological step. This is because in general the fractional rate of tissue protein synthesis is proportional to the total amount of RNA, which in most tissues is ribosomal.[159] It follows that decreases in RNA content reduce the potential or capacity of the tissues for protein synthesis. We have recently demonstrated that experimental chronic alcohol feeding causes a rapid and sustained decrease in muscle RNA content.[73,86] Muscle RNA content of ethanol-fed rats were significantly lower (i.e., by 23%) than pair-fed controls after only 7 d of treatment and slightly more marked reductions, i.e., 28%, were observed after 2 weeks.[86] At 6 weeks the RNA was reduced by 35%.[86] The dramatic reductions in the first week and gradual decrements thereafter suggest that some partial adaptation or attenuation in the sensitivity of RNA turnover also occurred.

We also have evidence that translation is altered in skeletal muscle. The efficiency of translation is essentially measured as the amount of protein synthesis per unit ribosome or RNA activity. This is obtained by dividing the fractional rate of protein synthesis by the protein synthetic capacity (i.e., RNA/protein ratio).[158] In acute studies, RNA activities in skeletal muscle are reduced by approximately 20 to 35%.[88] In chronic ethanol-feeding experiments, muscle RNA activities are also impaired, though not as much as in acute studies.[84] For example, the RNA activities in the gastrocnemius muscle of young rats fell by 17% from 16.5 ± 0.7 to 13.7 ± 0.5 mg protein per day per mg of RNA ($p < 0.05$).[160] This comparatively small change arises because over the long term ethanol also reduces the RNA capacity. Thus translational and transcriptional mechanisms appear to be involved in the development of the myopathy. We do not know the mechanisms of either of these processes in acute or chronic alcohol toxicity. Defects in peptide-chain initiation may be one possible mediating factor for the reductions in translational activities.[161,162] In this regard, Harbitz et al.[161] have shown that when ethanol reduced liver valine incorporation *in vitro*, it induced a redistribution of polysomes toward the small units, indicative of a defect in initiation. Ethanol inhibited the formation of ^{35}S-Met-tRNA$_f$-40S initiation complexes[161,162] which were also associated with an enhanced phosphorylation of the α-subunit of eukaryotic initiation factor-2 and inhibition of its recycling.[162] However, inhibition of acetaldehyde formation with 4-methylpyrazole prevented inhibitory effects of the ethanol on hepatic tissue.[161] This is a different pattern than the results on heart muscle, where 4-methylpyrazole did not ameliorate the effects of ethanol (Table 7). As far as we are aware no detailed studies exist on the effects of ethanol toxicity on initiation processes in skeletal muscle.

In addition to the above cellular mechanisms other, more physiological processes may be important, i.e., nutrition. Some alcoholics are undoubtedly malnourished and a variety of nutritional deficiencies are known to induce major effects on protein turnover.[1,2,163] However, some studies have indicated that heavy drinking may also be associated with a superior diet.[164] Presumably the ability to pay for alcoholic beverages may also be equated with the ability to finance the cost of other food items. Dietary surveys are difficult to interpret unless they are carried out on the same group of individuals in whom the pathological effects of alcohol were also investigated. Duane and Peters[81] showed that an indirect indicator of protein nutrition (i.e., serum alkaline ribonuclease activities) was higher in chronic alcoholic patients when compared to controls, essentially confirming the commonly held assumption that chronic alcoholics may be nutritionally compromised. However, they were unable to determine any distinction between nonmyopathic and myopathic patients.[81] Furthermore, no differences were found in serum vitamin B_{12}, red cell folate, and the following vitamin B-dependent erythrocyte enzymes: transketolase (B_1), glutathione reductase (GSH; B_2), and aspartate aminotransferase activities (B_6) between myopathic and nonmyopathic alcoholics.[81] Hickish et al.[165] have also excluded vitamin D as a precipitating factor for alcoholic muscle disease, and similar conclusions were drawn by Urbano-Marquez et al.[78] in the assessment of general nutritional intake in myopathic patients. Decrements in blood flow may also alter protein turnover by reducing nutritional supply at the cellular level via changes in cardiac output or a selective redistribution of flow to specific tissues. No relevant clinical studies in chronic myopathy have been done, although reviews of the acute ethanol dosage experiments in man have shown that blood flow to skeletal muscle is either unaltered, slightly decreased, or increased by as much as one third.[164] In the chronic ethanol-fed rats blood flow rates to skeletal muscle are identical to those of control animals.[149] Thus, myopathic alterations, and by implication the changes in protein metabolism, can arise independently of local or systemic nutritional changes. This was confirmed by our extensive laboratory studies on skeletal muscle in which both control and ethanol rats received identical diets, skeletal muscle mass is reduced, and muscle protein synthesis decreased.

Finally, we shall consider one other mechanism that may be involved in mediating reductions in protein turnover — plasma hormones. These are probably the most well-researched factors involved in the regulation of skeletal muscle protein synthesis.[1] Alcohol ingestion also induces various endocrine abnormalities involving androgens, thyroid and parathyroid hormones, as well as pituitary and pancreatic hormone.[166] Type II fiber atrophy and other skeletal muscle abnormalities are common in many of these endocrine defects.[167] It is tempting to raise the question of whether the alcohol-induced changes in muscle are secondary to these hormonal adjustments. For the purpose of brevity we have decided to exemplify this with reference to the steroid hormones and insulin. The relationship between glucocorticosteroids and alcoholic myopathy was comprehensively studied by Duane and Peters,[168] who showed that the diurnal serum concentration of cortisol and its urinary excretion in myopathic alcoholics was identical to nonmyopathic alcoholics. Thus, the possibility that clinical alcoholic myopathy may be a form of pseudo-Cushing's syndrome can be confidently excluded. At present we have not measured steroid levels in ethanol-treated rats, but we have assayed insulin levels in animals in which muscle protein metabolism is perturbed. Insulin levels are increased in acutely and chronically treated rats, which temptingly precludes this hormone in the development of the myopathy.[85,89] The inherent reservations in this statement relate to the possibility that alcohol may enhance the muscle sensitivity to steroids and other hormones.

CONCLUSIONS

Weight loss is a common problem in chronic alcoholism, and is partly due to perturbations in protein metabolism. The concomitant inefficient protein deposition may be exacerbated by the activation of the MEOS system of ethanol oxidation, which is also energetically inefficient. In very simple terms, it is apparent that alcoholics have increased requirements for dietary protein. The etiological mechanisms of this are poorly understood. However, the role of impaired nutritional intake can be excluded and the evidence suggests a direct effect of ethanol (or its ensuing metabolites or metabolic changes) on protein synthesis and degradation.

ACKNOWLEDGMENTS

We wish to thank Cheryl Riley for secretarial assistance and Dr. George Grimble for advice. The contribution of Jaspaul Marway, Elisabeth Cook, and Tahir Siddiq is acknowledged for providing us with data from their unpublished work. The patience and support of Jo-Ann Pinney throughout the writing of this review is personally acknowledged.

REFERENCES

1. Waterlow, J. C., Garlick, P. J., and Millward, D. J., *Protein Turnover in Mammalian Tissues and in the Whole-Body*, North-Holland, Amsterdam, 1978.
2. Waterlow, J. C., Protein turnover with special reference to man, *Q. J. Exp. Physiol.*, 69, 409, 1984.

3. Millward, D. J., Garlick, P. J., Stewart, R. J. C., Nnanyelugo, D., and Waterlow, J. C., Skeletal muscle growth and protein turnover, *Biochem. J.,* 150, 235, 1975.

4. Rabinowitz, M. and Zak, R., Biochemical and cellular changes in cardiac hypertrophy, *Annu. Rev. Med.,* 23, 245, 1972.

5. Jeejeebhoy, K. N., Energy metabolism in the critically ill, in *Substrate and Energy Metabolism,* Garrow, J. S. and Halliday, D., Eds., John Libbey, London, 1985, 93.

6. Morrison, W. L., Gibson, J. N. A., and Rennie, M. J., Skeletal muscle and whole body protein turnover in cardiac cachexia: influence of branched-chain amino acid administration, *Eur. J. Clin. Invest.,* 18, 648, 1988.

7. Preedy, V. R. and Peters, T. J., Alcohol and skeletal muscle disease, *Alcohol Alcohol.,* 25, 177, 1990.

8. Hodges, D., Kumar, V. N., and Redford, J. B., Effects of alcohol on bone, muscle and nerve, *Am. Family Phys.,* 34, 149, 1986.

9. Persson, J., Berg, N. O., Sjolund, K., Stenling, R., and Magnusson, P. H., Morphologic changes in the small intestine after chronic alcohol consumption, *Scand. J. Gastroenterol.,* 25, 173, 1990.

10. Schreiber, S. S., Evans, C. D., Reff, F., Oratz, M., and Rothschild, M. A., Prolonged feeding of ethanol to the young growing guinea pig. II. A model to study the effects of severe ischemia on cardiac protein synthesis, *Alcohol. Clin. Exp. Res.,* 8, 54, 1984.

11. Kato, S., Murawaki, Y., and Hirayama, C., Effects of ethanol feeding on hepatic collagen synthesis and degradation in rats, *Res. Commun. Chem. Pathol. Pharmacol.,* 47, 163, 1985.

12. Bengtsson, G., Smith-Kielland, A., and Morland, J., Ethanol effects on protein synthesis in nonparenchymal liver cells, hepatocytes, and density populations of hepatocytes, *Exp. Mol. Pathol.,* 41, 44, 1984.

13. Koch, F. and Koch, G., Reversible inhibition of macromolecular synthesis in HeLa cells by ethanol, *Res. Commun. Chem. Pathol. Pharmacol.,* 9, 614, 1974.

14. Preedy, V. R., Pain, V. R., and Garlick, P. J., The metabolic state of muscle in the isolated perfused rat hemicorpus in relation to rates of protein synthesis, *Biochem. J.,* 218, 429, 1984.

15. Preedy, V. R. and Garlick, P. J., Protein synthesis in skeletal muscle of the perfused rat hemicorpus compared with rates in the intact animal, *Biochem. J.,* 214, 433, 1983.

16. Preedy, V. R., Smith, D. M., Kearney, N. F., and Sugden, P. H., Rates of protein turnover *in vivo* and *in vitro* in ventricular muscle of hearts from fed and starved rats, *Biochem. J.,* 222, 395, 1984.

17. Preedy, V. R., Smith, D. M., Kearney, N. F., and Sugden, P. H., Regional variation and differential sensitivity of rat heart protein synthesis *in vivo* and *in vitro, Biochem. J.,* 225, 487, 1985.

18. Preedy, V. R., Smith, D. M., and Sugden, P. H., A comparison of rates of protein turnover in rat diaphragm *in vivo* and *in vitro, Biochem. J.,* 233, 297, 1985.

19. Jefferson, L. S., Koehler, J. O., and Morgan, H. E., Effect of insulin on protein synthesis in skeletal muscle of an isolated perfused preparation of rat hemicorpus, *Proc. Natl. Acad. Sci. U.S.A.,* 69, 816, 1972.

20. Kaplan, J. H. and Pitot, H. C., The regulation of intermediary amino acid metabolism in animal tissues, in *Mammalian Protein Metabolism*, Vol. 4, Munro, H. N., Ed., Academic Press, New York, 1970, 387.

21. Fern, E. B. and Garlick, P. J., The specific radioactivity of the tissue free amino acid pool as a basis of measuring the rate of protein synthesis in the rat *in vivo*, *Biochem. J.*, 142, 413, 1974.

22. Bandyopadhyay, A. K. and Deutscher, M. P., Complex of aminoacyl-transfer RNA synthetase, *J. Mol. Biol.*, 60, 113, 1971.

23. Watt, P. W., Stenhouse, M. G., Corbett, M. E., and Rennie, M. J., tRNA charging in pig muscle during fasting and infusion of amino acids, *Clin. Nutr.*, 8, 47, 1989.

24. Fern, E. B. and Garlick, P. J., The specific radioactivity of the precursor pool for estimates of the rate of protein synthesis, *Biochem. J.*, 134, 1127, 1973.

25. Hagan, S. N. and Scow, R. O., Effect of fasting on muscle proteins and fat in young rats of different ages, *Am. J. Physiol.*, 188, 91, 1957.

26. Read, W. W., Read, M., Rennie, M. J., Griggs, R. C., and Halliday, D., Preparation of CO_2 from blood and protein bound amino acid carboxyl groups for quantitation of ^{13}C-isotope enrichments, *Biochem. Mass Spectrom.*, 11, 348, 1984.

27. McNurlan, M. A., Tomkins, A. M., and Garlick, P. J., The effect of starvation on the rate of protein synthesis in rat liver and small intestine, *Biochem. J.*, 178, 373, 1979.

28. Garlick, P. J., McNurlan, M. A., and Preedy, V. R., A rapid and convenient technique for measuring the rate of protein synthesis in tissues by injection of [³H]phenylalanine, *Biochem. J.*, 192, 719, 1980.

29. Garlick, P. J., Protein turnover in the whole animal and specific tissues, *Comp. Biochem.*, 19B, 77, 1980.

30. Hasselgren, P.-O., Pedersen, P., Sax, H. C., Warner, B. W., and Fischer, J. E., Methods for studying protein synthesis and degradation in liver and skeletal muscle, *J. Surg. Res.*, 45, 389, 1985.

31. Siddiq, T., Richardson, P. J., Hashim, I. A., and Preedy, V. R., Effect of acute anaesthesia on synthesis of contractile and non-contractile proteins of heart muscle and mixed proteins of type I and II fibre rich skeletal muscles of rat, *Cardiovasc. Res.*, 25, 314, 1991.

32. Preedy, V. R., Paska, L., Sugden, P. H., Schofield, P. S., and Sugden, M. C., The effects of surgical stress and short-term fasting on protein synthesis *in vivo* in diverse tissues of the mature rat, *Biochem. J.*, 250, 179, 1988.

33. Martinez, J. A., Validation of a fast, simple and reliable method to assess protein synthesis in individual tissues by intraperitoneal injection of a flooding dose of [³H]phenylalanine, *J. Biochem. Biophys. Methods*, 14, 349, 1987.

34. Jepson, M. M., Pell, J. M., Bates, P. C., and Millward, D. J., The effects of endotoxaemia on protein metabolism in skeletal muscle and liver of fed and fasted rats, *Biochem. J.*, 235, 329, 1986.

35. Preedy, V. R. and Peters, T. J., Changes in protein, RNA and DNA and rates of protein synthesis in muscle containing tissues of the mature rat in response to ethanol feeding: a comparative study of heart, small intestine and gastrocnemius muscle, *Alcohol Alcohol.*, 25, 489, 1990.

36. Peters, T. and Peters, J. C., The biosynthesis of rat serum albumin, *J. Biol. Chem.*, 247, 3858, 1972.

37. Garlick, P. J., Wernerman, J., McNurlan, M. A., Essen, P., Lobley, G. E., Milne, E., Calder, G. A., and Vinnars, E., Measurement of the rate of protein synthesis in muscle of postabsorptive young men by injection of a flooding dose of [1-^{13}C]leucine, *Clin. Sci.*, 77, 329, 1989.

38. Buse, M. G. and Reid, S. S., Leucine: a possible regulator of protein turnover in muscle, *J. Clin. Invest.*, 58, 1250, 1975.

39. Preedy, V. R. and Garlick, P. J., The influence of restraint and infusion on rates of muscle protein synthesis in the rat: effect of altered respiratory function, *Biochem. J.*, 251, 577, 1988.

40. Garlick, P. J., Fern, M., and Preedy, V. R., The effect of insulin infusion and food intake on muscle protein synthesis in postabsorptive rats, *Biochem. J.*, 210, 669, 1983.

41. Pomposelli, J. J., Palombo, J. D., Hamawy, K. J., Bistrian, B. R., Blackburn, G. L., and Moldawer, L. L., Comparison of different techniques for estimating rates of protein synthesis *in vivo* in healthy and bacteraemic rats, *Biochem. J.*, 226, 37, 1985.

42. Samarel, A. M., *In vivo* measurements of protein turnover during muscle growth and atrophy, *FASEB J.*, 5, 2020, 1991.

43. Preedy, V. R. and Peters, T. J., unpublished data.

44. Preedy, V. R. and Peters, T. J., unpublished data.

45. Marway, J. S. and Preedy, V. R., unpublished data.

46. Preedy, V. R., Hammond, B., Bottiglier, T. G., Marway, J. S., and Peters, T. J., Measurement of protein synthesis by the flooding dose technique: effect of phenylalanine and anaesthesia on plasma electrolytes, enzyme and metabolite levels, *J. Pharm. Pharmacol.*, 42, 851, 1990.

47. Preedy, V. R. and Garlick, P. J., The response of muscle protein synthesis to nutrient intake in postabsorptive rats: the role of insulin and amino acids, *Biosci. Rep.*, 6, 177, 1986.

48. Preedy, V. R. and Garlick, P. J., The effect of glucagon administration on protein synthesis in skeletal muscles, heart and liver *in vivo*, *Biochem. J.*, 228, 575, 1985.

49. Preedy, V. R. and Garlick, P. J., Inhibition of protein synthesis by glucagon in different rat muscles and protein fractions *in vivo* and in the perfused rat hemicorpus, *Biochem. J.*, 251, 727, 1988.

50. Young, V. R., Alexis, S. D., Baliga, B. S., Munro, H. N., and Muecke, W., Metabolism of administered 3-methylhistidine. Lack of muscle transfer ribonucleic acid charging and quantitative excretion as 3-methylhistidine and its N-acetyl derivative, *J. Biol. Chem.*, 247, 3592, 1972.

51. Asatoor, A. M. and Armstrong, M. D., 3-Methylhistidine, a component of actin, *Biochem. Biophys. Res. Commun.*, 26, 168, 1967.

52. Johnson, P., Harris, C. I., and Perry, S. V., 3-Methylhistidine in actin and other muscle proteins, *Biochem. J.*, 105, 361, 1967.

53. Young, V. R. and Munro, H. N., N^T-Methylhistidine (3-methylhistidine) and muscle protein turnover: an overview, *Fed. Proc.*, 37, 2291, 1978.

54. Tomas, F. M., Munro, H. M., and Young, V. R., Effect of glucocorticoid administration on the rate of muscle protein breakdown *in vivo* in rats, as measured by urinary excretion of N^T-methylhistidine, *Biochem. J.*, 178, 139, 1979.

55. Millward, D. J., Bates, P. C., Grimble, G. K., Brown, J. G., Nathan, M., and Rennie, M. J., Quantitative importance of non-skeletal muscle sources of N^T-methylhistidine in urine, *Biochem. J.*, 190, 225, 1980.

56. Preedy, V. R., McNurlan, M. A., and Garlick, P. J., Protein synthesis in skin and bone of the young rat, *Br. J. Nutr.*, 49, 517, 1983.

57. McNurlan, M. A. and Garlick, P. J., Contribution of rat liver and gastro-intestinal tract to whole-body synthesis in the rat, *Biochem. J.*, 180, 381, 1980.

58. Preedy, V. R. and Garlick, P. J., Rates of protein synthesis in skin and bone, and their importance in the assessment of protein degradation in the perfused rat hemicorpus, *Biochem. J.*, 194, 373, 1981.

59. Afting, E. G., Bernhardt, W., Janzen, R. W. C., and Rothig, H. J., Quantitative importance of non-skeletal muscle N^T-methylhistidine and creatinine in human urine, *Biochem. J.*, 200, 449, 1981.

60. Robins, S. P., Turnover and cross-linking of collagen, in *Collagen in Health & Disease*, Weiss, J. B. and Jayson, M. I. V., Eds., Churchill Livingstone, Edinburgh, 1982, 160.

61. Black, D., Duncan, A., and Robins, S. P., Quantitative analysis of the pyridinium crosslinks of collagen in urine using ion-paired, reversed-phase, high-performance liquid chromatography, *Anal. Biochem.*, 169, 197, 1988.

62. Preedy, V. R. and Peters, T. J., The effect of chronic ethanol ingestion on synthesis and degradation of soluble, contractile and stromal protein fractions of skeletal muscles from immature and mature rats, *Biochem. J.*, 259, 261, 1989.

63. Goldspink, D. F. and Lewis, S. E. M., Age- and activity-related changes in three proteinase enzymes of rat skeletal muscle, *Biochem. J.*, 230, 833, 1985.

64. Tiernan, J. M. and Ward, L. C., Acute effects of ethanol on protein synthesis in the rat, *Alcohol Alcohol.*, 21, 171, 1986.

65. Cook, E. A., Preece, J. A., Robin, S. D. M., Sugden, M. C., Cox, D. J., and Palmer, T. N., Acute inhibition by ethanol of intestinal absorption of glucose and hepatic glycogen synthesis on glucose refeeding after starvation in the rat, *Biochem. J.*, 254, 59, 1988.

66. Jauhonen, V. P. and Hassinen, I. E., Metabolic and hormonal changes during intravenous infusions of ethanol, acetaldehyde and acetate in normal and adrenalectomized rats, *Arch. Biochem. Biophys.*, 191, 358, 1978.

67. Lieber, C. S., Jones, D. P., and DeCarli, L. M., Fatty liver, hyperlipemia and hyperuricaemia produced by prolonged alcohol consumption despite adequate dietary intake, *Trans. Assoc. Am. Phys.*, 76, 289, 1963.

68. Preedy, V. R., Duane, P., and Peters, T. J., Biological effects of chronic ethanol consumption. A re-appraisal of the Lieber-De Carli liquid diet model with reference to skeletal muscle, *Alcohol Alcohol.*, 23, 151, 1988.

69. Halsted, C. H. and Keen, C. I., Alcoholism and micronutrient metabolism and deficiencies, *Eur. J. Gastroenterol. Hepatol.*, 2, 399, 1990.

70. Thomson, A. D., Vitamin deficiency and its role in alcoholic tissue damage, *Eur. J. Gastroenterol. Hepatol.*, 2, 411, 1990.

71. Thompson, R. P. H., Alcohol, nutrition and the liver, *Eur. J. Gastroenterol. Hepatol.*, 2, 417, 1990.

72. World, M. J., Ryle, P. R., and Thomson, A. D., Alcoholic malnutrition and the small intestine, *Alcohol Alcohol.*, 20, 89, 1985.

73. Preedy, V. R., Marway, J. S., and Peters, T. J., Use of the Lieber-DeCarli liquid feeding regime with specific reference to the effects of ethanol on rat skeletal muscle RNA, *Alcohol Alcohol.*, 24, 439, 1989.

74. Preedy, V. R., Hammond, B., Illes, R. A., Davies, S. E. C., Gandy, J. D., Chalmers, R. A., and Peters, T. J., Urinary excretion of nitrogenous and non-nitrogenous compounds in the chronic ethanol-fed rat, *Clin. Sci.*, 80, 393, 1991.

75. Hanid, A., Slavin, G., Mair, W., Sowter, C., Ward, P., Webb, J., and Levi, A., Fibre type changes in striated muscle of alcoholics, *J. Clin. Pathol.*, 34, 991, 1981.

76. Martin, F. C., Slavin, G., Levi, A. J., and Peters, T. J., Investigation of the organelle pathology of skeletal muscle in chronic alcoholism, *J. Clin. Pathol.*, 37, 448, 1984.

77. Martin, F. C., Ward, K., Slavin, G., Levi, A. J., and Peters, T. J., Alcoholic skeletal myopathy, a clinical and pathological study, *Q. J. Med.*, 55, 233, 1985.

78. Urbano-Marquez, A., Estruch, R., Navarro-Lopez, F., Grau, J. M., Mont, L., and Rubin, E., The effect of alcoholism on skeletal and cardiac muscle, *N. Engl. J. Med.*, 320, 409, 1989.

79. Worden, R. E., Pattern of muscle and nerve pathology in alcoholism, *Ann. N.Y. Acad. Sci.*, 273, 351, 1976.

80. Faris, A. A., Reyes, M. G., and Abrams, B. M., Subclinical alcoholic myopathy: electromyographic and biopsy study, *Trans. Am. Neurol. Assoc.*, 92, 102, 1967.

81. Duane, P. and Peters, T. J., Nutritional status in alcoholics with or without skeletal muscle myopathy, *Alcohol Alcohol.*, 23, 271, 1988.

82. Pacy, P. J., Preedy, V. R., Peters, T. J., Read, M., and Halliday, D., The effect of chronic alcohol ingestion on whole body and muscle protein synthesis—a stable isotope study, *Alcohol Alcohol.*, 26, 505, 1991.

83. Martin, F. C. and Peters, T. J., Assessment *in vitro* and *in vivo* of muscle protein degradation in chronic skeletal muscle myopathy of alcoholism, *Clin. Sci.*, 68, 693, 1985.

84. Preedy, V. R. and Peters, T. J., The effect of chronic ethanol ingestion on protein metabolism in Type I and Type II fibre-rich skeletal muscles of the rat, *Biochem. J.*, 254, 631, 1988.

85. Preedy, V. R. and Peters, T. J., The effect of chronic ethanol feeding on body and plasma composition and rates of skeletal muscle protein turnover in the rat, *Alcohol Alcohol.*, 23, 217, 1988.

86. Marway, J. S., Preedy, V. R., and Peters, T. J., Experimental alcoholic skeletal muscle myopathy is characterised by a rapid and sustained decrease in muscle RNA content, *Alcohol Alcohol.*, 25, 401, 1990.

87. Preedy, V. R., Bateman, C. J., Salisbury, J. R., Price, A. B., and Peters, T. J., Ethanol-induced skeletal muscle myopathy: biochemical and histochemical measurements on Type I and Type II fibre-rich muscles in the young rat, *Alcohol Alcohol.*, 24, 533, 1989.

88. Preedy, V. R. and Peters, T. J., The acute effects of ethanol on protein synthesis in different muscles and muscle protein fractions of the rat, *Clin. Sci.*, 74, 461, 1988.

89. Preedy, V. R., Duane, P., and Peters, T. J., Comparison of the acute effects of ethanol on liver and skeletal muscle protein synthesis in the rat, *Alcohol Alcohol.*, 23, 155, 1988.

90. Ward, R. J., Venkatesan, S., Swe, T. N., Preedy, V. R., Price, A. B., and Peters, T. J., An animal model of alcohol-induced myopathy, *Clin. Sci.*, 73(Suppl. 17), 53p, 1987.

91. Tiernan, J. M. and Ward, L. C., N^T(3)methylhistidine excretion by ethanol-fed rats, *IRCS Med. Sci.*, 12, 945, 1984.

92. Cook, E., Palmer, T. N., Peters, T. J., and Preedy, V. R., unpublished data.

93. Robles, E. A., Mezey, E., Halsted, C. H., and Schuster, M. M., Effect of ethanol on motility of the small intestine, *John Hopkins Med. J.*, 135, 17, 1974.

94. Berenson, M. M. and Avner, D. L., Alcohol inhibition of rectosigmoid motility in humans, *Digestion*, 22, 210, 1981.

95. Willson, C. A., Bushnell, D., and Keshavarzian, A., The effect of acute and chronic ethanol acministration on gastric emptying in cats, *Dig. Dis. Sci.*, 35, 444, 1990.

96. Preedy, V. R. and Peters, T. J., Protein metabolism in the small intestine of the ethanol-fed rat, *Cell. Biochem. Funct.*, 7, 235, 1989.

97. Preedy, V. R. and Peters, T. J., Protein synthesis of muscle fractions from the small intestine in alcohol-fed rats, *Gut*, 31, 305, 1990.

98. Preedy, V. R., Duane, P., and Peters, T. J., Acute ethanol dosage reduces the synthesis of smooth muscle contractile proteins in the small intestine of the rat, *Gut*, 29, 1244, 1988.

99. Marway, J. S. and Preedy, V. R., unpublished data.

100. Marway, J. S. and Preedy, V. R., unpublished data.

101. Marway, J. S. and Preedy, V. R., unpublished data.

102. Bode, J. C., Alcohol and the gastrointestinal tract, *Adv. Intern. Med.*, 45, 1, 1980.

103. Pares, X., Moreno, A., Cederlund, E., Hoog, J.-O., and Jornvall, J., Class IV mammalian alcohol dehydrogenase, *FEBS Lett.*, 277, 115, 1990.

104. Puszkin, S. and Rubin, E., Adenosine diphosphate effect on contractility of human actomyosin. Inhibition by ethanol and acetaldehyde, *Science*, 188, 1319, 1975.

105. Rossi, M. A., Alcohol and malnutrition in the pathogenesis of experimental alcoholic cardiomyopathy, *Pathology*, 130, 105, 1980.

106. Preedy, V. R. and Peters, T. J., Synthesis of subcellular protein fractions in the rat heart *in vivo* in response to chronic ethanol feeding, *Cardiovasc. Res.*, 23, 730, 1989.

107. Preedy, V. R. and Peters, T. J., The acute and chronic effects of ethanol on cardiac muscle protein synthesis in the rat *in vivo*, *Alcohol*, 7, 97, 1990.

108. Deitrich, R. A., Troxell, P. A., and Worth, W. S., Inhibition of aldehyde dehydrogenase in brain and liver by cyanamide, *Biochem. Pharmacol.*, 25, 2733, 1976.

109. Lieber, C. S. and DeCarli, L. M., The role of hepatic microsomal ethanol oxidizing system (MEOS) for ethanol metabolism *in vivo*, *J. Pharmacol. Exp. Ther.*, 181, 279, 1972.

110. Siddiq, T. and Preedy, V. R., unpublished data.

111. Siddiq, T. and Preedy, V. R., unpublished data.

112. Saville, P. D., Changes in bone mass with age and alcoholism, *J. Bone Jt. Surg.*, 47, 492, 1965.

113. Diamond, T., Stiel, D., Lunzer, M., Wilkinson, M., and Posen, S., Ethanol reduces bone formation and may cause osteoporosis, *Am. J. Med.*, 86, 282, 1989.

114. Crilly, R. G., Anderson, C., Hogan, D., and Delaquerriere-Richardson, L., Bone histomorphometry, bone mass and related parameters in alcoholic males, *Calc. Tissue Int.*, 43, 269, 1988.

115. Feitelberg, S., Epstein, S., Ismail, F., and D'Amanda, C., Deranged bone mineral metabolism in chronic alcoholism, *Metab. Clin. Exp.*, 36, 322, 1987.

116. Preedy, V. R. and Peters, T. J., unpublished data.

117. Preedy, V. R., Baldwin, D. R., Keating, J. W., and Salisbury, J. R., Bone collagen, mineral and trace element composition, histomorphometry and urinary hydroxyproline excretion in chronically-treated alcohol-fed rats, *Alcohol Alcohol.*, 26, 39, 1991.

118. Preedy, V. R., Sherwood, R. A., Akpoguma, C. I. O., and Black, D., The urinary excretion of the collagen degradation markers pyridinoline and deoxypyridinoline in an experimental rat model of alcoholic bone disease, *Alcohol Alcohol.*, 26, 191, 1991.

119. Lieber, C. S., Alcohol, protein metabolism and liver injury, *Gastroenterology*, 79, 373, 1980.

120. Achord, J. L., Nutrition, alcohol and the liver, *Am. J. Gastroenterol.*, 83, 244, 1988.

121. Mitchell, M. C. and Herlong, H. F., Alcohol and nutrition: caloric value, bioenergetics, and the relationship to liver damage, *Annu. Rev. Nutr.*, 6, 457, 1986.

122. Keyser, J. W., Secretory liver proteins in disease, in *Plasma Protein Secretion by the Liver*, Glaumann, H., Peters, T., and Redman, C., Eds., Academic Press, London, 1983, 453.

123. Baraona, E., Leo, M. A., Borowsky, S. A., and Lieber, C. S., Alcoholic hepatomegaly: accumulation of protein in the liver, *Science*, 190, 794, 1975.

124. Lieber, C. S. and DeCarli, L. M., Hepatotoxicity of ethanol, *J. Hepatol.*, 12, 394, 1991.

125. Leblond-Francillard, M., Augereau, C., Nalpas, B., Trinchet, J. C., Hartmann, D. J., Beaugrand, M., and Brechot, C., Liver collagen mRNA and serum amino-terminal peptide of type III procollagen (PIIINP) levels in patients with alcoholic liver disease, *J. Hepatol.*, 9, 351, 1989.

126. Hartmann, D. J., Trinchet, J. C., Ricard-Blum, S., Beaugrand, M., Callard, P., and Ville, G., Radioimmunoassay of type I collagen detects mainly degradation products in human serum. Application to patients with liver disease, *Clin. Chem.*, 36, 421, 1990.

127. Rohde, H., Vargas, L., Hahn, E., Kalbfleisch, H., Bruguera, M., and Timpl, R., Radioimmunoassay for type III procollagen peptide and its application to human liver disease, *Eur. J. Clin. Invest.*, 9, 451, 1979.

128. Wallin, B., Bessesen, A., Fikke, A.-M., Aarbakke, J., and Morland, J., No effect of acute ethanol administration on hepatic protein synthesis and export in the rat *in vivo, Alcohol. Clin. Exp. Res.*, 8, 191, 1984.

129. Smith-Kielland, A., Blom, G. P., Bessesen, A., and Morland, J., A study of hepatic protein synthesis, three subcellular enzymes, and liver morphology in chronically ethanol-fed rats, *Acta Pharmacol. Toxicol.*, 53, 113, 1983.

130. Donohue, T. M., Sorrell, M. F., and Tuma, D. J., Hepatic protein synthetic activity *in vivo* after ethanol administration, *Alcohol. Clin. Exp. Res.*, 11, 80, 1987.

131. Preedy, V. R. and Peters, T. J., An investigation into the effects of chronic ethanol feeding on hepatic mixed protein synthesis in immature and mature rats, *Alcohol Alcohol.*, 24, 311, 1989.

132. McDonald, J. M. T. and Margen, S., Wine versus ethanol in human nutrition. I. Nitrogen and calorie balance, *Am. J. Clin. Nutr.*, 29, 1093, 1976.

133. Atwater, W. D. and Benedict, F. G., An experimental inquiry regarding the nutritive value of alcohol, *Mem. Natl. Acad. Sci.*, 8, 235, 1902.

134. Bunout, D., Petermann, M., Ugarte, G., Barrera, G., and Iturriage, H., Nitrogen economy in alcoholic patients without liver disease, *Metabolism*, 36, 651, 1987.

135. Gruchow, H. W., Sobocinski, K. A., Barboriak, J. J., and Scheller, J. G., Alcohol consumption, nutrient intake and relative body weight among USA adults, *Am. J. Clin. Nutr.*, 42, 289, 1985.

136. Colditz, G. A., Giovannucci, E., Rimm, E. B., Stampfer, M. J., Rosner, B., Speizer, F. E., Gordis, E., and Willett, W. C., Alcohol intake in relation to diet and obesity in women and men, *Am. J. Clin. Nutr.*, 54, 49, 1991.

137. Romieu, I., Willett, W. C., Stampfer, M. J., Colditz, G. A., Sampson, L., Rosner, B., Hennekens, C. H., and Speizer, F. E., Energy intake and other determinants of relative weight, *Am. J. Clin. Nutr.*, 47, 406, 1988.

138. Pirola, R. C. and Lieber, C. S., The energy cost of the metabolism of drugs, including ethanol, *Pharmacology*, 7, 185, 1972.

139. Jones, B. R., Barrett-Connor, E., Criqui, M. H., and Holdbrook, M. J., A community study of calorie and nutrient intake in drinkers and non-drinkers of alcohol, *Am. J. Clin. Nutr.*, 35, 135, 1982.

140. Pirola, R. C. and Lieber, C. S., Hypothesis. Energy wastage in alcoholism and drug abuse: possible role of hepatic microsomal enzymes, *Am. J. Clin. Nutr.*, 29, 90, 1976.

141. Israel, Y., Kalant, H., Orrego, J. H., Khanna, L., Videla, L., and Phillips, J. M., Experimental alcohol-induced hepatic necrosis: suppression by propylthiouracil, *Proc. Natl. Acad. Sci. U.S.A.*, 72, 1137, 1975.

142. Blachley, J. D., Johnson, J. H., and Knochel, J. P., The harmful effects of ethanol on ion transport and cellular respiration, *Am. J. Med. Sci.*, 289, 22, 1985.

143. Reinus, J. F., Heymsfield, S. B., Wiskind, R., Casper, K., and Galambos, J. T., Ethanol: relative fuel value and metabolic effects *in vivo, Metabolism,* 38, 125, 1989.

144. Mathews, D. E. and Cobelli, C., Leucine metabolism in man: lessons from modeling, *J. Parenteral Enteral Nutr.*, 15, 86S, 1991.

145. Rodrigo, C., Antezana, C., and Baraona, E., Fat and nitrogen balance in rats with alcohol-induced fatty live, *J. Nutr.*, 101, 1307, 1971.

146. Klatskin, G., The effect of ethyl alcohol on nitrogen excretion in the rat, *Yale J. Biol. Med.*, 34, 124, 1961.

147. Newsholme, E. A. and Leech, A. R., *Biochemistry for the Medical Sciences,* John Wiley & Sons, Chichester, U.K., 1983, 481.

148. Preedy, V. R., Marway, J. S., Salisbury, J. R., and Peters, T. J., Protein synthesis in bone and skin of the rat are inhibited by ethanol: implication for whole-body metabolism, *Alcohol. Clin. Exp. Res.*, 14, 165, 1990.

149. Preedy, V. R., Venkatesan, S., Peters, T. J., Nott, D. M., Yates, J., and Jenkins, S. A., Effect of chronic ethanol ingestion on tissue RNA and blood flow in skeletal muscle with comparative reference to bone and tissues of the gastrointestinal tract of the rat, *Clin. Sci.*, 76, 243, 1989.

150. Nott, D. M., Yates, J., Preedy, V. R., Venkatesan, S., Peters, T. J., and Jenkins, S. A., Effect of chronic ethanol administration on hepatic hae-modynamics and reticuloendothelial function in the rat, *Br. J. Surg.*, 77, A703, 1990.

151. Cook, E., Preedy, V. R., Peters, T. J., and Palmer, T. N., unpublished data.

152. Ward, L. C., Carrington, L. E., and Daly, R., Ethanol and leucine oxidation. I. Leucine oxidation by the rat *in vivo, Int. J. Biochem.*, 17, 187, 1985.

153. Lundquist, F., Sestoft, L., Damgaard, S. E., Clausen, J. P., and Trap-Jensen, J., Utilization of acetate in the human forearm during exercise after ethanol ingestion, *J. Clin. Invest.*, 52, 3231, 1973.

154. Karlsson, N., Fellenius, E., and Kiessling, K. H., The metabolism of acetate in the perfused hind-quarter of the rat, *Acta Physiol. Scand.*, 93, 391, 1975.

155. Suokas, A., Forsander, O., and Lindros, K., Distribution and utilization of alcohol-derived acetate in the rat, *J. Stud. Alcohol.*, 45, 381, 1984.

156. Garcia-Brunel, L., Lipid peroxidation in alcoholic myopathy and cardio-myopathy, *Med. Hypoth.*, 13, 217, 1984.

157. Ward, R. J., Jutla, J., Duane, P. D., and Peters, T. J., Reduced anti-oxidant status in patients with chronic alcoholic myopathy, *Biochem. Soc. Trans.*, 16, 581, 1988.

158. Sugden, P. H. and Fuller, S. J., Regulation of protein turnover in skeletal and cardiac muscle, *Biochem. J.*, 273, 21, 1991.

159. Young, V. R., Role of skeletal and cardiac muscle in the regulation of body protein metabolism, in *Mammalian Protein Metabolism,* Vol. 4, Munro, H. N., Ed., Academic Press, New York, 1970, 585.

160. Preedy, V. R. and Peters, T. J., unpublished data.

161. Harbitz, I., Wallin, B., Hauge, J. G., and Morland, J., Effect of ethanol metabolism on initiation of protein synthesis in rat hepatocytes, *Biochem. Pharmacol.*, 33, 3465, 1984.

162. Cox, S. and Proud, C. G., The effect of ethanol on polypeptide chain initiation in reticulocytes. Inhibition of recycling of initiation factor eIF-2, *Biochem. Pharmacol.*, 37, 2045, 1988.

163. Stein, T. P., Nutrition and protein turnover: a review, *J. Parenteral Enteral Nutr.*, 6, 444, 1982.

164. Preedy, V. R. and Peters, T. J., Alcohol, nutrition and muscle disease, *Eur. J. Gastroenterol. Hepatol.*, 2, 426, 1990.

165. Hickish, T., Colston, K. W., Bland, J. M., and Maxwell, J. D., Vitamin D deficiency and muscle strength in male alcoholics, *Clin. Sci.*, 77, 171, 1989.

166. Van Thiel, D. H. and Gavaler, J. S., Endocrine consequences of alcohol abuse, *Alcohol Alcohol.*, 25, 341, 1990.

167. Hudgson, P. and Hall, R., Endocrine myopathies, in *Skeletal Muscle Pathology*, Mastaglia, F. L. and Walton, J., Eds., Churchill Livingstone, Edinburgh, 1982, 393.

168. Duane, P. and Peters, T. J., Glucocorticosteroid status in chronic alcoholics with and without skeletal muscle myopathy, *Clin. Sci.*, 73, 601, 1987.

8 Effects of Dietary Fatty Acids and Alcohol on Fatty Acid Composition in Cellular Membranes

INTRODUCTION

The consumption of ethanol has been shown to exert profound effects on cellular membranes which result in damage and/or adaptation. Both membrane lipids and proteins are affected, but because of the physico-chemical properties of ethanol, many of the membrane effects are directly related to the interaction of ethanol with the lipid component of the membrane. In addition to the direct lipid-ethanol interaction, ethanol has been shown to dramatically alter lipid metabolism. This chapter focuses on the fatty acyl components of cellular membranes. Because the polyunsaturated fatty acids (PUFA) of these membranes must be supplied in the diet, the author also considers dietary fatty acids and their role in the overall relationships between ethanol and membrane acyl groups.

One of the major problems with many of the comparisons which we try to make with respect to the effects of ethanol on membrane and/or tissue fatty acid compositions is that several variables are in evidence that are difficult to control. No general consensus exists with respect to diet composition or the level or duration of exposure to ethanol. Each researcher has their own particular needs and designs their experiments accordingly. Many species of animal have been used, and each seem to have their own utility, but comparisons across species do present difficulties. There are several modes of ethanol delivery, but inhalation and liquid diet seem to be the most common. However, given all of the above-mentioned problems and differences in experimental approach many valid generalizations can be made which will probably stand the test of further research.

ISBN 0-8493-7933-4
© 1992 by CRC Press, Inc.

EFFECT OF ETHANOL ON
MEMBRANE FATTY ACYL GROUPS

What do we know about the effects of ethanol on the fatty acid composition of cellular membranes? Probably the most consistent finding has been that an increase occurs in linoleate (18:2n-6) and a decrease occurs in arachidonate (20:4n-6).[1-9] These changes are not confined to the PUFA of the n-6 family, but alterations also have been observed in the n-3 family.[6-9] Further, the diets with a medium to high fat content seem to accentuate these changes in 18:2n-6 and 20:4n-6, which almost always result in a decrease in the 20:4n-6/18:2n-6 ratio. Changes have been reported in both the C_{16} and C_{18} saturated and monoenoic fatty acids, but these fatty acids can be synthesized *de novo,* and it is not clear that the alterations actually reflect changes in dietary sources.

The increase in 18:2n-6 and the decrease in 20:4n-6 suggest that ethanol has altered the metabolic conversion of 18:2n-6 to 20:4n-6. The general consensus is that because the elongation reactions, which increase the chain length of the fatty acids, are much faster reactions compared to the desaturases, the acyl-CoA desaturases are the rate-limiting reactions in the biosynthesis of the C_{20} and C_{22} PUFA. *In vitro* studies with rats[10-12] have demonstrated that ethanol inhibits both the Δ^5- and Δ^6-desaturases (Figure 1). The Δ^6-desaturase converts both 18:2n-6 and α-linolenic acid (18:3n-3) to γ-linolenic acid (18:3n-6) and 18:4n-3, respectively. After chain elongation, the Δ^5-desaturase converts dihomo-γ-linolenic acid (20:3n-6) to 20:4n-6 and 20:4n-3 to eicosapentaenoic acid (20:5n-3). Chain elongation must again take place followed by desaturation with the Δ^4-desaturase. Also shown in this figure is the comparable metabolism of stearic acid to acids of the n-9 family; however, desaturation and chain elongation of oleic acid (18:1n-9) only occurs during situations in which PUFA from the other two families, n-6 and n-3, are absent from the diet for prolonged periods of time. When this occurs the conditions of essential fatty acid (EFA) deficiency call for the cell to increase its amount of PUFA by synthesizing the n-9 PUFA. Thus, the Δ^6- and Δ^5-desaturases are key enzymes in the metabolic conversions of dietary C_{18} PUFA to C_{20} and C_{22} PUFA of both n-6 and n-3 families, and, in certain situations, the n-9 family. Because ethanol ingestion has been shown to decrease their activity, these two enzymes have been strongly implicated in many of the alterations observed in the acyl group composition of many cellular membranes after

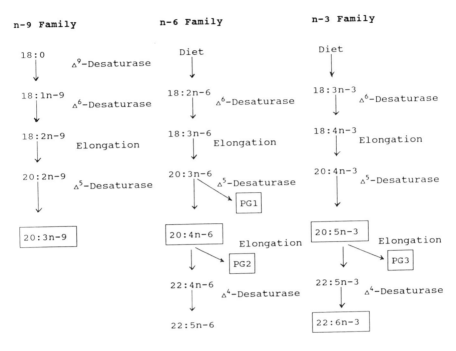

FIGURE 1. The fatty acids enclosed in boxes represent the major PUFA that are found to accumulate in membranes. Three of the fatty acids give rise to prostaglandins, and these conversions are represented by PG enclosed in boxes. Ethanol has been shown to have an effect on all of the desaturases except the Δ^4-desaturase.[10-12]

ethanol ingestion or inhalation. In support of the regulatory effects of the acyl-CoA desaturases, feeding diets containing oil of the evening primrose (10%), an oil rich in 18:3n-6, resulted in a doubling of the amount of 20:3n-6 in liver phospholipids of the Golden Syrian hamster after 4 weeks of feeding ethanol in the drinking water.[13] A similar finding was reported for platelets from rats on an 11% borage oil diet.[14] Borage oil contains 24% 18:3n-6 compared to 9% for evening primrose oil. The 18:3n-6 found in these two oils bypasses the Δ^6-desaturase and, thus, the effect of ethanol on the Δ^6-desaturase. Also shown in Figure 1 is another important use of the C_{20} PUFA, the conversion to various prostaglandins. Discussions relating to these metabolic pathways can be found elsewhere in this volume.

While the n-6 family of PUFA clearly has been established as EFAs, evidence is being accumulated to delineate the essential nature of the n-3 family of PUFA.[15-17] The biochemical indicators of EFA deficiency, i.e., the 20:3n-9/20:4n-6 ratio, have been noted to be amplified by ethanol in animals fed an EFA-deficient diet.[18] In noncirrhotic humans, an increase in PUFA derived from 18:2n-6 and 18:3n-3 has been observed, and cirrhosis resulted in an increase in PUFA. Further, alcoholism seemed to amplify this abnormal PUFA pattern by specifically resulting in an increase in the 20:3n-9 fatty acid.[19] Johnson et al.[19] noted that cirrhosis seemed to be required for the development of deficiencies of PUFA in serum phospholipids. The fact that ethanol seems to be related to increases in the EFA marker, 20:3n-9, suggests that the changes in PUFA, such as the increase in 18:2n-6 and the decrease in 20:4n-6, may not simply be the result of alterations to the desaturases. Both the Δ^5- and the Δ^6-desaturases are required for the synthesis of 20:3n-9; therefore, this fatty acid should not increase after the ingestion of ethanol if these two desaturases play such an important role in the fatty acid composition of membrane phospholipids. In synaptosomes from mice treated for 2 h via ethanol inhalation, the concentration of 18:2n-6 was increased and the concentrations of 20:4n-6 and 22:6n-3 docosqhexaenoic acid (DHA) were significantly decreased.[20] These data implicate mechanisms other than the desaturases. The half-life of the hepatic Δ^9-desaturase has been reported to be 3 to 4 h,[21] and even though no half-lives have been reported for the Δ^5- or Δ^6-desaturases, they are probably of about the same magnitude. Thus, these time frames are too short to implicate the desaturases. Other rapid mechanisms such as mobilization or removal of PUFA may take preference in response to alterations in membrane fluidity caused by the shear presence of ethanol.[22,23]

In addition to the Δ^5- and Δ^6-desaturases, Δ^9-desaturase reportedly decreased after chronic ethanol consumption;[11,24] however, decreases in oleate generally have not been reported, but the opposite.[7,13,25-28] This probably results from the fact that almost all dietary oils have oleate as a major component. The Δ^9-desaturase is influenced more significantly by dietary lipids than the other two desaturases;[21] thus, the alterations in oleate composition in membranes of ethanol-treated animals may reflect dietary availability rather than direct ethanol effects.

Other enzymes may be responsible for alterations in the unsaturated fatty acid composition of the various phospholipids in tissue membranes. These involve phospholipase A_2 and the acyl-CoA:phospholipid acyltransferases. The interplay of these two groups of enzymes is largely responsible for the incorporation of PUFA containing three or more double bonds during the retailoring process for the de novo synthesized phospholipids.

Jain and Cordes[29] have reported that phospholipase A_2 can be activated by various alcohols, and Arai et al.[30] have reported an increase in phospholipase A_2 after chronic ethanol consumption. In the isolated perfused heart, both phospholipase A_1 and A_2 were activated by ethanol.[31] Ethanol given *in vitro* has been shown to increase the release of 20:4n-6 from intracellular pools in macrophages, supporting the activation effects of ethanol on phospholipase A_2.[32] Gastaldi et al.[33] have demonstrated that erythrocytes from alcoholic patients incorporated 18:1 more readily into phosphatidylcholine (PC) and phosphatidylethanolamine (PE) than controls and that incorporation into PC was stimulated more than that into PE. Thus, both groups of enzymes responsible for the turnover of fatty acyl groups into the major phospholipids of cellular membranes are activated in some manner by ethanol. Tissue specificity for these changes in these two enzyme groups has not been measured. This would be useful to more clearly define the precise role that de- and reacylation play in altering the membrane fatty acyl groups of the various phospholipids.

Most studies report a general decrease in the PUFA fraction in membranes or in tissues. Due to the high concentrations of 18:2n-6 and 20:4n-6 in most membranes, the decreases in these two fatty acids usually account for the PUFA decreases. Further, a greater decrease in 20:4n-6 than 18:2n-6 generally occurs, leading to a decrease in the 20:4n-6/18:2n-6 ratio. In a few isolated papers, increases have been reported in the 22:6n-3 fatty acid after ethanol consumption,[7,13] but no mechanisms have been discussed for this observation.

ROLE OF DIETARY FAT

That different animals eliminate ethanol from the blood at different rates has been demonstrated repeatedly.[34-39] Thus, the possibility that the different effects of ethanol upon liver lipids may have been related to the use of different animals and their respective differences in rates of ethanol elimination. Further, the diets used by various researchers varied considerably. The normal chow diet for rats is a low-fat diet containing about 4.6% of calories as fat. Because the fat content of the typical U.S. diet is in the neighborhood of 40%, Lieber and DeCarli[40] designed the most widely used liquid diet for alcohol studies in animals. This liquid diet is a high-fat diet containing 36% of calories as fat. Using coconut and linseed oils, which contain fatty acids not normally present in the diet, Lieber et al.[41]

demonstrated that the fat content of the liver largely depended on dietary lipid. Lieber and DeCarli[42] further showed that maximum steatosis occurred when the dietary level of fat was 43% and minimum steatosis occurred at 10%. Zaki et al.[43] earlier noted that the severity of fatty liver disease seemed to be related to the amount of fat in the diet. Thus, it has been understood for quite some time that a direct relationship exists between dietary fat and the effects of ethanol on the liver.

With the development of a completely liquid diet,[4] the study of the effects of dietary lipids could be further expanded to include the use of high blood ethanol concentrations normally difficult to produce in the rat due to the high metabolic rate of ethanol oxidation by this animal. Using this dietary protocol, French and co-workers[44] have clearly shown that high blood alcohol levels could produce progressive steatosis and focal necrosis in rat liver when a low-fat diet was used. Further, they have shown that by increasing dietary fat from 5 to 25% they could induce hepatic fibrosis.[45] Thus, it can be concluded that high dietary fat is necessary for liver fibrosis to be induced by ethanol in the rat.

Not only is the level of fat of significance in producing deleterious effects upon the liver, but recent reports suggest that the kind of dietary fat is of equal importance. In fact, certain types of fat may be quite beneficial in protecting the liver against the damaging effects of ethanol. Nanji and French[46] conducted an epidemiological study of data from 17 countries and concluded that diets high in saturated fat and cholesterol seemed to protect against alcoholic cirrhosis while diets high in PUFA seemed to promote cirrhosis. In addition, the countries which have a high saturated fat intake also have been shown to have a strong correlation between mortality from cirrhosis and pork consumption.[47] These and other observations[45,48-50] suggested that different fats may affect the severity of alcoholic liver disease (ALD). Further experimentation has shown that beef tallow protected against the ethanol-induced liver disease.[51] The latter studies[51] provide a strong correlation between dietary 18:2n-6 and the histopathological abnormalities of ALD observed in this rat model.

Other studies have demonstrated that dietary fat and/or dietary fatty acids may alter ethanol-induced injury to a variety of cell types. The administration of arachidonic acid 30 or 60 min prior to ethanol provided protection to the gastric mucosa.[52] This protection was diminished by indomethacin pretreatment, thus implicating prostaglandins in the mechanism. In another set of experiments, this same group showed that a single oral dose of 37 mg of 20:4n-6 protected the liver against acute ethanol injury.[53] In other experiments, Rao's laboratory[54] showed that diets containing 7% of the 39.6% fat as 20:4n-6 reduced the ethanol-induced liver triacylglycerol levels, but later experiments using a pair-feeding protocol did not confirm this effect of 20:4n-6.[55] Stern et al.[56] also arrived at the conclusion that when using a pair-feeding protocol 20:4n-6 did not protect against the development of a fatty liver. If anything, 20:4n-6 seemed to accentuate the ethanol-induced fatty liver. Another study in mice[57] suggested that 20:4n-6 could protect against ethanol-induced fatty liver, but the level of protection was quite small. Using fish oil ω-3 fatty acids, the increases in liver and plasma cholesterol and triglyceride were blocked.[58] In addition, the effects of ethanol on plasma apolipoprotein A_1 and apolipoprotein E from HDL were reversed by the ω-3 fatty acids. It was concluded that ω-3 fatty acids can prevent and reverse some of the lipid and lipoprotein abnormalities caused by ethanol ingestion.

Many of the abnormalities noted above with respect to dietary fat and ethanol also reflect abnormalities in various membranes. Engler et al.[14] showed that feeding borage oil, an oil similar to that of evening primrose in that it contains a high level of 18:3n-6, increased the n-6 fatty acids (18:3n-6, 20:3n-6, 20:4n-6), and that feeding a mixture of linseed oil, an oil containing high levels of 18:3n-3, and safflower oil, an oil rich in 18:2n-6, increased the n-3 fatty acids (18:3n-3, 20:5n-3, 22:6n-3) in aorta and platelets. The effect of ethanol inhalation for 6 d was to mainly decrease 20:4n-6 in the platelet in the n-3 fatty acid diet. It was concluded that the diet rich in 18:3n-6 (borage oil) was able to protect against the ethanol-induced alterations in platelet fatty acid compositions. A decrease in the 20:4n-6/18:2n-6 ratio was observed with all three diets. Wainwright et al.[59] have presented evidence that using dietary n-3 fatty acids may reduce slightly some of the effects of ethanol on neurobehavioral development. In a companion paper,[50] they demonstrated that prenatal ethanol consumption altered the fatty acid composition of the developing brain, which lasted beyond the immediate period of drinking, and that dietary fatty acids could alter this effect. Cunnane et al.[13] have shown that ethanol altered the fatty acids of plasma and liver differently depending upon the type of dietary fatty acids (n-6 or n-3). They fed safflower oil (78% 18:2n-6), evening primrose oil (71% 18:2n-6, 9% 18:3n-6), and linseed oil (45% 18:3n-3, 21% 18:2n-6). Ethanol caused a decrease in liver phospholipid 18:2n-6 in all three diets, but an increase in 20:4n-6 was observed only in the primrose oil diet. Also observed only in the primrose oil diet was an ethanol-induced increase in 20:3n-6. An increase in 22:6n-3 was also observed in platelets from animals fed borage oil.[14] Ethanol caused an increase in 22:6n-3 in all three diets, but there was a greater increase after feeding the linseed oil diet. Further, feeding the linseed oil diet without ethanol reduced by half the amount of arachidonic acid and increased the amount of 22:6n-3 over three times. Thus, not only do dietary fatty acids significantly alter the fatty acid composition of tissues and membranes, but they alter the effect of ethanol upon the fatty acid composition of the same tissues and membranes.

EFFECTS ON SPECIFIC MEMBRANES

The following discussion focuses on a few studies that have isolated specific subcellular membrane fractions and determined the effects of ethanol on the fatty acid composition.

MICROSOMES

Microsomes from rats fed a diet for 308 d containing 8% fat (2% corn oil and 6% hydrogenated cottonseed oil[3]) had almost the same content of 18:2n-6 and 20:4n-6 as did rats fed a chow diet for only 30 d.[61] As a result of the dietary fat, the chow-fed animals had considerably more 22:6n-3 (12.6%) than did the animals fed the hydrogenated cottonseed oil (3%). Ethanol feeding resulted in increases in 18:2n-6 in both groups, but a greater decrease occurred in 20:4n-6 in the chow-fed animals. In another study,[62] the Lieber-DeCarli diet[40] was used, and this diet provided 35% of calories as a mixture of corn and olive oil fat. The dietary effects were quite similar to those of the corn oil/hydrogenated cottonseed oil,[3] but ethanol had little or no effect on the composition of any of the PUFA. Clearly the diet has modified the acyl composition, and ethanol feeding has resulted in selected effects, possibly depending upon the length of time on ethanol or the greater availability of dietary PUFA from the chow-fed animals. The dietary effects can also be seen by comparing a study using monkeys fed butter as fat for 12 months.[25] First, the butter diet resulted in a significant increase in the 18:2n-6 and a significant decrease in the 20:4n-6 and the 22:6n-3 content of the microsomes. Second, the ethanol effect was not nearly so dramatic as seen in the rats. Slight decreases occurred in all three of these fatty acids. Again, it appears that dietary lipid has modified the effects of ethanol. In addition, differences in animal species may also exert an influence.

In another study, the effects of chronic ethanol ingestion on the fatty acids of the four major phospholipids of liver microsomes were measured.[7] The dietary oil was the Lieber-DeCarli mixture noted above. Ethanol increased 18:2n-9 only in the PC and PE fractions. After ethanol, the 20:4n-6 was decreased in all fractions but the PE. The PE and the phosphatidylserine (PS) fractions have the largest amount of 22:6n-3, and ethanol decreased this acid in both of these fractions. Thus, ethanol has differential effects depending upon which phospholipid is being questioned.

MITOCHRONDRIA

Increasing dietary corn oil from about 5% of calories[63] to about 35%[4] resulted in a large increase in the content of 18:2n-6 in mitochondrial membranes. A slight decrease in 20:4n-6 was observed. Ethanol ingestion resulted in an increase in 18:2n-6 and a decrease in 20:4n-6 in only the low-fat diet. Changing the dietary fat composition to include 7.5% olive oil and 2% ethyl linoleate while keeping the total fat concentration at 35% of calories resulted in an 18:2n-6 content considerably lower and a 20:4n-6 content slightly higher than the low-fat corn oil diet.[62] Ethanol ingestion did not alter the 18:2n-6 content, but significantly decreased the 20:4n-6 content. In another paper,[3] the percent of calories as fat was lowered to 10%, and the composition consisted of 2% corn oil and 8% hydrogenated cottonseed oil. This diet produced mitochondrial membranes with a fatty acid composition fairly similar to the low-fat diet.[63] Also, the effect of ethanol was similar: 18:2n-6 was increased and 20:4n-6 was decreased. Thus, increasing the fat to a medium level and increasing the saturation did not alter the fatty acid composition nor the effects of ethanol, yet a large increase in fat without alteration of the fatty acid composition seemed to eliminate the ethanol effect. Monkeys fed a high-fat (28%) butter diet[25] had mitochondria with the highest level of 18:2n-6 and the lowest level of 20:4n-6 of any of the five groups being compared. Ethanol slightly lowered both of these fatty acids, thus producing an effect quite different than any of the other dietary treatments.

RBC MEMBRANES

The effects of dietary lipids on the acyl composition of the RBC membrane cannot be assessed due to a lack of data, but the effects of ethanol are different than those in microsomes. Three studies using three different animal species (rats,[26] golden Syrian hamster,[28] and human alcoholics[64]) have produced very similar results on the content of several unsaturated fatty acids. The percentage of 18:1n-9 was increased in all cases, the percentage of 18:2n-6 and 22:6n-3 was decreased in all cases, and no change occurred in the percentage of 20:4n-6 in all cases. Thus, the RBC membrane seems to respond to ethanol similarly without respect for the animal species.

PLATELETS

Feeding sesame oil, borage oil, or an equal mixture of these produced a small increase in the percent of 18:2n-6 and a significant decrease in the percent of 20:4n-6 only when the mixture was used.[14] When ethanol was added to the diet, an increase occurred in 18:2n-6 only in the sesame oil-fed animals, and decreases took place in 20:4n-6 in the sesame oil-fed animals and in the animals fed the mixture of oils. Thus, it appears that dietary borage oil plays a dominant role in controlling the effects of ethanol on 18:2n-6, while sesame oil seems to have a greater effect with respect to 20:4n-6. The effect of the large amount of dietary 18:3n-6 (24%) from the borage oil was interesting in that it caused a marked increase in 20:3n-6 after ethanol ingestion. This also may have influenced the conversion of this acid to 20:4n-6, resulting in no decrease in this acid after ethanol. Again, dietary fats seem to play very important roles in altering the effects of ethanol on membrane acyl compositions.

SUMMARY

Much of the research relating to the effects of ethanol on cellular membranes has simply focused on just this idea; however, data are beginning to accumulate that demonstrate that some of the effects of ethanol on the acyl composition of membranes can be modulated by dietary fats. There still are too few studies to make broad generalizations regarding which oils are capable of reversing or altering the detrimental effects of ethanol, but there is ample room for studies which will utilize different dietary lipids to alter the effects of ethanol. It is quite clear that the amount of dietary fat is critical with regard to ALD and fibrosis. Further, the correlation of 18:2n-6 with ethanol-induced liver abnormalities suggests that diets such as those utilizing evening primrose oil or borage oil, i.e., containing 18:3n-6, and those utilizing various fish oils, i.e., containing the n-3 family of fatty acids, should be studied in much more detail.

REFERENCES

1. Turchetto, E., Ottani, V., Zanetti, P., and Weiss, H., Hepatic fatty acids after ethanol ingestion, *Nutr. Diet Basal,* 10, 224, 1968.
2. French, S. W., Ihrig, T. J., and Morin, R. T., Lipid composition of RBC ghosts, liver mitochondria and microsomes of ethanol-fed rats, *Q. J. Stud. Alcohol,* 31, 801, 1970.
3. French, S. W., Ihrig, T. J., Shaw, G. P., Tanaka, T. T., and Norum, M. L., The effect of ethanol on the fatty acid composition of hepatic microsomes and inner and outer mitochondrial membranes, *Res. Commun. Chem. Pathol. Pharmacol.,* 2, 567, 1971.
4. Thompson, J. A. and Reitz, R. C., Effects of ethanol ingestion and dietary fat levels on mitochondrial lipids in male and female rats, *Lipids,* 13, 540, 1978.
5. Rao, G. A., Goheen, S. C., Manix, M., and Larkin, E. C., Enhanced ratio of linoleic acid to arachidonic acid in erythrocyte phosphatidylcholine in rats during withdrawal from ethanol, *Toxicol. Lett.,* 7, 37, 1980.
6. Foudin, L., Sun, G. Y., and Sun, A. Y., Changes in lipid composition of rat heart mitochondria after chronic ethanol administration, *Alcohol. Clin. Exp. Res.,* 10, 606, 1986.
7. Ellingson, J. S., Jones, N., Taraschi, T. F., and Rubin, E., The effect of chronic ethanol consumption on the fatty acid composition of phosphatidylinositol in rat liver microsomes as determined by gas chromatography and 1H-NMR, *Biochim. Biophys. Acta,* 1062, 99, 1991.
8. Rouach, H., Clement, M., Orfanelli, M.-T., Janvier, B., and Nordmann, R., Fatty acid composition of rat liver mitochondrial phospholipids during ethanol inhalation, *Biochim. Biophys. Acta,* 795, 125, 1984.
9. Reitz, R. C., Helsabeck, E., and Mason, D. P., Effects of chronic alcohol ingestion on the fatty acid composition of the heart, *Lipids,* 8, 80, 1973.
10. Nervi, A. M., Peluffo, R. O., and Brenner, R. R., Effect of ethanol administration on fatty acid desaturation, *Lipids,* 15, 263, 1980.
11. Wang, D. L. and Reitz, R. C., Ethanol ingestion and polyunsaturated fatty acids: effects on the acyl-CoA desaturases, *Alcohol. Clin. Exp. Res.,* 7, 220, 1983.
12. Reitz, R. C., Relationship of the acyl-CoA desaturases to certain membrane fatty acid changes induced by ethanol consumption, *Proc. West. Pharmacol. Soc.,* 27, 247, 1984.
13. Cunnane, S. C., Huang, Y.-S., Manku, M. S., and Horrobin, D. F., Influence of different dietary fatty acid sources on erythrocyte lipids and plasma and liver essential fatty acids in hamsters fed ethanol, *Ann. Nutr. Metab.,* 30, 81, 1986.
14. Engler, M. M., Karanian, J. W., and Salem, N., Jr., Ethanol inhalation and dietary N-6, N-3 and N-9 fatty acids in the rat: effect on platelet and aortic fatty acid composition, *Alcohol. Clin. Exp. Res.,* 15, 483, 1991.
15. Holman, R. T., Johnson, S. B., and Hatch, T. F., A case of human linolenic acid deficiency involving neurological abnormalities, *Am. J. Clin. Nutr.,* 35, 617, 1982.

16. Yamamoto, N., Saitoh, M., Moriuchi, A., Nomura, M., and Okyuama, H., Effect of dietary α-linolenic/linoleic balance on brain lipid compositions and learning ability in rats, *J. Lipid Res.*, 28, 144, 1987.

17. Lamptey, M. S. and Walker, B. L., A possible essential role for dietary linolenic acid in the development of the young rat, *J. Nutr.*, 106, 86, 1976.

18. Alling, C., Becker, W., Jones, A. W., and Anggard, E., Effects of chronic ethanol treatment on lipid composition and prostaglandins in rats fed essential fatty acid deficient diets, *Alcohol. Clin. Exp. Res.*, 8, 238, 1984.

19. Johnson, S. B., Gordon, E., McClain, C., Low, G., and Holman, R. T., Abnormal polyunsaturated fatty acid patterns of serum lipids in alcoholism and cirrhosis: arachidonic acid deficiency in cirrhosis, *Proc. Natl. Acad. Sci. U.S.A.*, 82, 1815, 1985.

20. Littleton, J. M., Synaptosomal membrane lipids of mice during continuous exposure to ethanol, *J. Pharm. Pharmacol.*, 29, 579, 1977.

21. Oshino, N. and Sato, R., The dietary control of the microsomal stearyl-CoA desaturation enzyme system in rat liver, *Arch. Biochem. Biophys.*, 149, 369, 1972.

22. Chin, J. H. and Goldstein, D. B., Effects of low concentrations of ethanol on the fluidity of spin-labelled erythrocytes and brain membranes, *Mol. Pharmacol.*, 13, 435, 1977.

23. Chin, J. H. and Goldstein, D. B., Drug tolerance in biomembranes: a spin-label study of the effects of ethanol, *Science*, 196, 684, 1977.

24. Reitz, R. C., Wang, L., Schilling, R. J., Starich, G. H., Bergstrom, J. D., and Thompson, J. A., Effects of ethanol ingestion on the unsaturated fatty acids from various tissues, *Prog. Lipid Res.*, 20, 209, 1981.

25. Cunningham, C. C., Botenus, R. E., Spach, P. I., and Rudel, L. C., Ethanol-related changes in liver microsomes and mitochondria from the monkey, *Macaca fascicularis*, *Alcohol. Clin. Exp. Res.*, 7, 424, 1983.

26. LaDroitte, P., Lamboeuf, Y., and de Saint Blanquat, G., Membrane fatty acid changes and ethanol tolerance in rat and mouse, *Life Sci.*, 35, 1221, 1984.

27. Cunnane, S. C., Manku, M. S., and Horrobin, D. F., Effect of ethanol on liver triglycerides and fatty acid composition in the Golden Syrian Hamster, *Ann. Nutr. Metab.*, 29, 246, 1985.

28. Cunnane, S. C., McAdo, K. R., and Horrobin, D. F., Long-term ethanol consumption in the hamster: effects on tissue lipids, fatty acids, and erythrocyte hemolysis, *Ann. Nutr. Metab.*, 31, 265, 1987.

29. Jain, M. H. and Cordes, E. H., Effect of n-alkanols on the rate of enzymatic hydrolysis of egg phosphatidylcholine, *J. Membr. Biol.*, 144, 101, 1978.

30. Arai, M., Gordon, E. R., and Lieber, C. S., Decreased cytochrome oxidase activity in hepatic mitochondria after chronic ethanol consumption and the possible role of decreased cytochrome AA₃ content and changes in phospholipids, *Biochim. Biophys. Acta*, 797, 320, 1984.

31. Choy, P. C., O, K., Man, R. Y., and Chan, A. C., Phosphatidylcholine metabolism in isolated rat heart: modulation by ethanol and vitamin E, *Biochim. Biophys. Acta*, 1005, 225, 1989.

32. Moscat, J., Aracil, M., Diez, E., Garcia-Barreno, P., and Munico, A. M., Effect of ethanol on the arachidonic acid metabolism in mouse peritoneal macrophages, *Prostaglandins*, 34, 853, 1987.

33. Gastaldi, M., Lerique, B., Feugere, T., le Petit-Thevenin, J., Nobili, O., and Boyer, J., Altered acylation of erythrocyte phospholipids in alcoholism, *Alcohol. Clin. Exp. Res.,* 12, 356, 1988.

34. Pikkarinen, P. H. and Lieber, C. S., Concentration dependency of ethanol elimination rates in baboons: effect of chronic alcohol consumption, *Alcohol. Clin. Exp. Res.,* 4, 40, 1980.

35. Pieper, W. P. and Skeen, M. J., Changes in rate of ethanol elimination associated with chronic administration of ethanol to chimpanzees and rhesus monkey, *Drug Metab. Dispos.,* 1, 634, 1973.

36. Marshall, E. K., Jr. and Owens, A. H., Jr., Rate of metabolism of ethyl alcohol in the mouse, *Proc. Soc. Exp. Biol. Med.,* 89, 573, 1955.

37. Aull, J. C., Jr., Roberts, W. J., Jr., and Kinard, F. W., Rate of metabolism of ethanol in the rat, *Am. J. Physiol.,* 186, 380, 1956.

38. Widmark, E., *Die Theoretischen Grundlagen and die Praktische Verwendbarkeit der Gerichtlich-Medizinischen Alkoholbestimmung,* Urban & Schwarzenberg, Berlin, 1932.

39. Elbel, H. and Schleyer, F., *Blutalkohol. Die Wissenschaftlichen Grundlagen der Beurteilung von Blutalkoholbefinden bei Strassenverkehrsdelikten,* 2nd ed., Georg Thieme, Stuttgart, 1956.

40. Lieber, C. S. and DeCarli, L. M., Fatty liver in the rat after prolonged intake of ethanol with a nutritionally adequate new liquid diet, *J. Nutr.,* 91, 331, 1967.

41. Lieber, C. S., Spritz, N., and DeCarli, L. M., Role of dietary, adipose and endogenously synthesized fatty acids in the pathogenesis of the alcoholic fatty liver, *J. Clin. Invest.,* 45, 51, 1966.

42. Lieber, C. S. and DeCarli, L. M., quantitative relationship between the amount of dietary fat and the severity of the alcoholic fatty liver, *Am. J. Clin. Nutr.,* 23, 474, 1970.

43. Zaki, F. G., Brandt, C., and Hoffbauer, F. W., Fatty cirrhosis in the rat. IV. The influence of different levels of dietary fat, *Arch. Pathol.,* 75, 654, 1963.

44. Tsukamoto, H., French, S. W., Benson, N., Delgado, G., Rao, G. A., Larkin, E. C., and Largman, C., Severe and progressive steatosis and focal necrosis in rat liver induced by continuous intragastric infusion of ethanol and low fat diet, *Hepatology,* 5, 224, 1985.

45. French, S. W., Miyamoto, K., and Tsukamoto, H., Ethanol-induced hepatic fibrosis in the rat: role of the amount of dietary fat, *Alcohol. Clin. Exp. Res.,* 10, 13s, 1986.

46. Nanji, A. A. and French, S. W., Dietary factors and alcoholic cirrhosis, *Alcohol. Clin. Exp. Res.,* 10, 271, 1986.

47. Nanji, A. A. and French, S. W. Relationship between pork consumption and cirrhosis, *Lancet,* 1, 681, 1985.

48. French, S. W., Benson, N. C., and Sun, P. S., Centriolobular liver necrosis induced by hypoxia in chronic ethanol fed rats, *Hepatology,* 4, 912, 1984.

49. Tsukamoto, H., French, S. W., and Largman, C., Correlation of cyclical blood alcohol levels with progression of alcoholic liver injury, *Biochem. Arch.,* 1, 215, 1985.

50. Tsukamoto, H., Reidelberger, R., French, S. W., and Largman, C., Long-term cannulation model for blood sampling and intragastric infusion in the rat, *Am. J. Physiol.*, 247, R595, 1984.

51. Nanji, A. A., Mendenhall, C. L., and French, S. W., Beef fat prevents alcoholic liver disease in the rat, *Alcohol. Clin. Exp. Res.*, 13, 15, 1989.

52. Hollander, D., Tarnawski, A., and Ivey, K. J., Arachidonic acid protection of rat gastric mucosa against ethanol injury, *J. Lab. Clin. Med.*, 100, 296, 1982.

53. Tarnawski, A., Hollander, D., Krause, W. J., Stachura, J., and Sekhon, D., Can a dietary essential fatty acid (arachidonate) protect the liver against acute alcohol injury?, *Gastroenterology*, 86, 1343, 1984.

54. Goheen, S. C., Larkin, E. C., Manix, M., and Rao, G. A., Dietary arachidonic acid reduces fatty liver and increases diet consumption and weight gain in ethanol-fed rats, *Lipids*, 15, 328, 1980.

55. Goheen, S. C., Pearson, E. E., Larkin, E. C., and Rao, G. A., The prevention of alcoholic fatty liver using dietary supplements: dihydroxyacetone, pyruvate and riboflavin compared to arachidonic acid in pair-fed rats, *Lipids*, 16, 43, 1981.

56. Stern, Z., Korsten, M. A., DeCarli, L. M., and Lieber, C. S., Effects of arachidonic acid on hepatic lipids in ethanol-fed rats, *Alcohol. Clin. Exp. Res.*, 14, 127, 1990.

57. Karpe, F., Wejde, I., and Anggard, E., Dietary arachidonic acid protects mice against the fatty liver induced by a high fat diet and by ethanol, *Acta Pharmacol. Toxicol.*, 55, 95, 1984.

58. Lakshman, M. R., Chirtel, S. J., and Chambers, L. L., Roles of omega-3 fatty acids and chronic ethanol in the regulation of plasma and liver lipids and plasma apoproteins A1 and E in rats, *J. Nutr.*, 118, 1299, 1988.

59. Wainwright, P. E., Ward, G. R., Winfield, D., Huang, Y.-S., Mills, D. E., Ward, R. P., and McCutcheon, D., Effects of prenatal ethanol and long-chain n-3 fatty acid supplementation on development in mice. I. Body and brain growth, sensorimotor development, and water T-maze reversal learning, *Alcohol. Clin. Exp. Res.*, 14, 405, 1990.

60. Wainwright, P. E., Huang, Y.-S., Simmons, V., Mills, D. E., Ward, R. P., Ward, G. R., Winfield, D., and McCutcheon, D., Effects of prenatal ethanol and long-chain n-3 fatty acid supplementation on development in mice. II. Fatty acid composition of brain membrane phospholipids, *Alcohol. Clin. Exp. Res.*, 15, 413, 1990.

61. Reitz, R. C., unpublished results.

62. Cunningham, C. C., Filus, S., Bottenus, R. E., and Spach, P. I., Effects of ethanol consumption on the phospholipid composition of rat liver microsomes and mitochondria, *Biochim. Biophys. Acta*, 712, 225, 1982.

63. Thompson, J. A. and Reitz, R. C., Studies on the acute and chronic effects of ethanol ingestion on choline oxidation, *Ann. N.Y. Acad. Sci.*, 273, 194, 1976.

64. La Droitte, P., Lamboeuf, Y., de Saint Blanquat, G., and Bezaury, J.-P., Sensitivity of individual erythrocyte membrane phospholipids to changes in fatty acid composition in chronic alcoholic patients, *Alcohol. Clin. Exp. Res.*, 9, 135, 1984.

9 Metabolic Flux and the Role of Lipids in Alcohol Tolerance in *Drosophila*

INTRODUCTION

Ethanol is consumed primarily by humans for its social impact. While many people are only occasional drinkers, a significant number of individuals are chronic consumers of ethanol and are likely candidates for ethanol-induced modifications which may include cellular damage. Most dietary ethanol is degraded into metabolites within the vertebrate liver. If ethanol is not fully metabolized or eliminated from the body, ethanol or its derivative, acetaldehyde, may exert toxic effects at the cellular and organismic levels. The ability of the individual to physiologically withstand these toxic effects is alcohol tolerance, or more specifically, ethanol tolerance.

We have employed the insect *Drosophila melanogaster* as a model system in which to experimentally examine the biochemical and genetic systems that control alcohol elimination and tolerance. Because *D. melanogaster* has fed on fermenting plant materials during much of its evolution, it is able to efficiently use low to moderate levels of dietary ethanol (up to 4.5% v/v, or approximately 733 mM) as a nutrient.[1] Although wild-type *D. melanogaster* is able to tolerate the toxic effects of relatively high concentrations of ethanol, the elimination systems become saturated at 5 to 6% (814 to 977 mM) dietary ethanol, and the toxic effects of ethanol accumulation become evident. In this chapter the authors discuss the factors that interact to limit the flux of ethanol through the major metabolic pathway for ethanol elimination. We also review the biochemical changes associated with ethanol toxicity in *D. melanogaster* and consider the ways that the animal copes with the toxicity. Two other recent reviews have dealt with related aspects of ethanol utilization and elimination by *D. melanogaster*.[2,3]

THE ELIMINATION OF ALCOHOLS
IN *DROSOPHILA*

A key to ethanol tolerance is the conversion of the alcohol to nontoxic metabolites. The major pathway for ethanol elimination is initiated by alcohol dehydrogenase (ADH; EC 1.1.1.1). Since the ADH pathway degrades >90% of the total ethanol in *D. melanogaster* and in many vertebrates, the regulation of the pathway is an important component of ethanol tolerance.

DEVELOPMENT AND THE ECOLOGICAL NICHE

D. melanogaster exhibits complete metamorphosis. Females and males become sexually mature within 12 h after they reach the adult stage. An adult female usually mates once and stores enough sperm to last a normal life span. Embryonic development is completed in 18 to 24 h. The larva that emerges from the egg devotes this period of development to growth. When fed an optimal medium, the larval period lasts approximately 6 d. When raised on a defined, sterile culture medium, an experimental tool that is used by our laboratory, the larval period lasts about 8.5 d.

Twice during the growth period the larva molts or sheds its exoskeleton, allowing rapid growth. The molts separate the three larval instars. We have examined larvae midway through the third instar in our research. Molting is stimulated by an increase in titer of the hormone, ecdysone, but high levels of juvenile hormone maintain the larval state. During the third instar ecdysone levels increase while juvenile hormone levels drop. This causes the larva to crawl onto a dry surface, glue itself down, and form a pupal case around itself. During the pupal period, larval tissues are replaced by adult tissues which develop from a series of small disks known as imaginal disks. The pupal developmental period takes about 5 d. The adult then ecloses from the pupal case. Larvae are relatively immobile and must cope with the alcohols in their environment. Adult *D. melanogaster* may move to a site that is compatible with their degree of alcohol tolerance.

D. melanogaster females often lay their eggs on fermenting plant material. Consequently, the normal habitat of *D. melanogaster* contains a number of alcohols in which the predominant alcohol is ethanol.[4] *D. melanogaster* appear to have the same ethanol-metabolizing pathways as vertebrates.[2,3] ADH is present at all stages of the life cycle, and is an important part of the metabolic system that matches *D. melanogaster* to its ecological niche.

The weight of *D. melanogaster* adults that were fed ethanol during the larval period has been observed to be greater than that of adults fed an ethanol-free diet in numerous experiments in our laboratories.[3,5,6] The weight gain occurs when nonlethal concentrations of ethanol are consumed by larvae and may be an evolved adaptive response to an ethanol-rich environment. A large proportion of ethanol that is ingested by larvae is channeled into body lipids by the ADH pathway.[1] Evidence is available that natural selection can act on the genes that determine the capabilities of *D. melanogaster* to synthesize and store lipids, and that the selection largely affects the kinetic properties of the biosynthetic enzymes.[7,8] Since the stored lipids from the larval period are a primary energy source for pupal development,[9] differences in the abilities of larvae to convert ethanol into lipids could be of adaptive significance.[2,10]

ETHANOL TOLERANCE TESTS

Ethanol tolerance in *D. melanogaster* is a composite of the abilities to grow and to survive in the presence of ethanol, and it is a complex trait that depends heavily on the diagnostic conditions applied. Many tolerance tests have been performed by adding ethanol to the culture medium,[11-14] but different life stages have been tested. The diagnostic traits, survival of larvae to the pupal and adult stages, length of the larval development period, and adult male weight most likely depend upon the interaction of different metabolic pathways and may be the result of the toxicity of ethanol to specific tissues.[10,15] We have eliminated many of the variable factors that may affect the outcome of tolerance tests by carrying them out on *D. melanogaster* cultured on a controlled axenic defined medium, and by using strains that have a uniform genetic background.

The activity of the ADH pathway is important in the utilization of ethanol as a nutrient by *D. melanogaster* and for ethanol tolerance throughout development. Flies expressing a mutant null allele for *Adh* are much more sensitive to the toxic effects of ethanol than normal wild-type flies. For ADH-deficient larvae 2% dietary ethanol (v/v) (325 mM) is lethal, whereas wild-type larvae are killed by 6% (977 mM) ethanol.[10,16]

THE METABOLIC ROLES OF ALCOHOL DEHYDROGENASE AND ALDEHYDE DEHYDROGENASE

Ethanol is degraded by a number of enzyme systems to acetaldehyde, which in turn is converted to acetate and acetyl-CoA (Figure 1). Acetyl-CoA

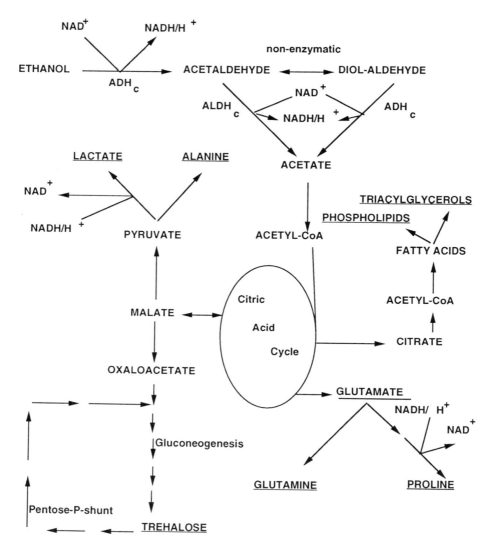

FIGURE 1. A scheme that depicts the intermediary metabolism of ethanol elimination in *Drosophila* larvae based upon ^{14}C-tracer and ^{13}C-NMR studies. ADH_c and $ALDH_c$ denote the cytosolic localization of alcohol dehydrogenase and aldehyde dehydrogenase, respectively. For clarity, no subcellular compartments of the different pathways have been indicated; these details are given in the text. Underlined are those (end)products that can be followed easily by means of proton-decoupled ^{13}C-NMR spectroscopy.[3,38,50]

may be channeled completely into the tricarboxylic acid (TCA) cycle, or be diverted by way of citrate into fatty acids. In *D. melanogaster* larvae, 91 to 93% of all ethanol is degraded by the ADH pathway.[1,15] The remainder is degraded by catalase and other minor pathways.[3,17]

The conversion of acetaldehyde to acetate is catalyzed in vertebrates by aldehyde dehydrogenase (ALDH, EC 1.2.1.3). For a number of years the role of ALDH in *D. melanogaster* was the subject of controversy, which the authors shall try to clarify.

The *Drosophila* ADH enzyme is located exclusively in the cytosolic fraction of the cells,[18,19] and is expressed primarily in the fat body, gut, and Malpighian tubules.[20] The catalytic mechanism of this oxidation reaction is thought to be either rapid equilibrium, random, or ordered as based upon kinetic studies that examined the purified enzyme at different pHs.[21,22] Whether an alcoholate-ion is involved in the reaction remains to be determined.[23] Kapoun et al.[24] conclusively demonstrated that the "rapid equilibrium" type of mechanism prevails *in vivo* by observing a large kinetic isotope effect in wild-type larvae fed deuterated ethanol as compared to the absence of the isotope effect in larvae lacking ADH activity.[25]

The product of the first reaction, acetaldehyde, is at equilibrium with its hydrated gem-diol form.[26] These two forms are substrates for two different *in vivo* enzymes that catalyze the dehydrogenation to acetate. Not only does *Drosophila* ADH catalyze the first reaction of the pathway, but it also oxidizes acetaldehyde to acetate.[18,27] For the latter reaction *Drosophila* ADH prefers the gem-diol form of acetaldehyde. While *Drosophila* ALDH also oxidizes acetaldehyde,[28,29] *Drosophila* ALDH prefers the unhydrated form of acetaldehyde.[20,26]

The relative importance of ADH and ALDH in the oxidation of ethanol-derived acetaldehyde was investigated in *D. melanogaster* larvae by Heinstra et al.[20] and in adults by Martinez-Leal and Barbancho[30] and Anderson and Barnett.[19] Heinstra et al.[20] inhibited *in vivo* ALDH activity by feeding larvae cyanamide, and then assessing the flux of label from ^{14}C-ethanol into lipids. ADH activity was mildly inhibited by cyanamide feeding, whereas all but 5% of wild-type ALDH activity was eliminated. Meanwhile, the flux of label into lipids was only mildly decreased.[20] This suggested that *Drosophila* ADH rather than the *Drosophila* ALDH-enzyme(s) is the main enzyme responsible for the oxidation of ethanol-derived acetaldehyde in larvae.

Through the use of cyanamide, Barbancho and co-workers[30,31] found that elimination of all but 15% of the adult wild-type ALDH activity greatly increased the sensitivity of adults to environmental ethanol. This indicates that in adults the second step of acetaldehyde oxidation is mediated mainly by *Drosophila* ALDH. Anderson and Barnett[19] arrived at a similar conclusion by exposing adults of different genotypes to acetaldehyde and measuring survival rates.

Mitochondrial and cytosolic ALDH isoenzymes exist in *D. melanogaster*.[19,20,29,30] The cytosolic isozyme in adults is approximately three times more active than the mitochondrial isozyme,[19] whereas the mitochondrial isozyme is predominant in larvae.[20] The ALDH isozymes have different *in vitro* sensitivities toward cyanamide inhibition. The larval mitochondrial form is susceptible to cyanamide inhibition, whereas the cytosolic form is largely insensitive to cyanamide.[20,30]

Since *D. melanogaster* larvae largely possess the less active, cyanamide-sensitive, mitochondrial ALDH isozyme, the authors hypothesize that the conversion of acetaldehyde into acetate is catalyzed by cytosolic ADH. Larvae simply do not possess enough of the more active cytosolic ALDH isozyme for the sequential action of ADH-ALDH enzymes (see Figure 1). Since adult flies possess higher levels of the cyanamide-insensitive, cytosolic form of ALDH, the conversion of ethanol into acetate may be catalyzed by the sequential action of ADH-ALDH enzymes (see Figure 1). This implies that ethanol metabolism may be regulated differently in *D. melanogaster* larvae and adults. In contrast to *D. melanogaster,* the conversion of acetaldehyde to acetate is almost exclusively mediated by the mitochondrial ALDH isozyme in mammals.[32]

As previously noted, *D. melanogaster* encounters alcohols other than ethanol in nature.[4] Primary alcohols are degraded to an aldehyde and subsequently to a carboxylic acid, while secondary alcohols are catalyzed in one step to a ketone end-product by ADH.[15,33] The ADH-mediated oxidation of saturated secondary alcohols eventually results in complete inhibition of ADH activity *in vivo* because of the formation of inactive ADH:NAD-ketone ternary complexes.

METABOLIC CONTROL THEORY AND FLUX THROUGH THE ADH PATHWAY

To understand how alcohol metabolism is modulated by the diet, the enzymes that control the flux through the degradative pathway must be identified. Theoretically an enzyme may catalyze a single step which is rate limiting for the entire pathway. Early work on the effects of ethanol on carbohydrate metabolism was directed at those enzymes that were already known to be rate limiting.[34] However, the "metabolic control theory" (MCT) that was developed by Kacser and Porteous[35] envisions that control of a steady-state biochemical pathway is not vested in a single step, but is shared among the enzymes of the pathway. The extent to which the control of the pathway is distributed among the individual steps is expressed in the "flux control coefficient". According to the MCT, the flux control coefficient of all the enzymes in a given biochemical pathway equals unity ($= 1$). Enzymes exerting no control have a coefficient of 0.0; those that exert some degree of control have higher values with their total sum $= 1.0$.

More analysis of mathematical equations/modeling has been done than empirical verifications of the MCT through investigations of intact metabolic systems. Enzymes possessing high flux control coefficients must be examined because their modifications would exert direct effects on flux through the pathway, for example, on ethanol degradation. Some efforts have been directed toward solving evolutionary problems by using *Drosophila* as a working model. To illustrate the experimental approaches that might be followed, the authors present a few examples.

Middleton and Kacser[36] compared the combined flux from ethanol into lipids and carbon dioxide in *D. melanogaster* adults that possessed several combinations of *Adh* alleles. Despite an appreciable *in vitro* range of ADH activity in adults expressing these alleles, no significant differences between the fluxes could be found. The flux control coefficient was 0.04 $\pm$ 0.10, indicating that the ADH does not represent a controlling step in the adult ethanol degrading pathways. According to the MCT, the rate of flux through the entire ADH pathway must be controlled by other enzymes, but other enzymes of the pathway were not examined. If the flux control coefficient for ADH is 0.04, then natural selection should not discriminate among *Adh* genotypes. Differences in fitness between individuals can only be generated when genotypes specify differences in metabolic-physiological processes. For further discussions of the evolutionary aspects of alcohol metabolism, see References 2 and 15.

We recently used a different approach to gain insight into the control of flux through the ADH pathway in third instar larvae. Comparisons were made between two sibling *Drosophila* species, *viz.*, *D. melanogaster* and

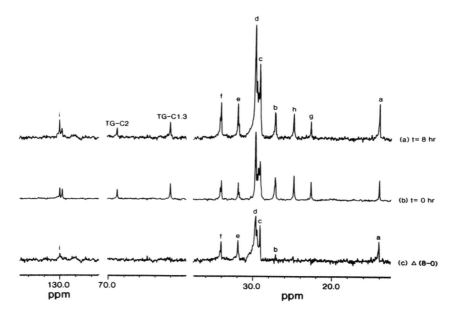

FIGURE 2. ^{13}C-NMR spectra of chloroform extracts of *Drosophila melanogaster* larvae homozygous for the Adh^F allele. (a) Fatty acid resonances after 8 h of [2-^{13}C]ethanol administration. In (b) the natural background level of fatty acids is shown. The $\Delta(8–0)$ h subtraction figure between (a) and (b) is shown in (c). For assignments of the peaks, see the first equation in the text. Peak b is $-CH_2*CH_2-CH=CH-$ and peak i, $-CH=*CH-CH_2-$ of monounsaturated fatty acids. TG-C2 and TG-C1,3 represent the carbon atoms of the glycerol backbone in endogenous triacylglycerols (see Reference 32).

D. simulans. D. simulans is more sensitive to environmental ethanol than *D. melanogaster*.[15] The activities of ADH and ALDH were modified in tandem by prefeeding the larvae, cyanamide. Subsequently, the flux from ethanol into lipids was determined by ^{14}C-tracer methods.[37] Cyanamide inhibition resulted in ADH activities that varied fourfold and ALDH activities that varied eightfold. For third instar larvae the flux control coefficient for ADH was 0.86 ± 0.12, and for ALDH 0.02 ± 0.07. Freriksen and co-workers[38] measured the specific enrichments in fatty acids from dietary [2-^{13}C]ethanol in larvae with ^{13}C nuclear magnetic resonance (NMR) spectroscopy in seven different strains possessing three *Adh* genotypes (see Figure 2). ADH activities were compared with summed enrichments in individual fatty acid peaks; the flux control coefficient for the ADH in this case was approximately 1.0. Thus, in larvae ADH seems to almost completely control the rate of flux through this pathway.

A number of reasons are possible for the apparent discrepancy between the control mechanisms of the ADH pathway in *D. melanogaster* larvae and adults:

1. Because of differences in the general metabolic physiology, larvae and adults are almost totally different organisms.[7]
2. As noted earlier, the first two oxidative steps in larvae are catalyzed by ADH, while the sequential action of the ADH-ALDH enzymes is required in adults. Plausibly, major control of the ADH pathway in adults is vested in ALDH. Nonetheless, this would be uncharacteristic of vertebrate systems. Acetaldehyde plays at most a minor role in controlling the rate of ethanol oxidation in rat liver,[39] and the rate of ethanol oxidation is the same in Japanese with the inactive $ALDH_2$ variant as in individuals with the common form.[40]
3. According to Koehn,[41] the strains used by Middleton and Kacser have a long selection history of ethanol exposure; therefore, modifier genes at loci other than *Adh* may have been selected.

Does this mean that every modulation in larval ADH activity influences flux? Based on extensive empirical data, the answer is no. Two examples illustrate this point:

1. ADH activity is significantly increased in *D. melanogaster* larvae by sucrose supplements to the diet.[16,48] However, the flux from ethanol to lipid is greatest at low dietary sucrose levels because sucrose and ethanol are alternate energy sources.
2. Also, dietary ethanol strongly increases ADH activity in third instar, wild-type larvae[16,24] (see the following section) with a concomitant increase in flux from ethanol into lipids ($r = 0.92$).[42]

DIETARY MODULATION OF THE *Adh* GENE

D. melanogaster ADH is encoded in a single structural gene (*Adh*) at 50.1 of chromosome 2^{43} and lies cytogenetically within bands 35B2-3.[27] The organization of the *Adh* gene in *D. melanogaster* and the control of its activity were recently reviewed.[3,23] The *Adh* gene is transcribed through the use of two promoters which are separated by 708 bp. The proximal (larval) promoter is active during the three larval instars, while the distal (adult) promoter is most active late during the third larval instar and the adult stage.[23]

McKechnie and Geer[16] found that ADH activity increased in both the fat body and gut of wild-type larvae that were fed a moderate concentration (2.5% (v/v), 400 mM) of ethanol. Induction of ADH activity by ethanol in third instar larvae is mainly due to the increased usage of the larval promoter.[42] An increase in *Adh* mRNA levels was evident within 2 h and an increase in ADH activity was noted within 5 h after ethanol feeding was initiated. All primary alcohols of four carbons or less were effective inducers of ADH activity in *D. melanogaster* larvae.[44] Because of the number of alcohols that serve as inducers, ADH with its broad substrate specificity is able to amplify and degrade the variety of alcohols that may be present in the environment of *D. melanogaster*. The relatively rapid induction of ADH activity allows larvae to adapt to changes in environmental alcohol content.

Examination of P-element-transformed strains of *D. melanogaster* that possessed deletions of part of their upstream *Adh* regulatory DNA indicated that a sequence between-110 and -187 of the proximal (larval) promoter start site is essential for the induction of *Adh* by ethanol.[24] A DNA sequence between -660 and about -5000 of the distal (adult) transcript start site is important for the down-regulation of the induction response.

THE METABOLIC FATE OF ETHANOL

Prolonged feeding on a diet containing ethanol allows time for the carbons of ethanol to be channeled into a variety of intermediates, some of which may be far removed metabolically from ethanol. Some of the derivatives of ethanol may be beneficial to the animal, whereas other derivatives may be toxic. This section is concerned with the metabolic fate of ethanol in *D. melanogaster* during longer periods of exposure to the alcohol.

OXIDATIVE ELIMINATION OF ETHANOL IN
DROSOPHILA

The metabolic pathways that radiate from ethanol metabolism have been studied in *D. melanogaster* by ^{14}C-tracer and ^{13}C-NMR methods. The degradation of ethanol forms cytosolic acetate which is converted into acetyl-CoA within mitochondria (Figure 1). In 2-h pulse-chase studies, which utilized adults of different *Adh* genotypes, lipids and carbon dioxide were found to be labeled, presumably by multiple cycles of the TCA cycle.

Unfortunately, no details were given on the relative contributions of lipogenesis or the TCA cycle.[36] Wild-type larvae were also shown to rapidly incorporate label from ethanol into lipids by means of long-term (24 to 48 h) tracer studies.[1] The administration of labeled glucose and ethanol to larvae indicated that the rate of glycolysis slowed to about one third of the rate that was observed when only glucose was fed.[1] Consequently, dietary glucose and ethanol serve as alternate substrates for lipid synthesis in *D. melanogaster* larvae.

Through the use of ^{13}C-NMR spectroscopy on perchloric acid extracts of larvae fed [2-^{13}C]ethanol, the fate of ethanol-derived carbons has been established (Figure 1). Our findings show that acetyl-CoA condenses with oxaloacetate (OAA) to form citrate, which is a branch point in ethanol metabolism. When excess citrate is formed, part of this citrate enters the cytoplasm and serves as the substrate for citrate lyase (EC 4.3.1.8), leading to the reformation of acetyl-CoA and OAA (Figure 1). The cytoplasmic acetyl-CoA provides a precursor for the synthesis of saturated fatty acids. Lipogenesis becomes most active in third instar larvae about 4 h after ethanol feeding is initiated.

Another branch point exists within the TCA cycle at the level of 2-oxoglutarate. TCA intermediates are channeled into glutamate, glutamine, and proline, through the Glu-Gln-Pro "triangle". The glutamate and proline concentrations were approximately equal, but the glutamine concentrations were found to be twofold greater than glutamate levels.[45] This Glu-Gln-Pro triangle allowed ^{13}C-NMR measurements of the carbon fluxes resulting from multiple cycles of the TCA cycle.[38,46,47] When [2-^{13}C]ethanol is degraded, only the C4-atom of glutamate is ^{13}C-enriched by the first cycle through the TCA cycle. However, in the second cycle, the C2, C3, C4-atoms in glutamate are ^{13}C-enriched. Through the analysis of multiplet isotope patterns, one can see if metabolic steady-state conditions apply. The absolute contribution of ethanol to the supply of acetyl-CoA that enters the TCA cycle may be calculated, and the relative flux through anaplerotic and citrate synthase pathways may be determined.[46,47] Multiplet analysis of larvae homozygous for the *Adh^s* allele indicated that dietary ethanol may provide 70% of the acetyl-CoA that enters the TCA cycle. The intermediary metabolism was shown to be at steady state,[45] whereas the anaplerotic pathway contributed 50% of the TCA intermediates.

^{13}C-NMR analysis also indicated that part of the malate derived in mitochondria from 2-oxoglutarate may enter the cytoplasm where it is

converted into pyruvate through the action of malic enzyme (EC 1.1.1.40). Malic enzyme (EC 1.1.1.40) activity increased by 50% in *D. melanogaster* larvae that were fed 2.5% (v/v) (400 m*M*) ethanol,[48] suggesting that malic enzyme supplies NADPH (reduced form of nicotinamide adenine dinucleotide) for the synthesis of fatty acids from ethanol.[49] The pyruvate that is formed may be converted into lactate via lactate dehydrogenase (EC 1.1.1.27), providing a way to maintain the NADH/NAD$^+$ balance in the cytoplasm during ethanol degradation. After 8 h of ethanol digestion and degradation, larvae accumulated appreciable levels of trehalose in which the coupling of C5- and C6-trehalose atoms was first evident (Figure 1).[3,45,50] After 24 h of ethanol degradation, larvae showed about 30% C-C coupling at the C1-, C5-, C2-, and C6-atoms of trehalose. These high levels of coupling indicated that trehalose turns over rapidly in *D. melanogaster* larvae.

Additional information was also deduced from the enrichment patterns of the C1- to C6-atoms of trehalose. First, the C2/C5 ratio of trehalose atoms represents the activity of the pentose-phosphate shunt.[51] Second, the C1-, C2-, C5-, and C6-atoms of trehalose are enriched after one cycle of the TCA cycle when [2-^{13}C]ethanol is degraded. Only through multiple TCA cycles do the C3- and C4-atoms of trehalose become enriched.[51,52] Consequently, the relative activity of the TCA cycle may be assessed. Finally, the C3/C4 ratio of trehalose is representative of the triose-phosphate-isomerase (EC 5.3.1.1) reaction during gluconeogenesis.[52] After 8 and 24 h of ethanol feeding, *D. melanogaster* larvae showed a trehalose-C2/C5 ratio of 0.80 ± 0.13 and 0.78 ± 0.02, respectively (n = 3).[3,45] About 20% of the glucose-6-phosphate enters the pentose-phosphate shunt in larvae that were fed ethanol, which is rather high as compared to rat hepatocytes.[51] The ratios indicate that TCA cycle activity was deduced to be 0.57 ± 0.06 at 8 h and 0.41 ± 0.02 (n = 3) at 24 h of ethanol exposure. This indicated that there was an increase in C3-C4 contribution to trehalose synthesis during the test period. Finally, the ratio thought to represent the triose-phosphate isomerase equilibrium was 1.22 ± 0.13 at 8 h, and 1.24 ± 0.09 (n = 3) at 24 h in contrast to the value of 1.0 for rat hepatocytes.[51] The equilibrium in *D. melanogaster* apparently favors the formation of dihydroxyacetone-phosphate, reflecting perhaps the demand for *sn*-glycerol-3-phosphate for lipid synthesis (Figure 1).

FATTY ACID SYNTHESIS IS AN IMPORTANT
COMPONENT OF ETHANOL ELIMINATION

Acetyl-CoA derived from the action of the cytosolic citrate lyase serves as a precursor for *de novo* synthesis of fatty acids (see the earlier section on MCT). This process was followed easily by means of ^{13}C-NMR spectroscopy of chloroform extracts of *D. melanogaster* larvae that were exposed to [2-^{13}C]ethanol.[50] Freriksen et al.[38] established the relationship of fatty acid/triacylglycerol synthesis to ethanol degradation in *D. melanogaster* third instar larvae using methods developed by Cohen.[53] [2-^{13}C]Ethanol degradation eventually will enrich only specific carbon atoms in saturated fatty acids. These atoms are marked by the symbol * in the scheme

$$^-OOC*CH_2CH_2(*CH_2CH_2)_n*CH_2CH_2*CH_3$$
$$\quad\ z\ \ f\quad\ h\qquad\ c/d\qquad\quad\ e\quad\ g\quad\ a$$

The operation of this scheme in fatty acid synthesis from ethanol was verified in *D. melanogaster* third instar larvae after an 8-h feeding period,[38] which is depicted in Figure 2. The net result of subtracting average control patterns of endogenous fatty acids/triacylglycerols from patterns obtained after 8 h was that intensities of the peaks (g), (h), (TG1,3) and (TG2) remained unenriched in contrast to the other strongly enriched peaks. These patterns are evidence of the extensive *de novo* production of fatty acids from ethanol, but also allow three other phenomena to be recorded:

1. Chain elongation of endogenous fatty acids from ethanol did not occur, because no spin-spin coupling at peak (h) could be observed. That the $\Delta f/\Delta a$ and $\Delta e/\Delta a$ ratios were found to be approximately 1.0 confirmed the thesis that chain elongation occurs only in fatty acids that were synthesized *de novo*.

2. The average chain length of the *de novo* synthesized fatty acids was apparently dependent on the activity of the ADH enzyme. Low activity resulted in fatty acids of shorter chain length; higher activity resulted in long-chain fatty acids. (Perhaps the feeding times of ethanol were too short to relate ADH activity directly to fatty acid chain length.)[38]

3. Monounsaturated fatty acids were also found to be synthesized *de novo* from those saturated fatty acids.^{13}C-NMR provides a versatile

tool to monitor those processes as well. In addition, the peaks of the glycerol backbone in triacylglycerols (TG1,3 and TG2) were increased by a factor of about 1.5 after 24 h of ethanol feeding. A large portion of the fatty acids produced from ethanol was stored as triacylglycerols, a finding earlier derived from ^{14}C-tracer studies.[1,3] Geer and co-workers[54] found that about 65% of the label from ethanol was in the triacylglycerol fraction, about 27% in phospholipids, and the remaining portion in diacylglycerol (4%), monoacylglycerol (2.5%), and in free fatty acids (FFA) (0.7%). The major site for diacylglycerol, triacylglycerol, and phospholipid synthesis in insects is the fat body.[55-58]

THE NONOXIDATIVE ELIMINATION OF ETHANOL IN *DROSOPHILA*

Collectively the minor pathways account for <10% of the ethanol elimination capacity in *D. melanogaster* larvae. The possible involvements of catalase, the microsomal ethanol-oxidizing system (MEOS), and glutathione-S-transferase (GST; EC 2.5.1.18) in alcohol elimination in *D. melanogaster* have recently been reviewed.[3] Therefore, the authors consider a minor system[58-60] for ethanol elimination that has only been reported in vertebrates.

The ^{13}C-NMR measurements of chloroform extracts of larvae exposed to ethanol for 24 h contained two novel peaks of 18.3 and 58.4 ppm. These peaks were not found in larvae that were fed ethanol for shorter periods of time (Figure 3a). By using the ethyl ester of lauric acid as a standard, the peak at 58.4 in Figure 3b was identified as an FFA ethyl ester (FFAEE). However, the peak at 18.3 ppm was not identified. The overall chemical structure of an FFAEE is depicted below. The asterisk represents the position of the ^{13}C-atom derived from [2-^{13}C]ethanol.

$$\text{CH}_3\text{CH}_2(\text{CH}_2)_n\text{CH}_2\overset{\displaystyle\overset{\text{O}}{\|}}{\text{C}} - \text{O*CH}_2\text{CH}_3$$

Based upon a quantitative assessment of the NMR data (as shown in Figure 3a), the contribution of this nonoxidative pathway to ethanol elimination may be appreciable in third instar larvae. In insects, FFAEEs may function as pheromones as well as storage molecules.[62,63]

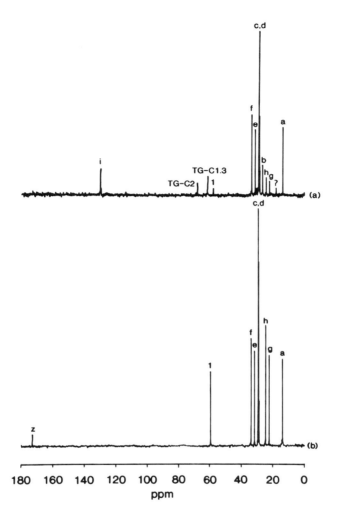

FIGURE 3. ^{13}C-NMR spectrum of chloroform extracts of (a) larvae administered [2-^{13}C]ethanol for 24 h, and of a test solution containing 2.5 M lauric acid ethyl ester (in b). The peak at 58.4 ppm in (a) corresponds to FFAEE as shown in the test solution. The peak at 18.3 in (a) has not been identified. (From Freriksen, A. et al., unpublished data.)

FFAEE were first observed in mammalian cardiac tissue that had been exposed to ethanol.[59] FFAEE have also been found in other human tissues where the levels seem to correlate with the pathological phenomena.[64] Lange and co-workers[60] suggested that human GST may be involved in the formation of FFAEEs, but the resolution of GST and FFAEE synthase activities during protein purification suggests that this may not be the case.[65] The enzyme(s) that forms FFAEE in *D. melanogaster* has not been identified.

ETHANOL EFFECTS ON PHOSPHOLIPIDS

D. melanogaster individuals that possess fully functional ADH systems may differ little in their abilities to eliminate ethanol. Differences in the fitness of these individuals when exposed to environmental alcohols may depend on differences in lipid composition, and subsequently, membrane characteristics.

MEMBRANE EFFECTS

In vertebrate systems, ethanol is known to destabilize membranes and increase membrane fluidity.[66-71] By monitoring the incorporation of 5- and 12-doxyl-stearic acid into mitochondrial membranes by electron spin resonance (ESR), our laboratory recently observed that ethanol, *n*-propanol, and *n*-butanol all increase mitochondrial membrane fluidity in third instar *D. melanogaster* larvae (Figures 4 and 5).[72] The 5-doxyl-stearic acid spin probe is incorporated into the outer regions of membranes, whereas the 12-doxyl-stearic acid spin probe is incorporated deeper into membranes. The 12-doxyl-stearic acid probe data showed that ethanol increases fluidity deep within the membrane in a dose-dependent manner, agreeing with observations of vertebrate membranes (Figure 4).[73,74]

Ethanol-induced alterations deep within the membrane may be more important to the ethanol tolerance of the animal than ethanol-induced lipid changes at the periphery of membranes. The ethanol tolerance of *D. melanogaster* larvae was determined by the percent of larvae that pupated under ethanol stress and was examined for association with membrane fluidity. Membrane fluidity as determined with the 5-doxyl-stearic acid probe was not significantly associated with ethanol tolerance ($r = 0.102$; $F = 0.22$, df $= 1, 21$; $p = 0.64$), whereas membrane fluidity as measured with the 12-doxyl-stearic acid probe was significantly correlated to ethanol tolerance ($r = 0.677$; $F = 16.898$, df $= 1,20$; $p < 0.0005$).[72] This suggests that a decrease in membrane fluidity within hydrophobic membrane domains is accompanied by greater sensitivity to the toxic effects of ethanol in *D. melanogaster*.

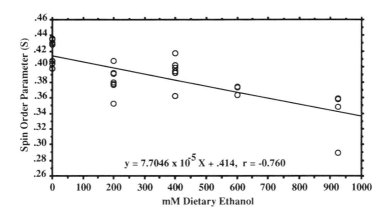

FIGURE 4. The effect of dietary ethanol on fluidity within hydrophobic domains of mitochondrial membranes. 4-d posthatch Canton-S larvae were exposed to various concentrations of dietary ethanol under axenic conditions. After a 48-h exposure to dietary ethanol, larvae were removed from test media, washed, and homogenized in 0.5 ml of 10 mM potassium phosphate buffer, pH 7.2; 2 mM Na$_2$H$_2$EDTA; 0.2 mM dithiothreitol; and 0.07 mM phenylthiourea. Insoluble material was removed by a 15-min centrifugation at 900 $\times$ g. Mitochondrial pellets were isolated by centrifugation for a 30-min spin at 15,000 $\times$ g. Mitochondrial membranes were then labeled with 12-doxyl-stearic acid (30 ng of probe in ethanol per microgram of mitochondrial protein) for 30 min on ice. Solvent was removed under N$_2$ and unincorporated probe removed by washing mitochondrial pellets with buffer. ESR spectra were then taken on a modified Varian (V4500) spectrometer with precautions guarding against spectral distortions due to power and modulation effects. Data from spectral scans were analyzed and expressed as spin order parameter (S), as reported by Gaffney.[75]

Increases in fluidity of the outer regions of the membrane may be related to changes in the amounts of phospholipid headgroups. A 48-h exposure to dietary ethanol significantly decreased the level of phosphatidylcholine (PC) in third instar larvae, and increased the level of phosphatidylethanolamine (PE).[76] Ethanol-induced increases in PE and decreases in PC have also been seen in other animal systems. Alling et al.[77] reported that 80% of human alcoholics suffering from liver damage display abnormally low levels of PC. Moscatelli and Demediuk[78] reported that exposure to ethanol increased the levels of ethanolamine-containing phospholipids in rat brains.

Ethanol-induced decreases in PC levels may be partially related to ethanol enhancement of phospholipase C (PLC; EC 3.1.4.3) and phospholipase D (PLD; EC 3.1.4.4) activities, and the ethanol-induced influx of Ca^{2+} into fat body cells.[76] Ethanol-induced decreases in PC are partially

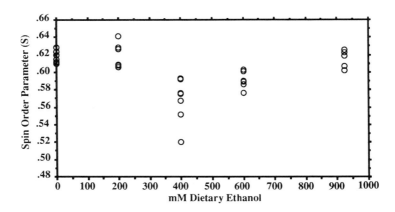

FIGURE 5. The effect of dietary ethanol on fluidity within hydrophilic domains of mito-chondrial membranes. 4-d posthatch Canton-S larvae were exposed to various concentrations of dietary ethanol under axenic conditions. After a 48-h exposure to dietary ethanol, larvae were removed from test media, washed, and homogenized in 0.5 ml of 10 mM potassium phosphate buffer, pH 7.2; 2 mM Na$_2$H$_2$ EDTA; 0.2 mM dithiothreitol; and 0.07 mM phenylthiourea. Insoluble material was removed by a 15-min centrifugation at 900 $\times$ g. Mitochondrial pellets were isolated by a 30-min spin at 15,000 $\times$ g. Mitochondrial mem-branes were then labeled with 5-doxyl-stearic acid (10 ng of probe in ethanol per microgram of mitochondrial protein) for 30 min on ice. Solvent was removed under N$_2$ and unincor-porated probe removed by washing mitochondrial pellets with buffer. ESR spectra were then taken on a modified Varian (V4500) spectrometer with precautions guarding against spectral distortions due to power and modulation effects. Data from spectral scans were analyzed and expressed as spin order parameter (S), as reported by Gaffney.[75]

related to ethanol-induced increases in PLC (r = -0.486, F = 10.497, df = 1, 34; p = 0.0027) and PLD (r = -0.55, F = 14.740, df = 1, 34; p = 0.0005) activities. Isopropanol (200 mM), methanol, n-propanol, and n-butanol also promoted decreased levels of PC along with higher activities of PLC and PLD.[76] The hydrolytic activities of PLC and PLD toward PC have been demonstrated in other systems.[79-82] Therefore, PLC and PLD activities are not directed solely to phosphatidylinositol-mediated forms of signal transduction.

The content of PC was significantly correlated to mitochondrial mem-brane fluidity as determined using the 5-doxyl-stearic acid probe (r = 0.504; F = 8.874; df = 1, 24; p = 0.0062). However, PC content was not significantly associated with membrane fluidity as measured using a 12-doxyl-stearic acid probe (r = 0.265; F = 1.624; df = 1, 22; p = 0.2158). Loss of PC within larval tissues may therefore be partially related to increases in fluidity in the periphery of mitochondrial membranes of *D. melanogaster*.

MECHANISMS OF ALCOHOL-INDUCED PHOSPHATIDYLCHOLINE CHANGES

At least three mechanisms for the alcohol-induced decreases in PC levels appear to be possible: (1) alcohols may enhance the enzymatic activities of phospholipases that hydrolytically degrade PC; (2) ethanol may inhibit the uptake of dietary choline into cells; (3) ethanol may inhibit the final stages of PC synthesis.

Phospholipases and Ca^{2+}

Alcohol-induced changes in the activities of PLC and PLD were correlated with a redistribution of Ca^{2+} in third instar larvae of *D. melanogaster*.[76] Dietary methanol, ethanol, isopropanol, *n*-propanol, and *n*-butanol all caused Ca^{2+} levels to decrease within larvae, while some tissues, such as the fat body and gut, demonstrated alcohol-induced increases in Ca^{2+} influx. Thus, a redistribution of Ca^{2+} was seen within alcohol-treated larvae. This redistribution of Ca^{2+} may be very important in ethanol tolerance as demonstrated by the correlation of endogenous levels of Ca^{2+} to survival to pupation under ethanol stress (r = 0.777; F = 39.492; df = 1, 26; p = 0.0001). The uptake of $^{45}Ca^{2+}$ into the fat body also was correlated to the survival of larvae under ethanol stress (r = -0.769; F = 33.369; df = 1, 23; p = 0.0001). This suggests that the level of intracellular Ca^{2+} may be related to ethanol tolerance in larvae.

This may also explain how Ca^{2+} ethanol enhances the hydrolytic activity of *Drosophila* PLC and PLD toward PC. *In vitro* assays have demonstrated that while the hydrolytic activities of *Drosophila* PLC and PLD are not dependent on Ca^{2+}, PLD and PLC activities can be enhanced through the addition of submicromolar concentrations of Ca^{2+}.[76]

The stimulatory and inhibitory effects of Ca^{2+} on PLD activity has been observed in other systems. Halenda and Rehm[83] recently demonstrated that the formation of phosphatidylethanol was not only catalyzed by PLD, but was also Ca^{2+}-dependent. Taki and Kanfer[84] have reported that increasing concentrations of $CaCl_2$ ranging from 0 to 5 μM stimulated the catalytic activity of rat brain PLD toward PC. This stimulatory effect did not appear to be Ca^{2+}-specific since rat brain PLD activity was also promoted by Fe^{2+}. In the same study, concentrations of $CaCl_2$, ranging from 5 to 40 μM were found to inhibit the activity of PLD that utilized PC as a substrate.

The stimulating effect of Ca^{2+} on PLD activity may explain the observations that Ca^{2+}-mobilizing agents, such as vasopressin, angiotensin

II, and epinephrine, all induced the formation of phosphatidylethanol by hepatic PLD.[85] This finding is particularly interesting since the transphosphatidylation activity of rat hepatic PLD was enhanced by GTP-γS [guanosine-5′-O-(3-thiotriphosphate)][80,85] and raises the possibility that PLD activity may be regulated by G-proteins. Like the hydrolytic activity of rat brain PLD toward PC, the transphosphatidylation of rat brain PLD was inhibited by high concentrations of divalent cations, and PC rather than PE was the best substrate for phosphatidylglycerol formation.[86]

Ethanol may also affect the distribution of Ca^{2+} in vertebrate tissues. It has been shown to inhibit the influx of Ca^{2+} through Ca^{2+}-channels in vertebrate neurons,[87-91] has been reported to reduce the levels of membrane-bound Ca^{2+} by 30 to 40% in rat aortas and portal veins,[92-95] and has stimulated the influx of Ca^{2+} into hepatocytes and enhanced the formation of Ca^{2+}-deposits within mitochondria and microsomal membranes.[96-98]

Choline Uptake and Ethanol

In vertebrates, dietary choline crosses cell membranes through carrier-mediated transport systems before being phosphorylated by choline kinase or in the case of liver or kidney cells, metabolized by the mitochondrial enzymes choline dehydrogenase (EC 1.1.99.1) and betaine aldehyde dehydrogenase (EC 1.2.1.8). Choline transport mechanisms are frequently described as low and high affinity, Na^+-dependent systems.[99]

Since choline is a rather small ligand for a receptor, it is not surprising to find that other ligands of similar size inhibit choline uptake. In a variety of vertebrate systems, ethanolamine and choline each are known to inhibit the high affinity uptake of the other.[100-103] Inhibition of high affinity choline uptake has also been demonstrated in ethanol-treated synaptosomes isolated from mouse[104] and rat.[105,106]

D. melanogaster has a strict requirement for dietary choline for development,[107,108] reproduction,[109] and ethanol tolerance.[110] Recent experiments in the authors' laboratory indicated that dietary ethanol inhibits the uptake of dietary ^{14}C-choline into third instar Canton-S larvae. When larvae were raised on a defined medium that lacked ethanol,[111] and K'_m for ^{14}C-choline uptake was 79.233 μM ± 19.262 with a V_{max} of 1.591 × 10^{-3} nmol/h/ng protein ± 1.4382 × 10^{-4}. When larvae were raised on 200 mM ethanol, the K'_m for ^{14}C-choline uptake was 132.074 μM ± 22.152 (t = 5.31; p <0.001). The V_{max} of 0 and 200 mM ethanol diets did not differ (Figure 6).[72] This indicates that low concentrations of dietary ethanol

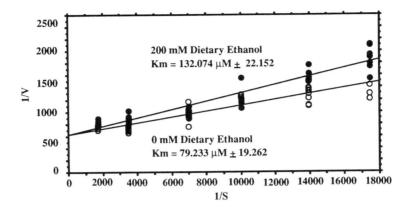

FIGURE 6. The effect of dietary ethanol on choline uptake. 4-d posthatch Canton-S larvae were placed on sterile media containing various concentrations of ethanol and choline (approximately 6725 drops per minute of ^{14}C-choline per milliliter of media [v/v] supplemented with various concentrations of nonradioactive choline). Total choline concentrations ranged from 28.7 to 574 μM, while dietary ethanol concentrations ranged from 0 to 600 mM. After 44 h on test media, larvae were removed, washed, and homogenized in 300 μl of 10 mM potassium phosphate buffer, pH 7.2; 2 mM Na$_2$H$_2$ EDTA; 0.2 mM dithiothreitol; and 0.07 mM phenylthiourea. Insoluble material was removed by a 10-min centrifugation at 15,000 $\times$ g. Homogenates were then assayed for protein and the incorporation of ^{14}C-choline.

act as competitive inhibitors in choline uptake. Since the study was performed at equilibrium, where K_m may approximate K_s, low concentrations of ethanol may be able to bind to the active site of the choline pump and lower the affinity for choline. Whether this binding initiates signal transduction is unknown.

At higher dietary concentrations ethanol acted as a noncompetitive inhibitor (Figure 7). The K_m' values at 400 and 600 mM ethanol were not different. Meanwhile, 600 mM concentrations of ethanol promoted a significant decrease in V_{max} when compared to 400 mM ethanol diets ($t = 3.524$; $p < 0.001$). The V_{max} for 400 mM ethanol diets was 1.385×10^{-3} nmol/h/ng protein $\pm 1.142 \times 10^{-4}$. The V_{max} in 600 mM ethanol diets was 1.105×10^{-3} nmol/h/ng protein $\pm 1.121 \times 10^{-4}$.[72] If K_m truly approximates K_s, then the data suggest that high concentrations of dietary ethanol may inhibit choline uptake by either binding to the choline transport system at a point removed from the active site, or reducing the efficiency of the transport system by increasing membrane fluidity. With increased membrane fluidity, the choline transport system may sink deeper into the membrane and have a lower affinity for choline.

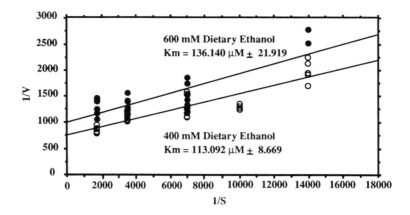

FIGURE 7. The effect of dietary ethanol on choline uptake. 4-d posthatch Canton-S larvae were placed on sterile media containing various concentrations of ethanol and choline (approximately 6725 drops per minute of ^{14}C-choline per milliliter of media [v/v] supplemented with various concentrations of nonradioactive choline). Total choline concentrations ranged from 28.7 to 574 μM, while dietary ethanol concentrations ranged from 0 to 600 mM. After 44 h on test media, larvae were removed, washed, and homogenized in 300 μl of 10 mM potassium phosphate buffer, pH 7.2; 2 mM Na$_2$H$_2$ EDTA; 0.2 mM dithiothreitol; and 0.07 mM phenylthiourea. Insoluble material was removed by a 10-min centrifugation at 15,000 $\times$ g. Homogenates were then assayed for protein and the incorporation of ^{14}C-choline.

The concept that high concentrations of ethanol inhibit choline uptake by increasing membrane fluidity is controversial. Mrak and North[105] reported that 50 mM ethanol reduced the uptake of ^{14}C-choline into rat synaptosomes *in vitro*. Ethanol (600 mM) not only inhibited ^{14}C-choline uptake, but also inhibited the uptake of [^{3}H]-γ-aminobutyric acid (GABA).[107] The ethanol-induced inhibition of choline and GABA occurred in the presence of 0.5% dimethylsulfoxide (DMSO). Since DMSO stabilizes membranes and decreases membrane fluidity,[112,113] Mrak and North[105] argued that the ethanol-induced inhibition of choline and GABA uptake cannot solely be due to ethanol-induced increases in membrane fluidity.

Other factors may contribute to a reduction in the level of choline in cells. Ethanol ingestion has been shown to enhance choline oxidation in rat liver, and this may result in choline deficiency.[114] The breakdown product, betaine, may serve as an important methylating agent when normal methylation pathways are impaired by ethanol.[115]

Ethanol and the Final Stages of
Phosphatidylcholine Synthesis

Since dietary ethanol stimulates the hydrolysis of PC by PLD and PLC and inhibits choline uptake, ethanol may impair the final stages of PC synthesis in *D. melanogaster* larvae. Although this question has not been addressed in *D. melanogaster,* a review of the vertebrate literature indicates that ethanol may inhibit the final stages of PC synthesis.

The synthesis of PC in many animal systems occurs by two different pathways. In the first pathway, the amino of PE is methylated in a three-step process which is catalyzed by phospholipid methyltransferase (PMTase). This pathway is active in vertebrate tissues. Although *Drosophila*-PMTase presumably has been isolated and partially characterized,[116] the *in vivo* methylation capabilities of *D. melanogaster* are at best poor, as evidenced by the absolute requirement for choline for development.[3,57,107]

The major pathway for PC synthesis is the Kennedy pathway,[117,118] a three-step pathway that begins with choline.[119] In the first step, the phosphorylation of choline is phosphorylated through the use of ATP (adenosine-5'-triphosphate) by choline kinase (ATP:choline phosphotransferase [CPT], EC 2.7.1.32) which has a strict requirement for Mg^{2+}.[99] Choline-phosphate cytidyl-transferase (CT, CTP; EC 2.7.7.15) catalyzes the formation of CDP-choline (cytidine-5'-diphosphate-choline) from phosphorylcholine. Once CDP-choline is formed, CDP-choline is then transferred to diacylglycerol through the use of CPT (EC 2.7.8.2).

CPT requires Mg^{2+} or Mn^{2+} as a cofactor and is inhibited by Ca^{2+}.[120] Ca^{2+}-induced inhibition of CPT and ethanolaminephosphotransferase (EPT; EC 2.7.8.1) has also been demonstrated in rat adipose tissue,[121] rat hepatocytes,[118,122-124] rat brain,[125] lung,[126-129] and skeletal muscle.[130] Ca^{2+}-induced inhibition has also been observed in shrimp,[131] indicating that even CPT and EPT from invertebrates may be regulated by Ca^{2+}.

Since the enzymes of the Kennedy pathway appear to universally require Mg^{2+} or Mn^{2+} as cofactors while being inhibited by Ca^{2+}, the ethanol-induced influx of Ca^{2+} into larval fat body cells[76] may inhibit the synthesis of PC in *D. melanogaster*. This reduction in PC content appeared to increase the fluidity of the outer edges of mitochondrial membranes when larvae were subjected to moderate to high concentrations of dietary ethanol[72] and may be in part explained by the loss of cylindrically shaped phospholipids coupled with a shift to the hexagonal$_{II}$ membrane configuration associated with increases in PE.[3,68,132,133]

While ethanol tolerance has been linked to ethanol-induced increases in membrane fluidity,[3,68,73,91,134,135] differences in ethanol tolerance cannot be explained solely on the basis of differences in ethanol-induced reductions in choline content within larvae. Ethanol-induced decreases in PC failed to significantly correlate to ethanol toxicity in larvae fed 573.71 μM dietary choline (r $=$ 0.162, F $=$ 1.624, df $=$ 1, 22; p $=$ 0.674).[72] However, ethanol-induced increases in membrane fluidity in deeper regions of larval mitochondrial membranes were correlated to ethanol tolerance (r $=$ 0.677, F $=$ 16.898, df $=$ 1, 20; p $=$ 0.0005). This may indicate that ethanol-induced changes within membrane fatty acids may be more important to ethanol tolerance and membrane fluidity than the presence or absence of the choline headgroup within PC residues.

LIPID COMPOSITION AND ALCOHOL TOLERANCE

Keys to the toxicity of ethanol in *D. melanogaster* have been derived from studies on the effects of dietary ethanol on the fat body cell ultra-structure of ADH-deficient larvae.[10] Ethanol caused a reduction of the interdigitating cell membrane. Mitochondria with abnormal structures were also observed, and the capacities to form glycogen rosettes, protein bodies, and lipid droplets were significantly diminished by dietary ethanol.[10] This suggests that at growth-limiting concentrations, dietary ethanol decreases the capacity of the fat body cells to absorb nutrients and to release metabolites, perhaps because of its effect on membrane structure.

In humans excessive ethanol consumption may affect the metabolism of key nutrients and vitamins in the liver and other parts of the body,[136] a situation that may be analogous to the cellular changes noted in the cells of the fat body of ADH-deficient *D. melanogaster*.[10] Although chronic exposure to ethanol may result in permanent damage to the liver and other tissues, the mechanism is unknown.[136,137] Acetaldehyde, which promotes lipid peroxidation, may be the agent that modifies mitochondrial and plasma membranes of the vertebrate liver.[137] Induction of MEOS by dietary ethanol may increase the capacity to form acetaldehyde from ethanol, but may also increase the capacity to form other toxic metabolites, xenobiotics, that contribute to cell damage.[136,137] This section is an attempt to establish the importance of the lipid composition of cell membranes to ethanol tolerance, as indicated by experiments with *D. melanogaster*.

THE PHYSIOLOGICAL STATE AND TOLERANCE

In studies of the effect of dietary supplements on physiological processes it often can be argued that a nutrient exerts its influence by improving the general physiological state of the organism. Thus, the individual is more vigorous and can better withstand stress. It has been postulated that resistance to a number of stress factors is accomplished via a single mechanism by *D. melanogaster*.[138,139] Some evidence exists that nutritional stress has a general effect on the physiological state of *D. melanogaster*. Adult *D. melanogaster* males raised on diets deficient for one of several vitamins and nutrients were found to be more sensitive to the mutagenic action of an alkylating agent compared to adult males raised on a proficient diet.[140] During times of environmental stress megadoses of required nutrients or the inclusion of nutrients in the diet that are not usually required may be beneficial to the animal. Sucrose improved ethanol tolerance to a moderate extent in *D. melanogaster* larvae.[6] Sucrose also prevented the development of fatty liver in rats that were chronic consumers of ethanol,[115] suggesting that the toxic effects of ethanol are greater when the animal is malnourished.[141]

Nonetheless, supplementation of the diet per se does not increase ethanol tolerance in *D. melanogaster* larvae.[6] Casein, L-threonine, and RNA supplements had little influence on the ethanol tolerance of larvae as compared to long-chain fatty acids.[6]

FATTY ACIDS AND ETHANOL TOLERANCE

Dietary ethanol, as well as other short-chain alcohols, promotes the appearance of shorter, more unsaturated fatty acids in the phospholipids[72] and total lipids of *D. melanogaster* larvae.[3,111] Since these studies were performed with defined sterile media, which lacked all lipids except cholesterol, the alcohol-induced changes seen within fatty acids are due to alcohol-induced changes in the *de novo* synthesis of fatty acids. A shift toward shorter, more unsaturated fatty acids in phospholipids has been linked to increased membrane fluidity in a variety of systems.[3,68,132,133] The percent of phospholipid-derived fatty acids that were short chain (^{10} to ^{14}C) was correlated with fluidity of the inner regions of mitochondrial membranes ($r = -0.70$; $F = 18.755$; $df = 1, 20$; $p = 0.0003$).[72] These data suggest that the ethanol-induced shift toward shorter fatty acids not only increases membrane fluidity within the hydrophobic regions of membranes, but also reduces ethanol tolerance.

Other lines of evidence suggest that the fatty acid compositions of lipids are important to ethanol tolerance. Exposure to ethanol has been shown to destabilize membrane order in vertebrate cells, which in turn promotes increased fluidity of membranes.[69,73,134,135,142] In contrast to membranes from animals not tolerant of ethanol, membranes isolated from alcohol-tolerant animals resist the membrane-disordering effects of ethanol.[69-71,143-145] Ethanol has been found to modify the lipids of a wide variety of cells.[146-148] These changes may be mediated by ethanol-stimulated changes in the specificities of enzymes that are involved in lipid synthesis. The maintenance of the normal membrane configuration in the presence of alcohol could be, at least in part, a product of the fatty acid composition of its lipid components.

THE ASSOCIATION OF LONG-CHAIN FATTY ACIDS WITH ETHANOL TOLERANCE

Although insects do not require saturated fatty acids in the diet, inclusion of these fatty acids in the diet improves growth.[149] Only certain Diptera, including D. melanogaster, have the ability to develop in the absence of polyunsaturated fatty acids.[150] McKechnie and Geer[6] found that the dietary inclusion of long-chain (14- to 18-carbon) saturated dietary fatty acids significantly altered the fatty acid content of larval lipids. Partial correlation analysis of this set of data indicated that the percent of larvae to pupate in an ethanol environment was positively associated with the levels of 18-carbon fatty acids in two wild-type strains. Although the 18-carbon fatty acids of E. melanogaster are rich in unsaturated fatty acids,[151] a less robust association was seen when the degree of unsaturated fatty acids was correlated to ethanol tolerance. This implies that ethanol-induced changes in fatty acid chain length are more important to ethanol tolerance in Drosophila larvae than ethanol-induced increases in fatty acid desaturation.[6]

Geer et al.[54] examined third instar larvae of seven isochromosomal lines with different second chromosomes and significantly different degrees of ethanol tolerance, but which also differed within their second chromosomes. They found that genetic factors influencing ethanol tolerance of larvae are located on chromosome 2, and analyzed the data for significant correlations between biochemical traits and ethanol tolerance. The correlations between ADH and *sn*-glycerol-3-phosphate dehydrogenase (GPDH; EC 1.1.1.8) activities and ethanol tolerance were weak, and the association of flux of ethanol into lipid was moderate. Larvae of the lines with the highest concentrations of long-chain fatty acids in their phospholipids were more resistant to the toxicity of ethanol. These correlations suggest that larvae of lines with the greater proportions of 18-carbon fatty acids, regardless of whether the fatty acids dietary or synthesized *de novo*, are more capable of surviving growth-limiting concentrations of ethanol.[3,6]

   sn-Glycerol-3-phosphate oxidase (GPO; EC 1.1.99.5) activity is related to the ethanol tolerance of *D. melanogaster* larvae,[151] and the association of GPO activity with survival in the experiments with isochromosomal lines of *D. melanogaster* was a consequence of the GPO-18-carbon fatty acid association.[54] Although the GPO enzyme has not been implicated directly in the metabolism of long-chain fatty acids, it may modify lipid metabolism by influencing the concentration of *sn*-glycerol-3-phosphate, an important lipid substrate, through its possible rate-limiting role in the *sn*-glycerol-3-phosphate cycle.[153,154] The *sn*-glycerol-3-phosphate cycle also facilitates the regeneration of cytoplasmic NAD^+, thus influencing the $NADH/NAD^+$ ratio.[155] This means GPO could mediate ethanol degradation by supplying NAD^+ for ADH activity.[1,48,156] Both enzymes of the *sn*-glycerol-3-phosphate cycle, GPO and GPDH, are induced by dietary ethanol in *D. melanogaster* larvae.[157,158] As mentioned, the reoxidation of NADH may at times be rate limiting.

   In addition to alcohols and carbohydrates the natural diet of *D. melanogaster* includes yeasts which are rich sources of fatty acids. Evidence indicates that 18- and 20-carbon polyunsaturated fatty acids are important to most, if not all, insect species.[159] In fact, long-chain, polyunsaturated fatty acids were preferentially incorporated into phospholipids over 16:0 and 18:0 in adults of housefly and the field cricket.[160-162] Selective incorporation of fatty acids into membrane phospholipids may allow the organism to regulate membrane fluidity under stress conditions.[163] If this mechanism is operating in the larvae of *E. melanogaster,* fatty acids that optimize membrane function may be selected from the intracellular fatty acid pool for incorporation into membrane lipids. The authors plan to test this hypothesis in future experiments.

ACKNOWLEDGMENTS

We would like to thank the many Knox College students who assisted in some of the research projects that are reported in this chapter, and who provided the stimulation that motivated us to complete this task. We are grateful to Christine Baumgardner and Amos Dare who provided leadership during the course of our research on nutrition and alcohol. We appreciate the assistance and advice of Robert Kooser in the ESR studies. We are indebted to Astrid Freriksen and Barbara de Ruiter for their support. We are especially grateful to Stephen McKechnie who stimulated our initial interest in alcohol dehydrogenase. Finally, we are grateful for the support of National Institutes of Health Grant AA06702.

REFERENCES

1. Geer, B. W., Langevin, M. L., and McKechnie, S. W., Dietary ethanol and lipid synthesis in *Drosophila melanogaster, Biochem. Genet.*, 23, 607, 1985.
2. Geer, B. W., Heinstra, P. W. H., Kapoun, A., and van der Zel, A., Alcohol dehydrogenase and alcohol tolerance in *Drosophila melanogaster,* in *Ecological and Evolutionary Genetics of Drosophila*, Barker, J. S. F. and Starmer, W. T., Eds., Plenum Press, New York, 1990, 231.
3. Geer, B. W., Miller, R. R., Jr., and Heinstra, P. W. H., Genetic and dietary control of alcohol degradation in *Drosophila,* in *Drug and Alcohol Abuse Reviews,* Vol. 2, *Liver Pathology,* Watson, R. R., Ed., Humana Press, Clifton, NJ, 1991, 325.
4. McKechnie, S. W. and Morgan, P., Alcohol dehydrogenase polymorphism of *Drosophila melanogaster:* aspects of alcohol and temperature variation in the larval environment, *Aust. J. Biol. Sci.,* 35, 85, 1982.
5. Hoffmann, A. A. and McKechnie, S. W., Heritable variation in resource performance and resource response in a winery population of *Drosophila melanogaster, Evolution,* 45, 1000, 1991.
6. McKechnie, S. W. and Geer, B. W., Long-chain dietary fatty acids affect the capacity of *Drosophila melanogaster,* to tolerate ethanol, *J. Nutr.,* submitted, 1992.
7. Clark, A. G. and Keith, L. G., Variation among extracted lines of *Drosophila melanogaster* in triacylglycerol and carbohydrate storage, *Genetics,* 119, 595, 1988.
8. Clark, A. G., Genetic components of variation in energy storage in *Drosophila melanogaster, Evolution,* 44, 637, 1990.
9. Green, P. R. and Geer, B. W., Changes in fatty acid composition of *Drosophila melanogaster* during development and ageing, *Arch. Int. Physiol. Biochim.,* 87, 485, 1979.

10. Geer, B. W., Dybas, L., and Shanner, L. J., Alcohol dehydrogenase and ethanol tolerance at the cellular level in *Drosophila melanogaster, J. Exp. Zool.*, 250, 22, 1989.

11. Gibson, J. B., Enzyme flexibility in *Drosophila melanogaster, Nature,* 227, 959, 1970.

12. Bijlsma-Meeles, E. and van Delden, W., Intra- and interpopulation selection concerning the alcohol dehydrogenase locus in *Drosophila melanogaster, Nature,* 247, 369, 1974.

13. McDonald, J. F., Chambers, G. K., David, J., and Ayala, F. J., Adaptive response due to changes in gene regulation: a study with *Drosophila, Proc. Natl. Acad. Sci. U.S.A.,* 74, 4562, 1977.

14. Cavener, D. R. and Clegg, M. T., Dynamics of correlated genetic systems. IV. Multilocus effects of ethanol stress environments, *Genetics,* 90, 629, 1978.

15. Heinstra, P. H. W., Scharloo, W., and Thorig, G. E. W., Physiological significance of the alcohol dehydrogenase polymorphism in larvae of *Drosophila, Genetics,* 117, 75, 1987.

16. McKechnie, S. W. and Geer, B. W., Regulation of alcohol dehydrogenase in *Drosophila melanogaster* by dietary alcohol and carbohydrate, *Insect Biochem.,* 14, 231, 1984.

17. van der Zel, A., Dadoo, R., Geer, B. W., and Heinstra, P. W. H., The involvement of catalase in alcohol metabolism in *Drosophila melanogaster* larvae, *Arch. Biochem. Biophys.,* 287, 121, 1991.

18. Heinstra, P. W. H., Eisses, K. Th., Schoonen, W. G. E. J., Aben, W., de Winter, A. J., van der Horst, D. J., van Marrewijk, W. J., Beenakkers, A. M. Th., Scharloo, W., and Thörig, G. E. W., A dual function of alcohol dehydrogenase in *Drosophila, Genetica,* 60, 129, 1983.

19. Anderson, S. M. and Barnett, S. E., The involvement of alcohol dehydrogenase and aldehyde dehydrogenase in alcohol/aldehyde metabolism in *Drosophila melanogaster, Genetica,* 83, 99, 1991.

20. Heinstra, P. W. H., Geer, B. W., Seykens, D., and Langevin, M. L., The metabolism of ethanol-derived acetaldehyde by alcohol dehydrogenase (EC 1.1.1.1.) and aldehyde dehydrogenase (EC 1.2.1.3.) in *Drosophila melanogaster* larvae, *Biochem. J.,* 259, 791, 1989.

21. Heinstra, P. W. H., Scharloo, W., and Thörig, G. E. W., Alcohol dehydrogenase polymorphism in *Drosophila:* enzyme kinetics of product inhibition, *J. Mol. Evol.,* 28, 145, 1988.

22. Winberg, J.-O. and McKinley-McKee, J. S., The ADH-S alloenzyme of alcohol dehydrogenase from *Drosophila melanogaster:* variation of kinetic parameters with pH, *Biochem. J.,* 255, 589, 1989.

23. Chambers, G. K., Minireview: gene expression, adaptation and evolution in higher organisms. Evidence from studies of *Drosophila* alcohol dehydrogenase, *Comp. Biochem. Physiol.,* 99B, 723, 1991.

24. Kapoun, A. M., Geer, B. W., Heinstra, P. W. H., Corbin, V., and McKechnie, S. W., Molecular control of the induction of alcohol dehydrogenase by ethanol in *Drosophila melanogaster* larvae, *Genetics,* 124, 881, 1990.

25. Heinstra, P. W. H. and Geer, B. W., unpublished data, 1988.
26. Eisses, K. T., On the oxidation of aldehydes by alcohol dehydrogenase of *Drosophila melanogaster:* evidence for the gem-diol as the reacting substrate, *Bioorg. Chem.,* 17, 268, 1989.
27. Moxom, L. N., Holmes, R. S., Parsons, P. A., Irving, M. G., and Doddrell, D. M., Purification and molecular properties of alcohol dehydrogenase from *Drosophila melanogaster:* evidence from NMR and kinetic studies for function as an aldehyde dehydrogenase, *Comp. Biochem. Physiol.,* 80B, 525, 1985.
28. Garcin, F. J., Côté, J., Radouco-Thomas, S., Kasenczuk, D., Chawl, S., and Radouco-Thomas, C., Acetaldehyde oxidation in *Drosophila melanogaster* and *Drosophila simulans:* evidence for the presence of an NAD$^+$-dependent aldehyde dehydrogenase, *Comp. Biochem. Physiol.,* 75B, 205, 1983.
29. Garcin, F. J., Hin, G. L. Y., Côté, J., Radouco-Thomas, C., Chawla, S., and Radouco-Thomas, C., Aldehyde dehydrogenase in *Drosophila:* development and functional aspects, *Alcohol,* 2, 85, 1985.
30. Martinez-Leal, J. F. and Barbancho, M., Acetaldehyde detoxification in *Drosophila melanogaster* adults involving ALDH (EC 1.2.1.3.) and ADH (EC 1.1.1.1.) enzymes, *Insect Biochem.,* submitted, 1992.
31. Barbancho, M., Effects of dietary ethanol, acetaldehyde, 2-propanol and acetone on the variation of several enzyme activities involved in alcohol metabolism of *Drosophila melanogaster* adults, *Insect Biochem.,* submitted, 1992.
32. Agarwal, D. P. and Goedde, H. W., Pharmacogenetics of alcohol dehydrogenase (ADH), *Pharmacol. Ther.,* 45, 69, 1990.
33. Heinstra, P. W. H., Aben, W. J. M., Scharloo, W., and Thörig, G. E. W., Alcohol dehydrogenase of *Drosophila melanogaster:* metabolic differences mediated through cryptic allozymes, *Heredity,* 57, 23, 1986.
34. Tejwani, G. A. and Duruibe, V. A., Effects of ethanol on carbohydrate metabolism, in *Regulation of Carbohydrate Metabolism,* Vol. 2, Beitner, R., Ed., CRC Press, Boca Raton, FL, 1985, 67.
35. Kacser, H. and Porteous, J. W., Control of metabolism: what do we have to measure?, *Trends Biochem. Sci.,* 12, 5, 1987.
36. Middleton, R. J. and Kacser, H., Enzyme variation, metabolic flux and fitness: alcohol dehydrogenase in *Drosophila melanogaster, Genetics,* 105, 633, 1983.
37. Heinstra, P. W. H. and Geer, B. W., Metabolic control analysis and enzyme variation: nutritional manipulation of the flux from ethanol to lipids in *Drosophila, Mol. Biol. Evol.,* 8(5), 8, 703, 1991.
38. Freriksen, A., Seykens, D., Scharloo, W., and Heinstra, P. W. H., Alcohol dehydrogenase controls the flux from ethanol into lipids in *Drosophila* larvae: a ^{13}C-NMR study, *J. Biol. Chem.,* 266, 21, 399, 1991.
39. Crabb, D., Bosron, W., and Li, T.-K., Steady-state kinetic properties of purified rat liver alcohol dehydrogenase: application to predicting alcohol elimination rates *in vivo, Arch. Biochem. Biophys.,* 224, 299, 1983.
40. Lindros, K. O., Stowell, L., Pikkarainen, P., and Salaspuro, M., Elevated blood acetaldehyde in alcoholics with accelerated ethanol elimination, *Pharmacol. Biochem. Behav.,* 13, 119, 1980.

41. Koehn, R. K., personal communication, 1991.

42. Geer, B. W., McKechnie, S. W., Bentley, M. M., Oakeshott, J. G., Quinn, E. M., and Langevin, M. L., Induction of alcohol dehydrogenase by ethanol in *Drosophila melanogaster, J. Nutr.,* 118, 398, 1988.

43. Lindsley, D. L. and Grell, E. H., *Genetic Variations of Drosophila melanogaster,* Publ. No. 627, The Carnegie Institute, Washington, D.C., 1968.

44. Trivinos, L. and Geer, B. W., The induction of alcohol dehydrogenase by primary alcohols in the fat body of *Drosophila melanogaster,* in preparation, 1992.

45. Freriksen, A., Scharloo, W., and Heinstra, P. W. H., manuscript in preparation, 1991.

46. Malloy, C. R., Sherry, A. D., and Jeffrey, F. M. H., Carbon flux through citric acid cycle pathways in perfused heart by ^{13}C NMR spectroscopy, *FEBS Lett.,* 212, 58, 1987.

47. Malloy, C. R., Sherry, A. D., and Jeffrey, F. M. H., Evolution of carbon flux and substrate selection through alternate pathways acid cycle of the heart by ^{13}C NMR spectroscopy, *J. Biol. Chem.,* 263, 6964, 1988.

48. Geer, B. W., McKechnie, S. W., and Langevin, M. L., Regulation of *sn*-glycerol-3-phosphate dehydrogenase in *Drosophila melanogaster* larvae by dietary ethanol and sucrose, *J. Nutr.,* 113, 1632, 1983.

49. Geer, B. W., Williamson, J. H., Cavener, D. R., and Cochrane, B. J., Dietary modulation of glucose-6-phosphate dehydrogenase and 6-phosphogluconate dehydrogenase in *Drosophila,* in *Current Topics in Insect Endocrinology and Nutrition,* Bhaskaran, G., Friedman, S., and Rodriguez, J., Eds., Plenum Press, New York, 1981, 253.

50. Heinstra, P. W. H., Seykens, D., Freriksen, A., and Geer, B. W., Metabolic physiology of alcohol degradation and adaptation in *Drosophila* larvae as studied by means of carbon-13 nuclear magnetic resonance spectroscopy, *Insect Biochem.,* 20, 343, 1990.

51. Cohen, S. M., Ogawa, S., and Shulman, R. G., ^{13}C NMR studies of gluconeogenesis in rat liver cells: utilization of labeled glycerol by cells from euthyroid and hyperthyroid rats, *Proc. Natl. Acad. Sci. U.S.A.,* 76, 1603, 1979.

52. den Hollander, J. A. and Shulman, R. G., ^{13}C NMR studies of *in vivo* kinetic rates of metabolic processes, *Tetrahedron,* 39, 3529, 1983.

53. Cohen, S. M., Enzyme regulation of metabolic flux, in *Methods in Enzymology,* Vol. 177, Oppenheimer, N. J. and James, T. L., Eds., Academic Press, San Diego, 1989, 417.

54. Geer, B. W., McKechnie, S. W., Heinstra, P. W. H., and Pyka, M. J., Heritable variation in ethanol tolerance and its association with biochemical traits in *Drosophila melanogaster, Evolution,* 45, 1107, 1991.

55. Williams, M. L., Bygrave, F. L., and Birt, L. M., Phospholipid synthesis in developing flight muscle of *Lucilia, Insect Biochem.,* 4, 161, 1974.

56. Tietz, A., Weintraub, H., and Peled, Y., Utilization of 2-acyl-*sn*-glycerol by locust fat body microsomes, *Biochem. Biophys. Acta,* 388, 165, 1975.

57. Downer, R. G. H., Functional role of lipids in insects, in *Biochemistry of Insects,* Rockstein, M., Ed., Academic Press, New York, 1978, 57.

58. Rizki, T. M., Fat body, in *The Genetics and Biology of Drosophila*, Vol. 2b, Ashburner, M. and Wright, T., Eds., Academic Press, New York, 1978, 561.

59. Lange, L. G., Nonoxidative ethanol metabolism: formation of fatty acid ethyl esters by cholesterol esterase, *Proc. Natl. Acad. Sci. U.S.A.*, 79, 3954, 1982.

60. Bora, P. S., Spilburg, C. A., and Lange, L. G., Metabolism of ethanol and carcinogens by glutathione transferase, *Proc. Natl. Acad. Sci. U.S.A.*, 86, 4470, 1980.

61. Lin, T.-N., Sun, A. Y., and Sun, G. Y., Effects of ethanol on arachidonic acid incorporation into lipids of a plasma membrane fraction isolated from brain cerebral cortex, *Alcohol. Clin. Exp. Res.*, 12, 795, 1988.

62. Ikan, R., Bergmann, E. D., Yinon, U., and Shulov, A., Identification, synthesis and biological activity of an "assembling scent" from the beetle *Trogoderma granarium, Nature*, 223, 317, 1969.

63. Calam, D. H., Species and sex-specific compounds from the heads of male bumblebees *(Bombus* spp.), *Nature*, 221, 856, 1969.

64. Laposata, E. A. and Lange, L. G., Presence of nonoxidative ethanol metabolism in human organs commonly damaged by ethanol abuse, *Science*, 231, 497, 1986.

65. Sharma, R., Gupta, S., Singhal, S. S., Ahmad, H., Haque, A., and Awasthi, Y. C., Independent segregation of glutathione S-transferase and fatty acid ethyl ester synthase from pancreas and other human tissues, *Biochem. J.*, 275, 507, 1991.

66. Waring, A. J., Rottenberg, H., Ohnishi, T., and Rubin, E., Membranes and phospholipids of liver mitochondria from chronic alcoholic rats are resistant to membrane disordering by ethanol, *Proc. Natl. Acad. Sci. U.S.A.*, 78, 2582, 1981.

67. Polokoff, M. A., Simon, T. J., Harris, R. A., Simon, F. R., and Iwahashi, M., Chronic ethanol increases liver plasma membrane fluidity, *Biochemistry*, 24, 3114, 1985.

68. Sun, G. Y. and Sun, A. Y., Ethanol and membrane lipids, *Alcohol. Clin. Exp. Res.*, 9, 164, 1985.

69. Taraschi, T. F. and Rubin, E., Biology of disease: effects of ethanol on the chemical and structural properties of biologic membranes, *Lab. Invest.*, 52, 120, 1985.

70. Taraschi, T. F., Ellingson, J. S., Wu, A., Zimmerman, R., and Rubin, E., Membrane tolerance is rapidly lost after withdrawal: a model for studies of membrane adaptation, *Proc. Natl. Acad. Sci. U.S.A.*, 83, 3669, 1986.

71. Taraschi, T. F., Ellingson, J. S., Wu, A., Zimmerman, R., and Rubin, E., Phosphatidylinositol from ethanol-fed rats confers membrane tolerance to ethanol, *Proc. Natl. Acad. Sci. U.S.A.*, 83, 9398, 1986.

72. Miller, R. R., Jr., Dare, A., Kooser, R. G., and Geer, B. W., The effects of ethanol on lipid metabolism in *Drosophila:* the role of the choline head-group and fatty acids in membrane fluidity, in preparation, 1992.

73. Chin, J. H. and Goldstein, D. B., Effects of alcohols on membrane fluidity and lipid composition, in *Membrane Fluidity in Biology*, Vol. 3, Aloia, R. C. and Boggs, J. M., Eds., Academic Press, New York, 1985, 1.

74. Taraschi, T. F., Wu, A., and Rubin, E., Phospholipid spin probes measure the effects of ethanol on the molecular order of liver microsomes, *Biochemistry,* 24, 7096, 1985.

75. Gaffney, B. J., Practical considerations for the calculation of order parameters for fatty acid or phospholipid spin labels in membranes, in *Spin Labeling: Theory and Applications,* Berliner, L. J., Ed., Academic Press, New York, 1976, 567.

76. Miller, R. R., Jr., Yates, J. W., and Geer, B. W., The effects of ethanol on phospholipids in *Drosophila melanogaster* larvae: the role of phospholipase C, phospholipase D, and Ca^{+2}, *Biochim. Biophys. Acta,* submitted, 1991.

77. Alling, C., Ballsin, J., Kahlson, K., and Olsson, R., Decreased linoleic acid in serum lecithin after chronic alcohol abuse, *Subst. Alcohol. Act. Mis.,* 1, 557, 1980.

78. Moscatelli, E. A. and Demediuk, P., Effects of chronic consumption of alcohol and low thiamin, low protein diets on the lipid composition of rat whole brain and rat membranes, *Biochim. Biophys. Acta,* 596, 331, 1980.

79. Besterman, J. M., Duronio, V., and Cuatrecasas, P., Rapid formation of diacylglycerol from phosphatidylcholine: a pathway for generation of a second messenger, *Proc. Natl. Acad. Sci. U.S.A.,* 83, 6785, 1986.

80. Qian, Z. and Drewes, L. R., Muscarinic acetylcholine receptor regulates phosphatidylcholine phospholipase D in canine brain, *J. Biol. Chem.,* 264, 21720, 1989.

81. Billah, M. M., Eckel, S., Mullmann, T. J., Egan, R. W., and Siegel, M. I., Phosphatidylcholine hydrolysis by phospholipase D determines phosphatidate and diglyceride levels in chemotactic peptide-stimulated human neutrophils, *J. Biol. Chem.,* 264, 17069, 1989.

82. Exton, J. H., Signaling through phosphatidylcholine breakdown, *J. Biol. Chem.,* 265, 1, 1990.

83. Halenda, S. P. and Rehm, A. M., Evidence for the calcium-dependent activation of phospholipase D in thrombin-stimulated erythroleukemia cells, *Biochem. J.,* 267, 479, 1990.

84. Taki, T. and Kanfer, J. N., Partial purification and properties of a rat brain phospholipase D, *J. Biol. Chem.,* 254, 9761, 1979.

85. Bocckino, S. B., Wilson, P. B., and Exton, J. H., Ca^{+2}-mobilizing hormones elicit phosphatidylethanol accumulation via phospholipase D activation, *FEBS Lett.,* 225, 201, 1987.

86. Chalifour, R. J., Taki, T., and Kanfer, J. N., Phosphatidylglycerol formation via transphosphatidylation by rat brain extracts, *Can. J. Biochem.,* 58, 1189, 1980.

87. Harris, R. A. and Hood, W. F., Inhibition of synaptosomal calcium uptake by ethanol, *J. Pharmacol. Exp. Ther.,* 213, 562, 1980.

88. Leslie, S. W., Barr, E., Chandler, J., and Farrar, R. P., Inhibition of fast and slow phase depolarization-dependent synaptosomal calcium uptake by ethanol, *J. Pharmacol. Exp. Ther.,* 225, 571, 1983.

89. Hoffman, P. L., Rabe, C. S., Moses, F., and Tabakoff, B., N-Methyl-D-aspartate receptors and ethanol: inhibition of calcium flux and cyclic GMP production, *J. Neurochem.,* 52, 1937, 1989.

90. Tabakoff, B. and Hoffman, P. L., Adaptive responses to ethanol in the central nervous system, in *Alcoholism: Biomedical and Genetic Aspects,* Goedde, H. W. and Agarwal, D. P., Eds., Pergamon Press, New York, 1989, 91.

91. Littleton, J. M., Effects of ethanol on membranes and their associated functions, in *Human Metabolism of Alcohol,* Vol. 3, Crow, K. E. and Batt, R. D., Eds., CRC Press, Boca Raton, FL, 1989, 161.

92. Turlapaty, P. D. M. V., Altura, B. T., and Altura, B. M., Ethanol reduces Ca^{+2} concentrations in arterial and venous smooth muscle, *Experientia,* 35, 639, 1979.

93. Turlapaty, P. D. M. V., Altura, B. T., and Altura, B. M., Interactions of Tris buffer and ethanol on agonist-induced responses of vascular smooth muscle and on calcium-45 uptake, *J. Pharmacol. Exp. Ther.,* 211, 59, 1979.

94. Altura, B. M. and Altura, B. T., Pharmacology of venules: some current concepts and clinical potential, *J. Cardiovasc. Pharmacol.,* 3, 1413, 1981.

95. Altura, B. M. and Altura, B. T., Cardiovascular functions in alcoholism and after acute administration of alcohol: heart and blood vessels, in *Alcoholism: Biomedical and Genetic Aspects,* Goedde, H. W. and Agarwal, D. P., Eds., Pergamon Press, New York, 1989, 167.

96. Rubin, R. and Hoek, J. B., Ethanol-induced stimulation of phosphoinositide turnover and calcium uptake in isolated hepatocytes, *Biochem. Pharmacol.,* 37, 2461, 1988.

97. French, S. W., Role of mitochondrial damage in alcoholic liver disease, in *Biochemistry and Pharmacology of Ethanol,* Majchrowicz, E. and Noble, E. P., Eds., Plenum Press, New York, 1979, 409.

98. Ponnappa, B. C., Waring, A. J., Hoek, J. B., Rottenberg, H., and Rubin, E., Chronic ethanol ingestion increases calcium uptake and resistance to molecular disordering by ethanol in liver microsomes, *J. Biol. Chem.,* 257, 10141, 1982.

99. Ishidate, K., Choline transport and choline kinase, in *Phosphatidylcholine Metabolism,* Vance, D. E., Ed., CRC Press, Boca Raton, FL, 1989, 9.

100. Jernigan, H. M., Kador, P. F., and Kinoshita, J. H., Carrier-mediated transport of choline in rat lens, *Exp. Eye Res.,* 32, 709, 1981.

101. Zelinski, T. A. and Choy, P. C., Ethanolamine inhibits choline uptake in the isolated hamster heart, *Biochim. Biophys. Acta,* 794, 326, 1984.

102. Yorek, M. A., Dunlap, J. A., Spector, A. A., and Ginsberg, B. H., Effect of ethanolamine on choline uptake and incorporation into phosphatidylcholine in human Y79 retinoblastoma cells, *J. Lipid Res.,* 27, 1205, 1986.

103. Lipton, B. A., Yorek, M. A., and Ginsberg, B. H., Ethanolamine and choline transport in cultured bovine aortic endothelial cells, *J. Cell. Physiol.,* 137, 571, 1988.

104. Beracochea, D., Durkin, T. P., and Jaffard, R., On the involvement of the central cholinergic system in memory deficits induced by long term ethanol in mice, *Pharmacol. Biochem. Behav.,* 24, 519, 1986.

105. Mrak, R. E. and North, P. E., Ethanol inhibition of synaptosomal high-affinity choline uptake, *Eur. J. Pharmacol.,* 151, 51, 1988.

106. North, P. E. and North, R. E., Synaptosomal uptake of choline and of gamma-aminobutyric acid: effects of ethanol and dimethylsulfoxide, *Neurotoxicology,* 10, 569, 1989.

107. Geer, B. W. and Vovis, G. F., The effects of choline and related compounds on the growth and development of *Drosophila melanogaster, J. Exp. Zool.,* 158, 223, 1965.
108. Geer, B. W., Vovis, G. F., and Yund, M. A., Choline activity during the development of *Drosophila melanogaster, Physiol. Zool.,* 41, 280, 1968.
109. Geer, B. W. and Dolph, W. W., A dietary choline requirement for egg production in *Drosophila menalogaster, J. Reprod. Fertil.,* 21, 9, 1970.
110. Tilghman, J. A. and Geer, B. W., The effects of choline deficiency on the lipid composition and ethanol tolerance of *Drosophila melanogaster, Comp. Biochem. Physiol.,* 90C, 439, 1988.
111. Geer, B. W., McKechnie, S. W., and Langevin, M. L., The effect of dietary ethanol on the composition of lipids of *Drosophila melanogaster* larvae, *Biochem. Genet.,* 24, 51, 1986.
112. Lyman, G. H., Papahadjopoulos, D., and Presiler, H. D., Membrane action of DMSO and other chemical inducers of Friend leukemic cell differentiation, *Nature,* 262, 360, 1976.
113. Lyman, G. H., Preisler, H. D., and Papahadjopoulos, D., Phospholipid membrane stabilization by dimethylsulfoxide and other inducers of Friend leukemia cell differentiation, *Biochem. Biophys. Acta,* 448, 460, 1976.
114. Roa, G. A. and Larkin, E. C., Role of nutrition in causing the effects attributed to chronic alcohol consumption, *Med. Sci. Res.,* 16, 53, 1988.
115. Rao, G. A., Larkin, e. C., Beckenhauer, H. C., and Barak, A. J., Chronic alcohol ingestion and hepatic methionine metabolism in rats: role of adequate nutrition, *Biochem. Arch.,* 3, 437, 1987.
116. de Sousa, S. M., Krishnan, K. S., and Kenkare, U. W., Phospholipid methyltransferase from *Drosophila melanogaster:* purification and properties, *Insect Biochem.,* 18, 377, 1988.
117. Kennedy, E. P. and Weiss, S. B., Cytidine diphosphate choline: a new intermediate in lecithin biosynthesis, *J. Am. Chem. Soc.,* 77, 250, 1955.
118. Kennedy, E. P. and Weiss, S. B., The function of cytidine coenzymes in the biosynthesis of phospholipides, *J. Biol. Chem.,* 222, 193, 1956.
119. Tijburg, L. B. M., Geelen, M. J. H., and van Golde, L. M. G., Regulation of the biosynthesis of triacylglycerol, phosphatidylcholine, and phosphatidylethanolamine in the liver, *Biochim. Biophys. Acta,* 1004, 1, 1989.
120. Cornell, R., Cholinesphosphotransferase, in *Phosphatidylcholine Metabolism,* Vance, D. E., Ed., CRC Press, Boca Raton, FL, 1989, 47.
121. Coleman, R. and Bell, R. M., Phospholipid synthesis in isolated fat cells, *J. Biol. Chem.,* 252, 3050, 1977.
122. Weiss, S. B., Smith, S. W., and Kennedy, E. P., The enzymatic formation of lecithin from cytidine diphosphate choline and D-1,2 diglyceride, *J. Biol. Chem.,* 231, 53, 1958.
123. Liteplo, R. G. and Sribney, M., Inhibition of rat liver CDP ethanolamine:1,2 diacylglycerol ethanolamine phosphotransferase activity by ATP and pantothenic acid derivatives, *Can. J. Biochem.,* 55, 1049, 1977.
124. Alemany, S., Varea, I., and Mato, J. M., Inhibition of phosphatidylcholine synthesis by vasopressin and angiotensin in rat hepatocytes, *Biochem. J.,* 208, 453, 1982.

125. McCaman, R. E. and Cook, K., Intermediary metabolism of phospholipids in brain tissue. III. Phosphocholine-glyceride transferase, *J. Biol. Chem.*, 241, 3390, 1966.

126. Zachman, R. D., The enzymes of lecithin biosynthesis in human newborn lungs. III. Phosphorylcholine-glyceride transferase, *Pediatr. Res.*, 7, 632, 1973.

127. van Heusden, G. P. H., Ruestow, B., van der Mast, M. A., and van den Bosch, H., Synthesis of disaturated phosphatidylcholine by cholinesphosphotransferase in rat lung microsomes, *Biochim. Biophys. Acta*, 666, 313, 1981.

128. Stith, I. E. and Das, S. K., Development of cholinephosphotransferase in guinea pig lung mitochondria and microsomes, *Biochim. Biophys. Acta*, 714, 250, 1982.

129. Post, M., Schurmans, E. A. J. M., Batenburg, J. J., and van Golde, L. M. G., Mechanisms involved in the synthesis of disaturated phosphatidylcholine by alveolar type II cells isolated from adult rat lung, *Biochim. Biophys. Acta*, 750, 68, 1983.

130. Pennington, R. J. and Worsfold, M., Biosynthesis of lecithin by skeletal muscle, *Biochim. Biophys. Acta*, 176, 774, 1969.

131. Ewing, R. D. and Finamore, F. J., Phospholipid metabolism during development of the brine shrimp *Artemia salina*, *Biochim. Biophys. Acta*, 218, 474, 1970.

132. Jain, M. K., *The Biomolecular Lipid Membrane*, Van Nostrand Reinhold, New York, 1972, 25.

133. Cullis, P. R. and De Kruijff, B., Lipid polymorphism and functional roles of lipids in biological membranes, *Biochim. Biophys. Acta*, 559, 399, 1979.

134. LeBourhis, B., Beaugé, F., Aufrere, G., and Nordmann, R., Membrane fluidity and alcohol dependence, *Alcohol. Clin. Exp. Res.*, 10, 337, 1986l

135. Goldstein, D. B., Alcohol and biological membranes, in *Alcoholism: Biomedical and Genetic Aspects*, Goedde, H. W. and Agarwal, D. P., Eds., Pergamon Press, New York, 1989, 87.

136. Palmer, T. N., Fuel homeostasis and alcohol abuse, *Eur. J. Gastroenterol. Hepatol.*, 2, 406, 1990.

137. Lieber, C. S., Mechanism of ethanol induced hepatic injury, *Pharmacol. Ther.*, 46, 1, 1990.

138. Hoffmann, A. A. and Parsons, P. A., An integrated approach to environmental stress tolerance and life-history variation: dessication tolerance in *Drosophila*, *Biol. J. Linn. Soc.*, 37, 117, 1989.

139. Hoffmann, A. A. and Parsons, P. A., Selection for increased dessication resistance in *Drosophila menalogaster:* additive genetic control and correlated responses for other stresses, *Genetics*, 122, 837, 1989.

140. Geer, B. W., Reno, D., and Anderson, C., Nutrient deficiency and the sensitivity of *Drosophila melanogaster* to an alkylating agent, *Nutr. Res.*, 1, 169, 1981.

141. Rao, G. A., Larkin, E. C., and Derr, R. F., Effect of chronic alcohol ingestion: role of nutritional factors, *Biochem. Arch.*, 5, 289, 1989.

142. Goldstein, D. B., Ethanol-induced adaptation in biological membranes, *Ann. N.Y. Acad. Sci.*, 7, 103, 1985.

143. Rottenberg, H., Robertson, D., and Rubin, E., The effect of ethanol on the temperature dependence of respiration and ATPase activities of rat liver mitochondria, *Lab. Invest.,* 42, 318, 1980.

144. Rottenberg, H., Waring, A., and Rubin, E., Tolerance and cross-tolerance in chronic alcoholics: reduced membrane binding of ethanol and other drugs, *Science,* 213, 583, 1981.

145. Wood, W. G., Gorka, C., and Schroeder, F., Acute and chronic effects of ethanol on transbilayer membrane domains, *J. Neurochem.,* 52, 1925, 1989.

146. Herrero, A. A., Gomez, R. F., and Roberts, M. F., Ethanol-induced changes in the membrane lipid composition of *Clostridium thermocellum, Biochim. Biophys. Acta,* 693, 195, 1982.

147. Goto, M., Banno, Y., Umeki, W., Kameyama, Y., and Nozawa, Y., Effects of chronic ethanol exposure on composition and metabolism of *Tetrahymena* membrane lipids, *Biochim. Biophys. Acta,* 751, 286, 1983.

148. Hoek, J. B. and Tarschi, T. F., Cellular adaptation to ethanol, *Trends Biochem. Sci.,* 13, 269, 1988.

149. Downer, R. G. H., Lipid metabolism, in *Comprehensive Insect Physiology, Biochemistry, Pharmacology,* Vol. 10, Kerkut, G. A. and Gilbert, L. I., Eds., Pergamon Press, Oxford, 1985, 77.

150. Stanley-Samuelson, D. W., Jurenka, R. A., Cripps, C., Bloomquist, G. J., and de Renobales, M., Fatty acids in insects: composition, metabolism, and biological significance, *Arch. Insect. Biochem. Physiol.,* 9, 1, 1988.

151. Geer, B. W. and Perille, T. T., Effects of dietary sucrose and environmental temperature on fatty acid synthesis in *Drosophila melanogaster, Insect Biochem.,* 7, 371, 1977.

152. McKechnie, S. W. and Geer, B. W., *sn*-Glycerol-3-phosphate oxidase and alcohol tolerance in *Drosophila melanogaster* larvae, *Biochem. Genet.,* 24, 859, 1986.

153. Beenakkers, A. M. T., Van Der Horst, D. J., and Van Marrewijk, W. J. A., Biochemical processes directed to flight muscle metabolism, *Comp. Insect Physiol. Biochem. Pharmacol.,* 10, 451, 1985.

154. McKechnie, S. W., Ross, J. L., and Turney, K. L., Environmental modulation of alpha-glycerol-3-phosphate oxidase (GPO) activity in larvae of *Drosophila melanogaster,* in *Ecological and Evolutionary Genetics of Drosophila,* Barker, J. S. F., Starmer, W. T., and MacIntyre, J. R., Eds., Plenum Press, New York, 1990, 253.

155. MacIntyre, R. J. and Davis, M. B., A genetic and molecular analysis of the alpha-glycerophosphate cycle in *Drosophila melanogaster, Isozymes: Curr. Topics Biol. Med. Res.,* 14, 195, 1987.

156. Kricka, J. W. M. and Clark, P. M. S., *Biochemistry of Alcohol and Alcoholism,* John Wiley & Sons, New York, 1979.

157. Ross, J. L. and McKechnie, S. W., Micro-spatial population differentiation in the activity of alpha-glycerol-3-phosphate oxidase (GPO) from mitochondria of *Drosophila melanogaster, Genetica,* 84, 145, 1991.

158. Lissemore, J. L., Baumgardner, C. A., Geer, B. W., and Sullivan, D. T., Effect of dietary carbohydrates and ethanol on expression of genes encoding glycerol-3-phosphate dehydrogenase, aldolase, and phosphoglycerate kinase in *Drosophila* larvae, *Biochem. Genet.,* 28, 615, 1990.

159. Stanley-Samuelson, D. W., Jurenka, R. A., Cripps, C., Blomquist, G. J., and de Renobales, M., Fatty acids in insects: composition, metabolism, and biological significance, *Arch. Insect Biochem. Physiol.*, 9, 1, 1988.

160. Stanley-Samuelson, D. W., Jurenka, R. A., Blomquist, G. J., and Loher, W., *De novo* biosynthesis of prostaglandins by the Australian field cricket *Teleogryllus commodus, Comp. Biochem. Physiol.*, 85C, 303, 1986.

161. Stanley-Samuelson, D. W., Loher, W., and Blomquist, G. J., Biosynthesis of polyunsaturated fatty acids by the Australian field cricket, *Teleogryllus commodus, Insect Biochem.*, 16, 387, 1986.

162. Wakayama, E. J., Dillwith, J. W., and Blomquist, G., Occurrence and metabolism of prostaglandins in the housefly, *Musca domestica* (L.), *Insect Biochem.*, 16, 895, 1986.

163. Sinensky, M., Homeoviscous adaptation — a homeostatic process that regulates the viscosity of membrane lipids in *Escherichia coli, Proc. Natl. Acad. Sci. U.S.A.*, 71, 522, 1974.

10 Riboflavin Status of Alcoholics

INTRODUCTION

The riboflavin status of mild and moderate drinkers varies with their intake of dairy foods as well as with their intake of nutrient supplements containing riboflavin. Riboflavin deficiency has been reported in a number of studies of alcoholics.[1] Alcoholics are particularly at risk for riboflavin deficiency, in part, because they tend not to drink milk, which is a major source of riboflavin for many in the U.S. An aversion to milk may arise in alcoholics because they associate milk drinking with a delay in achieving the desired effects of alcohol, due to slower absorption.[2,3] However, in those alcoholics who have alcohol-induced lactose intolerance, gassy diarrhea with or without abdominal pain is experienced when they drink milk, and they usually develop these same symptoms when they eat lactose-containing foods. Thus, the aversion to milk may be linked to their alcohol abuse or be symptom related.

Very low levels of milk consumption by alcoholics is also explained by the fact that alcohol is their principal beverage, and by the fact that negative health behaviors frequently include poor dietary habits as well as heavy alcohol consumption. Even in alcoholics who consume dairy as well as other dietary sources of riboflavin, deficiency of this vitamin may occur because of impaired vitamin absorption or utilization.[2]

This review of studies of the riboflavin status of alcoholics examines the effects of alcohol on riboflavin uptake, metabolism, and excretion. It also focuses on the postulated and known risks of chronic riboflavin deficiency in alcoholics. The differential diagnosis of riboflavin deficiency in alcoholics is discussed, with particular emphasis on differentiation from other nutritional deficiencies which may have similar clinical signs. This

ISBN 0-8493-7933-4
© 1992 by CRC Press, Inc.

is important in alcoholics in whom the correct nutritional diagnosis is the prerequisite of appropriate nutritional intervention.

FUNCTIONS OF RIBOFLAVIN: ROLE IN ALCOHOL AND DRUG METABOLISM

Riboflavin in its coenzyme forms, flavin mononucleotide (FMN) and flavin adenine dinucleotide (FAD), functions in oxidation reduction reactions in energy production, in the respiratory chain, and in drug as well as alcohol metabolism.[4] Support for the role of riboflavin in drug metabolism is largely based on observed changes in riboflavin depleted and repleted rats. In this study, a significant decrease of N-demethylation of aminopyrine, ethylmorphine, and N-methylaniline as well as a decreased hydroxylation of aniline and acetanilide occurred in animals of both sexes. Levels of flavin, the reduced form of nicotinamide adenine dinucleotide phosphate (NADPH) cytochrome c reductase, cytochrome P-450, and cytochrome b_5 were decreased in the riboflavin-depleted rats, and with repletion, levels were restored. The riboflavin depletion did not inhibit induction of drug-metabolizing enzymes by phenobarbital.[5] The latter is of interest in the present context because it suggests that alcohol induction of drug-metabolizing enzymes, which variably increases the alcoholic's tolerance of certain drugs, may not be influenced by their riboflavin status. However, interpretation of the results of this study needs to be very cautious with respect to the attribution of the changes in drug-metabolizing enzymes to riboflavin depletion. In fact, a striking finding was the progressive loss of weight in the riboflavin-depleted animals and a restoration of weight in the animals that were repleted. Since results of this study clearly indicate that the riboflavin depletion caused protein-energy malnutrition (PEM), it may well be asked whether the observed changes in the activities and levels of drug-metabolizing enzymes are actually due to PEM. Perhaps a comment by the authors that administration of the riboflavin antagonist, galactoflavin, reduced levels of cytochrome P-450 is relevant in supporting their claim that riboflavin deficiency per se inhibits the capacity for drug metabolism; since no data are provided to support this observation, no such conclusion can be made.

Riboflavin is involved in a number of vitamin-vitamin interactions that are of interest in that possibly the state of riboflavin nutriture in the alcoholic affects their risk of developing other B vitamin deficiencies. Riboflavin as well as niacin are required for the interconversion of the vitamers of pyridoxine.[6] Also, riboflavin is necessary for the conversion of folic acid to a coenzyme form.[7,8]

FOOD SOURCES OF RIBOFLAVIN IN THE U.S. DIET: COMPARISON OF ALCOHOLICS AND NONALCOHOLICS

Riboflavin-rich foods which contribute largely to the total dietary intake of nonalcoholics in the U.S. include milk, cheese, and yogurt. For nonalcoholics, other important sources of the vitamin include enriched bread and fortified breakfast cereals, as well as vegetables and meats. Liver and yeast, although very rich sources of the vitamin, are not eaten in large amounts and therefore contribute little to total intake.[9] In the alcoholic who avoids breakfast, whose meal pattern is erratic, and who has an aversion to milk and other dairy foods, most of the riboflavin intake is derived from enriched bread and beer.[2,4]

The frequent association of smoking with heavy alcohol use may contribute to the risk that alcoholics eat erratically. This is explained both by the appetite-reducing effects of the smoking habit, and by association of two negative health behaviors which are not conducive to selection of health-promoting dairy foods. In a longitudinal nutritional survey of community elderly in the U.K., those found to have lower riboflavin intakes and who showed biochemical evidence of riboflavin depletion were more likely to be smokers and to be men, who had chronic bronchitis and emphysema, the diseases of smokers. Low intakes of riboflavin were also reported by those who did not eat regularly cooked meals. Unfortunately, no information is provided in the survey report as to whether the malnourished elderly group were heavy drinkers.[10]

INTAKE OF RIBOFLAVIN RELATIVE TO DRINKING STATUS

When reviewing studies that have examined nutrient intake in relation to the level of alcohol intake, it is important to bear in mind that heavy drinkers confabulate. For example, if questioned in a diet history about the type of cereal they eat for breakfast, they will describe in quite a convincing manner not only the type of cereal, but even the variety of fruits that are added. This description is of a fictitious breakfast, and is provided either as a defense, or in response to a leading question which suggests that a positive answer is required. If heavy drinkers are asked to complete a semiquantitative food frequency questionnaire in which milk drinking habits are assessed, it is notably that milk is either avoided or only occasionally used in cooking. Riboflavin intake is usually low due to low dairy food intake. However, riboflavin may be consumed in vitamin supplements, taken by alcoholics in the belief that the nutrients contained in the pills may protect their livers.

Any generalization about the effect of increasing alcohol intake on the nutrient content of the daily diet must be qualified because gender, age, ethnic, regional, and sociocultural differences exist in the way that drinkers may modify their food choices and consumption patterns.

In a cohort study of 89,538 women and 48,493 men, it was found that alcohol was added to food-energy intake in men but that in women, energy from alcohol displaced energy from sugar.[11] These differences in the effect of drinking on eating patterns may be mirrored by gender differences in intake of riboflavin-rich foods.

Studies examining the riboflavin intake of moderate drinkers have not usually found a significant difference between subgroups of drinkers classified by grams of alcohol consumed per day. In a study of elderly men and women in the Boston area, in which riboflavin intake was determined by analysis of 3-d food records, those who reported drinking 15 g or more of alcohol per day had similar intakes of the vitamin vs. those who reported either that they did not consume alcohol, or that they consumed a lesser amount.[12] However, the riboflavin status of those who reported drinking 15 g or more of alcohol per day indicated a mild depletion that was not present in those who consumed less alcohol. In this study, where riboflavin status was determined using the erythrocyte glutathione reductase assay, the possibility exists that either moderate drinking did lead to a less satisfactory riboflavin nutriture or possibly that there was a group difference in the accuracy of reporting intake of dietary sources of riboflavin.

RIBOFLAVIN ABSORPTION, DISTRIBUTION, AND EXCRETION: EFFECTS OF ALCOHOL INTAKE

Riboflavin is mainly absorbed by an active transport process from a saturable site in the proximal small intestine. Absorption also occurs from the large intestine, although this is less efficient. The major stages in epithelial transport of the vitamin are uptake at the luminal membrane, intracellular disposition including metabolism, and basolateral release.[13] In studies of transmural transport of riboflavin in the rat, it has been shown that at physiologically relevant concentrations, a carrier-mediated saturable mechanism of riboflavin uptake predominates; at higher concentrations, simple diffusion is the predominant means of absorption.[14]

Riboflavin uptake by isolated enterocytes has been studied in guinea pigs.[15] However, it is clear that the isolated enterocyte is not ideal for studying the mechanisms by which riboflavin absorption occurs in the intact animal or in humans. In alcohol-fed animals, riboflavin absorption is reduced. Malabsorption of riboflavin may also occur in alcoholics due to changes in small intestine function and structure, as well as due to changes in gastrointestinal (GI) motility.[16]

After absorption, riboflavin is taken up and stored in the liver in its coenzyme forms. It has been shown in rats that severe riboflavin depletion, induced by feeding a riboflavin-free diet, is associated with marked depression of hepatic flavokinase activity and a lesser decrease in the activity of FAD synthetase.[17] This is of interest since flavokinase is the physiologically rate-limiting enzyme in the biosynthesis of flavin coenzymes. In alcoholics, conversion of this vitamin to its coenzyme forms is impaired.

Riboflavin excretion is increased in all catabolic states. Thus, alcoholics who have protein-energy malnutrition show hyper-riboflavinuria despite low intake of the vitamin.

ETIOLOGY AND SIGNS OF RIBOFLAVIN DEFICIENCY IN THE ALCOHOLIC

Riboflavin deficiency in alcoholics may be due to low intake, malabsorption, impaired utilization, or increased excretion of the vitamin. Several of these causes are usually contributory. Alcoholics who have fatty infiltration, alcoholic hepatitis, or cirrhosis have decreased concentrations of riboflavin in their livers.[18,19] It has been emphasized that riboflavin deficiency in alcoholics may be due to a specific action of alcohol and/or its metabolite, acetaldehyde, on riboflavin metabolism.[20] While no direct evidence exists that high alcohol intake increases renal losses of riboflavin, hyperexcretion of riboflavin may occur not only in alcoholics who have protein-energy malnutrition, but also in those who have muscle wasting due to alcoholic myopathy.[21]

Alcoholics with severe riboflavin deficiency may show seborrheic dermatitis of the nasolabial folds and of other flexural areas; angular stomatitis, cheilitis, and glossitis; and they may exhibit photophobia. Because other nutritional deficiencies are frequently present, signs of these other deficiencies may complicate the clinical picture. While protein-energy malnutrition is the most frequent of these nutritional disorders, other B vitamin deficiencies are not uncommon, including folate and niacin deficiency. Indeed, in areas of the world such as India, where endemic pellagra is prevalent among alcoholics, the seborrheic dermatitis of the face and the flexural dermatitis of the extremities which is seen in severe riboflavin deficiency may coexist with the phototoxic dermatosis of pellagra. On the other hand, in the U.S. where pellagra is rare even among severe alcoholics, the differential diagnosis of cutaneous lesions is usually between those of zinc (Zn) and riboflavin deficiency.[22]

Zn deficiency in alcoholics can present with a facial dermatitis and angular stomatitis which are similar (if not identical) to those seen in the riboflavin-deficient state.[23] Clinical differentiation of these two nutritional disorders is complicated by the fact that taste loss and slowed wound healing may be present in both. However, if riboflavin administration does not produce prompt healing of the cutaneous lesions, laboratory tests for Zn deficiency should be promptly carried out. If this is not feasible, a trial of Zn supplementation should be used as a diagnostic as well as a therapeutic measure.

RIBOFLAVIN DEFICIENCY AND ALCOHOL-RELATED DISEASE

Liver Disease

In subhuman primates it has been demonstrated that alcoholic liver disease (ALD) can be induced by chronic feeding of an alcohol-containing liquid diet that contains levels of nutrients, including riboflavin, that are believed to meet the animals' requirements.[24] However, multiple nutritional deficiencies, including riboflavin as well as vitamin A excess, may contribute to or modify the pathology of the liver.[25] While the hepatotoxicity of alcohol is now generally accepted, hepatic lesions in alcoholics may be influenced by other chemical hepatotoxins, by the hepatitis B virus, or by protein-energy malnutrition.[26] Whether severe riboflavin deficiency can also affect liver disease in alcoholics is unclear.

Risk of Hemolytic Anemia in Alcoholics

It has been shown that there is a decrease in fluidity of the red cell membrane in riboflavin-deficient rats. This change in the red cells is accompanied by an increase in activity of the membrane-bound enzyme, cholinesterase. Because of these changes the red cells have a diminished ability to resist oxidative damage and are more subject to hemolysis. Whether these changes in the red cells contribute to the pathogenesis of hemolytic anemia seen in alcoholics has not yet been explored. However, it is known that hypophosphatemia is the major disorder underlying Zieve's hemolytic anemia in alcoholics.[27]

RIBOFLAVIN DEFICIENCY AND CANCER

Whether riboflavin deficiency in alcoholics contributes to their cancer risk has been hotly debated. Epidemiological evidence suggested that cancer of the esophagus is more prevalent in areas of the world, such as parts of China, where there is severe riboflavin deficiency.[28] However, in these areas the cause of the deficiency is low intake, which may be independent of drinking status. The central Asian esophageal cancer belt includes sections of China, Afghanistan, and Russia. Although in these areas severe riboflavin deficiency is not uncommon, evidence to either define the etiological association between heavy alcohol intake with riboflavin deficiency or to link alcohol-related riboflavin deficiency to esophageal cancer has not been successful. Relative to the proposed etiological role of chronic riboflavin deficiency in esophageal cancer, epidemiological studies in the high-prevalence Linxian province of China showed that although 97% of the population had biochemical evidence of riboflavin depletion, no association was detected between the existence or severity of riboflavin deficiency and the occurrence of esophageal cancer. The investigators nevertheless proposed that the nutritional pathology of the esophagus associated with severe riboflavin deficiency might increase the vulnerability of the mucosa relative to the effects of environmental carcinogens.[29] Studies using animal models have not greatly clarified the issue.

In the case of azo dye carcinogenesis, riboflavin deficiency enhances the effect of the carcinogen on tumor development; however, a number of studies have indicated that riboflavin deficiency inhibits tumor growth in experimental animals.[30] The question of interest in the present context is whether riboflavin deficiency in alcoholics contributes to cancer risk. Another way of stating the problem is to ask whether in those cancers that are more prevalent in alcoholics (e.g., pharyngeal, laryngeal, and esophageal cancer), riboflavin deficiency explains the cancer development. The complexity of this question has been indicated by the findings of a study that was designed to show whether alcohol-induced riboflavin deficiency had a promotional effect on the development of 7,12-dimethylbenz[a]anthracene DMBA-induced pouch tumors in hamsters. Riboflavin deficiency was induced in these animals either by diet restriction, by alcohol feeding, or by a combination of both modalities. In the alcohol-fed animals, alcohol provided 35% of the calories in a liquid diet.

Nonalcohol-fed hamsters received a liquid diet in which the alcohol calories were replaced by carbohydrate. Groups of hamsters receiving the alcohol-containing diet showed slower development of the first pouch tumor. However, once the tumors appeared, tumor growth was accelerated in the hamsters fed alcohol. Riboflavin deficiency, whether in the alcohol or nonalcohol-fed groups, was associated with suppression of growth of the pouch tumors. Furthermore, the experiment showed that at least in this animal model system, the effect of alcohol on neoplastic growth was independent of alcohol-induced riboflavin deficiency.[31,32]

Riboflavin deficiency has been shown to promote the development of esophageal tumors induced by the chemical carcinogen methylbenzylnitrosamine in rats. In this study it was shown that riboflavin deficiency per se increased tumor invasiveness.[33]

These studies suggest that alcohol and riboflavin deficiency may independently affect development of cancers of the upper GI tract. However, no evidence presently exists that either the vitamin deficiency or the alcoholic state initiates neoplastic development. Furthermore, extrapolation of animal experiments relative to the effects of alcohol-induced riboflavin deficiency on chemical carcinogenesis to humans must be done in an extremely cautious manner. The human condition of alcohol abuse and the potential carcinogens and cancer-promoting factors to which the alcoholic is exposed are highly dissimilar from those existing in the chemical environment of the animal room. In addition, rodent or even subhuman primate models may not closely mimic the change in immunological defenses and susceptibilities relative to cancer imposed by alcohol abuse and riboflavin deficiency in human populations. It is hoped, however, that from current and ongoing long-term cancer intervention trials, it will be possible to evaluate the single and combined effects of control of alcohol abuse and increase in dietary riboflavin on upper GI cancer incidence.[34]

CONCLUSIONS AND SUMMARY OF NEEDS FOR FUTURE RESEARCH

Conclusions based on the studies cited in this review, or based on experience of alcoholics or of animals that simulate alcoholics in their ethanol consumption, are as follows:

1. That alcohol abuse increases the risk of riboflavin deficiency because of low intake of riboflavin-rich foods, because of malabsorption and

impaired utilization of the vitamin, and because renal excretion of the vitamin may be increased.

2. That protein-energy malnutrition in alcoholics increases the risk and alters the outcomes of riboflavin deficiency relative to morbidity.

3. That riboflavin deficiency may be misdiagnosed in alcoholics or conversely that Zn deficiency may be mistaken for riboflavin deficiency.

4. That both severe riboflavin deficiency and alcohol (or acetaldehyde) toxicity independently cause hepatic lesions.

5. That the effect of riboflavin deficiency on alcohol-related illnesses has not been well investigated in recent years, but may include a link to hemolytic, megaloblastic, and sideroblastic anemias of alcoholics because of vitamin-vitamin interactions.

6. That riboflavin deficiency may adversely effect the alcoholic's tolerance of therapeutic drugs.

7. That at the present time riboflavin deficiency cannot be claimed as a major etiological factor in the risk of upper GI cancer in the alcoholic.

Future research should include studies of the relationships between riboflavin deficiency and specific adverse drug reactions in alcoholics. Also, effects on riboflavin intervention trials on alcohol-related diseases should be studied in Third World countries where severe riboflavin deficiency is still prevalent.

REFERENCES

1. Leevy, C. M. and Baker, H., Vitamins and alcoholism, *Am. J. Clin. Nutr.*, 21, 1325, 1968.
2. Roe, D. A., *Alcohol and the Diet*, AVI Publishing, Westport, CT, 1979, 185.
3. Roe, D. A., Ariboflavinosis, in *Hunter's Tropical Medicine*, Strickland, G. T., Ed., W. B. Saunders, Philadelphia, 1991, 934.
4. Bates, C. J., Human riboflavin requirements, and metabolic consequences of deficiency in man and animals, *World Rev. Nutr. Diet.*, 50, 215, 1987.
5. Patel, J. M. and Pawar, S. S., Riboflavin and drug metabolism in adult male and female rats, *Biochem. Pharmacol.*, 23, 1467, 1974.
6. Rasmussen, K. M., Barsa, P. M., McCormick, D. B., and Roe, D. A., Effect of strain, sex and dietary riboflavin on pyridixone (Pyridoxine)-5'-phosphate oxidase activity in rat tissues, *J. Nutr.*, 110, 1940, 1980.

7. Cooperman, J. M. and Lopez, R., Riboflavin, in *Handbook of Vitamins,* Machlin, L. J., Ed., Marcel Dekker, New York, 1984, 299.

8. Machlin, L. J. and Langseth, L., Vitamin-vitamin interactions, in *Nutrient Interactions,* Bodwell, C. E. and Erdman, J. W., Eds., Marcel Dekker, New York, 1988, 287.

9. Hunt, S. M., Nutritional intake of riboflavin, in *Riboflavin,* Rivlin, R. S., Ed., Plenum Press, New York, 1975, 199.

10. Anon., *Nutrition and Health in Old Age,* Department of Health and Social Security, Her Majesty's Stationery Office, London, 1979, 129.

11. Colditz, G. A., Giovannucci, E., Rimm, E. B., Stampfer, M. J., Rosner, B., Speizer, F. E., Gordis, E., and Willett, W. C., Alcohol intake in relation to diet and obesity in men and women, *Am. J. Clin. Nutr.,* 54, 49, 1991.

12. Jacquez, P. F., Sulsky, S., Hartz, S. C., and Russell, R. M., Moderate alcohol intake and nutritional status in non-alcoholic elderly subjects, *Am. J. Clin. Nutr.,* 50, 875, 1989.

13. Bowman, B. B., McCormick, D. B., and Rosenberg, I. H., Epithelial transport of water soluble vitamins, *Annu. Rev. Nutr.,* 9, 187, 1989.

14. Daniel, H., Wille, U., and Rehner, G., *In vitro* kinetics of the intestinal transport of riboflavin in rats, *J. Nutr.,* 113, 636, 1983.

15. Hegazy, E. and Schwenk, M., Riboflavin uptake by isolated enterocytes of guinea pigs, *J. Nutr.,* 113, 1702, 1983.

16. Lindenbaum, J. and Lieber, C. S., Effects of chronic alcohol administration in man in the absence of nutritional deficiency, *Ann. N.Y. Acad. Sci.,* 252, 228, 1975.

17. Lee, S.-S. and McCormick, D. B., Effect of riboflavin status on hepatic activities of flavin-metabolizing enzymes in rat, *J. Nutr.,* 113, 2274, 1983.

18. Jusko, W. J. and Lewis, G. P., Effect of hepatic disease on liver flavin and protein levels, *Am. J. Clin. Nutr.,* 25, 265, 1972.

19. Morgan, M. Y., Alcohol and nutrition, *Br. Med. Bull.,* 38, 21, 1982.

20. Pinto, J., Huang, Y. P., and Rivlin, R. S., Mechanisms underlying the differential effects of ethanol on the bioavailability of riboflavin and flavin adenine dinucleotide, *J. Clin. Invest.,* 79, 1343, 1987.

21. Pinto, J. T. and Rivlin, R. S., Drugs that promote renal excretion of riboflavin, *Drug-Nutr. Interact.,* 5, 143, 1987.

22. Roe, D. A., Nutrition and the skin in historical perspective, in *Nutrition and the Skin,* Roe, D. A., Ed., Alan R. Liss, New York, 1986, 65.

23. Prasad, A. S., Zinc in growth and development and the spectrum of human zinc deficiency, *J. Am. Coll. Nutr.,* 7, 377, 1988.

24. Lieber, C. S. and DeCarli, L. M., An experimental model of alcohol feeding and liver injury in the baboon, *J. Primatol.,* 3, 153, 1974.

25. Lieber, C. S., The influence of alcohol on nutritional status, *Nutr. Rev.,* 46, 241, 1988.

26. Lieber, C. S. and DeCarli, L. M., Hepatotoxicity of ethanol, *J. Hepatol.,* 12, 394, 1991.

27. Levin, G., Cogan, U., Levy, Y., and Mokady, S., Riboflavin deficiency and the function and fluidity of rat erythrocyte membranes, *J. Nutr.,* 120, 857, 1990.

28. Day, N. E., The geographic pathology of cancer of the esophagus, *Br. Med. Bull.,* 40, 329, 1984.

29. Thurnham, D. I., Rathakette, P., Hambidge, K. M., Munoz, N., and Crespi, M., Riboflavin, vitamin A and zinc status in Chinese subjects in a high risk area for esophageal cancer in China, *Hum. Nutr. Clin. Nutr.*, 36c, 337, 1982.

30. Rivlin, R. S., Riboflavin and cancer, in *Riboflavin*, Rivlin, R. S., Ed., Plenum Press, New York, 1975, 369.

31. Park, C.-I., Riboflavin Deficiency and Alcohol as Interactive Factors in Chemical Carcinogenesis in Hamster Cheek Pouch, Ph.D. thesis, Cornell University, Ithaca, NY, 1986.

32. Roe, D. A., Alcohol, drugs and nutrition, in *Current Problems in Nutrition, Pharmacology and Toxicology*, McLean, A. J. and Wahlquist, M. L., Eds., John Libbey, London, 1988, 191.

33. Conner, M. W., Xie, Y., and Newberne, P. M., Riboflavin effects on esophageal cancer, *Fed. Proc.*, 46 (Abstr. 2534), 750, 1987.

34. Greenwald, P., The future of nutrition research in cancer prevention, in *Vitamins and Cancer Prevention*, Laidlaw, S. A. and Swenseid, M. M. E., Eds., Wiley-Liss, New York, 1991, 111.

11 Folate Metabolism in Alcoholism

INTRODUCTION

Folates are a family of water-soluble vitamins found predominantly in leafy vegetables, legumes, yeast, and liver, as well as in more commercial multivitamin preparations. The recommended dietary allowance for folate is 3 μg/kg body weight for adult men and nonpregnant or lactating women, while the minimum daily requirement for an average-sized adult is estimated at 50 μg.[1]

Folates occur in the diet and perform intracellular metabolic functions as pteroylpolyglutamates (PteGlu$_n$) but circulate in the blood and bile as reduced and methylated pteroylglutamate (PteGlu). Complex regulatory mechanisms include the following. During intestinal absorption, dietary PteGlu$_n$ are hydrolyzed to PteGlu by brush-border folate hydrolase (BBFH), a zinc (Zn)-dependent exopeptidase on the jejunal mucosal surface, followed by binding to folate-binding protein (FBP) and transport into the enterocyte. Intracellular events in the absorbing enterocyte probably include resynthesis from PteGlu to PteGlu$_n$ for metabolic reactions, hydrolysis of PteGlu$_n$ by intracellular folate hydrolase, and transport of PteGlu to the portal circulation.[2] A similar sequence occurs at the liver, with transport of PteGlu across the plasma membrane to the hepatocyte, synthesis of PteGlu$_n$ for intracellular reactions, protein binding and storage,[3,4] and probable intracellular hydrolysis to PteGlu for transport to the systemic circulation or the bile. Approximately 10% of the folate pool cycles through the bile for reabsorption in the proximal jejunum,[5] and <0.1% of the body pool of folate is lost in the feces per day.[6] PteGlu in the systemic circulation is filtered at the glomerulus and is conserved by efficient renal tubular reabsorption[7] so that daily excretion in the urine is <1.0% of the folate pool.[6]

ISBN 0-8493-7933-4
© 1992 by CRC Press, Inc.

The intracellular biochemical folate function of greatest clinical significance is the transfer of a methyl group from 5-methyltetrahydrofolate via vitamin B_{12} during the synthesis of methionine from homocysteine. As a result, intracellular tetrahydrofolate is available for conversion to 5,10-methylenetetrahydrofolate, the cofactor for thymidylate synthesis and production of DNA. Therefore, deficiency of either folate or vitamin B_{12} results in decreased availability of DNA for rapidly regenerating tissues, in particular, the bone marrow and intestinal mucosa. The common clinical expression of these deficiencies is megaloblastic anemia and, less well appreciated, intestinal dysfunction with diarrhea and malabsorption.

CLINICAL FOLATE DEFICIENCY IN ALCOHOLISM

INCIDENCE

Folate deficiency is assessed by measurements of the serum folate level, a relatively labile index of folate balance; by the red cell folate level, an index of tissue stores and depletion; and by evaluation of bone marrow morphology, the ultimate index of folate deficiency.[8] In addition to the measurement employed, the reported incidence of folate deficiency in alcoholism depends upon socioeconomic class and the presence or absence of alcoholic liver disease.[9] Studies of alcoholic patients admitted to municipal hospitals in the U.S. described low serum folate levels in about 80% of recent binge drinkers,[10] whereas low red cell folate levels were found in 40% of a similar population of alcoholics.[11] Other studies indicated a 35% incidence of megaloblastic bone marrow changes in anemic alcoholics.[12,13]

CLINICAL EFFECTS OF FOLATE DEFICIENCY IN ALCOHOLISM

Anemia

Folate deficiency in the alcoholic patient is characterized by anemia with low serum and red-cell folate levels, macrocytic red cells and hypersegmented polymorphonuclear neutrophils, megaloblastic bone marrow changes, and a normal or elevated serum vitamin B_{12} level (Table 1). Folate deficiency can be distinguished from vitamin B_{12} deficiency by the presence of an elevated serum level of homocysteine and a normal serum level of serum methylmalonic acid.[14]

TABLE 1
Clinical Consequences of Folate Deficiency in Alcoholism

Consequence	Mechanism	Ref.
Recognized effects		
Megaloblastic anemia	Delayed red cell maturation due to insufficient DNA	9–13
Diarrhea and malabsorption	Altered enterocyte proliferation and function due to insufficient DNA	15–20
Possible effects		
Decreased hepatic DNA	Insufficient hepatic regeneration	21
Decreased methionine and glutathione	Insufficient folate substrate, alcohol inhibition of methionine synthetase	22–24
Cellular dysplasia/neoplasia	Chromosomal fragility, DNA strand breaks	25–28

Diarrhea and Intestinal Malabsorption

The rapidly regenerating small intestinal mucosa is also a target organ for folate deficiency. Jejunal biopsies from folate-deficient alcoholics with megaloblastic bone marrows demonstrated macrocytosis of absorbing enterocytes.[15,16] Experimental folate deficiency in rats causes macrocytosis of enterocytes and intestinal malabsorption of fluids.[17,18] In human studies, volunteer subjects fed low-folate diets developed diarrhea with decreased absorption of water and electrolytes from the perfused jejunum.[19] When alcohol exposure was added to experimental folate deficiency in alcoholic patient volunteers, malabsorption of glucose and ^{3}H-PteGlu was observed in addition to fluid malabsorption.[20] These studies suggest a generalized effect of folate deficiency on the intestinal epithelium, with altered cellular morphology and transport of several water-soluble substances and nutrients. From a practical and clinical standpoint, the binge-drinking alcoholic patient who presents to a hospital with chronic diarrhea and weight loss is probably folate deficient. This diagnosis is best confirmed by measurement of the red cell folate level, an index of tissue folate stores that is more reliable than the labile serum folate level.

Other Possible Effects

Hepatic repair following alcoholic liver injury may be influenced by the availability of folate. An *in vitro* study using liver slices from alcoholic hepatitis patients demonstrated a decreased uptake of ^{3}H-thymidine, while increased DNA synthesis followed the addition of folic acid.[21] The availability of hepatic folate could influence the supply of methionine and its product glutathione, which plays a significant role in protection against oxidant injury to the liver.[22] Chronic alcohol exposure in the rat model may further restrict the hepatic supply of methionine, while folate metabolism is perturbed by inhibition of the enzyme methionine synthetase.[23,24] Folate deficiency is also associated with chromosomal fragility and DNA strand breaks,[25] and clinical studies showed that folate deficiency contributes to dysplasia in certain tissues.[26-28] Folate supplementation was associated with a lower incidence of bronchial dysplasia in smokers,[26] less cervical dysplasia in women taking oral contraceptives,[27] and a lower incidence of colonic neoplasia in patients with ulcerative colitis.[28] Whether the potential for tissue folate deficiency contributes to the increased incidence of cancer of the gastrointestinal tract in alcoholics has not been proven.

CAUSES OF FOLATE DEFICIENCY IN ALCOHOLISM

The etiology of folate deficiency in alcoholism is complex, involving the three universal causes of nutritional deficiency: inadequate diet, intestinal malabsorption, and increased requirement due to decreased stores and/or increased turnover. In addition, acute and chronic alcoholism appear to have differing effects on folate physiology and metabolism. Thus, the acute administration of an intoxicating dose of alcohol lowers the serum folate level,[29] and daily consumption of moderate amounts of alcohol prevented the hematopoietic response to folic acid in patients with megaloblastic anemia.[30] On the other hand, chronic alcoholic patients with liver disease have less than half the normal hepatic folate levels.[31] Even in the absence of liver disease, chronic alcoholics develop megaloblastic anemia more rapidly than normal when placed on experimental folate-deficient diets.[32] Assuming a similar minimum daily folate requirement of 50 μg in normal and alcoholic adults, hepatic folate stores were calculated from the time required to develop experimental megaloblastic anemia by deficient diet — 140 d in a normal subject vs. 70 d in an alcoholic — to be one-half normal or less in chronic alcoholic patients.[33] The causes of deficient stores are considered below (see also Table 2).

DIETARY INADEQUACY

When alcoholics substitute alcohol for >50% of dietary calories, they frequently deprive themselves of the typical sources of dietary folate.[12]

TABLE 2
Causes of Folate Deficiency in Alcoholism

Cause	Ref.
Dietary deficiency of folate	12, 34
Intestinal malabsorption of folate	
Clinical studies	20, 35, 36
Animal experiments	37–39
Altered hepatobiliary metabolism	41–44
Increased urinary excretion and turnover	6, 45–49

Furthermore, with the exception of malt liquors,[34] alcoholic beverages are essentially devoid of folate.

INTESTINAL MALABSORPTION

To date, clinical studies of folate absorption in alcoholics have focused on the jejunal uptake of PteGlu, the hydrolytic derivative of dietary PteGlu$_n$. An initial study of recently drinking alcoholics demonstrated a lesser rise of radioactivity in plasma following an oral dose of ^{3}H-PteGlu as compared to normal subjects.[35] Subsequently, the technique of intestinal perfusion through a triple-lumen tube demonstrated a significantly lower uptake of ^{3}H-PteGlu from the jejunum of malnourished and folate-deficient alcoholics than from well-nourished alcoholics and improved uptake with abstinence, yet unchanged uptake after 2 weeks' administration of alcohol with a nutritious hospital diet.[36] A synergistic effect of folate deficiency and exposure to alcohol was demonstrated in a subsequent prospective study in which decreased jejunal uptake of ^{3}H-PteGlu, glucose, sodium, and water followed the induction of folate deficiency by the combination of deficient diet and daily alcohol ingestion in two patients; the jejunal uptakes of each substance were unaffected by either folate deficiency or alcohol given separately to two other patients.[20] To summarize, these clinical studies demonstrated malabsorption of ^{3}H-PteGlu in malnourished binge-drinking alcoholics and suggested a relationship of the intestinal malabsorption defect to the synergism of chronic alcohol exposure and folate deficiency.

Animal models of alcoholism have been used to define the effect of chronic alcohol exposure on intestinal absorption under conditions that permit accurate control over diet and alcohol administration. Comparing findings in a group of monkeys (*Macaca radiata*) fed control diets or diets containing 50% of calories as alcohol for 2 years, alcohol feeding resulted in decreased hepatic folate levels together with decreased absorption of orally administered ^{3}H-PteGlu, as shown by decreased urinary and increased fecal excretion of tritium.[37] Subsequently, minipigs were used to study the effect of chronic alcohol feeding on the two initial stages of folate absorption, hydrolysis of PteGlu$_n$ and uptake of the hydrolytic product PteGlu.[38,39] After 1 year of controlled alcohol feeding, jejunal perfusion through indwelling tubes in awake animals showed decreased hydrolysis of PteGlu$_n$ but unchanged uptake of PteGlu.[38] A companion study using isolated jejunal brush-border vesicles showed significantly lower activity of jejunal BBFH in vesicles from alcohol-fed compared to control-fed animals, but similar vesicle uptake of PteGlu.[39] To summarize, the animal studies suggest that folate malabsorption and deficiency can be induced by chronic exposure to alcohol and that alcohol inhibition of BBFH may be the initial intestinal defect.

ALTERED HEPATOBILIARY METABOLISM

The finding of decreased hepatic folate levels in chronic alcoholic patients[31] and in experimental animals fed alcohol[37,38] suggests inhibitory effects of alcoholism on the hepatic uptake and/or metabolism of folate. Data from acute experiments conflict with those from experiments using chronic exposure to alcohol. Thus, in isolated rat hepatocytes, acute alcohol exposure enhanced the uptake of methyl-PteGlu.[40] In rats fed 10% alcohol for 3 d, hepatic folate was increased together with decreased biliary folate excretion.[41] On the other hand, two studies in which alcohol was fed to rats for >12 weeks showed unchanged liver folate levels and unchanged *de novo* synthesis of labeled ^{3}H-PteGlu$_n$ from parenterally administered ^{3}H-PteGlu.[42,43] Recent studies demonstrated that chronic alcohol feeding to rats perturbs folate metabolism by inhibition of methionine synthetase, the enzyme required for conversion of methyltetrahydrofolate to tetrahydrofolate during methionine synthesis.[23,24] In monkeys fed alcohol or control diets for 2 years, decreased hepatic folate levels in the alcohol group correlated with a decreased hepatic uptake of parenterally administered ^{3}H-PteGlu, but did not alter *de novo* hepatic synthesis of ^{3}H-PteGlu$_n$ and patterns of endogenous folates.[44] The studies in monkeys suggested that chronic exposure to alcohol decreases folate uptake by the liver but does not appreciably affect hepatic folate metabolism.

TABLE 3
Possible Cellular Mechanisms of Folate Deficiency in Alcoholism

Mechanism	Ref.
Oxidant destruction of folate molecule	52, 53
Altered membrane hydrolysis, binding, or transport of folate	
Intestinal brush border	39
Hepatocyte	40, 44
Renal tubule	6, 45–49

INCREASED URINARY EXCRETION AND TURNOVER

As indicated, the kidneys are the major route of folate excretion via a process of glomerular filtration and tubular reabsorption.[7] The excretion of folate in the urine was increased by the administration of alcohol to human subjects[45,46] and to rats.[45,47] Further studies showed that the alcohol effect on folate excretion is specific for endogenous forms of PteGlu.[48] The mechanism is uncertain, but may relate to an effect of alcohol or an alcohol metabolite on the folate binding and transport mechanism in the brush border of the renal tubule.[49]

Folate turnover was measured in monkeys fed alcohol for 4 years by following daily urinary and fecal excretion of the label for 30 d after parenteral ^{3}H-PteGlu.[6] Compared to control-fed monkeys, excretion of the label in both urine and feces and the calculated turnover of body folate stores was greater during the first 3 d in the alcohol group, whereas long-term folate elimination rates were similar in both groups. Since hepatic folate levels were lower in the alcohol group, the data can be interpreted to show both decreased hepatic uptake as well as increased urinary and fecal excretion of the exogenous dose of labeled PteGlu in the chronic alcohol group.[6]

CELLULAR AND MOLECULAR BASES FOR FOLATE DEFICIENCY IN ALCOHOLISM

Two possible mechanisms, molecular oxidant damage and altered membrane properties or functions, may account for the separate effects of acute and chronic alcoholism on the induction of low folate levels and folate deficiency (Table 3).

OXIDANT DAMAGE TO THE
FOLATE MOLECULE

The observed acute effect of alcohol on lowering serum folate levels[29] and on decreasing the availability of circulating folate to the recovering bone marrow[30] may be caused by oxidant destruction of the folate molecule. It is generally accepted that the alcohol metabolite, acetaldehyde, stimulates the production of superoxide and hydroxyl radicals in the presence of free iron and xanthine oxidase.[50] Other data indicate that exposure to alcohol reduces hepatic glutathione[22] and α-tocopherol,[51] both antioxidant compounds. *In vitro,* the addition of acetaldehyde to a mixture of methylated PteGlu, xanthine oxidase, and iron resulted in cleavage of the folate to pteridine and *p*-aminobenzoic acid, while this effect was prevented by the addition of the antioxidant enzyme superoxide dismutase.[52] This observation, suggesting an oxidant-mediated catabolic effect of acetaldehyde on the folate molecule, was supported by another *in vitro* study,[53] but has not been quantitatively confirmed *in vitro*.

ALTERED MEMBRANE COMPOSITION
AND FUNCTION

Folate homeostasis is regulated by various enzymes, including hydrolases and synthetases, and also by passage of the PteGlu form across several membranes utilizing specific binding proteins and transport systems (Figure 1). To summarize, intestinal absorption requires the functions of two brush-border membrane proteins, BBFH and FBP, as well as a carrier transport system; hepatic metabolism requires presumed binding and transport across the hepatocyte plasma membrane and exit across the basolateral membrane; and urinary folate excretion is regulated by a folate binding and transport system at the renal tubular brush-border membrane. Folate homeostasis could be perturbed in chronic alcoholism by generalized effects on membrane composition or by specific effects on the synthesis of membrane hydrolases and binding proteins involved in folate transport.

Considerable evidence indicates that acute and chronic alcohol exposure alters the phospholipid composition and fluidity of membranes, but these effects are not uniform and may differ among membranes. Thus, in rat intestinal membranes, acute alcohol exposure increased brush-border vesicle fluidity while decreasing sodium transport,[54] whereas another study showed opposing effects of chronic alcohol exposure on the fluidity of brush-border and basolateral membranes.[55] In rat liver, chronic alcohol feeding increased plasma membrane fluidity[56] but decreased mitochondrial

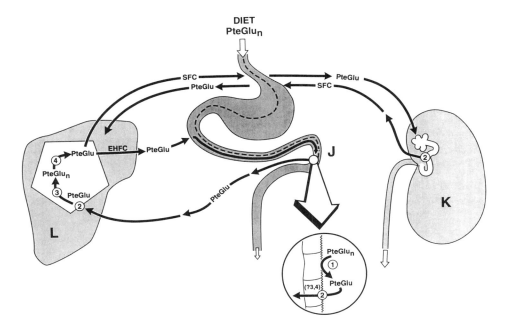

FIGURE 1. Folate homeostasis and enzyme and binding proteins potentially affected by chronic alcoholism. J: jejunum, major site for folate absorption; insert shows events at mucosal surface. L: liver, major site of folate storage (7 to 10 mg) and metabolism; insert shows events in hepatocyte. K: kidneys; insert shows events at renal tubule. EHFC: enterohepatic folate circulation, approximately 10% of total folate pool; <0.1% excreted in feces per day. SFC: systemic folate circulation from liver to other organs; <1% excreted in urine per day. (1) Jejunal BBFH, required for initial digestion of dietary polyglutamyl folates (PteGlu$_n$). (2) FBP and transport mechanism, probably required at intestinal brush border, hepatocyte plasma membrane, and renal tubular brush border for transport of monoglutamyl folate (PteGlu). (3) Folate synthetase, required for synthesis of intracellular PteGlu$_n$ from PteGlu. (4) Intracellular folate hydrolase, required for conversion of PteGlu$_n$ to PteGlu prior to efflux from the cell. See text for further details.

membrane fluidity.[57] Alcohol-induced changes in membrane fluidity and function could result from altered phospholipid metabolism due to inhibition of fatty-acid desaturases.[58] In recent studies from our laboratory, 1 year of alcohol feeding to minipigs had no demonstrable effect on brush-border membrane vesicle fluidity, fatty-acid composition, or PteGlu transport, whereas acute exposure of the vesicles to alcohol increased fluidity and decreased the activities of several brush-border hydrolases, including BBFH.[39] Translating to a clinical setting, these data suggest that frequent acute exposure of the intestine to large concentrations of alcohol, as occurs in binge drinkers,[59] could decrease the hydrolysis and hence absorption of folates simultaneously ingested in the diet.

In addition to its potential effects on membrane composition, fluidity, and function, alcohol exposure could affect the synthesis of membrane-bound proteins and enzymes involved in folate homeostasis. Such an effect could explain our additional finding that the activity of intestinal BBFH was decreased in minipigs fed alcohol for 1 year, in the absence of changes in membrane fluidity or lipid composition.[39] A mechanism for alcohol inhibition of protein synthesis is not defined. However, it is known that oxidant stress activates nucleases with resultant breaking of DNA strands.[60] Thus, a fundamental alcohol-induced oxidant attack on the genes that control folate-dependent proteins could have profound effects on folate homeostasis.

REFERENCES

1. National Research Council, Folic acid, in *Recommended Dietary Allowances,* 10th ed., National Academy Press, Washington, D.C., 1989, 150.
2. Halsted, C. H., Jejunal brush-border folate hydrolase — a novel enzyme, *West. J. Med.,* 155, 605, 1991.
3. Shane, B., Folylpolyglutamate synthesis and role in the regulation of one-carbon metabolism, *Vitam. Horm.,* 45, 263, 1989.
4. Wagner, C., Cellular folate binding proteins; function and significance, *Annu. Rev. Nutr.,* 2, 229, 1982.
5. Steinberg, S. E., Campbell, C. L., and Hillman, R. S., Kinetics of the normal folate enterohepatic cycle, *J. Clin. Invest.,* 64, 83, 1979.
6. Tamura, T. and Halsted, C. H., Folate turnover in chronically alcoholic monkeys, *J. Lab. Clin. Med.,* 101, 623, 1983.
7. Williams, W. M. and Hueng, K. C., Renal tubular transport of folic acid and methotrexate in the monkey, *Am. J. Physiol.,* 242, F484, 1982.
8. Herbert, V., Development of folate deficiency, in *Folic Acid Metabolism in Health and Disease,* Picciano, M. F., Stokstad, E. L. R., and Gregory, J. F., Eds., Wiley-Liss, New York, 1990, 195.
9. Halsted, C. H. and Tamura, T., Folate deficiency in liver disease, in *Problems in Liver Disease,* Davidson, C. S., Ed., Stratton Intercontinental Medical Books, New York, 1978, 91.
10. Herbert, V., Zalusky, R., and Davidson, C. S., Correlates of folate deficiency with alcoholism and associated macrocytosis, anemia, and liver disease, *Ann. Intern. Med.,* 58, 977, 1963.
11. Hines, J. D. and Cowan, D. H., Anemia in alcoholism, in *Drugs and Hematopoietic Reactions,* Dimitrov, N. V. and Nodine, J. H., Eds., Grune & Stratton, New York, 1974, 141.
12. Eichner, E. R. and Hillman, R. S., The evolution of anemia in alcoholic patients, *Am. J. Med.,* 50, 218, 1971.

13. Savage, D. and Lindenbaum, J., Anemia in alcoholics, *Medicine (Baltimore)*, 65, 322, 1986.

14. Lindenbaum, J., Healton, E. B., Savage, D. G., Brust, J. C. M., Garrett, T. J., Podell, E. R., Marcell, P. D., Stabler, S. P., and Allen, R. H., Neuropsychiatric disorders caused by cobalamin deficiency in the absence of anemia or macrocytosis, *N. Engl. J. Med.*, 318, 1720, 1988.

15. Bianchi, A., Chipman, D. W., Dreskia, A., and Rosensweig, N., Nutritional folic acid deficiency with megaloblastic changes in the small bowel epithelium, *N. Engl. J. Med.*, 282, 859, 1970.

16. Hermos, J. A., Adams, W. H., Lin, Y. K., and Trier, J., Mucosa of the small intestine in folate deficient alcoholics, *Ann. Intern. Med.*, 76, 951, 1972.

17. Klipstein, F. A., Lipton, S. D., and Schenk, E. A., Folate deficiency of the intestinal mucosa, *Am. J. Clin. Nutr.*, 26, 728, 1973.

18. Goetsch, C. A. and Klipstein, F. A., Effect of folate deficiency of the intestinal mucosa on jejunal transport in the rat, *J. Lab. Clin. Med.*, 89, 1002, 1977.

19. Mekhjian, H. S. and May, E. S., Acute and chronic effects of ethanol on fluid transport in the human small intestine, *Gastroenterology*, 72, 1280, 1977.

20. Halsted, C. H., Robles, E. A., and Mezey, E., Intestinal malabsorption in folate-deficient alcoholics, *Gastroenterology*, 64, 526, 1973.

21. Leevy, C. M., Abnormalities of hepatic DNA synthesis in man, *Medicine*, 45, 423, 1966.

22. Shaw, S., Jayatilleke, E., Ross, A., Gordon, E. R., and Lieber, C. S., Ethanol induced lipid peroxidation: potentiation by long-term alcohol feeding and attenuation by methionine, *J. Lab. Clin. Med.*, 98, 417, 1982.

23. Barak, A. J., Beckenhauer, H. C., and Tuma, D. J., Effects of prolonged ethanol feeding on methionine metabolism in rat liver, *Biochem. Cell. Biol.*, 65, 230, 1987.

24. Koblin, D. D. and Everman, B. W., Vitamin B12 and folate status in rats after administration of ethanol and acute exposure to nitrous oxide, *Alcohol. Clin. Exp. Res.*, 15, 543, 1991.

25. Yunis, J. J. and Soreng, A. L., Constitutive fragile sites and cancer, *Science*, 226, 1199, 1984.

26. Heimberger, D. C., Alexander, B., Birch, R., Butterworth, C. E., Bailey, W. C., and Krumdieck, C. L., Improvement in bronchial squamous metaplasia in smokers treated with folate and vitamin B12, *JAMA*, 259, 1525, 1988.

27. Butterworth, C. E., Hatch, K. D. S., Gore, H., Meuller, H., and Krumdieck, C. L., Improvement in cervical dysplasia with folic acid therapy in users of oral contraceptives, *Am. J. Clin. Nutr.*, 35, 73, 1982.

28. Lashner, B. A., Heidenreich, P. A., Su, G. L., Kane, S. V., and Hanauer, S. B., Effect of folate supplementation on the incidence of dysplasia and cancer in chronic ulcerative colitis, *Gastroenterology*, 97, 255, 1989.

29. Eichner, E. R. and Hillman, R. S., Effect of alcohol on serum folate level, *J. Clin. Invest.*, 52, 584, 1973.

30. Sullivan, L. W. and Herbert, V., Suppression of hematopoiesis by ethanol, *J. Clin. Invest.*, 43, 2048, 1964.

31. Baker, H., Frank, O., Ziffer, H., Goldfarb, S., Leevy, C. M., and Sobotka, H., Effect of hepatic disease on liver B-complex vitamin titers, *Am. J. Clin. Nutr.,* 14, 1, 1964.

32. Eichner, E. R., Pierce, H. I., and Hillman, R. S., Folate balance in dietary induced megaloblastic anemia, *N. Engl. J. Med.,* 284, 933, 1971.

33. Herbert, V., Predicting nutrient deficiency by formula, *N. Engl. J. Med.,* 284, 976, 1971.

34. Darby, W. J., The nutrient contributions of fermented beverages, in *Fermented Food Beverages in Nutrition,* Gastineau, C. F., Darby, W. J., and Turner, T. B., Eds., Academic Press, New York, 1979, 61.

35. Halsted, C. H., Griggs, R. C., and Harris, J. W., The effect of alcoholism on the absorption of folic acid (H³-PGA) evaluated by plasma levels and urine excretion, *J. Lab. Clin. Med.,* 69, 116, 1967.

36. Halsted, C. H., Robles, E. A., and Mezey, E., Decreased jejunal uptake of labeled folic acid (³H-PGA) in alcoholic patients: roles of alcohol and malnutrition, *N. Engl. J. Med.,* 285, 701, 1971.

37. Romero, J. J., Tamura, T., and Halsted, C. H., Intestinal absorption of [³H] folic acid in the chronic alcoholic monkey, *Gastroenterology,* 80, 99, 1981.

38. Reisenauer, A. M., Buffington, C. A. T., Villanueva, J. A., and Halsted, C. H., Folate absorption in alcoholic pigs: *in vivo* intestinal perfusion studies, *Am. J. Clin. Nutr.,* 50, 1429, 1989.

39. Naughton, C. A., Chandler, C. J., Duplantier, R. B., and Halsted, C. H., Folate absorption in alcoholic pigs: *in vitro* hydrolysis and transport at the brush border membrane, *Am. J. Clin. Nutr.,* 50, 1436, 1989.

40. Horne, D. W., Briggs, W. T., and Wagner, C., Studies on the transport mechanism of 5-methyltetrahydrofolic acid in freshly isolated hepatocytes: effect of ethanol, *Arch. Biochem. Biophys.,* 196, 557, 1979.

41. Hillman, R. S., McGuffin, R., and Campbell, C., Alcohol interference with the folate enterohepatic cycle, *Trans. Assoc. Am. Phys.,* 90, 145, 1977.

42. Keating, J. N., Weir, D. G., and Scott, J. M., The effect of ethanol consumption on folate polyglutamate biosynthesis in the rat, *Biochem. Pharmacol.,* 34, 1913, 1985.

43. Wilkinson, J. and Shane, B., Folate metabolism in the ethanol-fed rat, *J. Nutr.,* 112, 604, 1982.

44. Tamura, T., Romero, J. J., Watson, J. E., Gong, E. J., and Halsted, C. H., Hepatic folate metabolism in the chronic alcoholic monkey, *J. Lab. Clin. Med.,* 97, 654, 1981.

45. McMartin, K. E., Collins, T. D., Shiao, C. Q., Vidrine, L., and Redefski, H. M., Study of dose-dependence and urinary folate excretion produced by ethanol in humans and rats, *Alcohol. Clin. Exp. Res.,* 10, 419, 1986.

46. Russell, R. M., Rosenberg, I. M., Wilson, P. D., Iber, F. L., Oaks, E. V., Giovetti, A. C., Otradovec, C. L., Karwoski, P. A., and Press, A. W., Increased urinary excretion and prolonged turnover time of folic acid during ethanol ingestion, *Am. J. Clin. Nutr.,* 38, 64, 1983.

47. McMartin, K. E. and Collins, T. D., Relationship of alcohol metabolism to folate deficiency produced by ethanol in the rat, *Pharmacol. Biochem. Behav.,* 18, 257, 1983.

48. Eisenga, B. H., Collins, T. D., and McMartin, K. E., Effects of acute ethanol on urinary excretion of 5-methyltetrahydrofolic acid and folate derivatives in the rat, *J. Nutr.,* 119, 1498, 1989.

49. Bhandari, S. D., Fortney, T., and McMartin, K. E., Analysis of the pH dependence of folate binding and transport by rat kidney brush border membrane vesicles, *Proc. Soc. Exp. Biol. Med.,* 196, 451, 1991.

50. Lieber, C. S., Biochemical and molecular forms of alcohol-induced injury to liver and other tissue, *N. Engl. J. Med.,* 319, 1639, 1988.

51. Kawase, T., Kato, S., and Lieber, C. S., Lipid peroxidation and antioxidant defense system in rat liver after chronic ethanol feeding, *Hepatology,* 10, 815, 1989.

52. Shaw, S., Jayatilleke, E., Herbert, V., and Colman, N., Cleavage of folates during ethanol metabolism. Role of xanthine oxidase-generated superoxide dismutase, *Biochem. J.,* 257, 277, 1989.

53. Taber, M. M. and Lakshmaiah, N., Studies on hydroperoxide-dependent folic acid degradation by hemin, *Arch. Biochem. Biophys.,* 257, 100, 1987.

54. Hunter, C. L., Treanor, L. L., Gray, J. B., Halter, S. A., Hoyumpa, A., and Wilson, F. A., Effects of ethanol *in vitro* on rat intestinal brush-border membranes, *Biochim. Biophys. Acta,* 732, 256, 1983.

55. Harris, R. A., Burnett, R., McQuilkin, S., McClard, A., and Simon, F. R., Effects of ethanol on membrane order: fluorescent studies, *Ann. N.Y. Acad. Sci.,* 492, 125, 1987.

56. Kim, C., Leo, M. A., Lowe, N., and Lieber, C. S., Effects of vitamin A and ethanol on liver plasma membrane fluidity, *Hepatology,* 8, 735, 1988.

57. Waring, A. J., Rottenberg, H., Ohnishi, T., and Rubin, E., Membranes and phospholipids of liver mitochondria from chronic alcoholic rats are resistant to membrane disordering by alcohol, *Proc. Natl. Acad. Sci. U.S.A.,* 78, 2582, 1981.

58. Wang, D. L. and Reitz, R. C., Ethanol ingestion and polyunsaturated fatty acids: effects on the acyl-CoA desaturases, *Alcohol. Clin. Exp. Res.,* 7, 220, 1983.

59. Halsted, C. H., Robles, E., and Mezey, E., Distribution of ethanol in the human gastrointestinal tract, *Am. J. Clin. Nutr.,* 26, 831, 1973.

60. Halliwell, B. and Aruoma, O. I., DNA damage by oxygen-derived species. Its mechanism and measurement in mammalian systems, *FEBS Lett.,* 281, 9, 1991.

12 The Effects of Ethanol on Vitamin A and β-Carotene Nutriture

INTRODUCTION

The importance of vitamin A to vision, growth, cellular differentiation, and sexual development has been well documented since the early part of this century.[1-3] The role of vitamin A in immuno-potentiation, the interaction of vitamin A with DNA, and the effectiveness of vitamin A as an antioxidant have become the foci of more recent studies.[4-5] The biological importance of β-carotene was initially attributed to its convertability to vitamin A. It is now widely recognized that β-carotene is a potent antioxidant in its own right.[6-7] Numerous epidemiological studies have also shown that both retinoid and carotenoid ingestion (through the consumption of large quantities of leafy green vegetables) have significant protective effects against certain epithelial cancers in humans.[8-10] Any effects that alcohol ingestion may have on vitamin A or β-carotene absorption and/or metabolism must now be viewed in the light of this most recent research. In addition, the possibility that some of the toxic effects of ethanol on the liver may be mediated by the interactions of ethanol with vitamin A and the metabolites of vitamin A requires further investigation.

Alcoholism is a primary cause of protein-calorie malnutrition and micronutrient deficiency, including vitamin A deficiency, among American and European populations. Vitamin A deficiency is reported in 15% of alcoholics without liver disease and in 50% of those with liver cirrhosis.[11-13] In advanced stages of alcoholism, poor dietary intake, anorexia, impaired intestinal absorption, and chronic liver injury are the most important factors in the development of vitamin A deficiency. However, evidence has been accumulating which demonstrates that ethanol has a

ISBN 0-8493-7933-4

direct effect on the metabolism of vitamin A in the liver and in other tissues. This effect is observed even in the presence of normal absorption and adequate vitamin A intake.[14-17]

VITAMIN A NUTRITURE AND ETHANOL

Circulating vitamin A levels may actually be higher in heavy, non-cirrhotic alcohol drinkers than in nonalcoholic subjects or in subjects who drink only occasionally.[18] However, high or normal plasma levels may mask severe hepatic vitamin A losses. Symptoms of vitamin A deficiency, such as night blindness or hypogonadism, are still prevalent in alcoholics.[19] Despite low hepatic vitamin A levels, supplementation of alcoholics with vitamin A may be hepatotoxic[20] and, therefore, careful clinical follow-up with sequential liver function tests is indicated.

The administration of acute doses of ethanol has been shown to increase serum levels of vitamin A and to decrease hepatic vitamin A in various mammals.[21-24] The decline in hepatic vitamin A stores has been attributed mainly to the release or leakage of retinyl esters from the liver.[25] Concomitant increases of tissue vitamin A levels, in the kidneys and in adipose tissue, have also been demonstrated.[25] However, it also appears that alcohol can enhance the metabolism of vitamin A. This may occur as a result of increased conversion of retinyl esters to retinol through stimulation of retinyl ester hydrolase (EC 3.1.1.21).[26] Retinol may then be released or catabolized further to polar metabolites and conjugates and excreted in the bile.

CHRONIC ETHANOL INTAKE AND HEPATIC VITAMIN A

Hepatic vitamin A levels continue to decline with chronic alcohol intake.[27-29] Sato and Lieber have shown that ethanol given in large doses (36 to 50% of total calories) to rats (for 3 to 9 weeks) and baboons (for 4 to 84 months) under strict dietary control caused marked mobilization of vitamin A from the liver while increasing the vitamin A content of other tissues.[14] These authors suggest that hepatic vitamin A depletion after chronic alcohol ingestion is secondary to enhanced activity of microsomal cytochrome P-450 enzymatic activity. *In vitro* studies have shown that this enzyme system is able to metabolize retinol to 4-hydroxyretinol and to convert retinoic acid to other polar metabolites.[30-31] However, in a study of chronic ethanol feeding in rats using similar quantities of ethanol but lower quantities of dietary fat and higher amounts of dietary carbohydrate, Grummer and Erdman found no change in the activity of cytochrome C reductase, but still noted that the hepatic vitamin A concentration was reduced.[15]

Reduction of hepatic vitamin A levels may also be accompanied by changes in the ratio of retinol to retinyl esters. Under normal conditions, vitamin A is first taken up by the parenchymal cells, but it is eventually transferred to the stellate cells for storage.[32] More than 90% of the liver vitamin A, in parenchymal and nonparenchymal cells, is present in the form of retinyl esters. In vitamin A-deficient rats, the proportion of vitamin A as retinol, as well as the percentage of vitamin A recovered in the parenchymal cells, appears to increase.[33-34] Rasmussen et al. have shown that, although chronic ethanol intake in rats (36% of total calories for 6 weeks) does not significantly retard the transport of vitamin A from parenchymal to nonparenchymal cells, it does increase the proportion of hepatic vitamin A as retinol.[17] This may take on added significance if the concentration of the retinol binding proteins is not increased (or if retinol binding affinities are not enhanced), since it appears that free retinol may be toxic to cell membranes.[35-36] When supplemental vitamin A (five times the RDA) is given along with ethanol administration over a period of 2 to 9 months, significant hepatic cell injury is seen, with the appearance of giant mitochondria or frank liver cell necrosis and fibrosis.[37-38]

THE EFFECTS OF AGING

The rate of ethanol metabolism decreases with aging in humans and animals.[39-41] Other changes seen with aging include a decline in the rate of serum vitamin A clearance[42] and a rise in liver vitamin A concentration and content.[43] The increase in liver vitamin A concentration is almost linear with age,[43] although it has also been shown that hepatic vitamin A may plateau and even begin to decline with continued aging (after 6 months of age in mice).[44] In any case, the depleting effects of ethanol are less evident in older than in younger animals due to their larger reserves of vitamin A. Liver concentrations of vitamin A in humans also appear to increase with age, as has been observed in autopsy studies of accident victims and other subjects who died from chronic diseases.[45]

THE RETINOL-BINDING PROTEINS

We have recently shown that cellular retinol-binding protein (cRBP) activity levels in the liver decrease with advanced age.[46] Ethanol enhances this decline in older rats but does not affect the cRBP levels in younger animals.[46] The exact metabolic function of cRBP continues to be debated.[47] Some researchers have suggested that cRBP is essential for the interaction of vitamin A with DNA, thus playing a pivotal role in genomic expression. Other possible functions include the transport of retinol between the parenchymal and stellate cells of the liver and protection of cells and cell membranes from possible toxic effects of unbound retinol.

Effects of ethanol on the plasma levels of retinol-binding protein (pRBP), which is essential for the transport of retinol from the liver stores to the circulation, have also been reported.[14] Circulating pRBP levels were increased in ethanol-fed baboons with fatty liver, but were not different between control apes and ethanol-fed baboons with fibrosis or cirrhosis. In a corollary study, no differences were seen in the circulating pRBP of ethanol-fed rats compared to controls, but pRBP levels were higher in the liver (in whole homogenates and in the uncontaminated microsomal fractions) of the ethanol-fed animals.[14] This means that more pRBP should be available in the ethanol-fed animals to aid in the release of retinol from the liver.

The relative dose response test is a clinical method which is useful in the determination of vitamin A status.[48] The normal dose response is small, because serum vitamin A levels are already adequate and surplus pRBP required for a higher response is not available. In zinc-adequate, vitamin A-depleted alcoholics with cirrhosis, the relative dose response is elevated, but decreases significantly after 4 weeks of supplementation with vitamin A. The response is higher prior to vitamin A repletion because the synthesis of pRBP in the liver is apparently not affected by vitamin A deficiency per se and is therefore available for transport of the challenge dose.[48]

OTHER NUTRIENT INTERACTIONS

Synthesis of pRBP is affected by zinc deficiency. Hyperzincuria has also been noted in many alcoholics along with low serum zinc levels.[13] Treatment of vitamin A deficiency has occasionally proved intractable to vitamin A supplementation. In some cases, however, administration of zinc has proved effective in ameliorating the symptoms of vitamin A deficiency (e.g., in correcting abnormal dark adaptation) and in increasing serum vitamin A levels.[49] It is uncertain whether holo-pRBP (pRBP with an attached retinol molecule) requires zinc for the actual transport of vitamin A from the liver or if zinc acts indirectly, correcting adverse effects of zinc deficiency on plasma membranes or on animal growth and protein synthesis (including pRBP) and the subsequent reduction in body demand for vitamin A.[50] Increased dietary protein and energy intake has also been shown to raise serum retinol and pRBP levels in children with severe protein-energy malnutrition, even in the absence of vitamin A supplementation.[51]

The effects of fat in the diet may also alter the effects of ethanol on vitamin A metabolism. In a series of studies with corn oil, lard, and tallow, it has been shown that the presence of linoleic acid (18:2) is required for ethanol to exert its vitamin A depleting effects on the livers of rats. The absence of linoleic acid from the diet also appears to protect rats (and presumably humans) from some of the toxic effects of ethanol on liver tissue.[52] With a high fat diet, the number of Ito (stellate) cells seen in centrilobular scars is increased and the retinyl palmitate and RBP concentrations in these "activated" cells are decreased.[53]

β-CAROTENE NUTRITURE AND ETHANOL

Because the β-carotene levels in blood plasma of alcoholics are usually depressed prior to any decline in circulating retinol levels, Majumdar et al. proposed the use of β-carotene as a marker for risk of malnutrition in alcoholic subjects.[54] Serum β-carotene is more dependent on recent intake than serum vitamin A, which is under fairly strict homeostatic control. Yet the use of serum β-carotene levels for evaluation of patient nutritional status is presently fraught with difficulties due to large individual variability. Besides a seasonal variation in β-carotene intake, it appears that the range in the absorptive capacities of different subjects is very wide and may be sensitive to age, sex, and macronutrient composition of the diet.

In a 3-year, multiple risk factor intervention trial, Russell-Briefel et al. reported a correlation of 0.25 ($r^2 = 0.06$) between total blood carotenoids and carotene intake in 187 men.[55] In 330 melanoma study controls, Stryker et al. found the correlation between plasma β-carotene and dietary carotene intake to be 0.27 ($r^2 = 0.07$) for men and 0.37 ($r^2 = 0.14$) for women prior to adjustment for caloric intake and plasma lipids.[56] After adjustment the overall correlation for men and women was 0.43 ($r^2 = 0.18$).[56] Thus, in these regression models from two different surveys, carotene intake accounted for only 6 to 18% of the variation in plasma β-carotene. Alcohol drinking (10 g or more per day) tended to reduce the regression coefficients correlating carotene intake and plasma β-carotene, but not as much as smoking.[56] There is still little evidence that alcohol interferes with β-carotene absorption.[15,56]

Women generally have higher levels of β-carotene than men.[56-61] Nierenberg et al. speculate that, in comparison to men, women have lower amounts of the intestinal enzyme, β-carotene 15,15′-dioxygenase (EC 1.13.11.21), that converts β-carotene to retinol.[57] According to this hypothesis, more β-carotene should be available to women to absorb in the intact form. They also point out that women have lower levels of alcohol dehydrogenase, and therefore, higher bioavailability of alcohol. Interestingly, while a negative association between alcohol and serum β-carotene levels has been reported,[54-59,61-63] the effects of alcohol drinking on β-carotene levels appear to be stronger in men than in women.[56,61]

We have performed two different studies on the effects of aging on serum β-carotene.[65-65] In the first study, older women absorbed more β-carotene than younger women when the 24-h dietary intake was low (500 kcal).[64] In the second study, younger men absorbed more β-carotene than older men when the caloric intake was 1500 kcal/day or greater.[65] Higher fat diets may also increase β-carotene absorption in younger subjects,[66] but they also potentiate the adverse effects of ethanol on growing rats.[67]

We have recently shown that, in normal young subjects previously made hypocarotenemic, serum lipid peroxide levels are decreased after daily repletion with 15 or 120 mg of β-carotene for 3 weeks,[68] and that this decrease is dose-dependent.[69] In reviewing the effects of alcohol on testicular injury. Rosenberg et al. suggest that testicular peroxidation injury may be attenuated by dietary vitamin A or β-carotene supplementation.[70] Although direct *in vivo* evidence is lacking, it would be surprising, indeed, if vitamin A or β-carotene could not moderate the peroxidative injury produced by alcohol ingestion in other tissues with low oxygen pressures (e.g., the liver) as well.

CONCLUSION

It is quite clear that alcohol intake has dramatic effects on vitamin A metabolism: decreasing liver stores; increasing oxidation of retinol; and increasing the extra-hepatic vitamin A. Many of the symptoms associated with alcoholism, such as night blindness and azospermia, may be secondary to changes in vitamin A status. Because supplementation with vitamin A may be toxic, administration of β-carotene may be more useful as a treatment for alcoholics with depleted vitamin A stores.

Despite the difficulties in interpretation of serum β-carotene values, the abundance of studies showing an association between β-carotene intake and reduction of cancer risk make this an important part of any nutritional evaluation. The effect of alcohol on β-carotene metabolism needs to be assessed more carefully and the toxic interactions of alcohol and vitamin A should be more thoroughly researched. Because alcoholic behavior is also frequently associated with cigarette smoking, the toxic effects of tobacco must be controlled in any clinical study of alcohol and vitamin A or β-carotene.

REFERENCES

1. McCullom, E. V., Simmonds, N., and Pitz, W., The relation of the unidentified dietary factors, the fat-soluble A, and water-soluble B, of the diet to the growth promoting properties of milk, *J. Biol. Chem.*, 27, 33, 1916.
2. Wohlbach, B. and Howe, P. R., Tissue changes following deprivation of fat-soluble vitamin A, *J. Exp. Med.*, 42, 753, 1925.
3. Patek, A. J. and Haig, C., The occurrence of abnormal dark adaptation and its relation to vitamin A metabolism in patients with cirrhosis of the liver, *J. Clin. Invest.*, 18, 609, 1939.
4. Bendich, A., A role for carotenoids in immune function, *Clin. Nutr.*, 7, 113, 1988.
5. Liau, G., Ong, O. E., and Chytil, F., Interaction of the retinol/cellular retinol binding protein complex with isolated nuclei and nuclear components, *J. Cell Biol.*, 91, 63, 1981.
6. Krinsky, N. I. and Deneke, S. M., Interaction of oxygen and oxy-radicals with carotenoids, *J. Natl. Cancer Inst.*, 69, 205, 1982.
7. Burton, G. W. and Ingold, K. U., β-Carotene: an unusual type of lipid antioxidant, *Science*, 224, 569, 1984.
8. Peto, R., Doll, R., Buckley, J. D., and Sporn, M. B., Can dietary beta-carotene materially reduce human cancer rates?, *Nature*, 290, 201, 1981.
9. Nomura, A. M. Y., Stemmermann, G. N., Heilbrun, L. K., Salkeld, R. M., and Vuilleumier, J. P., Serum vitamin levels and the risk of cancer in specific sites in men of Japanese ancestry in Hawaii, *Cancer Res.*, 45, 2369, 1985.
10. Weisburger, J. H., Nutritional approach to cancer prevention with emphasis on vitamins, antioxidants and carotenoids, *Am. J. Clin. Nutr.*, 53, 226S, 1991.
11. Halsted, C. H., Alcoholism and malnutrition: introduction to the symposium, *Am. J. Clin. Nutr.*, 33, 2705, 1980.
12. Mezey, E., Alcoholic liver disease: roles of alcohol and malnutrition, *Am. J. Clin. Nutr.*, 33, 2709, 1980.
13. Russell, R. M., Vitamin A and zinc metabolism in alcoholism, *Am. J. Clin. Nutr.*, 33, 2741, 1980.

14. Sato, M. and Lieber, C. S., Hepatic vitamin A depletion after chronic ethanol consumption in baboons and rats, *J. Nutr.,* 111, 2015, 1981.
15. Grummer, M. A. and Erdman, J. W., Effect of chronic alcohol consumption and moderate fat diet on vitamin A status in rats fed either vitamin A or beta carotene, *J. Nutr.,* 113, 350, 1983.
16. Mobarhan, S., Layden, T. J., Friedman, H., Kunigk, A., and Donahue, P. E., Depletion of liver and esophageal epithelium vitamin A after chronic moderate ethanol consumption in rats: inverse relation to zinc nutriture, *Hepatology,* 6(4), 615, 1986.
17. Rasmussen, M., Rune, B., Helgerud, P., Solberg, L. A., Berg, T., and Norum, K. R., Retinol and retinyl esters in parenchymal and nonparenchymal rat liver cell fractions after long term administration of ethanol, *J. Lipid Res.,* 26, 1112, 1985.
18. Ferro-Luzzi, A., Mobarhan, S., Maiani, G., Scaccini, C., Sette, S., Nicastro, A., Ranaldi, L., Polito, A., Azzini, E., Torre, S. D., and Jama, M. A., Habitual alcohol consumption and nutritional status of the elderly, *Eur. J. Clin. Nutr.,* 42, 5, 1988.
19. McClain, C. J., Van Thiel, D. H., Parker, S., Badzin, L. K., and Gilbert, H., Alterations in zinc, vitamin A, and retinol-binding protein in chronic alcoholics: a possible mechanism for night blindness and hypogonadism, *Alcoholism Clin. Exp. Res.,* 3, 135, 1979.
20. Leo, M. A. and Lieber, C. S., Interaction of ethanol with vitamin A, *Alcoholism Clin. Exp. Res.,* 7, 15, 1983.
21. Miller, R. W., Hemken, R. W., Waldo, D. R., and Moore, L. A., Effect of alcohol on the vitamin A status of holstein heifers, *J. Dairy Sci.,* 52, 1998, 1969.
22. Lee, M. and Lucia, S. P., Effect of ethanol on the mobilization of vitamin A in the dog and in the rat, *Stud. Alcohol,* 28, 1, 1965.
23. Frank, O., Luisada Opper, A. L., Sorrell, M. F., Zetterman, R., and Baker, H., Effects of a single intoxicating dose of ethanol on the vitamin profile of organelles in rat liver and brain, *J. Nutr.,* 106, 606, 1976.
24. Clausen, S. W., Breez, B. B., Baum, W. S., McCoord, A. B., and Rydeen, J. O., Effect of alcohol on vitamin A content of blood in human subjects, *Science,* 93, 21, 1941.
25. Sato, M. and Lieber, C. S., Changes in vitamin A status after acute ethanol administration in the rat, *J. Nutr.,* 112, 1118, 1982.
26. Friedman, H., Mobarhan, S., Hupert, J., Henderson, C., Luchessi, D., and Layden, T. J., *In vitro* stimulation of rat liver retinyl ester hydrolase by ethanol, *Arch. Biochem. Biophys.,* 269, 69, 1989.
27. Bauman, C. A., Foster, E. G., and Moore, P. R., The effect of dibenzathracene, alcohol and other agents on vitamin A in the rat, *J. Biol. Chem.,* 142, 597, 1941.
28. Bloomstrand, R., Lof, A., and Ostling, H., Studies on the metabolic effects of long term administration of ethanol and 4 methylpyrazole in the rat: vitamin A depletion in the liver, *Nutr. Metab.,* 21(Suppl. 1), 148, 1977.
29. Nadkarni, G. D., Deshpande, U. R., and Pahuja, D. N., Liver vitamin A stores in chronic alcoholism in rats: effects of propylthiouracil treatment, *Experientia,* 35, 1059, 1979.

30. Sato, M. and Lieber, C. S., Increased metabolism of retinoic acid after chronic ethanol consumption in rat liver microsomes, *Arch. Biochem. Biophys.*, 213, 557, 1982.

31. Leo, M. A. and Lieber, C. S., New pathway for retinol metabolism in liver microsomes, *J. Biol. Chem.*, 260, 5228, 1985.

32. Blaner, W. S., Dixon, J. L., Moriwaki, H., Martino, R. A., Stein, O., Stein, Y., and Goodman, DeW. S., Studies on the *in vivo* transfer of retinoids from parenchymal to stellate cells in rat liver, *Eur. J. Biochem.*, 164, 301, 1987.

33. Blomhoff, R., Berg, T., and Norum, K. R., Distribution of retinol in rat liver cells: effect of age, sex and nutritional status, *Br. J. Nutr.*, 60, 233, 1988.

34. Batres, R. O. and Olson, J. A., A marginal vitamin A status alters the distribution of vitamin A among parenchymal and stellate cells in rat liver, *J. Nutr.*, 117, 874, 1987.

35. Dingle, A. D. and Lucy, J. A., Studies on the mode of action of excess vitamin A. 5. The effect of vitamin A on the stability of the erythrocyte membrane, *Biochem. J.*, 84, 611, 1962.

36. Dingle, J. T., Fell, H. B., and Goodman, DeW. S., The effect of retinol and retinol-binding protein on embryonic skeletal tissue in organ culture, *J. Cell Sci.*, 2, 393, 1972.

37. Leo, M. A., Arai, M., Sato, M., and Lieber, C. S., Hepatotoxicity of vitamin A and ethanol in the rat, *Gastroenterology*, 82, 194, 1982.

38. Leo, M. A. and Lieber, C. S., Hepatic fibrosis after long-term administration of ethanol and moderate vitamin A supplementation in the rat, *Hepatology*, 3, 1, 1983.

39. Schmucker, D. L., Age related changes in drug disposition, *Pharmacol. Rev.*, 30, 445, 1979.

40. Vestal, R. E., McGuire, E. A., Tobin, J. D., Andres, R., Norris, A. H., and Mezey, E., Aging and ethanol metabolism, *Clin. Pharmacol. Ther.*, 21, 343, 1977.

41. Hahn, H. K. J. and Burch, R. E., Impaired ethanol metabolism with advancing age, *Alcoholism Clin. Exp. Res.*, 7, 299, 1983.

42. Krasinsi, S. D., Cohn, J. S., Scaefer, E. J., and Russell, r. M., Postprandial plasma retinyl ester response is greater in older subjects compared with younger subjects: evidence for delayed plasma clearance of intestinal lipoproteins, *J. Clin. Invest.*, 85, 883, 1990.

43. Hollander, D. and Morgan, D., Aging: its influence on vitamin A intestinal absorption *in vivo* by the rat, *Exp. Gerontol.*, 14, 301, 1979.

44. Sundboom, J. and Olson, J. A., Effect of aging on the storage and catabolism of vitamin A in mice, *Exp. Gerontol.*, 19, 257, 1984.

45. Mitchell, G. V., Young, M., and Seward, C. R., Vitamin A and carotene levels of a selected population in metropolitan Washington, D.C., *Am. J. Clin. Nutr.*, 26, 992, 1973.

46. Mobarhan, S., Seitz, H. K., Russell, R. M., Mehta, R., Hupert, J., Friedman, H., Layden, T. J., Meydani, M., and Langenberg, P., Age-related effects of chronic ethanol intake on vitamin A status in Fisher 344 rats, *J. Nutr.*, 121, 510, 1991.

47. Chytil, F., Liver and cellular vitamin A binding proteins, *Hepatology, 2*, 282, 1982.

48. Mobarhan, S., Russell, R. M., Underwood, B., Wallingford, J., Mathieson, R. D., and Al-Midani, H., Evaluation of the relative dose response test for vitamin A nutriture in cirrhotics, *Am. J. Clin. Nutr.,* 34, 2264, 1981.

49. Shingwekar, A. G., Mohanram, M. M., and Reddy, V., Effect of zinc supplementation on plasma levels of vitamin A and retinol-binding protein in malnourished children, *Clin. Chem. Acta,* 93, 97, 1979.

50. Carney, S. M., Underwood, B. A., and Loerch, J. D., Effects of zinc and vitamin A deficient diets on the hepatic mobilization and urinary excretion of vitamin A in rats, *J. Nutr.,* 106, 1773, 1976.

51. Smith, F. R., Goodman, DeW. S., Zaklama, M. S., Gabr, M. K., El Maraghy, S., and Patwardhan, V. N., Serum vitamin A, retinol-binding protein, and prealbumin concentrations in protein-calorie malnutrition. I. A functional defect in hepatic retinol release, *Am. J. Clin. Nutr.,* 26, 973, 1973.

52. French, S. W., Nanji, A. A., and Mobarhan, S., Dietary fats modulate the effect of ethanol on hepatic vitamin A, *Hepatology,* 10 (Abstr. 535), 702, 1989.

53. Tsukamoto, H., Matsuoka, M., and French, S. W., Experimental models of hepatic fibrosis: a review, *Semin. Liver Dis.,* 10, 56, 1990.

54. Majumdar, S. K., Shaw, G. K., and Thomson, A. D., Blood beta-carotene status in chronic alcoholics — a good biochemical marker for malnutrition, *Drug Alcohol Depend.,* 12, 111, 1983.

55. Russell-Briefel, R., Bates, M. W., and Kuller, L. H., The relationship of plasma carotenoids to health and biochemical factors in middle-aged men, *Am. J. Epidemiol.,* 122, 741, 1985.

56. Stryker, W. S., Kaplan, L. A., Stein, E. A., Stampfer, M. J., Sober, A., and Willett, W. C., The relation of diet, cigarette smoking, and alcohol consumption to plasma β-carotene and α-tocopherol levels, *Am. J. Epidemiol.,* 127, 283, 1988.

57. Nierenberg, D. W., Stukel, T. A., Baron, J. A., Dain, B. J., and Greenberg, E. R., Skin Cancer Prevention Study Group, Determinants of increase in plasma concentration of β-carotene after chronic oral supplementation, *Am. J. Clin. Nutr.,* 53, 1443, 1991.

58. Aoki, K., Ito, Y., Sasaki, R., Ohtani, M., Hamajima, N., and Asano, A., Smoking, alcohol drinking and serum carotenoid levels, *Jpn. J. Cancer Res. (Gann),* 78, 1049, 1987.

59. Herbeth, B., Didelot-Barthelemy, L., LeDevehat, C., and Lemoine, A., Retinol, carotenoides et tocopherols plasmatiques: facteurs de variation biologique entre 18 et 45 ans, *Ann. Nutr. Metab.,* 32, 297, 1988.

60. Stacewicz-Sapuntzakis, M., Bowen, P. E., Kikendall, J. W., and Burgess, M., Simultaneous determination of serum retinol and various carotenoids: their distribution in middle-aged men and women, *J. Micronutr. Anal.,* 3, 27, 1987.

61. Shibata, A., Sasaki, R., Ito, Y., Hamajima, N., Suzuki, S., Ohtani, M., and Aoki, K., Serum concentration of beta-carotene and intake frequency of green-yellow vegetables among healthy inhabitants of Japan, *Int. J. Cancer,* 44, 48, 1989.

62. Suzuki, S., Sasaki, R., Ito, Y., Hamajima, N., Shibata, A., Tamakoshi, A., Otani, M., and Aoki, K., Changes in serum concentrations of β-carotene and changes in the dietary intake frequency of green-yellow vegetables among healthy male inhabitants of Japan, *Jpn. J. Cancer Res.,* 81, 463, 1990.

63. Ito, Y., Minohara, M., and Otani, M., Effects of alcohol drinking and cigarette smoking on serum α- and β-carotene concentrations in healthy adults, *Jpn. J. Hyg.,* 44, 607, 1989.

64. Maiani, G., Mobarhan, S., Ceccanti, M., Ranaldi, L., Gettner, S., Bowen, P., Friedman, H., DeLorenzo, A., and Ferro-Luzzi, A., Beta-carotene serum response in young and elderly females, *Eur. J. Clin. Nutr.,* 43, 749, 1989.

65. Sugerman, S. B., Mobarhan, S., Bowen, P., Stacewicz-Sapuntzakis, M., Langenberg, P., Henderson, C., Kiani, R., Friedman, H., and Lucchesi, D., Serum time curve characteristics of a fixed dose of β-carotene in young and old men, *J. Am. Coll. Nutr.,* 10, 297, 1991.

66. Shiau, A., Mobarhan, S., Stacewicz-Sapuntzakis, M., Bowen, P., Ford, C., Liao, Y., and Benya, R., Effects of diet on absorption of beta-carotene, *J. Am. Coll. Nutr.,* 9(5) (Abstr. 44), 533, 1990.

67. Grummer, M. A. and Erdman, J. W., Jr., Effect of chronic ethanol consumption and moderate or high fat diet upon tissue distribution of vitamin A in rats fed either vitamin A or β-carotene, *Nutr. Res.,* 6, 61, 1986.

68. Mobarhan, S., Bowen, P., Andersen, B., Evans, M., Stacewicz-Sapuntzakis, M., Sugerman, S., Simms, P., Lucchesi, D., and Friedman, H., Effects of β-carotene repletion on β-carotene absorption, lipid peroxidation, and neutrophil superoxide formation in young men, *Nutr. Cancer,* 14, 195, 1990.

69. Zarling, E. J., Mobarhan, S., Friedman, H., Bowen, P., and Sugerman, S., Beta-carotene supplementation reduces expired levels of pentane, *J. Am. Coll. Nutr.,* 10(5) (Abstr. 85), 562, 1991.

70. Rosenblum, E. R., Gavaler, J. S., and Van Thiel, D. H., Lipid peroxidation: a mechanism for alcohol-induced testicular injury, *Free Radical Biol. Med.,* 7, 569, 1989.

13 Zinc and Alcohol

INTRODUCTION

Zinc is a IIb trace metal which has only one valence state. Zinc is necessary for the function of over 200 metalloenzymes, it plays a role in gene expression, and it is important for membrane stability. In certain situations, zinc may act as a second messenger or a neurotransmitter, and it may play a role in protecting against cellular oxidant injury.[1,2] Major alterations in zinc metabolism can occur with alcoholism and/or alcoholic liver disease. The purpose of this chapter is to review normal human zinc metabolism, the effects of alcohol and alcoholic liver disease on zinc metabolism, clinical and biochemical manifestations of zinc deficiency, and the role of zinc in cellular integrity and in protection against hepatocellular injury.

NORMAL ZINC METABOLISM

Total body zinc stores in humans are approximately 2.3 g (about half that of iron). The recommended daily dietary intake of zinc for healthy adults in this country is 15 mg for males and 12 mg for females.[3] Spencer and co-workers have shown that zinc intake correlates directly with protein intake.[4] Thus, high protein foods are generally rich in zinc. However, only about 25% of ingested zinc is absorbed.[1,5] Indeed, studies in stable adults receiving total parenteral nutrition (TPN) suggest that about 3 mg per day is required intravenously, and this is the recommendation that has been put forth by the Nutrition Advisory Committee to the American Medical Association.[6] The amount of ingested zinc that is absorbed varies with a variety of factors including competing influences such as phytic acid, the overall zinc status of the subject, and intestinal diseases which may impair zinc absorption.[5,7] Zinc is mainly absorbed from the small intestine, and colonic absorption of zinc is minimal.[5,8] A variety of factors including certain amino acids (e.g., histidine) and prostaglandins have been suggested to enhance zinc absorption.[5] Zinc absorption in the small intestine appears to be regulated to a great degree by the zinc binding protein, metallothionein, in a classic homeostatic regulatory feedback loop.[9] During periods of excess zinc intake, intestinal metallothionein is induced and zinc absorption is blocked at the intestinal level. Thus, zinc bound to metallothionein does not enter the portal circulation and is lost in the feces with intestinal cell turnover. During periods of zinc deficiency, there is lower intestinal metallothionein and therefore more zinc is absorbed in an adaptive response.

Excretion of zinc is mainly through the feces, with pancreatic juice having large amounts of zinc.[5] There is an enteropancreatic circulation of zinc.[10] Thus, zinc endogenously excreted from the pancreas into the intestine can be absorbed further downstream in the GI tract. Urinary excretion of zinc normally is modest, usually less than 500 μg/24 h.[11] Under normal conditions, renal zinc losses play only a minor role in overall zinc homeostasis. In periods of zinc deficiency, urinary zinc excretion decreases in an adaptive attempt to maintain total body zinc stores.[12] However, this adaptive response is overcome in a variety of disease processes in which increased urinary zinc loss occurs even in the face of zinc deficiency. Thus, in these disease processes (including alcoholic liver disease), increased urinary zinc loss occurs despite zinc deficiency.[11,13]

Zinc exists in the plasma almost exclusively in the bound state, with approximately 60 to 70% bound to albumin, 25% to α_2-macroglobulin, and approximately 5% to amino acids.[7,14] Normal plasma/serum zinc concentrations in our laboratory range from 70 to 120 μg/dl. The plasma zinc concentration is the most frequently used indicator of zinc status. However, factors other than low total body zinc stores cause a decrease in the plasma zinc concentration. Especially relevant to patients with alcoholic liver disease are the effects of inflammatory mediators such as Interleukin-1 (IL-1) and tumor necrosis factor (TNF). Both of these cytokines cause a depression in plasma zinc concentration and an internal redistribution of total body zinc stores.[15] Urine zinc excretion decreases under conditions of diet-induced zinc deficiency. As noted previously, however, stress, tissue injury, inflammation, and multiple disease processes cause increased urinary zinc losses.[11,13] This renders the 24-h urine zinc excretion an unreliable marker of zinc status in many patients. Cellular zinc concentration such as that found in platelets, monocytes, lymphocytes, etc. are used on a research basis for evaluating zinc status.[16] However, these tests are not practical for clinical use because of the complexity in cell separation with subsequent zinc analysis. Thus far, no easily measurable enzyme has proven to be a clinically applicable indicator of zinc status. The thymus-derived nonapeptide, thymulin, has been successfully used by several research laboratories as a marker of zinc deficiency, but this test is available only in research settings.[17] Other investigators are studying cellular or plasma metallothionein as a marker of zinc status.[18] In summary, there are alterations in serum and tissue zinc concentrations related to disease activity or inflammation and unrelated to total body zinc status that make zinc assessment difficult in many clinical settings.

ZINC IN CHRONIC ALCOHOLISM AND ALCOHOLIC LIVER DISEASE

Chronic alcohol use and alcoholic liver disease frequently are complicated by zinc deficiency.[19,20] Both chronic alcoholics without obvious liver disease and animals fed alcohol in their diet developed zinc deficiency.[19-22] Alcoholic liver disease regularly is complicated by zinc deficiency.[23-26] It was recognized over three decades ago that alcoholic liver disease consistently is accompanied by hypozincemia, and this has been confirmed by multiple investigators.[23-26] Not only are low serum zinc concentrations noted in alcoholic liver disease, but depressed zinc concentrations have been reported in white blood cells, pancreatic juice, liver, and testes.[19,27-31] Recent studies by Bode et al. demonstrated low hepatic zinc concentrations not only in severe alcoholic liver disease, but also in mild fatty liver.[31] Subcellular liver fractions from this study showed significant reductions in nuclear and membrane fractions, and in microsomes from alcohol-induced cirrhotic livers. Studies by Schölmerich et al. have suggested that cirrhotics with shunting have more compromised zinc levels than those without evidence of shunting.[26] The well-documented zinc deficiency of alcoholism may have implications for continued ethanol abuse. Rats fed a zinc deficient diet voluntarily drink more ethanol than zinc sufficient controls.[32] When zinc deficient rats were then supplemented with zinc, alcohol intake became similar to zinc sufficient controls.

There are many mechanisms for the zinc deficiency and altered zinc metabolism in chronic alcoholism and alcoholic liver disease. Chronic alcoholics have very depressed zinc intake. As reported by our group, approximately 90% of alcoholics with or without liver disease have inadequate dietary zinc intake.[33] As noted in other chapters, chronic alcoholics consume approximately 50% of their calories as alcohol, which has virtually no zinc. Chronic alcoholics regularly have poor protein intake. As noted previously, zinc intake correlates directly with dietary protein intake. Thus, an inadequate dietary intake of zinc is a major reason for the zinc deficiency noted in chronic alcoholism.

Impaired zinc absorption is another likely cause of zinc deficiency in alcoholics with or without liver disease. Ethanol administration in experimental animals has been shown to decrease zinc absorption.[34] Zinc absorption, as assessed by the zinc tolerance test, is depressed in alcoholics with liver disease and patients with nonalcoholic liver disease.[35-37] Radioisotope studies also have confirmed the presence of impaired zinc absorption in patients with alcoholic liver disease.[38] Impaired zinc absorption also has been documented in patients with chronic pancreatitis and pancreatic insufficiency due to alcoholism.[39] The mechanisms for this impaired absorption in alcoholics are not well defined. As noted previously, zinc absorption is regulated to a great extent by intestinal metallothionein, a low molecular weight zinc binding protein.[9] During periods of zinc deficiency, there is less intestinal metallothionein induced, and more zinc should be absorbed. Thus, it is a paradox that zinc deficient alcoholics should have impaired zinc absorption. One possible explanation for this paradox is the observation that many substances other than zinc also induce metallothionein; examples being stress hormones such as glucocorticoids or cytokines such as IL-1 and TNF.[40,41] Thus, stress hormones or cytokines (elevated in alcoholism or alcoholic liver disease) may induce metallothionein and further worsen underlying zinc deficiency. One study also reported that acute ethanol administration to rats induces hepatic metallothionein (but apparently not intestinal metallothionein).[42] At this point, however, it is only speculation that these stress factors induce intestinal metallothionein, and no studies of intestinal metallothionein have been performed in humans or rats chronically fed alcohol. Recent work in rats from Cousins' laboratory demonstrated that while both metals, such as zinc, and a variety of inflammatory mediators, such as IL-1, stimulated hepatic metallothionein, only zinc and not the inflammatory mediators induced intestinal metallothionein.[43] Thus, further work is required to clarify factors (especially metallothionein) that regulate zinc absorption in chronic alcoholics or patients with alcoholic liver disease.

Increased cytokine activity may play a role in the altered zinc metabolism observed in alcoholic liver disease.[44] Cytokines such as IL-1, Interleukin-6 (IL-6), and TNF produce many diverse biochemical and clinical effects including anorexia, fever, neutrophilia, synthesis of acute phase reactants (such as C-reactive protein), decreased albumin production, increased endothelial permeability, expression of endothelial adhesion molecules, hypertriglyceridemia, and hypozincemia.[44] Many of these changes occur during the course of alcoholic liver disease. Endotoxin is a major stimulus for cytokine production.[44] It has been recognized for several decades that patients with liver disease frequently have endotoxemia. For example, Bode et al. observed endotoxemia in 59 of 88 patients with alcoholic cirrhosis, 19 of 42 patients with nonalcoholic liver disease, and 11 of 24 alcoholics without evidence of chronic liver disease.[45] These observations stimulated us to question whether there may be detectable cytokine levels in patients with alcoholic hepatitis. We initially took serum from patients with alcoholic hepatitis, removed endotoxin using absorbent columns, and injected alcoholic hepatitis serum into rats. Serum from healthy volunteers did not cause the serum zinc concentration to drop in experimental animals, but serum from alcoholic hepatitis patients caused significant hypozincemia, demonstrating that there was a factor in alcoholic hepatitis serum that induced hypozincemia. We next assayed serum from alcoholic hepatitis patients for IL-1 using a bioassay and found decreased IL-1 levels in selected patients with very severe disease.[46] We then demonstrated that monocytes, major producers of cytokines, released more TNF both spontaneously and after lipopolysaccharide (LPS) stimulation from alcoholic hepatitis patients compared to healthy volunteers.[44] Subsequently, several groups have shown increased plasma IL-1α, TNF, and IL-6 levels in alcoholic hepatitis patients.[47-50] Other patients with liver disease, such as those having chronic active hepatitis, viral hepatitis, and primary biliary cirrhosis, also have been shown to have elevated serum TNF concentrations and/or increased monocyte cytokine production.[50] Monocytes from patients having viral liver disease also have been shown to have increased TNF receptor density.[51] Thus, there is considerable evidence to support the hypothesis of increased/altered cytokine activity in multiple types of liver disease, especially alcoholic liver disease. One well-established biologic activity of IL-1, IL-6, and TNF is induction of hypozincemia.[15,44] With increased cytokine activity there is a decrease in zinc concentrations from some body components such as plasma, with an internal redistribution to other parts of the body.[9,15] Thus, certain tissues may develop a relative zinc deficiency during periods of stress or inflammation (as seen in alcoholic liver disease). We suggest that one important reason for the hypozincemia observed in alcoholic liver disease is increased cytokine activity, with subsequent altered zinc metabolism.

As noted earlier, albumin is the major zinc-binding protein in the plasma. Giroux et al. demonstrated that albumin from decompensated cirrhotics has less affinity for zinc than albumin from normal subjects.[52] Thus, patients with alcoholic liver disease not only have decreased levels of the major zinc-binding protein, albumin, but this albumin also binds zinc less avidly.

Alcoholics with or without liver disease have increased urinary excretion of zinc.[37] Patients with alcoholic liver disease tend to have the greatest zinc losses, with losses greatest in those with the most severe disease.[25,37] In healthy subjects, urinary zinc excretion is usually less than 500 to 700 μg/24 h. Chronic alcoholics frequently excrete 1000 μg or more per 24 h, and patients with alcoholic liver disease may lose 2000 to 5000 μg/24 h.[37] The mechanisms for this increased zinc loss are probably multifactorial.[53] Stress or trauma states are associated with increased urinary zinc loss and may contribute to total body zinc deficits.[11,13] Diuretics such as thiazides can lead to urinary loss of zinc.[54] Many alcoholic cirrhotics have ascites and are treated with diuretics. This may exacerbate underlying zinc deficiency. Intestinal loss of zinc has not been rigorously evaluated in chronic alcoholics with or without liver disease. However, it is well-documented that diarrheal states cause increased fecal zinc loss.[5] Diarrhea in chronic alcoholics could be an additive factor in the overall zinc deficiency.

In summary, there are multiple reasons for chronic alcoholics with and without liver disease to develop zinc deficiency. Many of the homeostatic regulatory mechanisms such as increased zinc absorption and renal conservation of zinc are not functional in the chronic alcoholic, thus worsening their overall zinc status.

FUNCTIONAL CONSEQUENCES OF ZINC DEFICIENCY

Zinc deficiency may present in multiple ways.[1] This section reviews the functional consequences of zinc deficiency as related to alcoholism (Table 1).

SKIN LESIONS

Much of the important information concerning functional consequences of zinc deficiency was first recognized in the hereditary disease of impaired zinc absorption, acrodermatitis enteropathica.[55] This disease process usu-

TABLE 1
Functional Consequences of Zinc Deficiency in Alcoholism

Skin lesions (acrodermatitis)
Hypogonadism
Impaired night vision, macular degeneration
Predisposition to portal systemic encephalopathy and impaired cognition
Anorexia, alterations in taste and smell
Depressed immune function
Poor wound healing and altered protein metabolism
Teratogenesis

ally manifests itself early in infancy with skin lesions presenting around the eyes, nose, mouth, and extremities, diarrhea, impaired immune function with frequent infections, growth retardation, and alopecia. The skin lesions of acrodermatitis are similar to those seen in diet-induced zinc deficiency in experimental animals and man. These skin lesions were next recognized with the advent of TPN.[56] Patients receiving TPN without added zinc developed these classic zinc deficiency skin lesions, and they corrected with oral or intravenous zinc supplementation. Chronic alcoholics appear to be especially susceptible to the development of zinc deficiency during TPN. In our initial series of seven patients with acrodermatitis during TPN administration, three had the diagnosis of chronic alcoholism.[56] Several cases of acrodermatitis also have been reported in alcoholics with or without liver disease who were not receiving TPN.[57-59] These patients usually consumed large amounts of alcohol, were on diuretics, had diarrhea, or had previous gastric surgery. In spite of increased knowledge of zinc metabolism, we continue to see several patients each year with chronic alcohol abuse who develop mild cases of "spontaneous" acrodermatitis.

HYPOGONADISM

Chronic alcoholics, especially alcoholics with liver disease, frequently have hypogonadism.[60] The mechanisms for this process appear to be multiple, including hypothalamic pituitary and gonadal defects. Zinc deficiency is a well-recognized cause of hypogonadism in experimental animals, and diet-induced zinc deficiency in man causes decreased sperm counts and low testosterone levels.[61-63] Zinc deficiency has been postulated to play a role in the hypogonadism seen in a variety of disease processes including chronic alcoholism and in the hypogonadism observed in some underdeveloped countries.[62-66] Animals with dietary-induced zinc deficiency have a functionally intact hypothalamic pituitary axis and the hypogonadism appears to be a primary gonadal defect. Zinc deficient rats have impaired testosterone production and response to stimuli such as human chorionic gonadotropin (HCG) or luteinizing hormone releasing hormone (LHRH).[61,62] This suggests that zinc deficiency may impair testosterone steroidogenesis, a likely hypothesis in view of the metalloenzymes involved in steroid metabolism. Positive results with zinc supplementation have been noted in the hypogonadism seen in renal disease and in some patients with sickle cell anemia.[64,65] Billington et al. correlated high urinary zinc excretion and low testosterone with impotence in the elderly.[67] They also associated diuretic use with low testosterone levels, and suggested a diuretic-induced zinc loss as a cause of this hypogonadism. Leevy et al. reported decreased testosterone levels in alcoholic cirrhotics that improved with zinc supplementation.[66] However, no prospective, randomized studies have evaluated the effects of zinc supplementation on hypogonadism in chronic alcoholism.

IMPAIRED NIGHT VISION, RETINA FUNCTION, AND MACULAR DEGENERATION

The eye contains the highest concentration of zinc in the body, and zinc is necessary for normal vision. In 1939, Patek et al. initially[68] observed that alcoholic cirrhotics frequently had abnormal night vision that usually improved with vitamin A supplementation. Research by Morrison et al.[69] and McClain et al.[33] demonstrated that certain alcoholic cirrhotics also required zinc to correct their abnormalities in dark adaptation. Keeling and co-workers showed that alcoholic cirrhotics had abnormal electroretinography, and depressed B wave amplitude correlated with leukocyte zinc concentrations.[70] Studies from Prasad's research group showed impaired dark adaptation in zinc-deficient sickle cell patients.[71] McClain et al. reported impaired dark adaptation in a zinc deficient patient with Crohn's disease that improved with zinc therapy and then worsened with withdrawal of zinc therapy.[72] Animals placed on zinc-deficient diets had abnormal electroretinography, thus supporting the above clinical observations. In some of the cirrhotic patients and Crohn's patients, a prolonged rod-cone break still persisted even after zinc and vitamin A supplementation for over one year.[33,72] This implied that chronic zinc deficiency may be causing not only a biochemical but also an anatomic defect. Interestingly, Toskes and co-workers reported anatomic defects in the retina (presumably in the retinal pigmen epithelium) on fluorescein angiography in patients with alcohol-induced pancreatic insufficiency.[73] These investigators suggested zinc deficiency as one possible etiologic factor for these anatomic abnormalities of the retina.

To investigate the possibility of zinc deficiency induced anatomic defect in the retina, Leure-duPree first treated rats with the zinc chelating agents, dithizone and 1,10-phenanthroline.[74] Degenerative changes of the retinal pigment epithelium (RPE) and unusual osmiophilic inclusion bodies in RPE were observed. Next, Leure-duPree and McClain evaluated the effect of differing durations of dietary zinc deficiency upon the ultrastructure of the rat retina.[75] Essentially identical abnormalities were seen with diet-induced zinc deficiency as compared to administration of zinc chelating agents. Osmiophilic inclusion bodies in the RPE were seen early in zinc deficiency, while severe disruption of the outer segments were seen later in the course of zinc deficiency. Sinning et al. performed scanning electron microscopy of the retina of zinc-deficient rats and confirmed the presence of anatomic defects.[76] Cameron and McClain had the opportunity to study the eyes of a patient who expired with acrodermatitis enteropathica.[77] This patient had severe degeneration of the RPE, similar to that seen in zinc-deficient rats.

Zinc deficiency could affect the retina adversely through several different mechanisms. Zinc deficiency could interfere with vitamin A metabolism (necessary for retina function and integrity) by decreasing retinol-binding protein (RBP) production and/or release from the liver, as reported in experimental animals.[78] RBP is a rapid turnover protein with a half-life of 12 h. It was reported that severe zinc deficiency in man decreases the level of rapid turnover proteins such as RBP and prealbumin (PA), and that zinc repletion alone increased these levels.[79] Depressed conversion of *retinol* to *retinal,* due to depressed zinc metalloenzyme activity, could also prevent photoreceptors from obtaining the amount of retinal they require. This could result in increased synthesis of high affinity receptor for the uptake of vitamin A by the RPE, and therefore, an increase in vitamin A uptake. A ''futile cycle'' might continue for as long as there is insufficient retinal reaching the photoreceptors, manifested by an accumulation of retinyl esters in lipid inclusion bodies in the RPE. This process could interfere with the normal biosynthesis of the visual pigment and the metabolism of the RPE. It is also documented that vitamin A esters are toxic to cells and are membranolytic.[75] If the lipid-containing inclusion bodies in the RPE of zinc-deficient rats contain vitamin A derivatives, such as retinyl esters, they could cause lysosomal instability and the release of lytic enzymes. The release of proteolytic enzymes into the cytoplasm of the RPE could mediate the degenerative changes seen in the RPE of zinc-deficient rats. This damaging effect on membranes also could be augmented by zinc deficiency. Zinc plays a vital role in membrane stability (reviewed by Bettger and O'Dell).[80] Zinc deficiency enhances lipid peroxidation and damage to lipids in membranes and thus the combination of retinyl esters and zinc deficiency might produce a synergistic deleterious effect on the retina. *In vitro* studies demonstrated that zinc exerts a protective effect on peroxidation-induced damage in rod outer segments. A recent investigation by Newsome and co-workers[81] showed that zinc supplementation was helpful in preventing macular degeneration. One postulated mechanism for the observed therapeutic effect is the antioxidant properties of zinc. Zinc also is required for normal protein metabolism and tissue repair processes. Studies in rats suggested that the protein malnutrition which accompanies zinc deficiency depresses opsin synthesis in the rods, thus providing the major mechanisms for the impaired retina function observed with zinc deficiency. In summary, it is clear that zinc deficiency causes biochemical and functional abnormalities of the retina that later may translate to structural defects. The reversibility of these lesions remains to be determined.

PREDISPOSITION TO PORTAL SYSTEMIC ENCEPHALOPATHY AND IMPAIRED COGNITION

Supporting evidence for a role for zinc in impaired cognition and portal systemic encephalopathy comes from several lines of research. Prasad and co-workers reported that experimental zinc deficiency in rats and in humans causes an increase in the plasma ammonia level.[82,83] Zinc deficiency was shown to decrease activity of glutamate dehydrogenase and ornithine transcarbamylase, important in normal nitrogen metabolism.[82,84] Thus, it was speculated that zinc deficiency may augment hepatic encephalopathy through increasing ammonia levels.

Reding and co-workers performed a randomized trial of zinc supplementation in patients with chronic hepatic encephalopathy and demonstrated beneficial results with administration of zinc acetate at 600 mg/d.[85] Recently, a patient with severe recurrent encephalopathy was reported in whom zinc deficiency was artificially induced by oral histidine treatment.[86] Overt encephalopathy occurred that was identical to the patient's earlier episodes of encephalopathy, and which responded to oral zinc supplementation. Long term zinc supplementation improved the patient's encephalopathy and quality of life. We reported a patient with alcoholic cirrhosis, severe hypozincemia, and skin lesions typical of zinc deficiency who had encephalopathy that corrected with zinc supplementation.[87] Other investigators have shown that patients with more severe portal systemic shunting have more depressed zinc status.[26] In one model of experimental hepatic encephalopathy, decreased brain zinc content was reported and related to alterations in GABAergic neurotransmission.[88] On the other hand, a recent double-blind, randomized, crossover trial of zinc supplementation by Riggio and co-workers failed to demonstrate that zinc supplementation improves chronic hepatic encephalopathy.[89]

Zinc deficiency has also been associated with altered mental status in patients and experimental animals without liver disease. Studies in experimental animals show that dietary-induced zinc deficiency is associated with altered behavior and learning impairment as well as peripheral neuropathy in some cases.[90,91] Henkin et al. reported that zinc deficiency induced in humans by feeding histidine was accompanied by apathy and irritability which reversed with zinc supplementation.[92] Children with acrodermatitis enteropathica frequently display apathy or confusion which responds to zinc supplementation.[93]

There are multiple reasons why zinc might influence mental function. Zinc is widely distributed throughout the brain and spinal cord in both humans and experimental animals.[94-96] The functions of zinc in the brain have been clarified over the past decade and are diverse. Frederickson has recently reviewed the current understanding of zinc neurobiology and described 3 major zinc pools: (1) protein-bound zinc; (2) "free zinc"; and (3) zinc associated with synaptic vesicles.[97] Multiple structural proteins and enzymes bind zinc in the brain, similar to nonneural tissues. However, brain-specific structural proteins, such as the S-100 proteins and tubulin, specifically bind zinc which appears to be potentially important for cellular integrity.[98,99] In addition to these proteins which are unique to the brain, zinc also functions by binding to calmodulin and interacting directly with membrane ion channels. Thus, it is becoming increasingly apparent that alteration of cerebral zinc status could have wide-ranging effects on the structure and function of the brain.

The importance of vesicular-associated zinc in the brain was recognized first in the hippocampus, the region of the brain containing the highest concentration of zinc.[94-96] Vesicular zinc is selectively stained by a variety of histochemical methods such as the neo-Timm's, selenium, dithizone, and the quinoline fluorescent techniques.[97,100,101] Adaptation of these methods to the ultrastructural level has demonstrated that zinc is associated with synaptic vesicles,[102] data which are complemented by the direct demonstration of zinc uptake into synaptosomes.[103]

Zinc-containing pathways are not restricted to the hippocampus, but also have been demonstrated in cerebrocortical interneurons and association fibers, numerous tracts connecting the hippocampus to the limbic system, and the cochlear granule neurons.[97] These pathways are involved in sensory processing, memory, and cortical association. Also, zinc is colocalized with several neurotransmitters and appears to be coreleased as "free" zinc upon membrane depolarization. "Free zinc" interacts postsynaptically to modulate the function of a wide variety of receptors including the ones for opiate, benzodiazepine, GABA, glutamate, and aspartate.[104]

The functional interaction between zinc and glutamate has received the most attention. Choi's group has shown in cultures of cortical neurons that zinc can selectively block the action of glutamate at the N-methyl-D-aspartate (NMDA) receptor subtype.[105] Other studies have demonstrated that the neurotoxicity of excitatory amino acid neurotransmitters, working at the NMDA receptor, can be attenuated by zinc.[106] Therefore, it appears likely that zinc may shape the reactivity of brain circuitry, in part by modulating the function of neurotransmitter receptors and receptor subclasses. These basic functions of zinc in the brain support the possibility of altered cognition due to zinc deficiency such as that caused by alcoholism and alcoholic liver disease (especially with the emerging importance of GABA in encephalopathy).

DEPRESSED APPETITE AND TASTE SENSATION

Zinc plays an important role in appetite regulation. In rats, decreased food consumption is an early sign of zinc deficiency.[107] At present, the mechanisms by which zinc deficiency induces anorexia are unknown. Henkin and co-workers have suggested that alterations in taste acuity may play a role in the genesis of the anorexia of zinc deficiency.[108] Zinc deficiency in rats and rabbits produces major morphologic alterations of the tongue and other oral mucosa. Zinc-deficient animals also demonstrate altered intake of a variety of solutions such as quinine sulfate and saline used to assess taste acuity.[109,110] Henkin et al. described histidine-treated scleroderma patients who developed zinc deficiency and severe taste abnormalities which were reversed with zinc supplementation.[92]

Patients with acute liver disease frequently complain of unpleasant olfactory and gustatory sensations, and this usually improves in conjunction with resolution of their liver disease. Burch et al. reported decreased taste and small acuity in cirrhotics with hypozincemia.[111] Smith et al. demonstrated abnormal gustatory acuity in patients with viral hepatitis or chronic liver disease, with both groups of patients having hypozincemia.[112] However, neither of these investigators proved a causal relationship between the hypozincemia and taste disturbances. Weismann et al. performed a double-blind clinical trial of zinc supplementation in stable cirrhotics.[113] They reported moderate but significant improvement in taste sensation in the zinc-treated group. However, a double-blind randomized study by Henkin and co-workers demonstrated that zinc supplementation was generally ineffective in treating taste dysfunction of undefined etiology, a finding now supported by other randomized studies.[114,115] Also, it is unclear that gustation is a major determinant of dietary intake.[116] Thus, while zinc deficiency may play a role in some of the altered taste sensation seen in liver disease, it is unlikely to be a major cause of the anorexia of liver disease. A much more likely cause of this anorexia is the documented increased cytokine activity (IL-1, IL-6, TNF). Indeed, cytokines such as TNF/cachectin are potent anorexigenics.[117]

ZINC AND IMMUNE FUNCTION

Zinc deficiency is known to cause defects in immune function. Zinc-deficient animals have thymic and lymph node atrophy, decreased production of the thymic hormone thymulin, loss of cytotoxic T-lymphocyte response to tumor cells, impaired response to thymus-dependent antigens, and decreased natural killer cell activity.[118-124] Children with acrodermatitis enteropathica are an excellent clinical example of immune dysfunction due to zinc deficiency.[125] Leukocyte function and cell-mediated immunity have been reported to be depressed in these children and improved or corrected with zinc supplementation. We reported two patients who developed clinical zinc deficiency with TPN administration.[123] They had cutaneous anergy and a very depressed T-cell response to phytohemagglutinin. These abnormalities corrected with zinc supplementation. We also reported depressed natural killer activity in clinical zinc deficiency and in human lymphocytes treated with a zinc chelating agent.[124] These abnormalities, again, corrected with zinc supplementation. Thymulin is a nonapeptide that induces a host of important T-cell functions. This metallopeptide requires zinc for hormone activity and thymulin activity decreases with mild dietary induced zinc deficiency in man.[126] Chronic alcoholics and alcoholics with liver disease frequently have impaired immune function.[127-130] Two prospective studies evaluated the effects of zinc supplementation on immune function in alcoholic cirrhosis. Significant improvements in several parameters of immune function were noted in both studies.[131,132] Thus, it would appear from these prospective studies that a component of the immune dysfunction noted in chronic alcoholism may be due to zinc deficiency.

IMPAIRED GROWTH, PROTEIN METABOLISM, AND WOUND HEALING

A major manifestation of zinc deficiency in both man and experimental animals is severe growth retardation and poor utilization of food.[133] An early biochemical marker of zinc deficiency is decreased activity of thymidine kinase, an integral enzyme in DNA synthesis.[134,135] The mechanisms for growth retardation associated with zinc deficiency are probably multifactorial and include impaired synthesis of both nucleic acids and protein, increased protein catabolism, the previously described anorexia, and impaired food utilization.[133-136]

Because of the above noted role of zinc in nucleic acid metabolism, in the synthesis of structural proteins such as collagen, in various enzymatic pathways, and in polyamine metabolism, it seems logical that positive zinc balance would be important to wound healing and hepatic repair. The clinical role of zinc in wound healing was studied initially by Pories et al., with the observation of improved healing of pilonidal sinuses with zinc administration.[137] Subsequent controlled studies by Hallbook and Lanner demonstrated that zinc supplementation improved wound healing of venous leg ulcers in patients having decreased serum zinc concentrations.[138] Studies in rats showed that zinc deficiency slowed healing of excised and thermal injuries, but excess zinc in the diet did not enhance wound healing.[139] Thus, it appears that when subjects are zinc deficient, zinc supplementation improves wound healing. However, if patients are zinc sufficient, providing further zinc does not accelerate wound healing.

Zinc deficiency also has been shown to cause decreased levels of insulin-like growth factor-1 (IGF-1).[140] IGF-1 is an anabolic hormone that is required for normal growth and protein metabolism. Plasma IGF-1 levels were measured in 95 alcoholic cirrhotic men, with levels being markedly reduced in these alcoholic patients.[141] Biochemical indicators of protein calorie malnutrition and liver function tests correlated with IGF-1 levels. Whether zinc supplementation would enhance IGF-1 levels or improve lean body mass in these patients has not been tested.

ZINC, TERATOGENESIS, AND THE FETAL ALCOHOL SYNDROME

Initial studies by Warkany and Petering and by Hurley described severe congenital malformations in rats born to mothers who had been exposed to zinc-deficient diets during their pregnancy.[142-144] Severe zinc deficiency during pregnancy caused fetal wastage. Less severe zinc deficiency caused marked congenital abnormalities, especially of the central nervous system. The malformations seen in the offspring of zinc-deficient rats involved virtually every organ system, and these malformations could occur with only brief exposure to zinc deficiency during pregnancy. Moreover, experimental animals exposed to suboptimal zinc nutriture *in utero* exhibited mild deficits in memory.[145] This was thought to represent behavioral consequences of altered brain development and maturation. One potential mechanism for these malformations was thought to be the vital role of zinc in DNA synthesis and in a host of zinc metalloenzymes.[1] Zinc deficiency in humans also has been associated with congenital abnormalities. Women with acrodermatitis enteropathica frequently had spontaneous abortions and malformed infants.[146] Recently, however, zinc-supplemented patients with acrodermatitis enteropathica completed normal pregnancies.[147] Epidemiologic studies by Jameson in Sweden showed correlations between low serum zinc levels in pregnancy and immature infants, premature or postmature delivery, and congenital malformations.[148] In a study from London, zinc content in peripheral blood leukocytes was significantly lower in mothers giving birth to babies who were small for gestational age compared to those who were normal for gestational age.[149] Leukocyte zinc concentrations also correlated positively with muscle zinc levels. This study suggested that maternal tissue zinc depletion was associated with fetal growth retardation. Thus, there is considerable animal and human data to suggest that zinc deficiency causes congenital abnormalities, fetal wastage, and growth retardation.

In 1973, the term fetal alcohol syndrome was coined to describe a constellation of abnormalities observed in infants born to alcoholic mothers.

The fetal alcohol syndrome consists of growth retardation, central nervous system deficits, and characteristic facial abnormalities.[150] There is a spectrum of severity of disease with the fetal alcohol syndrome. Because of the high rate of malnutrition in alcoholic mothers, there was an initial concern whether malnutrition was the cause of fetal alcohol syndrome. Considerable evidence suggested that alcohol per se was a teratogen and that malnutrition did not have to be present for the development of fetal alcohol syndrome.[151] However, there has been considerable interest in the possible role of zinc deficiency in fetal alcohol syndrome because of the similarities of fetal alcohol syndrome and fetal abnormalities caused by zinc deficiency. Some studies showed lower fetal tissue zinc concentrations in the alcohol-exposed rats compared to control rats or impaired transfer of zinc across the placenta in alcohol-exposed rats. However, the data are quite conflicting.[152-159] Possibly the best animal study relating to this issue is the recent study from Johnson's laboratory using [65]Zn assays.[160] They showed that alcohol consumption caused neither a decrease in maternal organ zinc or fetal zinc accretion. They showed that placental zinc declined with developmental age, and this was not influenced by alcohol consumption. Only limited studies have been done concerning zinc status in infants with fetal alcohol syndrome. Assadi et al. reported lower plasma zinc concentrations and markedly increased 24-h urinary zinc excretion in infants with fetal alcohol syndrome compared to control infants.[161] They suggested that the high urinary zinc losses may contribute to overall total body zinc deficits in these infants.

In summary, the literature is clear that zinc deficiency causes low birth weights, growth retardation, and congenital abnormalities in both experimental animals and humans. The severity of fetal alcohol syndrome may be augmented by zinc deficiency, but zinc deficiency is not the underlying etiology of this fetal abnormality.

ZINC PROTECTION AGAINST CELLULAR/HEPATOCELLULAR INJURY

Zinc is an important component of membranes, and it is necessary for normal membrane stability.[1,2,80] Biochemists have long used zinc as a nonspecific stabilizer of membranes. Erythrocytes have been used widely to evaluate the effect of zinc on membrane stability and cell integrity. Initial studies showed increased osmotic fragility of red cells and decreased erythrocyte zinc concentrations in zinc deficient rats.[162-164] This increased osmotic fragility was restored to normal values during zinc repletion.[162] Zinc deficiency also resulted in an increase in the membrane cholesterol to phospholipid ratio in rat erythrocytes, further suggesting a role of zinc in membrane stabilization.[165] Studies from Pasternak's laboratory have shown that zinc protected against a host of membrane-mediated injurious agents such as *Staph aureus* α-toxin and Sendai virus.[166] Studies from our group have shown that zinc deficiency significantly increased erythrocyte ghost membrane fluidity in a dose dependent fashion. We also have shown that zinc deficiency caused impairment of endothelial barrier cell function. A variety of toxic substances such as TNF also disrupt endothelial barrier function. Unpublished studies from our group showed that zinc supplementation in physiologic ranges attenuated the endothelial barrier disruption caused by the toxic agent, TNF. Lastly, zinc administration also has been reported to protect against endotoxin lethality and lethality from bacterial infection.[167,168]

With this background, investigators questioned whether zinc may protect against a variety of forms of liver injury. Potential mechanisms of hepatoprotection included: (1) the previously noted effects of zinc on stabilization of membranes and inhibition of lipid peroxidation, (2) zinc induction of hepatic metallothionein, which is rich in SH groups and binds to certain toxic metals such as copper, and (3) zinc-induced decreases in certain forms of P450 that are important for generation of toxic drug metabolites. Zinc has been shown to protect *in vivo* against a variety of hepatotoxic agents including pyrrolizidine alkaloids, carbon tetrachloride, cadmium, bromobenzene, copper, and acetaminophen.[170-176] One of the most interesting mechanisms for attenuation of liver injury is the effect of zinc on hepatocellular copper toxicity. Zinc appears to work at two levels in Wilson's disease, a hereditary disease of copper toxicity. It decreases copper absorption by induction of intestinal metallothionein, and it induces hepatic metallothionein which attenuates copper hepatotoxicity.[176] Induction of hepatic metallothionein has been shown to attenuate copper liver toxicity in animals in both *in vivo* and *in vitro* liver culture systems.[175,176] As noted previously, liver zinc stores appear to be depleted in alcoholic liver disease. To our knowledge, hepatic metallothionein has not been measured in alcoholic liver disease. Inadequate hepatic metallothionein stores could theoretically worsen alcohol-induced liver disease, but this hypothesis has not been tested.

CONCLUSIONS

In summary, zinc deficiency is a frequent complication of chronic alcoholism and alcoholic liver disease. The mechanisms for this zinc deficiency and altered zinc metabolism are multifactorial. Zinc deficiency may manifest in many different ways in the alcoholic, and health-care workers need to be aware of the multiple presenting features of zinc deficiency. Zinc clearly plays a role in cellular and hepatocellular protection against a variety of toxins. Whether zinc deficiency exacerbates organ specific injury such as liver injury in alcohol abuse remains to be determined.

REFERENCES

1. McClain, C. J., Kasarskis, E. J., and Allen, J. J., Functional consequences of zinc deficiency, *Prog. Food Nutr. Sci.,* 9, 185, 1985.
2. Bray, T. M. and Bettger, W. J., The physiological role of zinc as an antioxidant, *Free Radical Biol. Med.,* 8, 281, 1990.
3. National Research Council, *Recommended Daily Allowances,* 10th ed., National Academy Press, Washington, D.C., 1989, 208.
4. Spencer, H., Osis, D., Kramer, L., and Norris, C., Intake, excretion, and retention of zinc in man, in *Trace Elements in Human Health and Disease,* Academic Press, New York, 1976, 345.
5. McClain, C. J., Zinc in malabsorption syndromes, *J. Am. Coll. Nutr.,* 4, 49,064, 1985.
6. Guidelines for essential trace element preparations for parenteral use, *J. Am. Med. Assoc.,* 241, 2051, 1979.
7. McClain, C. J., Adams, L., and Shedlofsky, S., Zinc and the gastrointestinal system, in *Trace Elements in Human Research,* Prasad, A. S., Ed., Alan R. Liss, New York, 1988, 55.
8. Sandstrom, B., Cederblad, A., Kivisto, B., Stenquist, B., and Andersson, H., Retention of zinc and calcium from the human colon, *Am. J. Clin. Nutr.,* 44, 501, 1986.
9. Dunn, M. A., Blalock, T. L., and Cousins, R. J., Minireview. Metallothionein (42525A), *Proc. Soc. Exp. Biol. Med.,* 185, 107, 1987.
10. Anon., On the entero-pancreatic circulation of endogenous zinc, *Nutr. Rev.,* 39, 162, 1981.
11. McClain, C. J., Twyman, D. L., Ott, L. G., Rapp, R. P., Tibbs, P. A., Norton, J. A., Kasarskis, E. J., Dempsey, R. J., and Young, B., Serum and urine zinc response in head-injured patients, *J. Neurosurg.,* 64, 224, 1986.
12. Latimer, J. S., McClain, C. J., and Sharp, H. L., Clinical zinc deficiency during zinc-supplemented parenteral nutrition, *J. Pediatr.,* 97, 434, 1980.

13. Boosalis, M. G., Solem, L. D., Cerra, F. B., Konstantinides, F., Ahrenholz, D. H., McCall, J. T., and McClain, C. J., Increased urinary zinc excretion after thermal injury, *J. Lab. Clin. Med.*, 118, 538, 1991.

14. McClain, C. J. and Marsano, L., Zinc and gastrointestinal diseases, in *Trace Elements in Clinical Medicine*, Tomita, H., Ed., Springer-Verlag, Tokyo, 1990, 93.

15. Goldblum, S. E., Cohen, D. A., Jay, M., and McClain, C. J., Interleukin-1-induced depression of iron and zinc; role of granulocytes and lactoferrin, *J. Physiol.*, 252, E27, 1987.

16. Prasad, A. S., Clinical spectrum and diagnostic aspects of human zinc deficiency, in *Essential and Toxic Trace Elements in Human Health and Disease*, Prasad, A. S., Ed., Alan R. Liss, New York, 1988, 3.

17. Bach, J.-F., Pleau, J.-M., Savino, W., Laussac, J.-P., Cung, M.-H., Lefrancier, P., and Dardenne, M., The role of zinc in the biological activity of thymulin, a thymic metallopeptide hormone, in *Essential and Toxic Trace Elements in Human Health and Disease*, Prasad, A. S., Ed., Alan R. Liss, New York, 1988, 125.

18. Sato, M., Mehra, R. K., and Bremner, I., Measurement of plasma metallothionein-I in the assessment of the zinc status of zinc deficient and stressed rats, *J. Nutr.*, 114, 1683, 1984.

19. McClain, C. J., Antonow, D. R., Cohen, D. A., and Shedlofsky, S. I., Zinc metabolism in alcoholic liver disease, *Alcoholism Clin. Exp. Res.*, 10, 582, 1986.

20. Sullivan, J. F. and Lankford, H. G., Zinc metabolism and chronic alcoholism, *Am. J. Clin. Nutr.*, 17, 57, 1965.

21. Wang, J. and Peirson, R. N., Jr., Distribution of zinc in skeletal muscle and liver tissue in normal and dietary controlled alcoholic rats, *J. Lab. Clin. Med.*, 85, 50, 1975.

22. Barak, A. J., Beckenhauer, H. C., and Kerrigan, F. J., Zinc and manganese levels in serum and liver after alcohol feeding and development of fatty cirrhosis in rats, *Gut*, 8, 454, 1967.

23. Vallee, B. L., Wacker, W. E. C., Bartholomay, A. F., and Robin, E. D., Zinc metabolism in hepatic dysfunction. I. Serum zinc concentrations in Laennec's cirrhosis and their validation by sequential analysis, *N. Engl. J. Med.*, 255, 403, 1956.

24. Sullivan, J. F. and Heaney, R. P., Zinc metabolism in alcoholic liver disease, *Am. J. Clin. Nutr.*, 23, 170, 1970.

25. Kahn, A. M., Helwig, H. L., Redeker, A. G., et al., Urine and serum zinc abnormalities in disease of the liver, *Am. J. Clin. Pathol.*, 44, 426, 1965.

26. Schölmerich, J., Becher, M.-S., Köttgen, E., Rauch, N., Häussinger, D., and Löhle, E., The influence of portosystemic shunting on zinc and vitamin A metabolism in liver cirrhosis, *Hepatogastroenterology*, 30, 143, 1983.

27. Keeling, P. W. N., Jones, R. B., Hilton, P. J., et al., Reduced leucocyte zinc in liver disease, *Gut*, 21, 561, 1980.

28. Trentini, G. P., Dalla Pria, A. F., Ferrari de Gaetani, C., et al., Cirrosi epatica e modificazioni del contenuto testicolare di zinco. Possibile ruolo della ipozincoemia nella patogenesi dell'ipogonadismo del cirrotico, *Arch. De Vecchi Anat. Patol. Med.*, 52, 658, 1968.

29. Boyett, J. D., and Sullivan, J. F., Zinc and collagen content of cirrhotic liver, *Dig. Dis. Sci.,* 15, 797, 1970.

30. Fredricks, R. E., Ranaka, K. R., Valentine, W. N., et al., Zinc in human blood cells: normal values and abnormalities associated with liver disease, *J. Clin. Invest.,* 39, 1651, 1960.

31. Bode, J. C., Hanisch, P., Henning, H., Koenig, W., Richter, F.-W., Bode, C., Hepatic zinc content in patients with various stages of alcoholic liver disease and in patients with chronic active and chronic persistent hepatitis, *Hepatology,* 8, 1605, 1988.

32. Collipp, P. J., Kris, V. K., Castro-Magana, M., et al., The effects of dietary zinc deficiency on voluntary alcohol drinking in rats, *Alcoholism Clin. Exp. Res.,* 8, 556, 1984.

33. McClain, C. J., Van Thiel, D. H., Parker, S., Badzin, L. K., and Gilbert, H., Alterations in zinc, vitamin A, and retinol-binding protein in chronic alcoholism: a possible mechanism for night blindness and hypogonadism, *Alcoholism Clin. Exp. Res.,* 3, 135, 1979.

34. Antonson, D. L. and Vanderhoof, J. A., Effect of chronic ethanol ingestion on zinc absorption in rat small intestine, *Dig. Dis. Sci.,* 28, 604, 1983.

35. Sullivan, J. F., Jetton, M. M., and Burch, R. E., A zinc tolerance test, *J. Lab. Clin. Med.,* 93, 485, 1979.

36. Karayalcin, S., Arcasoy, A., and Uzunalimoglu, O., Zinc plasma levels after oral zinc tolerance test in nonalcoholic cirrhosis, *Dig. Dis. Sci.,* 33, 1096, 1988.

37. Antonow, D. R. and McClain, C. J., Nutrition and alcoholism, in *Alcohol and the Brain,* Tarter, R. E. and Thiel, D. H., Eds., Plenum Press, New York, 1985, 81.

38. Valberg, L. S., Flanagan, P. R., Ghent, C. N., and Chamberlin, M. J., Zinc absorption and leukocyte zinc in alcoholic and nonalcoholic cirrhosis, *Dig. Dis. Sci.,* 30, 329, 1985.

39. Boosalis, M. G., Evans, G. W., and McClain, C. J., Impaired handling of orally administered zinc in pancreatic insufficiency, *Am. J. Clin. Nutr.,* 37, 268, 1983.

40. Anon., Interleukin-1 regulates zinc metabolism and metallothionein gene expression, *Nutr. Rev.,* 47, 285, 1989.

41. Cousins, R. J. and Leinart, A. S., Tissue-specific regulation of zinc metabolism and metallothionein genes by interleukin 1. *FASEB J.,* 2, 2884, 1988.

42. Waalkes, M. P., Hjelle, J. J., and Klaassen, C. D., Transient induction of hepatic metallothionein following oral ethanol administration, *Toxicol. Appl. Pharmacol.,* 74, 230, 1984.

43. Hempe, J. M., Carlson, J. M., and Cousins, R. J., Intestinal metallothionein gene expression and zinc absorption in rats are zinc-responsive but refractory to dexamethasone and interleukin 1α, *J. Nutr.,* 121, 1389, 1991.

44. McClain, C. J. and Cohen, D. A., Increased tumor necrosis factor production by monocytes in alcoholic hepatitis, *Hepatology,* 9, 349, 1989.

45. Bode, C., Kugler, V., and Bode, J. C., Endotoxemia in patients with alcoholic and non-alcoholic cirrhosis and in subjects with no evidence of chronic liver disease following acute alcohol excess, *J. Hepatol.,* 4, 8, 1987.

46. McClain, C. J., Cohen, D. A., Dinarello, C. A., Cannon, J. G., Shedlofsky, S. I., and Kaplan, A. M., Serum interleukin-1 (IL-1) activity in alcoholic hepatitis, *Life Sci.*, 39, 1479, 1986.

47. Bird, G. L. A., Sheron, N., Goka, A. K. J., Alexander, G. J., and Williams, R. S., Increased plasma tumor necrosis factor in severe alcoholic hepatitis, *Ann. Intern. Med.*, 112, 917, 1990.

48. Felver, M. E., Mezey, E., McGuire, M., Mitchell, M. C., Herlong, H. F., Veech, G. A., and Veech, R. L., Plasma tumor necrosis factor α predicts decreased long-term survival in severe alcoholic hepatitis, *Alcoholism Clin. Exp. Res.*, 14, 255, 1990.

49. Khoruts, A., Stahnke, L., McClain, C. J., Logan, G., and Allen, J. I., Circulating tumor necrosis factor, interleukin-1, and interleukin-6 concentrations in chronic alcoholics, *Hepatology*, 13, 267, 1991.

50. Shedlofsky, S. I. and McClain, C. J., Hepatic dysfunction due to cytokines, in *Cytokines and Inflammation*, Kimball, E. S., Ed., CRC Press, Inc., Boca Raton, FL, 1991, 235.

51. Lau, J. Y. N., Sheron, N., Nouri-Aria, K. T., Alexander, G. J. M., and Williams, R., Increased tumor necrosis factor-α receptor number in chronic hepatitis B virus infection, *Hepatology*, 14, 44, 1991.

52. Gioux, E., Schechter, P. J., Shoun, J., and Sjoerdsma, A., Reduced binding of added zinc in serum of patients with decompensated hepatic cirrhosis, *Eur. J. Clin. Invest.*, 7, 71, 1977.

53. McClain, C. J., Shedlofsky, S., and Marsano, L., Trace minerals and alcoholism, in *Essential trace elements in gastroenterology and clinical medicine. Proc. 4th Annu. Symp. Associazone*, Farini, R., Sturniolo, G. C., McClain, C. J., and Abdulla, M., Eds., Smith-Gordon, London, 1991, 53.

54. Reyes, A. J., Leary, W. P., Lockett, C. J. and Alcocer, L., Diuretics and zinc, *S. Afr. Med. J.*, 62, 373, 1982.

55. Moynahan, E. J., Acrodermatitis enteropathica: a lethal inherited human zinc deficiency disorder, *Lancet*, 1, 399, 1983.

56. McClain, C. J., Trace metal abnormalities in adults during hyperalimentation, *JPEN*, 5, 424, 1981.

57. Ecker, R. I. and Schroeter, A. L., Acrodermatitis and acquired zinc deficiency, *Arch. Dermatol.*, 114, 937, 1978.

58. Weismann, K., Roed-Petersen, J., Hjorth, N., and Kopp, H., Chronic zinc deficiency syndrome in a beer drinker with a Billroth II resection, *Int. J. Dermatol.*, 15, 757, 1976.

59. Weismann, K., Hoyer, H., and Christensen, E., Acquired zinc deficiency in alcoholic liver cirrhosis: report of two cases, *Acta Derm. Venereol. Stockholm*, 60, 447, 1980.

60. Van Thiel, D. H., Gavaler, J. S., and Schade, R. R., Liver disease and the hypothalamic pituitary gonadal axis, *Semin. Liver Dis.*, 5, 35, 1985.

61. Lei, K. Y., Abassi, A., and Prasad, A., Function of pituitary-gonadal axis in zinc-deficient rats, *Am. J. Physiol.*, 230, 1730, 1976.

62. McClain, C. J., Gavaler, J. S., and Van Thiel, D. H., Hypogonadism in the zinc-deficient rat: localization of the functional abnormalities, *J. Lab. Clin. Med.*, 6, 1007, 1984.

63. Abbasi, A. A., Prasad, A. S., Rabbani, P., and DuMouchell, E., Experimental zinc deficiency in man. Effect on testicular function, *J. Lab. Clin. Med.*, 96, 544, 1980.

64. Abbasi, A. A., Prasad, A. S., Ortega, J., Congco, E., and Oberleas, D., Gonadal function abnormalities in Sickle cell anemia: studies in adult male patients, *Ann. Int. Med.,* 85, 601, 1976.
65. Antoniou, L. D., Shalhoub, R. J., Sudhakar, T., and Smith, J. C., Jr., Reversal of uraemic impotence by zinc, *Lancet,* 2, 895, 1977.
66. Leevy, C. M., Kanagasundaram, N., and Smith, F., Treatment of liver disease of the alcoholic: a composite approach, *Semin. Liver Dis.,* 1, 254, 1981.
67. Billington, C. J., Shafer, R. B., Krezowski, P. A., Levine, A. S., and Morley, J. E., Zinc status and impotence, in *Geriatric Nutrition,* Morley, J. E., Ed., Raven Press, New York, 1990, 441.
68. Patek, A. J. and Haig, C., The occurrence of abnormal dark adaptation and its relation to vitamin A metabolism in patients with cirrhosis of the liver, *J. Clin. Invest.,* 18, 609, 1939.
69. Morrison, S. A., Russell, R. M., Carney, E. A., and Oaks, I. V., Zinc deficiency: a cause of abnormal dark adaptation in cirrhotics, *Am. J. Nutr.,* 31, 276, 1978.
70. Keeling, P. W. N., O'Day, J., Ruse, W., Thompson, R. P. H., Zinc deficiency and photoreceptor dysfunction in chronic liver disease, *Clin. Sci.,* 62, 109, 1982.
71. Warth, J. A., Prasad, A. S., Zwas, F., and Frank, F. N., Abnormal dark adaptation in Sickle cell anemia, *J. Lab. Clin. Med.,* 98, 189, 1981.
72. McClain, C. J., Su, L.-C., Gilbert, H., and Cameron, D., Zinc deficiency-induced retinal dysfunction in Crohn's disease, *Dig. Dis. Sci.,* 28, 85, 1983.
73. Toskes, P. P., Dawson, W., Curington, C., Levy, N. S., and Fitzgerald, C., Non-diabetic retinal abnormalities in chronic pancreatitis, *N. Engl. J. Med.,* 300, 942, 1979.
74. Leure-duPree, A. E., Electron-opaque inclusions in the rat retinal pigment epithelium after treatment with chelators or zinc, *Invest. Ophthalmol. Vis. Sci.,* 21, 1, 1981.
75. Leure-duPree, A. E. and McClain, C. J., The effect of severe zinc deficiency on the morphology of the rat retinal pigment epithelium, *Invest. Ophthalmol. Vis. Sci.,* 4, 425, 1982.
76. Sinning, A. R., Olson, M. D., and Sandstead, H. H., The effects of zinc deficiency on developing photoreceptors in the rat retina: a scanning electron microscopic study, *Scanning Electron Microsc.,* 2, 867, 1984.
77. Cameron, J. D. and McClain, C. J., Ocular histopathy of acrodermatitis enteropathica, *Br. J. Ophthalmol.,* 70, 662, 1986.
78. Smith, J. E., Brown, E. D., and Smith, J. C., Jr., The effect of zinc deficiency on the metabolism of retinol-binding protein in the rat, *J. Lab. Clin. Med.,* 84, 692, 1974.
79. Bates, J. and McClain, C. J., The effect of severe zinc deficiency on serum levels of albumin, transferrin, and prealbumin in man, *Am. J. Clin. Nutr.,* 34, 1655, 1981.
80. Bettger, W. J. and O'Dell, B. L., A critical physiological role of zinc in the structure and function of biomembranes, *Life Sci.,* 28, 1625, 1981.
81. Newsome, D. A., Swartz, M., Leone, N. C., Elston, R. C., and Miller, E., Oral zinc in macular degeneration, *Arch. Ophthalmol.,* 106, 192, 1988.

82. Rabbani, P. and Prasad, A. S., Plasma ammonia and liver ornithine transcarbamylase activity in zinc-deficient rats, *Am. J. Physiol.*, 235, E203, 1978.

83. Prasad, A. S., Rabbani, P., Abbasii, A., Bowersox, E., and Fox, M. R. S., Experimental zinc deficiency in humans, *Ann. Intern. Med.*, 89, 483, 1978.

84. Burch, R. E., Williams, R. V., Hahn, H. K. J., et al., Serum and tissue enzyme activity and trace-element content in response to zinc deficiency in the pig, *Clin. Chem.*, 21, 568, 1975.

85. Reding, P., Duchateau, J., and Bataille, C., Oral zinc supplementation improves hepatic encephlopathy. Results of a randomized controlled trial, *Lancet*, 2, 493, 1984.

86. Van der Rijt, C. C. D., Schalm, S. W., Schat, H., Foeken, K., and De Jong, G., Overt hepatic encephalopathy precipitated by zinc deficiency, *Gastroenterology*, 100, 1114, 1991.

87. McClain, C. J., Souter, C., Steele, N., Levine, A. S., and Silvis, S. E., Severe zinc deficiency presenting with acrodermatitis during hyperalimentation: diagnosis, pathogenesis and treatment, *J. Clin. Gastroenterol.*, 2, 125, 1980.

88. Baraldi, M., Caselgrandi, E., Borella, P., and Zeneroli, L., Decrease of brain zinc in experimental hepatic encephalopathy, *Brain Res.*, 258, 170, 1982.

89. Riggio, O., Ariosto, F., Merli, M., Matteoli, G., Zullo, A., Ziparo, V., Pedretti, G., Fiaccadori, F., Bottari, E., and Capocaccia, L., Oral zinc supplementation does not improve chronic hepatic encephalopathy. Results from a double blind crossover trial, *Dig. Dis. Sci.*, in press.

90. Sandstead, H. H., Fosmire, G. J., McKenzie, J. M., and Halas, E. S., Zinc deficiency and brain development in the rat, *Fed. Proc.*, 34, 86, 1975.

91. O'Dell, B. L., Conley-Harrison, J., Browning, J. D., Besch-Williford, C., Hempe, J. M., and Savage, J. E., Zinc deficiency and peripheral neuropathy in chicks, *Soc. Exp. Biol. Med.*, 194, 1, 1990.

92. Henkin, R. I., Patten, B. M., and Re, R. P., A syndrome of acute zinc loss. Cerebellar dysfunction, mental changes, anorexia, and taste and smell dysfunction, *Arch. Neurol.*, 32, 745, 1975.

93. Moynahan, E. J., Zinc deficiency and disturbance of mood and visual behavior, *Lancet*, 1, 91, 1976.

94. Kasarski, E. J., Zinc metabolism in normal and zinc-deficient rat brain, *Exp. Neurol.*, 85, 114, 1984.

95. Chan, A. W. K., Minski, M. J., and Lai, J. C. K., An application of neutron activation analysis to small biological sample: simultaneous determination of thirty elements in rat brain regions, *J. Neurosci. Meth.*, 7, 317, 1983.

96. Donaldson, J., St. Pierre, T., Minnich, J. L., and Barbeau, A., Determination of Na +, K +, Mg2 +, Cu2 +, and MN2 + in rat brain regions, *Can. J. Biochem.*, 51, 87, 1973.

97. Frederickson, C. J., Neurobiology of zinc and zinc-containing neurons, *Int. Rev. Neurobiol.*, 31, 145, 1989.

98. Baudier, J., Glasser, N., and Gerard, D., Ions binding to S 100 proteins. I. Zn^{2+} regulates Ca^{2+} binding on S 100 b protein, *J. Biol. Chem.*, 25, 8912, 1986.

99. Hesketh, J. E., Microtubule assembly in rat extracts. Further characterization of the effects of zinc on assembly and cold stability, *Int. J. Biochem.*, 16, 1331, 1984.

100. Frederickson, C. J., Kasarskis, E. J., Ringo, D., and Frederickson, R. E., A quinoline fluorescence method for visualizing and assaying the histochemically reactive zinc (bouton zinc) in the brain, *J. Neurosci. Meth.*, 20, 91, 1987.

101. Savage, D. D., Montano, C. Y., and Kasarskis, E. J., Quantitative histofluorescence of hippocampal mossy fiber zinc, *Brain Res.*, 496, 257, 1989.

102. Claiborne, B. J., Rea, M. A., and Terrian, D. M., Detection of zinc in isolated nerve terminals using a modified Timm's sulfide-silver method, *J. Neurosci. Meth.*, j30, 17, 1989.

103. Wensink, J., Molenaar, A. J., Worniecka, U. D., and Van den Hamer, C. J. A., Zinc uptake into synaptosomes, *J. Neurochem.*, 50, 782, 1988.

104. Slevin, J. T. and Kasarskis, E. J., Effects of zinc on markers of glutamate and aspartate neurotransmission in rat hippocampus, *Brain Res.*, 334, 281, 1987.

105. Peters, S., Koh, J., and Choi, D. W., Zinc selectively blocks the action of N-methyl-D-aspartate on corticla neurons, *Science,* 236, 589, 1987.

106. Koh, J. and Choi, D. W., Zinc alters excitatory amino acid neurotoxicity on cortical neurons, *J. Neurosci.*, 8, 2164, 1988.

107. Essatara, M'B., Levine, A. S., Morley, J. E., and McClain, C. J., Zinc deficiency and anorexia in rats: normal feeding patterns and stress induced feeding, *Physiol. Behav.*, 32, 469, 1984.

108. Henkin, R. I., Graziadei, P. P. G., and Bradley, D. F., The molecular basis of taste and its disorders, *Ann. Int. Med.*, 71, 791, 1969.

109. Chen, S.-Y., Morphologic alterations in oral mucosa in zinc deficient rabbits, *Arch. Oral Biol.*, 25, 377, 1980.

110. Catalanotto, F. A. and Nanda, R., The effects of feeding a zinc-deficient diet on taste acuity and tongue epithelium in rats, *J. Oral Pathol.*, 6, 211, 1977.

111. Burch, R. E., Sacklin, D. A., Ursick, J. A., Jetton, M. M., and Sullivan, J. F., Decreased taste and smell acuity in cirrhosis, *Arch. Int. Med.*, 138, 743, 1978.

112. Smith, F. R., Henkin, R. I., and Dell, R. B., Disordered gustatory acuity in liver disease, *Gastroenterology,* 70, 568, 1976.

113. Weismann, K., Christensen, E., and Dreyer, V., Zinc supplementation in alcoholic cirrhosis, *Acta Med. Scand.*, 205, 361, 1979.

114. Henkin, R. I., Schecter, P. J., Friedewald, W. T., Demets, D., and Raff, N., A double-blind study of the effects of zinc sulfate on taste and smell dysfunction, *Am. J. Med. Sci.*, 272, 285, 1976.

115. Anon., Ineffectiveness of zinc in treating ordinary taste and smell dysfunctions, *Nutr. Rev.*, 37, 283, 1979.

116. Mattes, R. D., Gustation as a determinant of ingestion: methodological issues, *Am. J. Clin. Nutr.*, 41, 672, 1985.

117. Hellerstein, M. K., Meydani, S. N., Meydani, M., Wu, K., and Dinarello, C., Interleukin-1 induced anorexia in the rat, *J. Clin. Invest.*, 84, 228, 1989.

118. Chandra, R. K. and Au, B., Single nutrient deficiency and cell-mediated immune responses. I. Zinc, *Am. J. Clin. Nutr.*, 33, 736, 1980.

119. Brummerstedt, E., Flagstad, T., Basse, A., and Andresen, E., The effect of zinc on calves with hereditary thymus hypoplasia (lethal trait A46), *Acta Pathol. Microbiol. Scand. Sect. A*, 79, 686, 1971.

120. Iwata, T., Incefy, G. S., Tanaka, T., Fernandes, G., Menendez-Botet, C. J., Pih, K., and Good, R. A., Circulatory thymic hormone levels in zinc deficiency, *Cell. Immunol.*, 47, 100, 1979.

121. Fraker, P. J., DePasquale-Jardieu, P., Zwickl, C. M., and Luecke, R. W., Regeneration of T-cell helper function in zinc-deficient adult mice, *Proc. Natl. Acad. Sci. U.S.A.*, 75, 5660, 1978.

122. Golden, M. H. N., Jackson, A. A., and Golden, B. E., Effect of zinc on thymus of recently malnourished children, *Lancet*, 2, 1057, 1977.

123. Allen, J. I., Kay, N. E., and McClain, C. J., Severe zinc deficiency in humans: association with a reversible T-lymphocyte dysfunction, *Ann. Int. Med.*, 95, 154, 1981.

124. Allen, J. I., Perri, R. T., McClain, C. J., and Kay, N. E., Alterations in human natural killer activity and monocyte cytotoxicity induced by zinc deficiency, *J. Lab. Clin. Med.*, 102, 577, 1983.

125. Weston, W. L., Hutt, J. C., Humbert, J. R., Hambridge, K. M., Neldner, K. H., and Walravens, P. A., Zinc correction of defective chemotaxis in acrodermatitis enteropathica, *Arch. Dermatol.*, 113, 422, 1977.

126. Prasad, A. S., Meftah, S., Abdallah, J., Kaplan, J., Brewer, G. J., Bach, J. F., and Dardenne, M., Serum thymulin in human zinc deficiency, *J. Clin. Invest.*, 82, 1202, 1988.

127. Kaplan, J., Hess, J. W., and Prasad, A. S., Impairment of immune function in the elderly: association with mild zinc deficiency, in *Essential and Toxic Trace Elements in Human Health and Disease*, Prasad, A. S., Ed., Alan R. Liss, New York, 1988, 125.

128. Anon., Malnutrition and anergy in liver disorders, *Nutr. Rev.*, 4, 105, 1982.

129. Van Epps, D. E., Strickland, R. G., and Williams, R. C., Jr., Inhibitors of leukocyte chemotaxis in alcoholic liver disease, *Am. J. Med.*, 59, 200, 1975.

130. Bernstein, I. M., Webster, K. H., and Williams, R. C., Reduction in circulating T lymphocytes in alcoholic liver disease, *Lancet*, 2, 488, 1974.

131. Labadie, H., Verneau, H., Irinchet, J. C., et al., Does oral zinc improve the cellular immunity of patients with alcoholic cirrhosis, *Gastroenterol. Clin. Biol.*, 10(12), 799, 1986.

132. Radriguez, F. L., Martin Santana, H., and Gutierrez, F. J. Z. M., Alterations de la inmunidad celular, estado de nutricion y deficit de zinc en la cirrosis hepatica etilica, *Rev. Clin. Esp.*, 180, 496, 1987.

133. Essatara, M'B., Levine, A. S., Morley, J. E., and McClain, C. J., Zinc deficiency and anorexia in rats: normal feeding patterns and stress induced feeding, *Physiol. Behav.*, 32, 469, 1984.

134. Prasad, A. S. and Oberleas, D., Thymidine kinase activity and incorporation of thymidine into DNA in zinc-deficient tissue, *J. Lab. Clin. Med.*, 83, 634, 1974.

135. Williams, R. B. and Chesters, J. K., The effects of early zinc deficiency on DNA and protein synthesis in the rat, *Br. J. Nutr.*, 24, 1053, 1970.

136. Hsu, J. M., Anthony, W. L., and Buchanan, P. J., Zinc deficiency and incorporation of ^{14}C-labelled methionine into tissue proteins in rats, *J. Nutr.*, 99, 425, 1969.

137. Pories, W. J., Henzel, J. H., Rob, C. G., and Strain, W. H., Acceleration of healing with zinc sulfate, *Ann. Surg.*, 165, 432, 1967.

138. Hallbook, T. and Lanner, E., Serum-zinc and healing of venous leg ulcers, *Lancet*, 2, 780, 1972.

139. Sandstead, H. H., Lanier, V. C., Jr., Shephard, G. H., and Gillespie, D. D., Zinc and wound healing, *Am. J. Clin. Nutr.*, 23, 514, 1970.

140. Bolze, M. S., Reeves, R. D., Lindbeck, F. E., and Elder, M. J., Influence of zinc on growth, somatomedin, and glycosaminoglycan metabolism in rats, *Am. J. Physiol.*, 252, E21, 1987.

141. Mendenhall, C. L., Chernausek, S. D., Ray, M. B., Gartside, P. S., Roselle, G. A., Grossman, C. J., and Chedid, A., VA Coop Study. The interactions of insulin-like growth factor I(IGF-1) with protein-calorie malnutrition in patients with alcoholic liver disease: VA Cooperative study on alcoholic hepatitis VI, *Alcohol Alcoholism*, 24, 319, 1989.

142. Warkany, J. and Petering, H. G., Congenital malformations of the brain produced by short zinc deficiencies in rats, *Am. J. Ment. Defic.*, 77, 645, 1973.

143. Warkany, J. and Petering, H. G., Congenital malformations of the central nervous system in rats produced by maternal zinc deficiency, *Teratology*, 5, 319, 1972.

144. Hurley, L. S., Trace elements and their interactions as causes of congenital defects, in *Prevention of Physical and Mental Congenital Defects, Part B: Epidemiology, Early Detection and Therapy, and Environmental Factors*, Alan R. Liss, New York, 1985, 377.

145. Halas, E. S., Behavioral changes accompanying zinc deficiency in animals, in *Neurobiology of the Trace Elements, Volume 1*, Dreosti, I. D. and Smith, R. M., Eds., Humana Press, Clifton, NJ, 1983, 213.

146. Hambidge, K. M., Neldner, K. H., and Walravens, P. A., Zinc, acrodermatitis enteropathica, and congenital malformations, *Lancet*, 1, 577, 1975.

147. Brenton, D. P., Jackson, M. J., and Young, A., Two pregnancies in a patient with acrodermatitis enteropathica treated with zinc sulphate, *Lancet*, 2, 500, 1981.

148. Jameson, S., Zinc nutrition and human pregnancy, in *Zinc Deficiency in Human Subjects*, Alan R. Liss, New York, 1983, 53.

149. Meadows, N. J., Ruse, W., Smith, M. F., et al., Zinc and small babies, *Lancet*, 2, 1135, 1981.

150. Jones, K. L. and Smith, D. W., Recognition of the fetal alcohol syndrome in early infancy, *Lancet*, 2, 999, 1973.

151. Randall, C. L., Alcohol as a teratogen. A decade of research in review, *Alcohol Alcoholism Suppl.*, 1, 125, 1987.

152. Tanaka, H., Nakazawa, K., Suzuki, N., and Arima, M., Prevention possibility for brain dysfunction in rats with the fetal alcohol syndrome: low zinc status and hypoglycemia, *Brain Dev.*, 4, 429, 1982.

153. Suh, S. M. and Firek, A. F., Magnesium and zinc deficiency and growth retardation in offspring of alcoholic rats, *J. Am. Coll. Nutr.*, 1, 193, 1982.

154. Keppen, L. D., Pysher, T., and Rennert, O. M., Zinc deficiency acts as a coteratogen with alcohol in fetal alcohol syndrome, *Pediatr. Res.*, 19, 944, 1985.

155. Yeh, L. C. and Cerklewski, F. L., Interaction between alcohol and low dietary zinc during gestation and lactation in the rat, *J. Nutr.*, 114, 2027, 1984.

156. Ghishan, F. K., Patwardhan, R., and Greene, H. L., Fetal alcohol syndrome: inhibition of placental zinc transport as a potential mechanism for fetal growth retardation in the rat, *J. Clin. Lab. Med.*, 100, 45, 1981.

157. Ghishan, F. K. and Greene, H. L., Fetal alcohol syndrome: failure of zinc supplementation to reserve the effect of ethanol on placental transport of zinc, *Pediatr. Res.*, 17, 529, 1983.

158. Zidenberg-Cherr, S., Rosenbaum, J., and Keen, C. L., Influence of ethanol consumption on maternal-fetal transfer of zinc in pregnant rats on day 14 of pregnancy, *J. Nutr.*, 118, 865, 1988.

159. Henderson, G. I., Hoyumpa, A. M., McClain, C. J., and Schenker, S., The effects of chronic and acute alcohol administration of fetal development in the rat, *Alcoholism Clin. Exp. Res.*, 3, 99, 1979.

160. Greeley, S., Johnson, W. T., Schafer, D., and Johnson, P. E., Gestational alcoholism and fetal zinc accretion in Long-Evans rats, *J. Am. Coll. Nutr.*, 9, 265, 1990.

161. Assadi, F. K. and Ziai, M., Zinc status of infants with Fetal Alcohol Syndrome, *Pediatr. Res.*, 20, 551, 1986.

162. O'Dell, B. L., Browning, J. D., and Reeves, P. G., Zinc deficiency increases the osmotic fragility of rat erythrocytes, *J. Nutr.*, 177, 1883, 1987.

163. Bettger, W. J., Fish, T. J., and O'Dell, B. L., Effects of copper and zinc status of rats on erythrocyte stability and superoxide dismutase activity, *Proc. Soc. Exp. Biol. Med.*, 158, 279, 1978.

164. Bettger, W. J. and Taylor, C. G., Effects of copper and zinc status of rats on the concentration of copper and zinc in the erythrocyte membrane, *Nutr. Res.*, 6, 451, 1986.

165. Johanning, G. L. and O'Dell, B. L., Effect of zinc deficiency and food restriction in rats on erythrocyte membrane zinc, phospholipid and protein content, *J. Nutr.*, 119, 1654, 1989.

166. Mahadevan, D., Ndirika, A., Vincent, J., et al., Protection against membrane-mediated cytotoxicity by calcium and zinc, *Am. J. Pathol.*, 136, 513, 1990.

167. Snyder, S. L. and Walker, R. I., Inhibition of lethality in endotoxin-challenged mice treated with zinc chloride, *Infect. Immun.*, 13, 998, 1976.

168. Tocco-Bradley, R. and Kluger, M. J., Zinc concentration and survival in rats infected with *S. typhimurium*, *Infect. Immun.*, 45, 332, 1984.

169. Szymanska, J. A., Swietlicka, E. A., and Piotrowski, J. K., Protective effect of zinc in the hepatotoxicity of bromobenzene and acetaminophen, *Toxicology*, 66, 81, 1991.

170. McMillan, D. A. and Schnell, R. C., Amelioration of bromobenzene hepatotoxicity in the male rat by zinc, *Fundam. Appl. Toxicol.*, 5, 297, 1985.

171. Clarke, I. S. and Lui, E. M. K., Interaction of metallothionein and carbon tetrachloride on the protective effect of zinc on hepatotoxicity, *Can. J. Physiol. Pharmacol.*, 64, 1104, 1986.

172. Miranda, C. L., Henderson, M. C., Reed, R. L., Schmitz, J. A., and Buhler, D. R., Protective action of zinc against pyrrolozidine alkaloid-induced hepatotoxicity in rats, *J. Toxicol. Environ. Health,* 9, 359, 1982.
173. Cagen, S. Z. and Klaassen, C. D., Protection of carbon tetrachloride-induced hepatotoxicity by zinc: role of metallothionein, *Toxicol. Appl. Pharmacol.,* 51, 107, 1979.
174. Chvapil, M., Ryan, J. N., Elias, S. L., and Peng, Y. N., Protective effect of zinc on carbon tetrachloride-induced liver injury in rats, *Exp. Mol. Pathol.,* 19, 186, 1973.
175. Schilsky, M. L., Blank, R. R., Czaja, M. J., Zern, M. A., Scheinberg, I. H., Stockert, R. J., and Sternlieb, I., Hepatocellular copper toxicity and its attenuation by zinc, *J. Clin. Invest.,* 84, 1562, 1989.
176. Lee, D.-Y., Brewer, G. J., and Wang, Y., Treatment of Wilson's disease with zinc. VII. Protection of the liver from copper toxicity by zinc-induced metallothionein in a rat model, *J. Lab. Clin. Med.,* 114, 639, 1989.

14 Animal Models Show Nutritional Modulation of Alcoholic Liver Disease

INTRODUCTION

Animal models play a pivotal role in the investigation of cellular pathophysiology and are important in the diagnosis, prevention, and treatment of diseases. They have been used in such diverse areas as excessive or inadequate ingestion of nutrients, aging, carcinogenesis, diabetes, drug addiction, and heart disease among others. Depending on the complexity of the disease etiology under study, a single model often may not be adequate. No single animal model exists at this point in time which incorporates the various aspects of human alcoholism. Ethanol (alcohol) is not only a nutrient but also a toxic drug. The dose in humans is variable and can be either acute or chronic. Moreover, the pattern of human consumption has not been reproduced in animals. The rat, a commonly used animal model, exhibits an aversion to ethanol. Despite this difficulty, many rat models have been used, primarily to produce physical dependence on ethanol. Involuntary methods include inhalation,[1] gastric infusion,[2] or sustained ethanol release tube,[3] which provide a continuous ethanol administration, and gastric intubation,[4] which provides a discontinuous exposure to ethanol. Semivoluntary methods include ethanol as part of the fluid or diet ingested daily by the animal.[5-8] A voluntary method for the oral self-administration of ethanol has been developed.[9] Voluntary oral self-administration of ethanol has been made possible by the selective breeding of an alcohol-preferring P line and a nonalcohol-preferring NP line of Wistar rats.[10] While these models exhibit physical dependency on ethanol and a withdrawal syndrome depending on the dose and duration of ethanol treatment, only a few have contributed to our knowledge of alcoholic liver disease, a major cause of death in human alcoholics. In this chapter, we show how these models have revealed a synergism between nutritional factors and alcohol on the production of alcoholic liver disease. Significant alcoholemia is considered to be a prerequisite for the induction of liver injury. Investigations using various models reveal that the nutritional status of the animal plays a major role in the regulation of blood alcohol levels (BAL).

ALCOHOLIC LIVER DISEASE

Alcoholic liver disease is not a single entity but comprises a continuum of fatty liver (steatosis), alcoholic hepatitis, and cirrhosis. These lesions are found alone or more frequently in combination in the liver biopsies of symptomatic or asymptomatic patients.[11] These pathologic changes were thought to be progressive stages of alcohol-induced liver damage. However, the results from human and animal studies suggest that cirrhosis may develop in the absence of any evidence of prior hepatitis.[12,13] Both fatty liver and alcoholic hepatitis are reversible with abstinence, whereas cirrhosis is not. Among heavy drinkers, 90 to 100% exhibit some features of fatty liver, 10 to 35% develop alcoholic hepatitis, and 10 to 20% exhibit cirrhosis.[14]

Fatty liver is characterized by an increase in the hepatic lipid content, primarily due to a severalfold accumulation of triacylglycerol as compared to the level found in the liver of controls maintained on a diet devoid of alcohol.[15] Alcoholic steatosis can be macrovesicular, which is characterized by the presence of one medium-sized to large fat droplet per hepatocyte with lateral displacement of the nucleus.[16] It can also be present as microvesicular steatosis characterized by a striking increase in the size of liver cells which are filled with small fat droplets.[16] Mixtures of macro- and microvesicular steatosis also occur.

Alcoholic hepatitis is also known as alcoholic steatonecrosis.[17] In its advanced form, it is termed sclerosing hyaline necrosis.[18] It is characterized by a constellation of lesions that vary in degree from patient to patient. In addition to fatty metamorphosis, there is ballooning degeneration of liver cells with Mallory body formation. Continued activity of the lesions of alcoholic hepatitis leads to progressive pericellular fibrosis in acinar zone 3 with a lattice-like or "chicken-wire" appearance in sections stained with connective tissue stains, periportal fibrosis, and occlusive lesions of terminal hepatic venules.[16]

Cirrhosis represents more advanced alcoholic liver disease. It is a complex chronic alteration of hepatocyte structure and function. Its features are hepatocellular damage, hepatofibrosis, and nodular regeneration.[19] With the progression of alcoholic hepatitis, fibrous septa begin to link the chicken-wire fibrosis, eventually leading to complete encirclement of islets of hepatic parenchyma.[16] In this stage of alcoholic liver disease, the clinical signs are related to portal hypertension and liver failure.

ANIMAL MODELS FOR ALCOHOLIC LIVER DISEASE

DRINKING WATER MODEL

Experimental evidence from the studies of the effect of chronic alcoholism on the livers of animals carried out up to 1934 did not show that alcohol is a direct cause of liver injury.[20] In dogs in which fatty liver was previously induced by feeding low-protein diets, fatty cirrhosis was produced by feeding alcohol.[21] However, these results could also be observed in the absence of alcohol by feeding a high-fat/low-protein diet.[22] Fatty cirrhosis developed in rats fed a low-protein, low-choline diet when the drinking fluid contained 20% ethanol.[23,24] Correction of the dietary deficiencies by supplementation of the diets with choline, methionine, and casein, singly or in combination, prevented the fatty changes and cirrhosis in the liver even when rats consumed alcohol. Thus, results of early studies with this model of experimental alcoholism showed that alcohol itself in the presence of an adequate food intake was not harmful to the liver.

It has been reported that rats developed fatty livers when they consumed alcohol from their drinking fluid for 2 months and also received additionally daily doses of alcohol by stomach tube.[25] In this model, rats were intoxicated and not infrequently comatose and the amount of food ingestion was low. A nutritionally inadequate state in the animals was evident from the fact that loss of weight occurred in both the alcohol and control groups.

Best et al. used the isocaloric pair-feeding procedure for the first time to study the effects of chronic alcoholism on the liver by feeding sucrose to the controls in amounts equivalent to the alcohol calories from the drinking water in the experimental group.[26] The basal diet contained just those amounts of all essential food factors, vitamins, and proteins sufficient to the protect the liver when it was consumed without any caloric supplement from ethanol or sucrose. The alcohol group consumed a 15% solution of ethanol from the drinking fluid in addition to the basal diet. Some controls received not only the same amount of basal diet and the same amount of alcohol but also a supplement of either choline, methionine, or casein. Other controls received the same amount of the basal diet with various lipotropic supplements along with additional calories from sucrose equivalent to those derived from ethanol. Ingestion of basal diet alone without any additional lipotropes did not cause any excessive hepatic fat accumulation or fibrous tissue, but these lesions were present in rats fed the basal diet diluted by calories from ethanol or sucrose. When additional lipotropes were present, ingestion of additional calories from ethanol or sucrose resulted in a normal structure and lipid content in the liver. These observations were confirmed by others[27] and it was suggested that the requirement for choline was increased due to ethanol consumption.[28] These studies showed that alcoholic liver damage occurred only if the diet ingested by rats was deficient in essential nutrients, supporting the concept that malnutrition plays a major role in alcohol-induced liver injury.[26]

LIEBER-DeCARLI LIQUID ETHANOL DIET MODEL

In earlier studies, chronic ethanol administration consisted of adding 10 to 20% ethanol to the drinking water and feeding a solid diet to rats. By this method, rats consumed only 20 to 30% of total calories from ethanol. Increasing the ethanol concentration to enhance the consumption of alcohol resulted in a marked decrease in the total caloric intake and growth rate. Even at the highest levels of alcohol intake achieved by the drinking water method, fatty liver did not develop if the solid diet fed to rats was normal and not deficient in nutrients.[29,30]

Lieber and associates developed an animal model with an alcohol consumption of clinical relevance by feeding ethanol as part of a totally liquid diet.[7] When rats were given nothing to eat or to drink but the ethanol-containing liquid diet formula, their intake was sufficient to sustain a high daily intake of ethanol (12 to 18 g/kg), 2 to 3 times more than achieved by the drinking water method.[7] These rats developed fatty liver and exhibited high blood alcohol levels of 100 to 150 mg/100 ml. The original liquid diet contained 36% of total calories from ethanol, 16% from protein, 43% from fat, and only 5% from sucrose. Porta et al.[31] challenged the contention that alcoholic fatty liver developed despite nutritional adequacy in the animal. The ratio of protein, fat, and carbohydrate in the ethanol diet was abnormal for rats. Not only was the protein somewhat lower than that considered adequate, but the content of fat was very high and the content of carbohydrate was very low. To ascertain whether the dietary ratio of macronutrients is important for the development or prevention of fatty liver, Porta and associates conducted many investigations and concluded that when the amount of protein was normal or borderline, the proportions of fat were more important than carbohydrate in the development of hepatic lesions.[32,33] In experiments to determine the preventive role of high-protein levels, it was found that when the amino acid mixture was incorporated at the 25% level and the fat was kept within normal amounts for rats (6%), fatty liver was prevented even though the levels of ethanol had been elevated to 50%.[34]

Rats maintained for 4, 8, 12, and 16 weeks, with a daily intake of alcohol similar to that ingested by those fed the Lieber-DeCarli ethanol diet (19.48 ± 0.4 g/kg, 14.18 ± 0.24 g/kg, 11.83 ± 0.5 g/kg, and 10.24 ± 0.33 g/kg, respectively), had low liver triacylglycerol content (9.7 to 21.2 mg/g) compared to controls fed a diet without alcohol.[15,35] This low triacylglycerol content was ascribed to not only an increased content of protein (25%) but also to a reduced content of fat (15%) in the ethanol diet. The composition of the Lieber-DeCarli ethanol diet was subsequently changed by increasing the level of protein to 18% of total calories and decreasing the content of fat to 35% of total calories. This resulted in an increase in carbohydrate calories to 11% of total calories in the diet. Even in rats fed the modified Lieber-DeCarli ethanol diet, fatty liver is produced only when the diet contains at least 35% of calories from fat. When the content of fat is reduced and carbohydrate is increased correspondingly in the ethanol diet fed to rats, fatty liver is prevented.[36] Moreover, alcoholic fatty liver results only when the fat in the diet is composed of long-chain fatty acids.[37]

The alleged nutritionally independent hepatotoxic effect of ethanol was brought into question by the demonstration that a properly supplemented and calorically balanced 36% ethanol liquid diet permitted the regression of cirrhosis of choline-deficient rats to the same degree as in comparable cirrhotic rats fed a similarly balanced liquid diet containing no ethanol.[38] In rats fed the 36% liquid ethanol diet, serious vitamin disturbances have also been observed.[39] Thus, many studies have shown the association of nutritional factors in the development or prevention of the alcoholic fatty liver caused by ingestion of the Lieber-DeCarli ethanol liquid diet.

PORTA'S SWEETENED
ALCOHOLIC SOLUTION MODEL

In order to increase ethanol consumption to levels higher than those achieved by the drinking water technique, Porta and associates introduced a sweetened alcohol solution method.[40] It consists of feeding an aqueous solution of 25% sucrose and 32% ethanol (w/v) in place of drinking water and a stock diet to rats. This procedure enabled rats to consume 45 to 50% of their calories as ethanol. The relative importance of various dietary factors in the progression, regression, and prevention of alcoholic hepatic changes were investigated using this method.[40-43] Rats ingesting 46% of their calories from ethanol in the sweetened fluid and given a solid semi-synthetic diet containing 18.5% protein, 31% fat, and 50% carbohydrate and an abundant amount of vitamins for 5 months did not develop any biochemical or histologic signs of fatty changes.[42] However, the pair-fed and *ad libitum*-fed controls developed fatty livers when the calories from the ethanol in the diet were replaced with either carbohydrate or fat. When the calories derived from ethanol were replaced by a balanced mixture of carbohydrate, fat, and protein so that the final ratio of calories was 62:24:14 respectively in the diet fed to rats, essentially normal liver resulted. These results demonstrated the importance of the ratio of macronutrients in the diet when consumed alone and particularly when accompanied by a high intake (46%) of ethanol over a prolonged period of time (5 months).

OTHER LIQUID ETHANOL DIET MODELS

Rats maintained on a Lieber-DeCarli ethanol diet develop fatty liver but do not show liver pathology similar to that observed in human alcoholics.[44] Hence this model was improved by including 4-methylpyrazole (4-MP), an inhibitor of alcohol dehydrogenase in the ethanol liquid diet.[45,46] When rats were fed a 35% ethanol diet containing 4-MP for 12 weeks, a marked fatty infiltration and degenerative or mild inflammatory changes including eosinophilic cytoplasmic degeneration in centrilobular cells and focal inflammatory changes with cell necrosis in the livers were observed:[45,46] a more extensive liver pathology than fatty liver alone. Since the diet was considered to be nutritionally and completely adequate and balanced,[45,46] it would appear that chronic alcohol consumption produced significant liver pathology other than fatty liver alone in spite of an ostensibly adequate nutritional status in the animals.

Another ethanol liquid diet (Shorey-AIN Diet) model used primarily to produce dependence and tolerance in rats provided 35% of the total calories from ethanol and met the recommendations of the American Institute of Nutrition.[8] This diet is also considered to be nutritionally complete and balanced.[8] Rats maintained on this diet for prolonged periods are not likely to develop fatty liver since the caloric contribution from fat is low (12%) compared to that in the Lieber-DeCarli diet model.

NUTRITIONAL INADEQUACY OF LIQUID ETHANOL DIET MODELS

Numerous investigations by Porta and associates have shown that chronic ingestion of ethanol by rats does not result in liver injury if the four major sources of calories, namely fat, carbohydrate, protein, and alcohol, are in proper balance and accompanied by adequate amounts of all other known vitamins and essential food factors.[33] This observation suggests that nutritional status plays an important role in alcoholic liver damage. However, this concept was ignored and the one accepted during recent decades considered that fatty liver was produced due to direct ethanol toxicity and resulted despite the ingestion of a nutritionally adequate diet.[7,47,48] In order to resolve these conceptual differences, we extensively investigated the claim of nutritional adequacy of the Lieber-DeCarli ethanol diet model which is commonly used to study the effects of chronic alcohol consumption.

A diet defined as adequate must be able to be ingested in sufficient quantity to support normal growth, breeding, gestation, lactation, behavior patterns, nutrient storage, enzyme activity, and gross and histological appearance of tissues and their content of nucleic acid and protein.[49] One operational criterion that has been applied that encompasses all of these parameters is that a mammalian species fed an adequate diet should be able to reproduce, grow, and function normally for three to four generations, in which case it is presumed that all of the above parameters are within limits that allow survival of the species.

It has been recommended that in studies designed to produce alcoholic fatty liver, rats be started on the ethanol diet once they have reached a weight of 125 to 150 g.[44] When young rats are fed a Lieber-DeCarli control diet *ad libitum* for 4 weeks, they show a growth rate of 6 to 8 g/day.[50] This gain is similar to that observed when young rats are fed other nutritionally adequate control diets *ad libitum* such as the Purina Chow, AIN-76 diet, or NIH-07 diet.[50] On the other hand, when young rats are fed the Lieber-DeCarli ethanol diet *ad libitum,* they exhibit a slow growth rate

(1.86 to 3.05 g/d).[50] The original formula of the Lieber-DeCarli diet has been revised and several changes have been made based on the recommendations of the National Academy of Science.[44] Fiber was introduced in the diet and the content of zinc was increased.[51] The vitamin A content was also increased to levels comparable to that proposed in the 1967 and 1970 formulations.[51] Although these changes improve the quality of the diet, they do not improve the nutritional adequacy provided to the growing rat. The slow growth rate (about 3 g/d) observed with the currently available improved diet[52] is similar to that reported in the studies conducted with the diet formula two decades ago.[48,53] The reduced growth rate compared to the *ad libitum*-fed controls is not due to alcohol toxicity but rather to diet restriction since those pair-fed the Lieber-DeCarli control liquid diet also exhibit a slow growth rate.[47,53] A 50 to 75% reduction in growth shows that the young rats fed the 36% ethanol diet are malnourished. Feeding the 36% ethanol diet to pregnant rats resulted in a lower weight gain, a markedly lower litter weight, fewer pups born, and fewer pups born alive compared to the controls.[54] The 36% ethanol diet did not support the increased demands of lactation, 77% of the pups died, and the rest were not growing after 4 d of lactation.[54] In other studies, cannibalism, poor survival of pups to weaning, and less than normal weaning weights resulted from feeding rats the 36% ethanol diet during lactation.[55] A high protein, 36% ethanol diet has been recommended for lactation, but it resulted in a 96% postnatal mortality.[56]

Malnutrition results due to substantial (40%) reduction in diet consumption produced by the inclusion of 36% calories from ethanol. When fed *ad libitum,* young rats consume about 90 ml of the Lieber-DeCarli control diet daily, but they consume only about 55 ml/day when fed the 36% ethanol diet.[54,57,58] The reduced diet intake causes a reduction in the daily intake not only of energy, but also of several important nutrients such as calcium, copper, iron, manganese, phosphorus, vitamin B_6, and choline than those required for normal growth rate.[59,60] The nutritional inadequacy is greater during the early stages of alcohol consumption even if rats are weaned to the ethanol diet slowly. In the initial week, rats fed the 36% ethanol diet *ad libitum* consume only about 40 ml/d and lose weight, while those fed the control diet *ad libitum* ingest 80 to 100 ml/d and gain 7.5 to 9.5 g/d.[53] During the initial 2 weeks, young rats gain only about 0.9 g/d while the controls gain about 5.4 g/d.[61] During this period, alcohol-fed rats consume less energy, protein, and 12 other nutrients than the recommended levels.[61] Pregnant rats fed the 36% ethanol diet *ad libitum* ingested less energy, protein, and 11 other nutrients than recommended currently by the National Research Council.[54] Lactating female rats ingested less energy, protein, and 19 other nutrients than recommended currently.[54] For these reasons, it is clear that the claim that the 36% ethanol liquid diet provides nutritional adequacy is unfounded since not enough nutrients can be ingested to support normal growth, gestation, or lactation and hence, the survival of the species.[60]

When 4-MP is included in the ethanol diet, the diet consumption is further depressed. Hence the degree of malnutrition caused by the ingestion of the ethanol diet is even greater when 4-MP is present in the diet.[62] Young rats fed the ethanol + 4-MP diet showed a slow growth of about 2 g/d.[62] In some studies, rats fed the ethanol diet did not gain weight and those fed the ethanol + 4-MP diet lost 10% of their body weight during the 11-week period.[62,63] When liver pathology was produced in the ethanol + 4-MP model, an extreme degree of malnutrition was present in the animals.

Even in the ethanol liquid diet model introduced by Miller et al.,[8] while the *ad libitum*-fed controls showed a growth rate of 6.3 g/d, those fed the ethanol diet gained only about 3.2 g/d.[50] The ethanol-treated rats voluntarily consumed only 65% of the energy and nutrients compared to the *ad libitum*-fed controls.[64] In other experiments using this model, rats fed the ethanol diet gained only about 9.5% and pair-fed controls gained about 11.5% of the initial body weight, while those having free access to the control diet gained about 48.6% of the initial body weight.[65] Hence, those ingesting the ethanol diet gained only one fourth as much as the *ad libitum*-fed controls. From these discussions, it is evident that malnutrition is present not only in the animals fed the Lieber-DeCarli ethanol diet but also other ethanol liquid diets.

NUTRITION AND ALCOHOLIC FATTY LIVER

Although alcohol itself was incriminated as the direct etiologic factor in the pathogenesis of alcoholic fatty liver,[47] it is now known that several nutritional characteristics must be satisfied for the hepatic accumulation of lipid in the animal. The content of fat in the ethanol diet must be at least 35% of the total calories. Rats maintained on a 36% ethanol diet containing less than 35% calories from fat do not develop fatty liver.[36,66] The fat must be composed of long-chain fatty acids.[37] It has been suggested that the inability of medium-chain fat to cause alcoholic fatty liver is due to the propensity of the acids for oxidation rather than esterification.[37] Medium-chain fat is also incapable of producing fatty liver since it does not contain substantial amounts of unsaturated fatty acids. Recently, linoleic acid was found to facilitate the development of alcoholic liver disease.[67] In the Lieber-DeCarli ethanol diet, fat contains about 87% unsaturated fatty acids — 62% oleic and 25% linoleic.[68] Alcoholic fatty liver was produced when rats were fed the Lieber-DeCarli diet containing either olive oil or corn oil.[69] Since olive oil, like corn oil, is composed of mostly unsaturated fatty acids (90%) but contains a relatively low level of linoleate (4.8% vs. 59.4%), it is clear that unsaturated fat and not only linoleate is related to the development of alcoholic fatty liver.[69]

A restricted caloric intake compared to *ad libitum*-fed controls and a low daily ingestion of carbohydrate also appear to be related to the development of alcoholic fatty liver. When fatty liver was produced due to chronic ethanol ingestion, rats consumed only 4 or 11% of total calories from carbohydrate, depending on the content of fat in the diet (43 or 35%). Both anorexia and a reduced carbohydrate content cause rats to ingest only about 1 g of carbohydrate per day, while the pair-fed or *ad libitum*-fed controls consume about 6 g/d and 10 g/d of this macronutrient, respectively. When the Lieber-DeCarli ethanol diet was supplemented with small amounts of carbohydrate or gluconeogenic precursors and fed to rats, fatty liver did not develop.[70-73] It has been suggested that many biochemical changes observed in alcoholic fatty liver may not be due to a specific effect of ethanol but rather to the nutritional inadequacy such as the reduced caloric and carbohydrate intake which accompanies the Lieber-DeCarli ethanol diet regimen.[74,75]

The requirement of a high intake of fat and a low intake of carbohydrate for the development of alcoholic fatty liver ascertained from the animal model can also be extended to human conditions. A high level of liver triacylglycerol was observed in nonalcoholic human volunteers only when they consumed 46% of total calories from ethanol, 36% of calories from fat, 16% of calories from protein, and only 2% of calories from carbohydrate.[76,77] Although it was concluded that in normal nonalcoholic people alcohol itself is hepatotoxic independent of nutritional factors,[76] many subjects did not develop fatty liver.[77] One subject had only a normal level of liver triacylglycerol despite ingesting a greater amount of alcohol than was needed to produce fatty liver in another individual.[77] These differences in the effect of ethanol consumption were suggested to be due to the changes in the nutritional status of the individuals.[77]

Alcoholic liver damage is confined only to the development of fatty liver in young rats fed the Lieber-DeCarli diet for a month. However, hepatic lesions such as necrosis, inflammation, and fibrosis occur when weanling rats are fed for 9 months the Lieber-DeCarli ethanol diet containing a 5-fold increase in the level of vitamin A.[78] Rats fed an ethanol-high vitamin A diet ingested about 20% less diet than those fed the ethanol-normal vitamin A diet[78] and hence were even more malnourished during development. It would appear that fibrosis was not caused by ethanol ingestion per se and required an extreme degree of malnutrition in the animal and ingestion of a high dose of vitamin A. Hepatotoxic potential of vitamin A in liver disease has been studied by Seifert et al.,[79] who showed a dual role of vitamin A in experimentally induced liver fibrosis. Depending on the time of administration, vitamin A potentiates or suppresses liver fibrosis.

Recent investigations of Bosma et al.[80] and Seifert et al.[81] show that rats fed the Lieber-DeCarli ethanol diet containing a high level of vitamin A do not necessarily develop liver fibrosis. When 3-month-old rats of 2 strains (BN and WAG) were fed the Lieber-DeCarli ethanol-high vitamin A diet for 16 months, they did not exhibit hepatic fibrosis. The absence of fibrosis may not be due to a specific species response since both BN and WAG rats have been shown to be as sensitive to the induction of liver fibrosis by agents such as CCl_4[79] as in the case of Sprague-Dawley rats used in the studies by Leo and Lieber.[78] The role of vitamin A as a major factor in the pathogenesis of alcoholic liver fibrosis needs to be reevaluated due to the effects of other factors such as the age and nutritional status of the animal.

PRIMATE MODELS

Rats show an aversion to ethanol and do not consume diets containing more than 36% of total calories from the drug. It was believed that if increased amounts of alcohol were ingested, not only fatty liver, but advanced liver pathology, as observed in human alcoholics, would be produced. For this reason, a baboon model was introduced in which a modified Lieber-DeCarli diet with 50% of total calories from ethanol was fed for several years.[82] The livers of all baboons fed the ethanol diet developed fatty changes after 1 to 2 months, detectable fibrosis in 1 to 2 years, and cirrhosis in approximately 1/3 of the animals in 2 to 3 years.[82] When *macaca radiata* was maintained on a 50% alcohol liquid diet for 2 years, fatty infiltration was observed but not necrosis, inflammation, or fibrosis.[83] *Macaca mulatta*, fed a diet containing 40 to 50% of calories from ethanol for 4 to 5 years, failed to develop hepatic fibrosis or cirrhosis.[84] The difference in the results from baboons to those from other primates has been suggested to be due to differences in the genus susceptibility or the difference in the lipotrope content of the diets.[83]

Nutritional factors also play a role in producing alcoholic liver damage in baboons since studies by Ainley et al.[85] have shown that even when they consume a larger amount of ethanol than possible by the Lieber-DeCarli model, they do not develop fibrosis or cirrhosis. These investigators administered an ethanol semiliquid diet (Mazuri diet) to baboons for up to 5 years. Adolescent baboons fed this diet gained weight normally and ingested 3 to 5 times more ethanol per kilogram of body weight than from the Lieber-DeCarli diet, 1.9 to 4.2 times more energy, and significantly more nutrients.[85] The amount of fat ingested daily by the baboons was similar (1.4 g/kg) with either the Lieber-DeCarli or Mazuri diets. However, while this nutrient contributed to about 21% of total calories in the Lieber-DeCarli diet, it was only 5.5% of total calories with the Mazuri diet.[86] Thus, as in the case of the rat models, a relatively low contribution of calories from fat may have been responsible for preventing alcoholic liver damage in the baboons.

Primates generally consume each day 2 to 4% of their body weight in chow with a caloric density of 4.2 kcal/g.[87] Therefore, a baboon weighing 10 kg ingests a 200- to 400-g diet per day, an average of 126 kcal/kg/d (range 84 to 168 kcal/kg/d). In the investigations when choline supplementation failed to prevent liver fibrosis in the baboons fed the Lieber-DeCarli ethanol diet, the daily food consumption was only 58.0 ± 1.8 kcal/kg.[88] When a sequential production of fatty liver, hepatitis, and cirrhosis was caused by alcohol consumption, baboons ingested 80.0 ± 2.24 kcal/kg/d.[89] Hence, baboons developed alcoholic liver disease when they were ingesting significantly less than the average amount of diet.

The effect of the reduced diet intake is reflected in the growth. Baboons of age 4 years and 6 years weigh 10 and 20 kg, respectively.[88] When 4-year old baboons weighing 10.6 ± 0.35 kg were fed the Lieber-DeCarli ethanol diet *ad libitum* for 15 months, they lost weight to 10.2 ± 0.46 kg.[89] Had they ingested chow instead during this period, a body weight of about 16 kg would have been observed. The lack of growth in ethanol-fed baboons cannot be due to ethanol alone, but also to a reduced intake of energy and nutrients. This is shown by the results from the pair-fed controls. When baboons weighing 10.6 ± 0.33 kg were pair-fed an iso-caloric control diet without ethanol for 15 months, they weighed 11.8 ± 0.33 kg, exhibiting only a marginal weight gain.[89]

In the studies by Ainley et al., baboons consumed a larger amount of calories (218 to 261 kcal/kg/d) and had a weight gain of about 2.35 kg/year.[85] The energy contribution from the macronutrients in the diet, fat (5.5 vs. 21%), and protein (7.1 vs. 18.0%) was less and the energy contribution of carbohydrate (17.4 vs. 11.0%) was more in the ethanol diet used by Ainley compared to the Lieber-DeCarli model.[86] However, the absolute amounts of fat and protein ingested by alcoholic baboons were similar and the amounts of carbohydrate were much greater than those ingested by baboons fed the Lieber-DeCarli ethanol liquid diet.[85] The experimental conditions used by Ainley et al. were vastly different from those of Lieber and Associates. The results of Ainley et al. are very significant since they demonstrate that even a dose of ethanol as high as 178 kcal/kg/d, far greater than the 30 to 60 kcal/kg/d with the Lieber-DeCarli model, need not cause alcoholic liver damage. The difference in liver damage caused by the two diets is very likely due to the difference in the concomitant nutrient intake.

In the Lieber-DeCarli baboon model, feeding of lecithin rich in po-lyunsaturated fatty acids slows ethanol-induced fibrosis, and its withdrawal is associated with an acceleration of the fibrotic process, leading to a rapid development of cirrhosis.[90] Whether this effect is specifically due to the ingestion of lecithin or due to the presence of polyunsaturated fatty acids in the phospholipid is not known. In the continuous intragastric model for ethanol administration in rats, dietary polyunsaturated fat has been incrim-inated as a permissive rather than a protective factor in alcoholic liver injury.[67] Further studies with the baboon model using dietary dioleyl lec-ithin are necessary to ascertain whether the phospholipid must be comprised of polyunsaturated fatty acids in order to cause a protective action against the fibrogenic effect of ethanol ingestion. The mechanism of the protective effect of dietary lecithin in alcoholic liver injury is not known at present.

INTRAGASTRIC INFUSION MODEL

In order to circumvent rats' aversion to ethanol, Tsukamoto et al. developed a new model in which a continuous intragastric administration of an alcohol diet was possible for long periods.[91-95] In this model, the intake of ethanol was progressively increased from 32 to 47% of total calories. This model demonstrated that even in rats, severe liver pathology progressing beyond the fatty liver stage was produced by chronic alcohol ingestion.[94,95] Rats infused with the alcohol diet containing high levels of fat had increased (3–4 +) fatty change, necrosis, and inflammation in the liver.[95] Rats developed centrilobular scarring similar to that seen in baboons and man chronically ingesting ethanol.[95] As in the case of the Lieber-DeCarli model, rats given a continuous intragastric administration of ethanol also obtain a low level of carbohydrate. The ingest only 3% of total calories as carbohydrate when the content of fat and alcohol is 25 and 47%, respectively.[94] Even when they consumed the diet containing 35% of calories from fat and 32% from ethanol, carbohydrate provided only 8% of the total calories. Thus, advanced liver pathology occurred in this model only when rats consumed high levels of alcohol and fat and a low level of carbohydrate. Whether a dietary supplementation with carbohydrate can abate advanced liver injury in this model remains to be investigated.

It has been suggested that while rats consume high levels of fat and ethanol, their dietary intake of lipotropes (choline, methionine, folate, and vitamin B_{12}) is less than that of those rats *ad libitum*-fed a nutritionally adequate diet.[96] The daily consumption of other essential nutrients such as magnesium, manganese, and selenium is also reduced. Nutritional inadequacy with respect to the ingestion of lipotropes is also evident from the results of the control animals which developed steatosis even when ethanol was not ingested.[95]

In the intragastric model, an advanced degree of liver pathology occurred when alcohol consumption was accompanied by the ingestion of a diet containing 25% of total calories arising from corn oil comprised of mostly unsaturated fatty acids (81% of total) and predominantly linoleate (56.6% of total).[67] Only minimal to moderate alcoholic liver disease was observed when the diet fed contained lard which consists most of saturated fatty acids (82% of total) and a small amount of linoleate (2.5% of total).[67] When fed a diet containing tallow, which contains mostly saturated fatty acids (79% of total) but a much smaller level of linoleate (0.7% of total), none of the features of alcoholic liver disease developed.[67] Therefore, it was suggested that the degree of histopathological abnormality of alcoholic liver disease correlated with the content of linoleic acid in the diet fat.

The intragastric infusion technique has been employed to investigate the role of nutritional factors on the effects of chronic ethanol consumption. Rats fed the Lieber-DeCarli 36% ethanol diet *ad libitum* and small amounts of either maltose dextrins or casein were infused intragastrically.[97] A high level of ethanol in the blood observed due to the ingestion of the Lieber-DeCarli 36% ethanol diet was prevented by the availability of additional macronutrients in the animal. Thus, BAL are regulated by the nutritional status of the animal even though they ingest doses of ethanol which are sufficient to cause alcoholemia.[97]

NUTRITIONALLY ADEQUATE DIETS FOR CHRONIC ETHANOL ADMINISTRATION

From our knowledge of the conditions associated with the Lieber-DeCarli 36% ethanol diet model, questions arose such as: (1) can the nutritional status of the alcoholic animals be improved by reducing the anorexic effect of the ethanol diet and still enable them to ingest sufficient amounts of alcohol and fat necessary for the development of fatty liver; (2) will increased caloric or nutrient intake abolish the effects observed from the ingestion of a 36% ethanol diet, and (3) will the improved dietary status be adequate during growth, pregnancy, or lactation despite the chronic intake of ethanol? To seek answers to these questions, investigations were initiated using a 26% ethanol diet which was made isocaloric to the Lieber-DeCarli 36% ethanol diet by reducing the level of ethanol to 26% of total calories and increasing the content of maltose-dextrins correspondingly.[98] The daily ingestion of this diet increased about 50% compared to the 36% ethanol diet and enabled the rats to consume more energy, carbohydrate, fat, protein, and other nutrients needed for normal growth rate.[58,98] Growing rats fed the 26% ethanol diet gained 6.9 g/d, proving that they ingested adequate nutrients.[98] Anorexia was reduced sufficiently such that the dose of ethanol ingested per kilogram of body weight was not significantly different from that ingested by rats fed the 36% ethanol diet.[98] Rats fed the 26% ethanol diet ingested 13.6 g of ethanol per kilogram of body weight, a value within the 12- to 18-g ethanol per kilogram range ingested by young rats fed the Lieber-DeCarli 36% ethanol diet.[60]

In addition to supporting normal breeding, the 26% ethanol diet reduced the anorexigenic effect of the alcohol diet sufficiently so that the currently recommended amounts of nutrients were ingested by pregnant female rats simultaneously with an alcohol dose which was not significantly different from that ingested with the 36% ethanol diet.[99] Comparing the pregnant female rats fed the 26% ethanol diet and those fed the Lieber-

DeCarli liquid control diet *ad libitum,* there was no significant difference in weight gain by the pregnant female, litter weight, number of pups born, or number of pups born alive.[99] Neither the 26% nor the 36% alcohol diets provided adequate nutrients for lactation because the anorexigenic effect of the ethanol diet is too high to permit sufficient diet intake.[54,99] Lactating female rats with eight or eleven pups ingested recommended amounts of all nutrients when the alcohol content of the liquid diet was reduced to 20 or 17% of total calories respectively by isocaloric substitution of maltose-dextrins for ethanol.[100] The weight of weaning pups averaged 58.7 g at 21 d of age, markedly exceeding that of 44 to 46 g suggested as normal by the National Research Council[49] and not significantly different from that of pups raised by mothers fed the Lieber-DeCarli liquid control diet *ad libitum.* Lactating mothers fed the 26, 20, or 17% ethanol diets ingested significantly more ethanol per kilogram of body weight than was ingested by rats fed the 36% ethanol diet.[100]

It has been repeatedly shown in studies of diets with marginal dietary deficiencies that it often takes three or four generations before the deficiencies can be observed. Hence, it is possible that although the nutrients ingested with the 26 and 17% alcohol diets overcame the effects of a toxic alcohol dose in acute experiments, they were only marginally adequate and would not be effective in chronic studies. However, rats fed the 26 and 17% diets for four generations exhibited no gross effects of the toxic ethanol dose.[101] Hence, the recommended amounts of nutrients were able to significantly reduce all of the deleterious effects of the toxic ethanol dose to the various tissues, so that the alcohol dose had no practical effect on the rats. Dietary ethanol did not act as a toxic drug but served as a source of energy during growth, pregnancy, and lactation.

Regardless of whether rats are fed a 36 or 26% ethanol diet *ad libitum,* they ingest a similar amount of ethanol daily and the same type and proportion of fat in the diet. However, only those fed the 36% and not the 26% ethanol diet develop fatty liver.[58] Lack of fatty liver in rats fed the 26% ethanol diet may be related to an increased daily ingestion of energy and carbohydrate compared to those fed the 36% ethanol diet. Dietary carbohydrate has a role in the production of alcoholic fatty liver.[15,102] When rats maintained for 4 weeks on a Lieber-DeCarli 36% ethanol diet to develop fatty liver were then fed the 26% ethanol diet for 4 weeks, fatty liver regressed despite continued chronic alcohol ingestion.[103] Hence, when animals ingest adequate nutrients, even existing fatty liver regresses despite continued alcohol consumption. These studies show that the inadequate intake of macronutrients has a major role in the production of fatty liver.[103]

Some of the effects of chronic alcohol consumption such as fatty liver, high BAL, and those effects observed during pregnancy[104] may be due to the synergistic action of alcohol ingestion and malnutrition. On the other hand, other effects may not be directly related to ethanol per se, but to the nutritional factors associated with the dietary regimen. For example, the reduced level of pancreatic amylase in rats fed the 36% ethanol diet is due to the depressed ingestion of carbohydrate.[105,106] The low level of glycogen and the enhanced activity of microsomal glucose 6-phosphatase found in rats fed the 36% ethanol diet are due to a decreased ingestion of energy and carbohydrate.[107] Changes in the hepatic metabolism of protein associated with fatty liver production as reflected by an enhanced level of circulating branched-chain amino acids are also due to a depressed ingestion of energy and carbohydrate.[108] Several changes in the metabolism of methionine occur in alcoholic fatty liver.[109] These are not due to alcohol ingestion per se but to the inadequate nutritional condition associated with the ingestion of a 36% ethanol diet.[110] These conclusions regarding the role of nutritional factors on the production or prevention of alcoholic fatty liver and other effects of chronic ethanol ingestion resulted from investigations using the nutritionally adequate 26% ethanol diet.

Another approach to feeding a nutritionally adequate diet during chronic alcohol consumption utilizes the intragastric infusion technique (Gastrostomy model). Rats were allowed to ingest a nutritionally adequate liquid diet *ad libitum* and increasing amounts of alcohol were infused through the gastrostomy tube continuously over a period of 8 to 10 weeks.[111] Unlike the Lieber-DeCarli ethanol diet and intragastric infusion models, the content of carbohydrate was not reduced to compensate for alcohol calories in the gastrostomy model. Infusion of as little as 1.3 g of ethanol per rat (about 4 g/kg of body weight) caused a significant reduction in food intake. Higher doses of ethanol up to 4.8 g (9.2 g/kg of body weight) produced a progressive decrease in food intake.[111] However, the growth rate of rats was normal and comparable to those fed chow diet *ad libitum*. These rats did not exhibit any BAL. It would appear that under these conditions, ethanol served as a source of energy complementing the nonalcohol calories despite reduced food intake. With doses greater than 4.8 g per rat (>9.2 g/kg of body weight) a profound decrease in food intake, high BAL, and depressed growth rate were observed. Histopathologic examination of the postmortem liver samples of rats that died in a comatose state revealed no fatty liver or other signs of liver damage despite the ingestion of a high level of fat (35% of calories) and alcohol (10.8 g/kg of body weight) over a period of 8 to 10 weeks. This is in contrast to rats which develop fatty liver due to the ingestion of the Lieber-DeCarli ethanol diet for 4 weeks. The absence of fatty liver in the gastrostomy model may be due to the macronutrient sufficiency since rats ingested a nutritionally adequate control diet. These results are in conformity with those of Yonekura et al.[102] who showed that carbohydrate caloric deficiency in the 36% ethanol diet directly correlated with the severity of fatty liver production.

ALCOHOLIC LIVER DAMAGE AND BLOOD ALCOHOL LEVELS

It has been generally accepted that alcoholic liver disease only occurs when the amount of ethanol ingested markedly exceeds metabolic capacity to dispose of the ethanol, resulting in elevated blood levels for prolonged periods of time.[112] For example, when rats develop fatty liver due to the consumption of the Lieber-DeCarli ethanol diet for 4 weeks, they exhibit high BAL.[44] On the other hand, when fatty liver is avoided despite the ingestion of a dose of ethanol sufficient to cause fatty liver and BAL, only insignificant BAL are observed.[58,61] Furthermore, rats fed the 36% ethanol diet containing less than 35% of the calories from fat[36,66] or with 35% of fat containing medium-chain fatty acids[37] do not develop fatty liver despite high BAL. In addition, depending on the nutritional condition, monkeys,[83,84] baboons,[85,90] and rats[67] do not develop severe liver pathology in spite of high BAL. Not only liver damage but also some extrahepatic effects of alcohol ingestion are not related to high BAL. For example, decreased levels of pancreatic amylase are observed in rats having high BAL.[113] However, it has been shown that in chronic alcoholic rats, despite high BAL, pancreatic amylase levels are influenced by the amount of carbohydrate ingested.[105,114,115]

As in the case of fatty liver production, inadequate intake of energy is involved in causing high BAL. When rats fed the 36% ethanol diet *ad libitum* are given small amounts of glucose intraperitoneally daily[114] or intragastrically infused with either maltose dextrins or casein,[97] only low or insignificant BAL result. Rats fed various liquid diets *ad libitum* containing 36, 30, or 26% of ethanol calories consume similar amounts of alcohol calories (13 to 15 g/kg/d).[116] However, in those receiving at least threefold greater amounts of total energy compared to energy derived from ethanol, BAL were significantly reduced in contrast to alcoholic rats ingesting less than threefold amounts of total energy.[97,116] Recently, it was shown that when rats fed the 36% ethanol diet for 4 weeks exhibiting high BAL were then fed the 26% ethanol diet for one day, only insignificant BAL were observed.[117] An increase in macronutrient intake not only reverses high BAL rapidly but also maintains insignificant BAL in rats consuming doses of ethanol sufficient to cause alcoholemia.[117] Thus, not only the development of alcoholic liver disease but also the capacity of liver to metabolize ethanol is controlled by the nutritional status of the animal.

CONCLUSIONS

A critical examination of the results from the various animal models used to study alcoholic liver damage shows that the interaction of ethanol and nutritional factors plays an important role in producing various effects which were previously ascribed to ethanol per se. A dose of ethanol for a specific duration need not always result in high BAL, fatty liver, or advanced liver pathology, fetal alcohol syndrome, low hepatic glycogen content, or other effects unless some nutritional abnormalities are also present in the animal. Some effects appear to be due to the synergism of alcohol and nutrition while others are due to the nutritional anomalies which accompany ethanol ingestion.

It has been concluded from the results of the Lieber-DeCarli model that alcoholics cannot fully prevent the development or aggravation of liver injury by maintaining an adequate diet unless they also control the degree of alcohol intake.[89] However, chronic consumption of ethanol adequate to produce high BAL and liver pathology does not result in liver damage in the Lieber-DeCarli, in the continuous intragastric infusion, or in the baboon models when the contribution of fat in the diet is low and carbohydrate is relatively high, when the type of fat is comprised of saturated fatty acids, or when the daily ingestion of energy is increased to levels generally seen in the *ad libitum*-fed controls. The results from several animal models show that while BAL and liver injury coexist in alcoholism, BAL need not be the sole causative factor for alcoholic liver damage.

Epidemiologic examination of alcoholic liver pathology has not placed due weight on the contributory role of various nutritional factors. The wide variability or discrepancy in the observations within the human population can be related not only to the dose and duration of ethanol intake but also to the differences in the nutritional conditions of the individuals. Although malnutrition is common in alcoholics, the type of nutrients ingested and the degree of nutritional inadequacy can vary from one individual to another. An understanding of the important role of nutrition can be beneficial in developing appropriate nutritional therapies for the abatement, prevention, or potential reversal of some of the effects of chronic ethanol ingestion.

ACKNOWLEDGMENTS

Investigations carried out in our laboratories and referred to in this chapter were supported by the U.S. Department of Veterans Affairs. The authors are indebted to Mr. Vivek A. Rao for his assistance in the preparation of this chapter.

REFERENCES

1. Goldstein, D. B. and Pal, N., Alcohol dependence produced in mice by inhalation of ethanol: grading the withdrawal reaction, *Science,* 172, 288, 1971.
2. Tsukamoto, H., French, S. W., Benson, N., Delgado, G., Rao, G. A., Larkin, E. C., and Largman, C., Severe and progressive steatosis and focal necrosis in rat liver induced by continuous intragastric infusion of ethanol and low fat diet, *Hepatology,* 5, 224, 1985.
3. Erickson, C. K., Koch, K. I., and McGinity, J. W., Subcutaneous silastic implants: maintenance of high blood ethanol levels in rats drinking a liquid diet, *Pharmacol. Biochem. Behav.,* 13, 781, 1980.
4. Majchrowicz, E., Induction of physical dependence upon ethanol and the associated behavioral changes in rat, *Psychopharmacologia,* 43, 245, 1975.
5. Richter, C. P., A study of the effect of moderate doses of alcohol on the growth and behavior of the rat, *J. Exp. Zool.,* 44, 397, 1926.
6. Freund, G., Alcohol withdrawal syndrome in mice, *Arch. Neurol. Chicago,* 21, 315, 1969.
7. Lieber, C. S., Jones, D. P., Mendelson, J., and DeCarli, L. M., Fatty liver, hyperlipemia and hyperuricemia produced by prolonged alcohol consumption despite adequate dietary intake, *Trans. Assoc. Amer. Physicians,* 76, 289, 1963.
8. Miller, S. S., Goldman, M. E., Erickson, C. K., and Shorey, R. L., Induction of physical dependence on and tolerance to ethanol in rats fed a new nutritionally complete and balanced liquid diet, *Psychopharmacology,* 68, 55, 1980.
9. Meisch, R. A. and Thompson, T., Rapid establishment of ethanol as a reinforcer for rats, *Psychopharmacologia,* 37, 311, 1974.

10. Lumeng, L., Hawkins, T. D., and Li, T.-K., New strains of rats with alcohol preference and non-preference, in *Alcohol and Aldehyde Metabolizing Systems*, Vol. 3, Thurman, R. G., Williamson, J. R., Drott, H., and Chance, B., Eds., Academic Press, New York, 1977, 537.

11. Derr, R. F., Porta, E. A., Larkin, E. C., and Rao, G. A., Is alcohol per se hepatotoxic?, *J. Hepatol.*, 10, 381, 1990.

12. Popper, H. and Lieber, C. S., Histogenesis of alcoholic fibrosis and cirrhosis in the baboon, *Am. J. Pathol.*, 98, 695, 1980.

13. Maddrey, W. C., Alcoholic hepatitis: clinicopathologic features and therapy, *Semin. Liver Dis.*, 8, 91, 1988.

14. Grant, B. F., Dufour, M. C., and Harford, T. C., Epidemiology of alcoholic liver disease, *Semin. Liver Dis.*, 8, 12, 1988.

15. Rao, G. A. and Larkin, E. C., Alcoholic fatty liver: a nutritional problem of carbohydrate deprivation and concomitant ethanol ingestion, *Nutr. Res.*, 4, 903, 1984.

16. Ishak, K. G., Zimmerman, H. J., and Ray, M. B., Alcoholic liver disease: pathologic, pathogenetic and clinical aspects, *Alcoholism Clin. Exp. Res.*, 15, 45, 1991.

17. Zimmerman, H. J., The evolution of alcoholic cirrhosis. Clinical, biochemical and histologic correlations, *Med. Clin. North Am.*, 39, 241, 1955.

18. Edmondson, H. A., Peters, R. L., Reynolds, T. B., and Kuzuma, C. T., Sclerosing hyaline necrosis of the liver in the chronic alcoholic, *Ann. Intern. Med.*, 59, 646, 1963.

19. Porta, E. A., Nutrition and diseases of the liver and gallbladder, *Prog. Food. Nutr. Sci.*, 1, 289, 1975.

20. Moon, V. H., Experimental cirrhosis in relation to human cirrhosis, *Arch. Path.*, 18, 381, 1934.

21. Connor, C. L. and Chaikoff, I. L., Production of cirrhosis in fatty livers with alcohol, *Proc. Soc. Exp. Biol. Med.*, 39, 356, 1938.

22. Chaikoff, I. L. and Connor, C. L., Production of cirrhosis of the liver of normal dog by high fat diets, *Proc. Soc. Exp. Biol. Med.*, 43, 638, 1940.

23. Daft, F. S., Sebrell, W. H., and Lillie, R. D., Production and apparent prevention of dietary liver cirrhosis in rats, *Proc. Soc. Exp. Biol. Med.*, 48, 228, 1941.

24. Lowry, J. V., Daft, F. S., Sebrell, W. H., Ashburn, L. L., and Lillie, R. D., Treatment of dietary liver cirrhosis in rats with choline and casein, *Public Health Rep.*, 56, 2216, 1941.

25. Ashworth, C. T., Production of fatty infiltration of liver in rats by alcohol in spite of adequate diet, *Proc. Soc. Exp. Biol. Med.*, 66, 382, 1947.

26. Best, C. H., Hartroft, W. S., Lucas, C. C., and Ridout, J. H., Liver damage produced by feeding alcohol or sugar and its prevention by choline, *Br. J. Med.*, 2, 1001, 1949.

27. Forbes, J. C. and Duncan, G. M., Effect of alcohol on liver lipids and on liver and heart glycogen, *Q. J. Stud. Alcohol*, 11, 373, 1950.

28. Klatskin, G., Krehl, W. A., and Corn, H., Effect of alcohol on choline requirement. I. Changes in rat liver following prolonged ingestion of alcohol, *J. Exp. Med.*, 100, 605, 1954.

29. Scheig, R., Alexander, N. M., and Klatskin, G., Effects of prolonged ingestion of glucose or ethanol on tissue lipid composition and lipid biosynthesis in rat, *J. Lipid Res.*, 7, 188, 1966.

30. Thorpe, M. E. C. and Shorey, C. D., Long term alcohol administration. Its effects on the ultrastructure and lipid content of the rat liver cell, *Am. J. Pathol.*, 48, 557, 1966.

31. Porta, E. A., Hartroft, W. S., and De La Iglesia, F. A., Hepatic changes associated with chronic alcoholism in rats, *Lab. Invest.*, 14, 1437, 1965.

32. Porta, E. A., Hartroft, W. S., Gomez-Dumm, C. L. A., De La Iglesia, F. A., and Turner, D., Role of dietary constituents in experimental chronic alcoholism, *Proc. 7th Int. Congr. Nutr.*, 5, 223, 1966.

33. Porta, E. A., Hartroft, W. S., Gomez-Dumm, C. L. A., and Koch, O. R., Dietary factors in the progression and regression of hepatic alterations associated with experimental chronic alcoholism, *Fed. Proc.*, 26, 1449, 1967.

34. Gomez-Dumm, C. L. A. and Porta, E. A., Protein and hepatic injury associated with experimental chronic alcoholism, *Fed. Proc.*, 25, 304, 1966.

35. Porta, E. A., Koch, O. R., Gomez-Dumm, C. L. A., and Hartroft, W. S., Effects of dietary protein on the liver of rats in experimental chronic alcoholism, *J. Nutr.*, 94, 437, 1968.

36. Lieber, C. S. and De Carli, L. M., Quantitative relationship between the amount of dietary fat and the severity of the alcoholic fatty liver, *Am. J. Clin. Nutr.*, 23, 474, 1970.

37. Lieber, C. S., Lefevre, A., Spritz, N., Feinman, L., and DeCarli, L. M., Difference in hepatic metabolism of long and medium chain fatty acids: the role of fatty acid chain length in the production of the alcoholic fatty liver, *J. Clin. Invest.*, 46, 1451, 1967.

38. Takada, A., Porta, E. A., and Hartroft, W. S., Regression of dietary cirrhosis in rats fed alcohol and a 'superdiet', evidence for the nonhepatotoxic nature of ethanol, *Am. J. Clin. Nutr.*, 20, 213, 1967.

39. Frank, O. and Baker, H., Vitamin profile in rats fed stock or liquid ethanol diets, *Am. J. Clin. Nutr.*, 33, 221, 1980.

40. Porta, E. A. and Gomez-Dumm, C. L. A., A new experimental approach in the study of chronic alcoholism. I. Effects of high alcohol intake in rats fed a commercial laboratory diet, *Lab. Invest.*, 18, 352, 1968.

41. Gomez-Dumm, C. L. A., Porta, E. A., Hartroft, W. S., and Koch, O. R., A new experimental approach in the study of chronic alcoholism. II. Effects of high alcohol intake in rats fed diets of various adequacies, *Lab. Invest.*, 18, 365, 1968.

42. Koch, O. R., Porta, E. A., and Hartroft, W. S., A new experimental approach in the study of chronic alcoholism. III. Role of alcohol versus sucrose or fat-derived calories in hepatic damage, *Lab. Invest.*, 18, 379, 1968.

43. Porta, E. A., Koch, O. R., and Hartroft, W. S., Recovery from chronic hepatic lesions in rats fed alcohol and a solid super diet, *Am. J. Clin. Nutr.*, 25, 881, 1972.

44. Lieber, C. S. and DeCarli, L. M., The feeding of alcohol in liquid diets: two decades of applications and 1982 update, *Alcoholism Clin. Exp. Res.*, 6, 523, 1982.

45. Lindros, K. O., Pikkarainen, P., Pekkanen, L., Sipponen, P., Vaananen, H., and Salaspuro, M., An improved animal model for production of alcoholic liver damage using a nutritionally adequate liquid diet containing ethanol and 4-methyl-pyrazole, in *Animal Models in Alcohol Research,* Eriksson, K., Sinclair, J. D., and Kiianmaa, K., Eds., Academic Press, New York, 1980, 445.

46. Lindros, K. O., Stowell, L., Vaananen, H., Sipponen, P., Lamminsivu, U., Pikkarainen, P., and Salaspuro, M., Uninterrupted prolonged ethanol oxidation as a main pathogenetic factor of alcoholic liver damage: evidence from a new liquid diet animal model, *Liver,* 3, 79, 1983.

47. Lieber, C. S., Jones, D. P., and DeCarli, L. M., Effects of prolonged ethanol intake: production of fatty liver despite adequate diets, *J. Clin. Invest.,* 44, 1009, 1965.

48. DeCarli, L. M. and Lieber, C. S., Fatty liver in the rat after prolonged intake of ethanol with a nutritionally adequate new liquid diet, *J. Nutr.,* 91, 331, 1967.

49. National Research Council, Nutritional requirements of the laboratory rat, in *Nutrient Requirements of Laboratory Animals,* No. 10, 3rd ed., National Academy of Sciences, Washington, D.C., 1978, 7.

50. Rao, G. A., Tsukamoto, H., Larkin, E. C., and Derr, R. F., Nutritional inadequacy of diets for young growing rats used in models of chronic alcohol ingestion, *Biochem. Arch.,* 1, 97, 1985.

51. Lieber, C. S. and DeCarli, L. M., The feeding of ethanol in liquid diets, *Alcoholism Clin. Exp. Res.,* 10, 550, 1986.

52. Lieber, C. S. and DeCarli, L. M., Effects of mineral and vitamin supplementation on the alcohol-induced fatty liver and microsomal induction, *Alcoholism Clin. Exp. Res.,* 13, 142, 1989.

53. Rao, G. A., Larkin, E. C., and Derr, R. F., Nutritional adequacy versus ethanol toxicity in chronic alcoholic rats: is the 36% ethanol liquid diet model nutritionally adequate?, *Biochem. Arch.,* 6, 1, 1990.

54. Derr, R. F., Draves, K., and Rao, G. A., Inadequate intake by female rats during gestation and lactation of essential nutrients from liquid diets used for alcohol studies: implication for the fetal alcohol syndrome, *Biochem. Acta,* 3, 137, 1987.

55. Yeh, L. C. and Cerklewski, F. L., Formulation of a liquid diet for ethanol studies involving gestation and lactation in the rat, *J. Nutr.,* 114, 634, 1984.

56. Sanchis, R., Sancho-Tello, M., and Guerri, C., The role of liquid diet formulation in the postnatal ethanol exposure of rats via mother's milk, *J. Nutr.,* 119, 82, 1989.

57. Singh, S. P. and Snyder, A. K., Ethanol ingestion during pregnancy: effects on pregnant rats and their offspring, *J. Nutr.,* 112, 98, 1982.

58. Rao, G. A., Riley, D. E., and Larkin, E. C., Dietary carbohydrate stimulates alcohol diet ingestion, promotes growth and prevents fatty liver in rats, *Nutr. Res.,* 7, 81, 1987.

59. Rao, G. A. and Larkin, E. C., Inadequate intake by growing rats of essential nutrients from liquid diets used for chronic alcohol consumption, *Nutr. Res.,* 5, 789, 1985.

60. Derr, R. F., The quantities of nutrients recommended by the NRC abate the effects of a toxic alcohol dose administered to rats, *J. Nutr.*, 119, 1228, 1989.

61. Rao, G. A., Sankaran, H., Nishimura, C. Y., and Larkin, E. C., High blood alcohol levels: association with malnutrition, *Biochem. Arch.*, 3, 363, 1987.

62. Rao, G. A., Larkin, E. C., and Derr, R. F., Inadequate nutrition in the model for alcoholic liver damage using an ethanol + 4-methylpyrazole liquid diet, *Biochem. Arch.*, 3, 325, 1987.

63. Lindros, K. O., Sipponen, P., Pikkarainen, P., Turunen, U., and Salaspuro, M., Alcoholic liver damage is provoked by 4-methylpyrazole which prolongs the influence of ethanol but reduces acetaldehyde levels, *Alcoholism Clin. Exp. Res.*, 3, 78, 1979.

64. Shorey, R. L., Pyle, B., McAllister, M., Miller, S. S., Erickson, C. K., and Thompson, G. A., Jr., Effects of ethanol on fatty acid composition of muscle phospholipids of rats fed nutritionally complete liquid diets, *Biochem. Pharmacol.*, 31, 2447, 1982.

65. Goldman, M. E., Miller, S. S., Shorey, R. L., and Erickson, C. K., Ethanol dependence produced in rats by nutritionally complete diets, *Pharmacol. Biochem. Behav.*, 12, 503, 1980.

66. Shoemaker, J. D. and Visek, W. J., Growth, liver lipid and blood amino acids in rats fed ethanol with an adequate diet, *Drug Alcohol Depend.*, 22, 49, 1988.

67. Nanji, A. A., Mendenhall, C. L., and French, S. W., Beef fat prevents alcoholic liver disease in the rat, *Alcoholism, Clin. Exp. Res.*, 13, 15, 1989.

68. Goheen, S. C., Larkin, E. C., Manix, M., and Rao, G. A., Dietary arachidonic acid reduces fatty liver, increases diet consumption and weight gain in ethanol-fed rat, *Lipids*, 15, 328, 1980.

69. Rao, G. A., Larkin, E. C., Deveney, C. W., and Sankaran, H., Is linoleate an essential factor to cause alcoholic liver disease?, *Alcoholism Clin. Exp. Res.*, 14, 331, 1990.

70. Stanko, R. T., Mendelow, H., Shinozuka, H., and Adibi, S. A., Prevention of alcohol-induced fatty liver by natural metabolites and riboflavin, *J. Lab. Clin. Med.*, 92, 228, 1978.

71. Goheen, S. C., Pearson, E. E., Larkin, E. C., and Rao, G. A., The prevention of alcoholic fatty liver using dietary supplements: dihydroxyacetone, pyruvate and riboflavin compared to arachidonic acid in pair-fed rats, *Lipids*, 16, 43, 1981.

72. Rao, G. A., Riley, D. E., and Larkin, E. C., Fatty liver caused by chronic alcohol ingestion is prevented by dietary supplementation with pyruvate or glycerol, *Lipids*, 19, 583, 1984.

73. Rao, G. A., Riley, D. E., and Larkin, E. C., Role of dietary carbohydrate in the prevention of alcohol induced fatty liver, *Biochem. Arch.*, 2, 261, 1986.

74. Rao, G. A., Larkin, E. C., and Derr, R. F., Biologic effects of chronic ethanol consumption related to a deficient intake of carbohydrates, *Alcohol Alcoholism*, 21, 369, 1986.

75. Rao, G. A. and Larkin, E. C., Role of nutrition in causing the effects attributed to chronic alcohol consumption, *Med. Sci. Res.*, 16, 53, 1988.

76. Rubin, E. and Lieber, C. S., Alcohol-induced hepatic injury in nonalcoholic volunteers, *N. Engl. J. Med.*, 278, 869, 1968.

77. Rao, G. A., Larkin, E. C., and Porta, E. A., Is alcohol itself hepatotoxic independent of nutritional factors in nonalcoholic humans?, *Biochem. Arch.*, 5, 1, 1989.

78. Leo, M. A. and Lieber, C. S., Hepatic fibrosis after long-term administration of ethanol and moderate vitamin A supplementation in the rat, *Hepatology*, 3, 1, 1983.

79. Seifert, W. F., Bosma, A., Hendriks, H. F. J., De Ruiter, G. C. F., Van Leeuwen, R. E. W., Knook, D. L., and Brouwer, A., Dual role of vitamin A in experimentally induced liver fibrosis, in *Cells of the Hepatic Sinusoid*, Vol. 2, Wisse, E., Knook, D. L., and Decker, K., Eds., Kupffer Cell Foundation, Rijswijk, The Netherlands, 1989, 43.

80. Bosma, A., Seifert, W. F., Wilson, J. H. P., Roholl, P. J. M., Brouwer, A., and Knook, D. L., Chronic administration of ethanol with high vitamin A supplementation in a liquid diet to rats does not cause liver fibrosis: 1. Morphological observations, *J. Hepatol.*, 13, 240, 1991.

81. Seifert, W. F., Bosma, A., Hendriks, H. F. J., Blaner, W. S., Van Leeuwen, R. E. W., Van Thiel-de Ruiter, G. C. F., Wilson, J. H. P., Knook, D. L., and Brouwer, A., Chronic administration of ethanol with high vitamin A supplementation in a liquid diet to rats does not cause liver fibrosis: 2. Biochemical observations, *J. Hepatol.*, 13, 249, 1991.

82. Lieber, C. S. and DeCarli, L. M., An experimental model of alcohol feeding and liver injury in the baboon, *J. Med. Primatol.*, 3, 153, 1974.

83. Mezey, E., Potter, J. J., French, S. W., Tamura, T., and Halsted, C. H., Effect of chronic ethanol feeding on hepatic collagen in the monkey, *Hepatology*, 3, 41, 1983.

84. Rogers, A. E., Fox, J. G., and Murphy, J. C., Ethanol and diet interactions in male rhesus monkeys, *Drug Nutr. Interact.*, 1, 3, 1981.

85. Ainley, C. C., Senapati, A., Brown, I. M. H., Iles, C. A., Slavin, B. M., Mitchell, W. D., Davies, D. R., Keeling, P. W. N., and Thompson, R. P. H., Is alcohol hepatotoxic in the baboon?, *J. Hepatol.*, 7, 85, 1988.

86. French, S. W., Alcoholic hepatotoxicity, *J. Hepatol.*, 9, 134, 1989.

87. *Purina Diet Manual. Monkey Chow 5038*, Purina Mills, Inc., Richmond, IN.

88. Lieber, C. S., Leo, M. A., Mak, K. M., DeCarli, L. M., and Sato, S., Choline fails to prevent liver fibrosis in ethanol-fed baboons but causes toxicity, *Hepatology*, 5, 561, 1985.

89. Lieber, C. S., DeCarli, L. M., and Rubin, E., Sequential production of fatty liver, hepatitis and cirrhosis in sub-human primates fed ethanol with adequate diets, *Proc. Natl. Acad. Sci. U.S.A.*, 72, 437, 1975.

90. Lieber, C. S., DeCarli, L. M., Mak, K. M., Kim, C. I., and Leo, M. A., Attenuation of alcohol-induced hepatic fibrosis by polyunsaturated lecithin, *Hepatology*, 12, 1390, 1990.

91. Tsukamoto, H., Reidelberger, R. D., French, S. W., and Largman, C., Long term cannulation model for blood sampling and intragastric infusion in the rat, *Am. J. Physiol.*, 247, R 595, 1984.

92. Tsukamoto, H., Lew, G., Larkin, E. C., Largman, C., and Rao, G. A., Hepatic origin of triglycerides in fatty livers produced by the continuous intragastric infusion of an ethanol diet, *Lipids,* 19, 419, 1984.

93. Tsukamoto, H., French, S. W., and Largman, C., Correlation of cyclical blood alcohol levels with progression of alcoholic liver injury, *Biochem. Arch.,* 1, 215, 1985.

94. Tsukamoto, H., Towner, S. J., Ciofalo, L. M., and French, S. W., Ethanol-induced liver fibrosis in rats fed high fat diet, *Hepatology,* 6, 814, 1986.

95. French, S. W., Miyamoto, K., and Tsukamoto, H., Ethanol-induced hepatic fibrosis in the rat: role of the amount of dietary fat, *Alcoholism Clin. Exp. Res.,* 10, 13s, 1986.

96. Rao, G. A., Larkin, E. C., and Derr, R. F., Continuous intragastric infusion model for chronic alcohol administration: a possible deficient intake of lipotropes, *Biochem. Arch.,* 3, 197, 1987.

97. Sankaran, H., Baba, G. C., Deveney, C. W., and Rao, G. A., Enteral macronutrients abolish high blood alcohol levels in chronic alcoholic rats, *Nutr. Res.,* 11, 217, 1991.

98. Rao, G. A., Riley, D. E., and Larkin, E. C., Lieber-DeCarli alcohol diet modification to enhance growth of young rats, *Nutr. Res.,* 6, 101, 1986.

99. Derr, R. F., Draves, K., and Rao, G. A., Modification of liquid alcohol diets used for alcohol studies to provide adequate nutrition during gestation, *Biochem. Arch.,* 3, 223, 1987.

100. Derr, R. F., Draves, K., and Rao, G. A., Liquid alcohol diets which provide recommended quantities of nutrients for lactation of the rat, *Nutr. Rep. Int.,* 38, 361, 1988.

101. Derr, R. F. and Draves, K., Adequate nutrition abates the effects of a toxic alcohol dose fed to rats for four generations, *Biochem. Arch.,* 4, 341, 1988.

102. Yonekura, I., Nakano, M., Nakajima, T., and Sato, A., Dietary carbohydrate intake as a modifying factor for the development of alcoholic fatty liver, *Biochem. Arch.,* 5, 41, 1989.

103. Larkin, E. C., Sankaran, H., Baba, G. C., Deveney, C. W., and Rao, G. A., Regression of fatty liver despite chronic ethanol consumption, *Alcoholism Clin. Exp. Res.,* 14, 308, 1990.

104. Rao, G. A., Larkin, E. C., and Derr, R. F., Chronic alcohol consumption during pregnancy: alleviation of untoward effects by adequate nutrition, *Nutr. Res.,* 8, 421, 1988.

105. Sankaran, H., Nishimura, C. Y., Lin, J. C., Desai, A., Deveney, C. W., Larkin, E. C., and Rao, G. A., Reversal by glucose of pancreatic amylase insufficiency in chronic alcoholic rats, *Pancreas,* 4, 107, 1989.

106. Sankaran, H., Nishimura, C. Y., Lin, J. C., Larkin, E. C., and Rao, G. A., Regulation of pancreatic amylase by dietary carbohydrate in chronic alcoholic rats, *Pancreas,* 4, 733, 1989.

107. Nguyen, T., Chi, C. W., Larkin, E. C., and Rao, G. A., Lower liver glycogen content in alcoholic rats due to depressed carbohydrate ingestion, *Biochem. Arch.,* 6, 217, 1990.

108. Rao, G. A. and Larkin, E. C., Branched chain amino acid and alpha-amino-N-Butyric acid levels in chronic alcoholic rats: role of nutrition, *Biochem. Arch.,* 7, 77, 1991.

109. Barak, A. J., Beckenhauer, H. C., Tuma, D. J., and Badakhsh, S., Effects of prolonged ethanol feeding on methionine metabolism in rat liver, *Biochem. Cell. Biol.*, 65, 230, 1987.

110. Rao, G. A., Larkin, E. C., Beckenhauer, H. C., and Barak, A. J., Chronic alcohol ingestion and hepatic methionine metabolism in rats: role of adequate nutrition, *Biochem. Arch.*, 3, 437, 1987.

111. Baba, G. C., Deveney, C. W., and Sankaran, H., Synergism between alcohol and non-alcohol caloric intake in chronic alcoholic rats: effects of intragastric alcohol infusion on diet intake and blood alcohol levels, *Eur. J. Gastroenterol. Hepatol.*, 3, 841, 1991.

112. Mezey, E., Animal models for alcoholic liver disease, *Hepatology*, 9, 904, 1989.

113. Singh, M., La Sure, M. M., and Bockman, D. E., Pancreatic acinar cell function and morphology in rats chronically fed an ethanol diet, *Gastroenterology*, 82, 425, 1982.

114. Rao, G. A., Nishimura, C. Y., Lin, J. C., Larkin, E. C., and Sankaran, H., Role of glucose in the regulation of blood alcohol-related extrahepatic effects in rats, *Med. Sci. Res.*, 15, 1051, 1987.

115. Sankaran, H., Deveney, C. W., Larkin, E. C., and Rao, G. A., Pancreatic enzyme content and secretion in chronic rats: insignificant role for high blood alcohol levels, *Pancreas*, 6, 718, 1991.

116. Rao, G. A., Nishimura, C. Y., Larkin, E. C., and Sankaran, H., Inverse relationship of blood alcohol levels to energy availability in chronic alcoholic rats, *Biochem. Arch.*, 4, 1, 1988.

117. Sankaran, H., Baba, G. C., Deveney, C. W., Larkin, E. C., and Rao, G. A., Rapid reversal of blood alcohol levels in chronic alcoholic rats: role of macronutrients, *Biochem. Arch.*, 7, 145, 1991.

15 Nutritional Factors in the Pathogenesis of Alcoholic Liver Disease

INTRODUCTION

Speculation regarding which nutritional factors contribute to the development of alcoholic liver disease (ALD) is common. This topic has been thoroughly debated in numerous reviews.[1-4] The validity of the different animal models is also contested.[5-8] With this background, how can the topic be meaningfully approached? The nutritional deficiency associated with ALD could be reviewed for their potential involvement of it in the pathogenesis of ALD. Another approach could be to review the dietary replacement therapy, which brings improvement in the patient with ALD. Lastly, the dietary measures which have prevented or facilitated the development of experimental ALD in animal models could be detailed. Unfortunately, none of these approaches has led to the resolution of the question in alcoholic patients.

The nutritional deficiencies that are observed in patients with ALD include calorie, protein, and vitamin deficiencies (for a review see Mendenhall[9]). Malnutrition clinically appears to precede the development of the liver injury, but may not be essential for the development of alcoholic hepatitis.[10] However, dietary supplements over the short term have not stopped the relentless course of the disease[11-16] as compared to the natural history of the disease.[17-27] ALD progresses to death at the same rate regardless of the stage of the liver disease (Figure 1).[26]

All the experimental models developed so far have failed to completely replicate ALD morphologically as it is seen in patients,[7,28-48] although alcoholic cirrhosis has been induced in rabbits, dogs, monkeys, and baboons.[7,30,36,40,48] Because no nutritional factors have definitely been identified in ALD pathogenesis, some have postulated that alcohol is toxic to

ISBN 0-8493-7933-4
© 1992 by CRC Press, Inc.

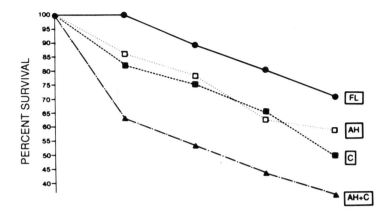

FIGURE 1. Percent survival per year over 4 years' followup of patients diagnosed clinically as having moderate to severe alcoholic hepatitis. Notice the mortality rate is parallel after the first year for all the histologic stages, i.e., about 10% per year. (From Chedid, A. et al., *Am. J. Gastroenterol.*, 86, 214, 1991. With permission.)

the liver, provided high blood-alcohol levels are achieved by the diet.[49] However, against this is the experimental evidence that ALD can be completely prevented by dietary manipulation,[50-53] despite the achievement of high blood-alcohol levels.[50]

It has been argued that the distinction between the role of toxic effects of alcohol and the effects of malnutrition in the pathogenesis of ALD is arbitrary since alcohol metabolism alters the metabolism of nutrients.[4] Therefore it is more important to emphasize the interaction of nutrients with alcohol metabolism since neither alcohol ingestion alone, nor nutritional aberrations alone, account for the development of ALD.

One exception is the experiment of nature where the histologic features of ALD are observed in nonalcoholic patients, a condition clinically referred to as nonalcoholic steatohepatitis (NASH). In this clinical entity, the problem is either an excess of calories ingested (obesity) or altered metabolism such as found in diabetics.[54-66] In this regard it should be pointed out that obesity in alcoholics increases the risk for alcoholic hepatitis and cirrhosis.[67] In both ALD and NASH the problem is neither undernutrition nor malnutrition in the sense that there may not be a deficiency of vitamins, minerals, or macronutrients. The problem seems to reside in an imbalance in the metabolism of nutrients such as fatty acids.[57-58]

In this review, the role that dietary fat, high blood-alcohol levels and vitamin A deficiency play in the pathogenesis of ALD will be emphasized.

The discussion is limited to the effect of nutritional factors which alter the histopathology of the liver.

ROLE OF DIETARY FAT

TYPE AND AMOUNT OF DIETARY FAT

Using an epidemiological approach has provided some leads regarding the role that dietary fat might play in the pathogenesis of ALD. Published data for per capita consumption of beef and pork as well as alcohol consumption for 1965 were analyzed for 16 countries. The correlation between ethanol consumption and mortality rate from cirrhosis was 0.64 ($p < 0.01$). The correlation between pork consumption and cirrhosis mortality was 0.40 ($p < 0.05$). There was no correlation between beef consumption and cirrhosis mortality. When the product of pork and alcohol consumption was correlated with cirrhosis mortality the correlation was highly significant (r = 0.98, $p < 0.001$).[68] These results suggested that pork may differ from beef in the type of fat because of the differences in the diet fed cattle and pigs, i.e., pigs often are fed corn whereas cattle graze on grasses of different types. Taking this epidemiologic approach a step further, per capita consumption of cholesterol, saturated fatty acids, and polyunsaturated fatty acids (grams per capita per day averaged over 1954 to 1965) were obtained for 17 countries where carrier rates for hepatitis B virus (HBV) were less than 2%. Deviations from the expected mortality rates for cirrhosis as predicted by the per capita alcohol consumption of each country during 1967 were utilized for actual and age-adjusted mortality rates. Correlation between dietary cholesterol and percent deviation from the expected cirrhosis mortality was at a significant level (r = -0.86, $p < 0.001$). Similarly, dietary saturated fatty acid consumption and percent deviation correlated (r = -0.80, $p < 0.001$). The results with polyunsaturated fatty acid consumption (grams per capita per day) and percent deviation were in the positive direction (r = 0.55, $p < 0.05$).[69] Thus, the data suggested that pork may be richer in polyunsaturated fatty acids than beef and that this could be the reason why pork appeared to support the development of cirrhosis in countries which have a higher per capita alcohol consumption. Of course, other interpretations of the data are possible since the alcohol consumption rates were dramatically increasing at the time that this sample was taken.[70]

When rats were pair-fed diets high in either beef fat, pork fat, or corn oil with or without ethanol by intragastric tube feeding for 6 months, the liver pathology was very different between groups.[71] Rats fed corn oil and alcohol developed severe fatty liver with focal fibrosis. Rats fed ethanol and lard developed less fatty change and fibrosis, whereas rats fed ethanol and tallow never developed any liver pathology over the 6 months studied. Controls fed each type of fat showed no significant pathologic changes. When the diets were analyzed for their fatty acid composition the main difference in the fats was in the linoleic acid content (i.e., tallow, 0.7%; lard, 2.5%; and corn oil, 56.6%). Thus the tallow diet, which did not support the development of ALD in the rats fed ethanol, was essential fatty acid deficient. When a diet containing alcohol and tallow was supplemented with linoleic acid so that the total 18:2 equaled that of lard (2.5%), the liver pathology achieved with lard and ethanol was reproduced.[72] These studies added credence to the epidemiological correlates which indicated that the high consumption rate of pork and polyunsaturated fatty acids support the development of cirrhosis. They also support the conclusion that ethanol, when given in large amounts to maintain high blood-alcohol levels (i.e., 200 to 300 mg percent), requires dietary linoleate in order to induce ALD. It implies that a product of linoleate metabolism is required in order for ethanol to cause liver damage. Speculation regarding the mechanisms involved in this liver damage will be discussed.

That polyunsaturated fats might augment ethanol-induced liver disease in man has not been noted in clinical studies. However, LeMarchand et al.[73] found that people who drank alcoholic beverages also consumed greater amounts of fat, particularly polyunsaturated fatty acids, compared with abstainers. The results correlated with the experimental findings reported by Zaki et al.[74] using a low protein, choline-deficient diet which induced cirrhosis. They studied red palm oil (18:2 = 10%), lard (18:2 = 10.8%), crisco (18:2 = 26.5%), cotton seed oil (18:2 = 53.6%), and safflower oil (18:2 = 75.4%). The frequency of cirrhosis was highest where the dietary fat increased the choline deficiency the most, i.e., red palm oil and lard. On the other hand Patek et al.[75] found that corn oil high in linoleate (56%) was more effective in producing cirrhosis than was coconut oil which is low in 18:2.

Recently Degli Esposti et al.[76] showed that a diet containing fish oil (rich in Omega 3 fatty acids) enhanced the liver damage caused by ethanol using the intragastric tube feeding rat model of ALD. With this source of dietary fat there was a marked increase in liver necrosis and fibrosis when compared to rats pair-fed corn oil and ethanol (Figure 2). On the other hand, the degree of fatty liver was less in the rats fed fish oil and ethanol. Perhaps more important from the point of view of the mechanism of the

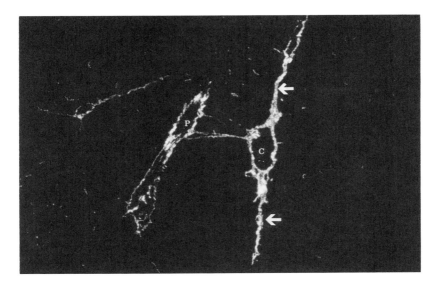

FIGURE 2. Centrilobular fibrosis (arrow) and bridging portal (P) and central (C) fibrosis are shown in a rat fed alcohol and fish oil as a source of dietary fat for 4 months using an intragastric cannula. (Sirius red stain of collagen visualized by polarized light. Original magnification × 165.)

liver injury and fibrosis is that it was found that fish oil increased the gene expression (mRNA levels) for collagen I, III, and IV, as well as the expression of cytokines such as TGF-β1 and TNF as well as fibronectin. Thus, fish oil derivatives stimulated the activity of Ito cells and macrophages involved in the mechanism of liver fibrogenesis when ethanol was also fed.

Lieber et al.[77] found that baboons fed a diet which normally supported the development of alcoholic cirrhosis failed to induce cirrhosis over an 8-year course of feeding when the diet was supplemented with polyunsaturated lecithin. Three of these animals developed cirrhosis when the phospholipid supplement was removed from the diet after 8 years of feeding it. The activation of Ito cells in these baboons correlated with the development of scarring. Thus both in rats fed corn oil or fish oil with alcohol and baboons fed ethanol without a phospholipid supplement, fibrosis of the liver is activated. It is intriguing to examine how the dietary lipids interact with alcohol metabolism in order to provoke fibrogenesis in the liver in these experiments.

The amount of fat in the diet, in terms of percent of dietary calories, may play an important role in the pathogenesis of ALD. Dietary surveys

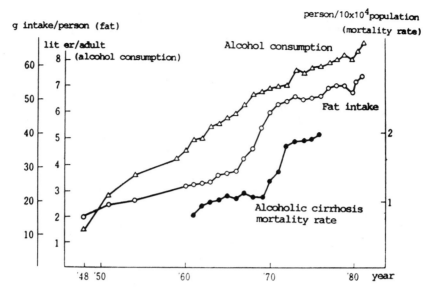

FIGURE 3. Temporal relationship between the increase in the per capita consumption of alcohol and fat and alcoholic cirrhosis mortality rate in Japan. (Published with the permission of Dr. A. Takada, Kanazawa Medical University, Japan.)

of drinkers indicate that dietary calories derived from fat range from 36 to 43%.[78] However, in patients with clinically severe alcoholic hepatitis this figure may drop to an average of 15%.[10] In an epidemiologic survey of per capita fat consumption, alcohol consumption and the mortality rate from cirrhosis, the increase in the frequency of cirrhosis followed the increase in fat consumption rather than the increase in the consumption of alcohol (Figure 3).

The amount of fat in the diet fed with ethanol influences the amount of fat that accumulates in the liver in the rat.[79] Using the intragastric tube-feeding model of ALD in the rat where alcohol was fed at levels which maintained a blood-alcohol level (BAL) of 200 mg percent, 5% calories as fat caused an 11-times increase in fat in the liver after 30 d and a 25-times increase in fat after 80 d of feeding.[80] Thus the amount of fat, the duration of feeding, and the BAL all are factors in the induction of fatty liver by alcohol. This model also caused liver necrosis. When the same model was changed so that the amount of calories derived from dietary fat was increased to 25% or more, fibrosis also developed.[44] The severity of the liver pathology was further accentuated when the diet was marginally deficient in nutrients such as choline and protein.[42]

The explanation for the induction of fibrosis by the high fat diet may be found in the fact that the high-fat diet with or without alcohol increases the basal production of collagen as well as increases the reponse of Ito cells to synthesize collagen when stimulated in tissue culture.[81] Other parameters besides fatty liver, necrosis, and fibrosis are altered by increasing the fat in the diet. For instance, it was shown that when 16 dogs were maintained on a high-fat/lean-meat diet, 4 developed cirrhosis when alcohol was added to the diet,[82] however, the same diet induced cirrhosis without alcohol even though the type of cirrhosis was different.[83] In rats fed a choline-deficient diet low or high in lard content cirrhosis was more advanced and more frequent in the rats fed 38% fat compared to 5% fat.[84] Thus cirrhosis is more likely when experimental animals are fed a diet high in fat with or without alcohol ingestion.

A high-fat diet fed with ethanol caused a reduction in the respiratory rate of mitochondria, whereas no change occurred when low dietary fat was fed.[85] Induction of hepatic γ-glutamyltransferase (GGT) activity following chronic ethanol intake in combination with a high-fat diet (37% of calories) was not seen when a diet low in fat (11% of calories) was fed with alcohol.[86]

The disappearance rate of alcohol in rats fed diets high in fat with alcohol was faster compared to rats fed a low-fat diet.[87] Likewise, the microsomal ethanol-oxidizing system (MEOS), aniline hydroxylase, and glucose-6-phosphatase were more active in the liver when rats were fed a high-fat diet with ethanol.[87] It was concluded that the high-fat diet accelerated ethanol metabolism by increasing MEOS activity. This conclusion was supported when pyrazole treatment was added to the alcohol/high-fat diet regimen.[88] A high-fat diet enhanced the induction of cytochrome P450 in the liver by ethanol feeding. This was first shown by Joly and Hetu[89] and Winston and Narayan,[90] although the induction was further increased by adding linoleate to the diet.[91] The ethanol-inducible P450 isozyme (apo CYP IIEI) was increased 20 times over controls if the dietary fat was corn oil compared to 10 times if the fat was tallow.[92] It is likely that both the amount and the type of dietary fat are important in the induction of microsomal enzymes by ethanol.

The amount of fat in the diet is also important for the same enzyme systems where induction is caused by high-fat diets in the absence of alcohol. For instance, a 20% corn oil enhances the induction of CYP 2EI as well as glutathione S transferase.[93,94] Obese rats overfed with a diet containing 60% fat had increased P450 content.[95] Microsomal ethanol oxidation was proportionately increased.[96] This may explain why obese humans are more susceptible to drugs such as halothane, acetaminophen, or ethanol, where a more active cytochrome P450 in microsomes accelerates drug metabolism, thus increasing toxic intermediates. This phenomenon could explain, in part, why obese patients are more apt to develop cirrhosis.

COMBINED HIGH BLOOD ALCOHOL LEVELS WITH INCREASED MEOS ACTIVITY DUE TO DISPLACEMENT OF DIETARY CARBOHYDRATES WITH FAT

Sato et al. have shown that the induction of cytochrome P450 by ethanol is prevented by a high-carbohydrate diet.[97] In the absence of carbohydrate in the diet, MEOS is maximally induced by alcohol and the addition of a high-protein or high-fat diet did not affect the increase in MEOS caused by the absence of carbohydrate in the diet.[98] Changes in cytochrome P450 run parallel to MEOS induction. Carbohydrate in the diet also reduces the accumulation of lipids in the diet caused by ethanol as assessed histologically or chemically.[98] It has been shown in rats that dietary carbohydrate, not protein, regulates the activity of hepatic drug-metabolizing enzymes.[99] Consistent with this, diets rich in carbohydrate are highly protective against CCl_4-induced liver injury, protracted duration of barbiturate-induced sleep, and decreased rate of metabolism of antipyrine and theophylline.[100] Starvation has the same effect as low-carbohydrate diet in this respect. Thus a low-carbohydrate diet plays a permissive role in the pathogenesis of fatty liver and increase in xenobiotic metabolism by cytochrome P450 isozymes and in this way facilitates liver damage by ethanol when blood-alcohol levels are high. In this way ethanol hepatotoxicity requires a low carbohydrate diet[101] as well as an essential fatty acid-rich diet.[92] What the three dietary factors have in common is they all enhance ethanol oxidation by the cytochrome P450 system. Thus, in humans, up to 63% of ethanol oxidation may be accomplished by MEOS at high blood-ethanol levels[102] and this could be the key to understanding how ethanol injures the liver as discussed below.

Lipid Peroxidation by Increased Ethanol-Induced Cytochrome P450 Free Radical Production: Role of Free Radical Scavengers

The significance of free radical damage as an important mechanism of alcohol-induced liver disease is debatable. Recent investigations where *in vivo* and *in vitro* spin traps were employed to detect free radicals by electron paramagnetic resonance spectroscopy have clearly documented the occurrence of free radicals such as α-hydroxymethyl radical and hydroxyl free radicals during ethanol metabolism as a result of cytochrome P450 mediated reaction.[103-109] α-Hydroxymethyl radical generation results from the oxidation of ethanol by the hydroxyl radical formed by hepatic microsomes during NADPH oxidation catalyzed by iron.[104,105] Lipid peroxidation damage may also result from the ethanol-induced increase in CYP IIEI which generates free radicals through its dioxygenase activity.[110] The rate of oxygen consumption and the formation of reactive oxygen species for this enzyme are severalfold higher than any other cytochrome P450 isozyme.[111]

We have reported a twofold greater increase in CYP IIEI after chronic ethanol feeding when a diet containing corn oil and ethanol was compared to one containing tallow and ethanol.[92] The twofold increase was associated with the development of severe ALD compared to normal liver histologic in the rats fed tallow and ethanol. Furthermore, the CYP IIEI induction is observed primarily in its normal centrilobular location where the pathology of ALD develops so that the localized increase in oxidative stress could be contributing to the development of ALD.[111] In a more recent study using the same intragastric tube-feeding model of ethanol and diet administration we showed that lipid peroxidation by hepatic microsomes was increased 42 times when ethanol was fed, and this was further increased to 68 times when isoniazid (INH) was added to the diet.[112] Severe focal fibrosis of the liver was encountered in these rats fed ethanol and INH.

Dioxygenase activity by CYP IIEI could account for the depletion of microsomal arachidonic acid[113-115] without lipid peroxidation resulting, but rather the biosynthesis of several bioactive eicosanoids such as epoxyeicosatrienoic acid (EETs) and certain hydroxyeicosatetraenoic acid (HETE) isomers may result.[116] The induction of this pathway is significantly modulated by the diet fed with ethanol as opposed to the induction of MEOS. When a diet containing corn oil as a source of fat was fed with ethanol, MEOS increased to the same level as seen when tallow was fed as the fat source. However, the level of induction of CYP IIEI was twice as high in the corn oil-fed rats fed ethanol.[92] This difference correlated with the presence of severe liver pathology in the corn oil-fed rats fed ethanol, whereas, the lower level of CYP IIEI induction in the tallow-fed rats fed ethanol correlated with the total absence of liver pathologic change.

A third mechanism of ethanol-induced liver injury which might result from the induction of MEOS by ethanol when high BAL is maintained is lipid peroxidation by the xanthine oxidase pathway of acetaldehyde oxidation.[117-121] Alcohol enhances this reaction at low concentrations, but inhibits it at high concentrations, because in high concentration ethanol acts as a free radical scavenger.[121] The hepatotoxicity that results is enhanced by ethanol under conditions of low oxygen supply[122-127] since hypoxic conditions favor conversion of xanthine dehydrogenase to xanthine oxidase through proteolysis. This hepatotoxicity was blocked by allopurinol, a xanthine oxidase inhibitor.[124] The hepatotoxicity has been adequately demonstrated to occur at high BAL,[121,126] indicating the importance of MEOS in generating acetaldehyde to act as substrate for this reaction.[119] The reaction is stimulated by ferritin.[118]

VITAMINS AND MINERALS: THEIR ROLE AS FREE RADICAL SCAVENGERS

Lipid peroxidation and free radical-induced liver injury in ethanol-fed animals may depend on the depletion of protective antioxidant nutrients and intermediates such as vitamin E,[128-135] β-carotene,[128,134] vitamin C,[128,136,137] glutathione,[138-146] uric acid,[128,147] coenzyme Q10,[134] linoleic acid,[148] superoxide dismutase (copper, zinc, manganese),[114,128,132,142,144,149,150] glutathione peroxidase (selenium),[114,128,130-132,134,151-153] catalase (iron),[128,132,142,151] and ceruloplasmin (copper),[128] as well as ethanol.[121]

Plasma vitamin E levels are often decreased in chronic alcoholics.[129-132] Vitamin E levels in the liver fall on a vitamin E-deficient diet fed with ethanol, and this is restored to normal with a vitamin E supplement.[133] Lipid peroxidation and increase in α-tocopherol quinone in microsomes, a metabolite of α-tocopherol by free radical reactions, increases in rats fed ethanol and a vitamin E-deficient diet. Like vitamin E, ascorbate depletion is worsened by chronic alcohol ingestion[136] and ascorbate inhibits lipid peroxidation by the liver.[137]

Glutathione (GSH) depletion enhances lipid peroxidation and the addition of GSH completely inhibits lipid peroxidation by liver homogenates.[138] GSH must reach a critical low of 20% of the initial hepatic content before an enhanced lipid peroxidation is seen.[139] Chronic ethanol feeding followed by overnight withdrawal from ethanol, followed by an acute dose of ethanol, decreases liver GSH and increases lipid peroxidation. This is attenuated by methionine administration, which is important as a precursor for GSH synthesis.[140] These changes were seen in patients with ALD.[141] In some studies however, liver GSH levels were increased by chronic ethanol ingestion.[142,145] Acute ethanol administration causes an increased loss of GSH from the liver into the plasma.[142] Pigs fed ethanol chronically developed reduced hepatic levels of GSH, but did not show evidence of increased lipid peroxidation.[143] In the baboon fed ethanol chronically, GSH levels in the liver were reduced and this depletion was corrected by the administration of S-adenosyl-L-methionine (AdoMet).[145] However, this treatment had little effect on the liver morphology of ALD. AdoMet was reduced in chronic ethanol-fed baboon livers and this was partially restored by oral AdoMet therapy. Decreased GSH was also attenuated by AdoMet therapy. Thus, AdoMet is more effective in restoring GSH synthesis than methionine because it bypasses the inhibition of the enzymes involved in AdoMet synthesis from methionine, i.e., decreased AdoMet synthetase and methyltransferase. For more details see the review by Lieber.[146]

Uric acid, which is often elevated in the serum of chronic alcoholics, is also a free radical scavenger.[128] In fact, the serum uric acid level correlated with the deviations from expected cirrhosis mortality and per capita protein intake in different countries, as was indicated by an epidemiologic study.[147] High serum uric acid and high intake of animal proteins ingested correlated with a lower than expected rate of cirrhosis, suggesting an inhibitory effect on lipid peroxidation in the liver in this study of various populations.

The role of dietary lipids as free radical scavengers which protect the liver from alcohol-induced lipid peroxidation includes fatty acids such as linoleic acid.[148] In fact, 95% of diene conjugation in human serum and tissues occurs as a nonperoxide isomer of linoleic acid. The concentration of this form of 18:2 is elevated in the lipid fraction in 75% of alcoholics.[148] It is the result of free radical attack, but it acts to block peroxidation. This could be the way that the lecithin dietary supplement protects the ethanol-fed baboon liver from the fibrogenesis caused by alcohol as reported by Lieber et al.[77] On the other hand, when fish oil instead of corn oil-lard (18:2 = 1.2% vs. 36.4%, respectively) is fed, lipid peroxidation was greater in the liver of rats fed n-3 fatty acids.[135] This may account for the enhanced liver pathology found in the liver of rats fed fish oil and alcohol compared with those fed corn oil and alcohol.[76]

Several metalloenzymes capable of removing free radicals are effected by dietary-derived minerals such as selenium, iron, copper, zinc, and manganese. For instance, superoxide dismutase (CuZn SOD) was reduced in the liver in pigs and monkeys fed ethanol, whereas, manganese SOD (Mn SOD) was increased.[114,144,149] SOD activity was reduced in the liver of rats fed ethanol.[142] CuZn SOD were increased in the serum of alcoholics when measured by enzyme-linked immunosorbent assay (ELISA).[150] However, the amount of both enzymes was reduced in the livers of these patients.[150]

Hepatic glutathione peroxidase (selenium) activity was decreased in pigs fed ethanol.[114] However, there was no increase in lipid peroxidation (malonaldehyde) and no histologic evidence of hepatic damage was found.[114] The activity of glutathione peroxidase is reduced by a selenium-deficient diet where increased lipid peroxidation results.[151] Liver glutathione peroxidase was not reduced in rats fed ethanol, even though lipid peroxidation was increased.[142] Lipid peroxidation and glutathione peroxidation inversely correlated with malonaldehyde production by liver tissue slices from rats fed different levels of selenium in the diet.[134] Serum glutathione peroxidase activity was not altered in alcoholic patients,[132] but serum levels of selenium were reduced in alcoholics in other studies.[130,131,152,153]

METHYL DONORS: CHOLINE

In the older literature, dietary levels of so-called lipotrophic factors were felt to be important in supporting phospholipid synthesis and lipoprotein export by the liver to prevent alcohol-induced fatty liver. Either dietary methionine, protein, or choline could provide the methyl groups for this purpose. One of the arguments against this mechanism of alcohol-induced liver injury operating in man was that primates have less choline oxidase activity in their livers, which would be expected to reduce the choline requirement, compared to rodents.[154] However, monkeys developed fatty liver and cirrhosis similar to ALD when they were fed a diet deficient in choline and protein and high in cholesterol.[155] Alcohol added to a high-fat (lard), low-choline, and low-protein diet did not worsen the cirrhosis and portal hypertension observed in monkeys.[30,39] More recently it has been established that choline is an essential nutrient for humans to make membrane phospholipids.[156] If excess methionine and folate were not available in the diet, decreased plasma phosphatidylcholine and increased serum alanine aminotransferase resulted.[156] This new finding has renewed the interest in examining the role of methyl donor deficiency in the development of ALD. This despite the observation that choline supplements failed to prevent fatty liver and fibrosis in the baboon fed ethanol.[157] Paradoxically, polyunsaturated lecithin (phosphatidyl choline) did prevent ethanol-induced fibrosis in the baboon.[77]

How could choline deficiency accentuate alcoholic liver injury? One way would be to enhance free radical injury induced by ethanol. It was first shown that a diet deficient in choline and methionine enhanced lipid peroxidation in nuclei.[158] The resultant lipid peroxidation of nuclear membrane lipids correlated with the ability of a choline-deficient diet to act as a potent promoter of liver cancer.[159] This phenomenon was enhanced by feeding a predominantly polyunsaturated fat in the diet (corn oil).[159] This may explain why corn oil enhances the development of choline deficiency cirrhosis.[160] Hydrogenated corn oil does not have this enhancing effect, suggesting that peroxidation of polyunsaturated fatty acids might be involved in the mechanism of liver injury.[160] It should be pointed out here that there are reports that dietary alcohol prevented or delayed choline deficiency cirrhosis.[161,162] A possible explanation for this phenomenon is that the induction of MEOS is inhibited by choline deficiency, possibly due to a decrease in available hepatic phosphatidyl choline due to choline deficiency.[163] Of course, other metabolic interactions between the effects of ethanol and choline may be involved, as reviewed by Barak et al.[164] and Thompson and Reitz.[165]

ROLE OF VITAMIN A IN HEPATIC FIBROSIS

Plasma and liver vitamin A levels as well as retinol-binding protein levels are reduced in patients with alcoholic hepatitis and cirrhosis.[166-170] Vitamin A plasma levels correlated negatively with the presence of Mallory bodies and necrosis in the liver,[169] as well as the activation of Ito cells responsible for liver fibrosis.[170,171] Rats fed ethanol develop decreased levels of liver retinol[172-176] and changes in Ito cells in the perisinusoid spaces which are consistent with activation, especially when associated with fibrosis.[42,43,171,177-185] See Figures 4 and 5.

Both the Ito cell activation and the decreased hepatic vitamin A levels are dependent on the type of dietary fat fed with ethanol.[178] A high level

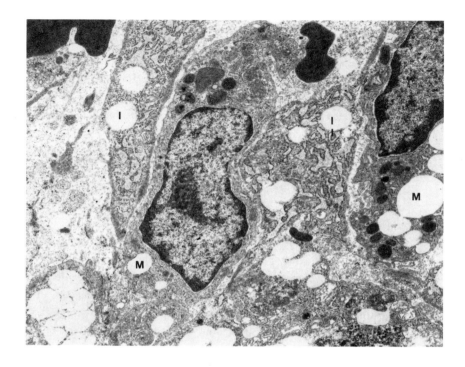

FIGURE 4.   Electron microscopic view of Ito cells (I) showing features of activation in the liver of a rat fed ethanol and corn oil as a source of dietary fat for one month by intragastric cannula. The Ito cells are closely applied to macrophages (M) in the early stages of necrosis prior to scar formation. (Original magnification × 10,875.)

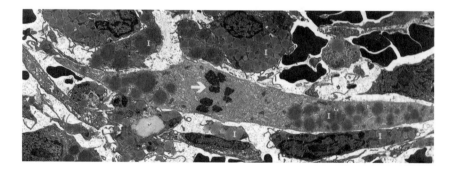

FIGURE 5.   Electron microscopic view of Ito cells (I) in an area of necrosis in a rat fed ethanol and sunflower oil as dietary fat for 6 months by intragastric cannula. Note that a large fat filled Ito cell is in mitoses (arrow). (Original magnification × 3,450.)

of linoleate in the diet decreases the hepatic vitamin A stores even when alcohol is not fed.[186] A high-fat diet enhances the depression of liver vitamin A stores in rats fed ethanol[187] and also sensitizes the Ito cells to TGFβ stimulation of collagen synthesis.[81] The decrease in vitamin A in the liver is the result of the increased metabolism of vitamin A by ethanol-induced cytochrome P450 and the mobilization of vitamin A from the liver.[143,173,175] Vitamin A is known to play a regulatory role in the activation of Ito cells and resultant scarring. For instance, vitamin A given parenterally prevents the fibrosis and cirrhosis induced by chronic poisoning with carbon tetrachloride[188] and diminishes type I and III collagen production in the liver.[189] On the other hand, toxic amounts of dietary vitamin A given with ethanol cause liver fibrosis in rodents.[190] This may be a result of its effect on membrane fluidity.[191]

REFERENCES

1. Jacobs, R. M. and Sorrell, M. F., The role of nutrition in the pathogenesis of alcoholic liver disease, *Semin. Liver Dis.*, 1, 244, 1981.
2. Rao, G. A., Larkin, E. C., and Porter, E. A., Two decades of chronic alcoholism research with the misconception that liver damage occurred despite adequate nutrition, *Biochem. Arch.*, 2, 223, 1986.
3. Derr, R. F., Larkin, E. C., and Rao, G. A., Is malnutrition necessary for the development of alcoholic fatty liver in the rat?, *Med. Hypothesis*, 27, 277, 1988.
4. Lieber, C. S., The influence of alcohol on nutritional status, *Nutr. Rev.*, 46, 241, 1988.
5. Rao, G. A., Sankaran, H., and Larkin, E. C., Rat models for chronic alcohol consumption, *J. Nutr.*, 118, 799, 1988.
6. Lieber, C. S., DeCarli, L. M., and Sorrell, M. F., Experimental methods of ethanol administration, *Hepatology*, 10, 501, 1989.
7. Lieber, C. S. and DeCarli, L. M., Liquid diet technique of ethanol administration: 1989 update, *Alcohol Alcoholism*, 24, 197, 1989.
8. Derr, R. F., The quantities of nutrients recommended by the NRC abate the effects of a toxic alcohol dose administered to rats, *J. Nutr.*, 119, 1228, 1989.
9. Mendenhall, C. L., Clinical and therapeutic aspects of alcoholic liver disease, in *Alcohol Related Disease in Gastroenterology*, Seitz, H. K. and Kommersell, B., Eds., Springer-Verlag, Berlin, 1985, 304.
10. Mendenhall, C. L., Anderson, S., Weisner, R. E., Goldberg, S. L., and Crolic, K. A., Protein-calorie malnutrition associated with alcoholic hepatitis, *Am. J. Med.*, 76, 211, 1984.

11. Achord, J. L., Malnutrition and the role of nutritional support in alcoholic liver disease, *Am. J. Gastroenterol.*, 82, 1, 1987.
12. Diehl, A. M., Boitnott, J. K., Herlong, H. F., Potter, J. J., Van Duyn, M. A., Chandler, E., and Mezey, E., Effect of parenteral amino acid supplementation in alcoholic hepatitis, *Hepatology*, 5, 57, 1985.
13. Mendenhall, C. L., Anabolic steroid therapy as an adjunct to diet in alcoholic hepatic steatosis, *Am. J. Dig. Dis.*, 13, 783, 1968.
14. Mendenhall, C. L., Bongiovanni, G., Goldberg, S., Miller, B., Moore, J., Rouster, S., Schneider, D., Tamburro, C., Tosch, T., and Weisner, R., V.A. cooperative study on alcoholic hepatitis III. Changes in protein-calorie malnutrition associated with 30 days of hospitalization with and without enteral nutritional therapy, *J. Parenteral Enteral Nutr.*, 9, 590, 1985.
15. Galambos, J. T., Alcoholic hepatitis: its therapy and prognosis, in *Progress in Liver Disease*, Vol. 4, Popper, H. and Schaffner, F., Eds., Grune and Stratton, New York, 1973, 567.
16. Soberon, S., Pauley, M. P., Duplantier, R., Fan, A., and Halted, C. H., Metabolic effects of enteral formula feeding in alcoholic hepatitis, *Hepatology*, 7, 1204, 1987.
17. Goldberg, S., Mendenhall, C., Anderson, S., Garcia-Pont, P., Kiernan, T., Seeff, L., Sorrell, M., Tamburro, C., Weisner, R., Zetterman, R., Chedid, A., Chan, T., and Rabin, L., VA cooperative study on alcoholic hepatitis IV. The significance of clinically mild alcoholic hepatitis — describing the population with minimal hyperbilirubinemia, *Am. J. Gastroenterol.*, 81, 1029, 1986.
18. Soterakis, J., Resnik, R. H., and Iber, F. L., Effect of alcohol abstinence on survival in cirrhotic portal hypertension, *Lancet*, July 14, 65, 1973.
19. Schenker, S., Alcoholic liver disease: evaluation of natural history and prognostic factors, *Hepatology*, 4, 36S, 1984.
20. Galambos, J. T., Natural history of alcoholic hepatitis III. Histologic changes, *Gastroenterology*, 63, 1026, 1972.
21. Galambos, J. T., Alcoholic hepatitis, in *The Liver and Its Diseases*, Schaffner, F., Sherlock, S., and Leevy, C. M., Eds., Intercontinental Medical Book Corp., New York, 1974, 255.
22. Sorensen, T. I. A., Orholm, M., Bentsen, K. D., Hoybye, G., Eghoje, K., and Christoffersen, P., Prospective evaluation of alcohol abuse and alcoholic liver injury in men as predictors of development of cirrhosis, *Lancet*, August 4, 241, 1984.
23. Patek, A. J., Jr. and Koff, R. S., Predicting clinical recovery from alcoholic liver disease, *J. Clin. Gastroenterol.*, 5, 303, 1983.
24. Maier, K. P., Seitzer, D., Haag, G., Peskar, B. M., and Gerok, W., Verlaufsformen alkoholischer Lebererkrankungen, *Klin. Wochenschr.*, 57, 311, 1979.
25. Borowsky, S. A., Strome, S., Lott, E., Continued heavy drinking and survival in alcoholic cirrhotics, *Gastroenterology*, 80, 1405, 1981.
26. Chedid, A., Mendehall, C. L., Gartside, P., French, S. W., Chen, T., and Rabin, L., Prognostic factors in alcoholic liver disease, *Am. J. Gastroenterol.*, 86, 210, 1991.
27. Lelbach, W. K., Cirrhosis in the alcoholic and its relation to the volume of the alcohol abuse, *Ann. N.Y. Acad. Sci.*, 252, 85, 1975.

28. Leathers, C. W., Bond, M. G., Bullock, B. C., and Rudel, L. L., Dietary ethanol and cholesterol in Malaca nemestrina serum lipid and hepatic changes, *Exp. Mol. Pathol.*, 35, 285, 1981.

29. Lindros, K. O., Storwell, L., Vaananen, H., Sipponen, P., Lamminsivu, U., Pikkarainen, P., and Salaspuro, M., Uninterrupted prolonged ethanol oxidation as a main pathogenetic factor of alcoholic liver damage: evidence from a new liquid diet animal model, *Liver*, 3, 79, 1983.

30. Cueto, J., Tajen, N., Gilbert, E., and Currie, R. A., Experimental liver injury in the rhesus monkey: effects of cirrhogenic diet and ethanol, *Ann. Surg.*, 166, 19, 1967.

31. Porta, E. A., Koch, O. R., and Hartroft, W. S., Recovery from chronic hepatic lesions in rats fed alcohol and a solid super diet, *Am. J. Clin. Nutr.*, 25, 881, 1972.

32. Ainley, C. C., Senapati, A., Brown, I. M. H., Iles, C. A., Slavin, B. M., Mitchell, W. D., Davies, D. R., Keeling, P. W. N., and Thompson, R. P. H., Is alcohol hepatotoxic in the baboon?, *J. Hepatol.*, 7, 85, 1988.

33. Mezey, E., Animal models for alcoholic liver disease, *Hepatology*, 9, 904, 1989.

34. Rubin, E. and Lieber, C. S., Experimental alcoholic hepatitis: a new primate model, *Science*, 182, 712, 1973.

35. Friedenwald, J., The pathologic effects of alcohol on rabbits, an experimental study, *J. Am. Med. Assoc.*, 45, 780, 1905.

36. Connor, C. L., Some effects of chronic alcohol poisoning in rabbits, *Arch. Pathol.*, 30, 165, 1940.

37. Ruebner, B. H., Brayton, M. A., Freedland, R. A., Kanayama, R., and Tsao, M., Production of a fatty liver by ethanol in Rhesus monkeys, *Lab. Invest.*, 27, 71, 1972.

38. Chey, w. Y., Kosay, S., Siplet, H., and Lorber, S. H., Observations on hepatic histology and function in alcoholic dogs, *Am. J. Dig. Dis.*, 16, 825, 1971.

39. Rogers, A. E., Fox, J. G., and Gottlieb, L. S., Effects of ethanol and malnutrition on nonhuman primate liver, in *Frontiers in Liver Disease*, Berk, P. D. and Chalmers, T. C., Eds., Thieme-Stratton, New York, 1981, 167.

40. Popper, H. and Lieber, C. S., Histogenesis of alcoholic fibrosis and cirrhosis in the baboon, *Am. J. Pathol.*, 98, 695, 1980.

41. Mezey, E., Potter, J. J., French, S. W., Tamura, T., and Halsted, C. H., Effect of chronic ethanol feeding on hepatic collagen in the monkey, *Hepatology*, 3, 41, 1983.

42. French, S. W., Miyamoto, K., and Tsukamoto, H., Ethanol-induced hepatic fibrosis in the rat: role of the amount of dietary fat, *Alcoholism Clin. Exp. Res.*, 10, 13S, 1986.

43. Tsukamoto, H., Gaal, K., and French, S. W., Insights into the pathogenesis of alcoholic liver necrosis and fibrosis: status report, *Hepatology*, 12, 599, 1990.

44. Tsukamoto, H., Towner, S. J., Cioffalo, L. M., and French, S. W., Ethanol-induced liver fibrosis in rats fed high fat diet, *Hepatology*, 6, 814, 1986.

45. French, S. W. and Costagna, J., Some effects of chronic ethanol feeding on Vitamin B_6 deficiency in the rat, *Lab. Invest.*, 16, 526, 1967.

46. Chaikoff, I. L., Enteman, C., Gillman, T., and Connor, C. L., Pathologic reaction in the livers and kidneys of dogs fed alcohol while maintained on a high protein diet, *Arch. Pathol.*, 45, 435, 1948.

47. Porto, L. C., Chevallier, M., and Grimaud, J. A., Morphometry of terminal hepatic veins. 2. Follow up in chronically alcohol-fed baboons, *Virchows Arch. A*, 414, 299, 1989.

48. Rogers, A. E., Fox, J. G., Murphy, J. C., Ethanol and diet interactions in male Rhesus monkeys, *Drug Nutr. Interact.*, 1, 3, 1981.

49. Lieber, C. S. and DeCarli, L. M., Recommended amounts of nutrients do not abate the toxic effects of an alcohol dose that sustains significant blood levels of alcohol, *J. Nutr.*, 119, 2038, 1989.

50. Nanji, A. A., Mendenhall, C. L., and French, S. W., Beef fat prevents alcoholic liver disease in the rat, *Alcoholism Clin. Exp. Res.*, 13, 15, 1989.

51. Rao, G. A., Riley, D. E., and Larkin, E. C., Lieber-DeCarli alcohol diet modification to enhance growth in young rats, *Nutr. Res.*, 6, 101, 1986.

52. Derr, R. F. and Draves, K., Adequate nutrition abates the effects of a toxic alcohol dose fed to rats for four generations, *Biochem. Arch.*, 4, 341, 1988.

53. Derr, R. F., The quantities of nutrients recommended by the NRC abate the effects of a toxic alcohol dose administered to rats, *J. Nutr.*, 119, 1228, 1989.

54. Lee, R. G., Nonalcoholic steatohepatitis. A study of 49 patients, *Human Pathol.*, 20, 594, 1989.

55. Wanless, I. R. and Lentz, J. S., Fatty liver hepatitis (Steatohepatitis) and obesity: an autopsy study with analysis of risk factors, *Hepatology*, 12, 1106, 1990.

56. Powell, E. E., Cooksley, W. G. E., Hanson, R., Searle, J., Halliday, J., and Powell, L. W., The natural history of nonalcoholic steatohepatitis: a follow-up study of forty-two patients patients for up to 21 years, *Hepatology*, 11, 74, 1990.

57. Wanless, I. R., Bargman, J. M., Oreopoulos, D. G., and Vas, S. I., Subcapsular steatonecrosis in obesity, *Mod. Pathol.*, 2, 69, 1989.

58. Mavrelis, P. G., Ammon, H. V., Gleysteen, J. J., Komorowski, R. A., and Charaf, U. K., Hepatic free fatty acids in alcoholic liver disease and morbid obesity, *Hepatology*, 3, 226, 1983.

59. Cueller, R. E., Tarter, R., Hays, A., and Van Thiel, D. H., The possible occurrence of ''alcoholic hepatitis'' in a patient with bulimia in the absence of diagnosable alcoholism, *Hepatology*, 7, 878, 1987.

60. French, S. W., Eidus, L. B., and Freedman, J., Nonalcoholic fatty hepatitis. An important clinical condition, *Can. J. Gastroenterol.*, 3, 189, 1989.

61. Batman, P. A. and Scheuer, P., Diabetic hepatitis preceding the onset of glucose intolerance, *Histopathology*, 9, 237, 1985.

62. Nagore, N. and Scheuer, P. J., The pathology of diabetic hepatitis, *J. Pathol.*, 156, 155, 1988.

63. Ludwig, J., Viggiano, T. R., McGill, D. B., and Oh, B. J., Nonalcoholic steatohepatitis, *Mayo Clin. Proc.*, 555, 434, 1980.

64. Diehl, A. M., Goodman, Z., and Ishak, K. G., Alcohol-like liver disease in nonalcoholics, *Gastroenterology*, 95, 1056, 1988.

65. Capron, J.-P., Delamarre, J., Dupas, J. L., Braillon, A., Degott, C., and Quenum, C., Fasting in obesity. Another cause of liver injury with alcoholic hyaline?, *Dig. Dis. Sci.*, 27, 265, 1982.

66. Alder, M. and Schaffner, F., Fatty liver hepatitis and cirrhosis in obese patients, *Am. J. Med.*, 67, 811, 1979.
67. Bunout, D., Gattas, V., Iturriaga, H., Perez, C., Pereda, T., and Ugarte, G., Nutritional status of alcoholic patients: its possible relationship to alcoholic liver damage, *Am. J. Clin. Nutr.*, 38, 469, 1983.
68. Nanji, A. A. and French, S. W., Relationship between pork consumption and cirrhosis, *Lancet,* March 23, 681, 1985.
69. Nanji, A. A. and French, S. W., Dietary factors and alcoholic cirrhosis, *Alcoholism Clin. Exp. Res.*, 10, 271, 1986.
70. Grant, B. F., Dufour, M. C., and Harford, T. C., Epidemiology of alcoholic liver disease, *Semin. Liver Dis.*, 8, 12, 1988.
71. Nanji, A. A., Mendenhall, C. L., and French, S. W., Beef fat prevents alcoholic liver disease in the rat, *Alcoholism Clin. Exp. Res.*, 13, 15, 1989.
72. Nanji, A. A. and French, S. W., Dietary linoleic acid is required for development of experimentally induced alcoholic liver injury, *Life Sci.*, 44, 223, 1989.
73. LeMarchand, L., Kolonel, L. N., Hankin, J. H., and Yoshizawa, C. N., Relationship of alcohol consumption to diet: a population based study in Hawaii, *Am. J. Clin. Nutr.*, 49, 567, 1989.
74. Zaki, F. G., Hoffbauer, F. W., and Grande, F., Fatty cirrhosis in the rat. VIII. Effect of dietary fat, *Arch. Pathol.*, 80, 323, 1965.
75. Patek, A. J., Jr., Defritsch, N. M., Kendall, F. E., and Hirsch, R. L., Corn and coconut oil effects in dietary cirrhosis in rats, *Arch. Pathol.*, 75, 264, 1963.
76. Degli Esposti, S., McKibbon, D., Wong, K., Jui, L., Zern, M. A., and French, S. W., Omega 3 fatty acids (W3FAs) induced liver fibrosis in a rat model of alcoholic liver disease (ALD), *Hepatology,* 12, 923, 1990.
77. Lieber, C. S., DeCarli, L. M., Mak, K. M., Kim, C.-I., and Leo, M. A., Attenuation of alcohol-induced hepatic fibrosis by polyunsaturated lecithin, *Hepatology,* 12, 1390, 1990.
78. Mitchell, M. C. and Herlong, H. F., Alcohol and nutrition: caloric value, bioenergetics, and relationship to liver damage, *Annu. Rev. Nutr.*, 6, 457, 1986.
79. Lieber, C. S. and DeCarli, L. M., Quantitative relationship between amount of dietary fat and severity of alcoholic fatty liver, *Am. J. Clin. Nutr.*, 23, 474, 1970.
80. Tsukamoto, H., French, S. W., Benson, N., Delgado, G., Rao, G. A., Larkin, E. C., and Largman, C., Severe and progressive steatosis and focal necrosis in rat liver induced by continuous intragastric infusion of ethanol and low fat diet, *Hepatology,* 5, 224, 1985.
81. Matsuoka, M., Zhang, M. Y., and Tsukamoto, H., Sensitization of hepatic lipocytes by high-fat diet to stimulatory effects of Kupffer cell-derived factors: implication in alcoholic liver fibrogenesis, *Hepatology,* 11, 173, 1990.
82. Connor, C. L. and Chaikoff, I. L., Production of cirrhosis in fatty livers with alcohol, *Proc. Soc. Exp. Biol. Med.*, 39, 356, 1938.
83. Chaikoff, I. L. and Connor, C. L., Production of cirrhosis of the liver of the normal dog by high fat diets, *Proc. Soc. Exp. Biol. Med.*, 43, 638, 1940.

84. Zaki, F. G., Bandt, C., and Hoffbauer, F. W., Fatty cirrhosis in the rat. IV. The influence of different levels of dietary fat, *Arch. Pathol.*, 75, 654, 1963.

85. Wahid, S., Khanna, J. M., Carmichael, F. J., and Israel, Y., Mitochondrial function following chronic ethanol treatment: effect of diet, *Res. Commun. Chem. Pathol. Pharmacol.*, 30, 477, 1980.

86. Misslbeck, N. G., Campbell, T. C., and Roe, D. A., Increase in hepatic gamma-glutamyltransferase (GGT) activity following chronic ethanol intake in combination with a high fat diet, *Biochem. Pharmacol.*, 35, 399, 1986.

87. Kanayama, R., Takase, S., Matsuda, Y., and Takada, A., Effect of dietary fat upon ethanol metabolism in rats, *Biochem. Pharmacol.*, 33, 3283, 1984.

88. Takada, A., Matsuda, Y., and Takase, S., Effects of dietary fat on alcohol-pyrazole hepatitis in rats: the pathogenetic role of the nonalcohol dehydrogenase pathway in alcohol-induced hepatic cell injury, *Alcoholism Clin. Exp. Res.*, 10, 403, 1986.

89. Joly, J.-G. and Hetu, C., Effects of chronic ethanol administration in the rat relative dependence on dietary lipids. I. Induction of hepatic drug metabolizing enzymes in vitro, *Biochem. Pharmacol.*, 24, 1475, 1975.

90. Winston, G. W. and Narayan, S., Alteration of liver microsomal monooxygenases and substrate competition with amiline hydroxylase from rats chronically fed low-fat and high-fat containing alcohol diets, *J. Biochem. Toxicol.*, 3, 191, 1988.

91. Joly, J.-G. and Hetu, C., Effects of chronic ethanol administration in the rat: relative dependency on dietary lipids. II. Paradoxical role of linoleate in the induction of hepatic drug-metabolizing enzymes in vitro, *Can. J. Physiol. Pharmacol.*, 55, 34, 1977.

92. Takahashi, H., Johansson, I., French, S. W., and Ingelman-Sundberg, M., Effects of dietary fat composition on activities of the microsomal ethanol oxidizing system and ethanol-inducible cytochrome P450 (CYP 2EI) in the liver of rats chronically fed ethanol, *Pharmacol. Toxicol.*, 70, in press, 1992.

93. Yoo, J.-S. H., Hong, J.-J., Ning, S. M., and Yang, C. S., Roles of dietary corn oil in the regulation of cytochrome P450 and glutathione S-transferases in rat liver, *J. Nutr.*, 120, 1718, 1990.

94. Kim, H. J., Choi, E. S., and Wade, A. E., Effect of dietary fat on the induction of hepatic microsomal cytochrome P450 isozymes by phenobarbital, *Biochem. Pharmacol.*, 39, 1423, 1990.

95. Matsumoto, R. M., Jusko, W. J. and Corcoran, G. B., Hepatic cytochrome P450 and in vitro drug metabolism in an overfed rat model of obesity, *Drug Nutr. Interact.*, 5, 237, 1988.

96. Salazar, D. E., Sorge, C. L., and Corcoran, G. B., Obesity as a risk factor for drug-induced organ injury. VI. Increased hepatic P450 concentration and microsomal ethanol oxidizing activity in the obese overfed rat, *Biochem. Biophys. Res. Commun.*, 157, 315, 1988.

97. Sato, A., Nakajima, T., and Koyama, Y., Interaction between ethanol and carbohydrate on the metabolism in rat liver of aromatic and chlorinated hydrocarbons, *Toxicol. Appl. Pharmacol.*, 68, 242, 1983.

98. Yonekura, I., Nakano, M., Nakajima, T., and Sato, A., Dietary carbohydrate intake as a modifying factor for the development of alcoholic fatty liver, *Biochem. Arch.*, 5, 41, 1980.

99. Nakajima, T., Koyama, Y., and Sato, A., Dietary modification of metabolism and toxicity of chemical substance with special reference to carbohydrate, *Biochem. Pharmacol.*, 31, 1005, 1982.

100. Sato, A. and Nakajima, T., Dietary carbohydrate and ethanol-induced alteration of the metabolism and toxicity of chemical substances, *Nutr. Cancer*, 6, 121, 1984.

101. Derr, R. F., Porta, E. A., Larkin, E. C., and Rao, G. A., Is ethanol per se hepatotoxic? *J. Hepatol.*, 10, 381, 1990.

102. Teschke, R. and Gellert, J., Hepatic microsomal ethanol oxidizing system (MEOS): metabolic aspects and clinical implications, *Alcoholism Clin. Exp. Res.*, 10, 20s, 1986.

103. Knecht, K. T., Thurman, R. G., and Mason, R. P., Free radical metabolism of ethanol by deermouse microsomes, *FASEB J.*, 5, A1209, 1991.

104. McCay, P. B., Reinke, L. A., and Rau, J. M., Hydroxyl radicals are generated by hepatic microsomes during NADPH oxidation: relation to ethanol metabolism, *FASEB J.*, 5, A1614, 1991.

105. Cederbaum, A. I., Oxygen radical generation by microsomes: role of iron and implications for alcohol metabolism and toxicity, *Free Radical Biol. Med.*, 7, 559, 1989.

106. Reinke, L. A., Lai, E. K., Dubose, C. M., and McCay, P. B., Reactive free radical generation in vivo in heart and liver of ethanol-fed rats: correlation with radical formation in vitro, *Proc. Natl. Acad. Sci. U.S.A.*, 84, 9223, 1987.

107. Albano, E., Tomasi, A., Goria-Gatti, L., Poli, G., and Dianzani, M. U., Spin trapping of ethanol derived free radicals in rat liver microsomes, *Adv. Biosci.*, 71, 17, 1988.

108. Albano, E., Tomasi, A., Goria-Gatti, L., and Dianzani, M. V., Spin trapping of free radical species produced during the microsomal metabolism of ethanol, *Chem. Biol. Interactions*, 65, 223, 1988.

109. Knecht, K. T., Bradford, B. V., Mason, R. P., and Thurman, R. G., In vivo formation of a free radical metabolite of ethanol, *Mol. Pharmacol.*, 838, 26, 1990.

110. Ingelman-Sundberg, M., Ekstrom, G., and Tindberg, N., Lipid peroxidation dependent on ethanol-inducible cytochrome P450 from rat liver, *Adv. Biosci.*, 71, 43, 1988.

111. Ekstrom, G. and Ingelman-Sundberg, M., Rat liver microsomal NADPH-supported oxidase activity and lipid peroxidation dependent on ethanol-inducible cytochrome P450, *Biochem. Pharmacol.*, 58, 1313, 1989.

112. French, S. W., Wong, K., McKibbon, D., Jui, L., and Ingelman-Sundberg, M., Effect on INH inhibition of ethanol-inducible cytochrome P450 on ethanol-induced liver damage, *FASEB J.*, 5, A1614, 1991.

113. French, S. W., Ihrig, T. J., and Morin, R. J., Lipid composition of liver mitochondrial and microsomes and erythrocyte ghosts after chronic ethanol feeding, *Q. J. Stud. Alcohol*, 31, 801, 1970.

114. Zidenberg-Cherr, S., Olin, K. L., Villanueva, J., Tang, A., Phinney, S. D., Halsted, C. H., and Keen, C. L., Ethanol-induced changes in hepatic free radical defense mechanisms and fatty acid composition in the miniature pig, *Hepatology*, 13, 1185, 1991.

115. Inomata, T., Rao, G. A., and Tsukamoto, H., Lack of evidence for increased lipid peroxidation in ethanol-induced centrilobular necrosis of rat liver, *Liver*, 7, 233, 1987.

116. Fitzpatrick, F. A. and Murphy, R. C., Cytochrome P450 metabolism of arachidonic acid: formation and biological actions of "epoxygenase"-derived eicosanoids, *Pharmacol. Rev.*, 40, 229, 1989.

117. Lewis, K. O. and Paton, A., Could superoxide cause cirrhosis, *Lancet*, July 24, 188, 1982.

118. Shaw, S. and Jayatilleke, E., Acetaldehyde-mediated hepatic lipid peroxidation: role of superoxide and ferritin, *Biochem. Biophys. Res. Commun.*, 143, 984, 1987.

119. Shaw, S., Lipid peroxidation, iron mobilization and radical generation-induced by alcohol, *Free Radical Biol. Med.*, 7, 541, 1989.

120. Fridovich, I., Oxygen radicals from acetaldehyde, *Free Radical Biol. Med.*, 7, 557, 1989.

121. Videla, L. A., Assessment of the scavenging action of reduced glutathione, (+)-cyanidanol-3 and ethanol by the chemiluminescent response of the xanthine oxidase reaction, *Experientia*, 39, 500, 1983.

122. Yamada, S., Fujiwara, K., Masaki, N., Ohta, Y., Sato, Y., and Oka, H., Evidence for potentiation of lipid peroxidation in the rat liver after chronic ethanol feeding, *Scand. J. Clin. Lab. Invest.*, 48, 627, 1988.

123. Younes, M., Wagner, H., and Strubelt, O., Enhancement of acute ethanol hepatotoxicity under conditions of low oxygen supply and ischemial reperfusion. The role of oxygen radicals, *Biochem. Pharmacol.*, 38, 3573, 1989.

124. Younes, M. and Strubelt, O., Enhancement of hypoxic liver damage by ethanol. Involvement of xanthine oxidase and the role of glycolysis, *Biochem. Pharmacol.*, 36, 2973, 1987.

125. Israel, Y., Kalant, H., Orrego, H., Khanna, J. M., Vidella, L., and Phillips, J. M., Experimental alcohol-induced hepatic necrosis: suppression by propylthiouracil, *Proc. Natl. Acad. Sci. U.S.A.*, 72, 1137, 1975.

126. French, S. W., Benson, N. C., and Sun, P. S., Centrilobular liver necrosis induced by hypoxia in chronic ethanol-fed rats, *Hepatology*, 4, 912, 1984.

127. Tsukamoto, H. and Xi. X. P., Incomplete compensation of enhanced oxygen consumption in rats with alcoholic centrilobular liver necrosis, *Hepatology*, 9, 302, 1989.

128. Machlin, L. J. and Bendich, A., Free radical tissue damage: protective role of antioxidant nutrients, *FASEB J.*, 1, 441, 1987.

129. Majumdar, S. K., Shaw, G. K., and Thompson, A. D., Plasma vitamin E status in chronic alcoholic patients, *Drug Alcohol Dep.*, 12, 269, 1983.

130. Tanner, A. R., Bantock, I., Hinko, L., Lloyd, B., Turner, N. R., and Wright, R., Depressed selenium and vitamin E levels in an alcoholic population. Possible relationship to hepatic injury through increased lipid peroxidation, *Dig. Dis. Sci.*, 31, 1307, 1986.

131. Ward, R. J., Duane, P. D., and Peters, T. J., Nutritional, selenium and α-tocopherol status of alcohol abusers with and without chronic skeletal muscle myopathy, *Adv. Biosci.*, 71, 93, 1988.

132. Bjornehoe, G.-E. A., Johnsen, J., Bjorneboe, A., Marklund, S. L., Skylu, N., Hoiseth, A., Bache-Wig, J.-E., Morland, J., and Drevon, C. A., Some aspects of antioxidant status in blood from alcoholics, *Alcoholism Clin. Exp. Res.*, 12, 806, 1988.

133. Kawase, T., Kato, S., and Lieber, C. S., Lipid peroxidation and antioxidant defense systems in rat liver after chronic ethanol feeding, *Hepatology*, 10, 815, 1989.

134. Leibovitz, B., Hu, M.-L., and Tappel, A. L., Dietary supplements of vitamin E, β-carotene, coenzyme Q10 and selenium protect tissues against lipid peroxidation in rat tissue slices, *J. Nutr.*, 120, 97, 1990.

135. Hu, M.-L., Frankel, E. N., Liebovitz, B. E., and Tappel, A. L., Effect of dietary lipids and vitamin E on in vitro lipid peroxidation in rat liver and kidney homogenates, *J. Nutr.*, 119, 1574, 1989.

136. Yunice, A. A., Hsu, J. M., Fahmy, A., and Henry, S., Ethanol-ascorbate interrelationship in acute and chronic alcoholism in the guinea pig, *Proc. Soc. Exp. Biol. Med.*, 177, 262, 1984.

137. Chen, L. H., Ascorbic acid-stimulated peroxidation in hepatocytes and inhibition by antioxidants, *Biochem. Arch.*, 4, 373, 1988.

138. Younes, M. and Siegers, C.-P., Lipid peroxidation as a consequence of glutathione depletion in rat and mouse liver, *Res. Commun. Chem. Pathol. Pharmacol.*, 27, 1119, 1980.

139. Younes, M. and Siegers, C.-P., Mechanistic aspects of enhanced lipid peroxidation following glutathione depletion in vivo, *Chem. Biol. Interact.*, 34, 257, 1981.

140. Shaw, S., Jayatilleke, E., Ross, W. A., Gordon, E. R., and Lieber, C. S., Ethanol-induced lipid peroxidation: potentiation by long-term alcohol feeding and attenuation by methionine, *J. Lab. Clin. Med.*, 98, 417, 1981.

141. Shaw, S., Rubin, K. P., and Lieber, C. S., Depressed hepatic glutathione and increased diene conjugates in alcoholic liver disease. Evidence of lipid peroxidation, *Dig. Dis. Sci.*, 28, 585, 1983.

142. Harata, J., Nagata, M., Sasaki, E., Ishiquro, I., Ohta, Y., and Murakami, Y., Effect of prolonged alcohol administration on activities of various enzymes scavenging activated oxygen radicals and lipid peroxide in the liver of rats, *Biochem. Pharmacol.*, 32, 1795, 1983.

143. Speisky, H., MacDonald, A., Gites, G., Orrego, H., and Israel, Y., Increased loss and decreased synthesis of hepatic glutathione after acute ethanol administration, *Biochem. J.*, 225, 565, 1985.

144. Zidenberg-Cherr, S., Halsted, C. H., Olin, K. L., Reisenauer, A. M., and Keen, C. L., The effect of chronic alcohol ingestion on free radical defense in the miniature pig, *J. Nutr.*, 120, 213, 1990.

145. Lieber, C. S., Casini, A., DeCarli, L. M., Kim, C.-I., Lowe, N., Sasaki, R., and Leo, M. A., S-adenosyl-L-methionine attenuates alcohol-induced liver injury in the baboon, *Hepatology*, 11, 165, 1990.

146. Lieber, C. S., Metabolic effects of ethanol and its interaction with other drugs, hepatotoxic agents, vitamins and carcinogens: a 1988 update, *Semin. Liver Dis.*, 8, 47, 1988.

147. Nanji, A. A. and French, S. W., Correlations between deviations from expected cirrhosis mortality and serum uric acid and dietary protein intake, *J. Stud. Alcohol*, 47, 253, 1986.

148. Dormandy, T. L., Diene conjugation in chronic alcoholics, *Adv. Biosci.*, 71, 55, 1988.
149. Keen, C. L., Tamura, T., Lonnerdal, B., Hurley, L. S., and Halsted, C. H., Changes in hepatic dismutase activity in alcoholic monkeys, *Am. J. Clin. Nutr.*, 41, 929, 1985.
150. Inagaki, T., Takiya, S., Ikuta, K., Sasaki, T., Kato, K., Shimizu, A., Suzuki, M., and Kato, K., Serum activity and hepatic localization of superoxide dismutase in alcoholics, *Gastroenterol. Jpn.*, 24, 277, 1989.
151. Simmons, T. W. and Jamall, I. S., Significance of alterations in hepatic antioxidant enzymes. Primacy of glutathione peroxidase, *Biochem. J.*, 251, 913, 1988.
152. Korpela, H., Kumpulainen, J., Luoma, P. V., Arranto, A. J., and Sotaniemi, E. A., Decreased serum selenium in alcoholics as related to liver structure and function, *Am. J. Clin. Nutr.*, 42, 147, 1985.
153. Valimaki, M. J., Harju, K. J., and Ylikahri, R. H., Decreased serum selenium in alcoholics — a consequence of liver dysfunction, *Clin. Chem. Acta,* 13, 291, 1983.
154. Lombardi, B. and Oler, A., Choline deficiency fatty liver. Protein synthesis and release, *Lab. Invest.*, 17, 308, 1967.
155. Ruebner, B. H., Moore, J., Rutherford, R. B., Selegman, A. M., and Zuidema, G. D., Nutritional cirrhosis in Rhesus monkeys: electron microscopy and histochemistry, *Exp. Mol. Pathol.*, 11, 53, 1969.
156. Zeisel, S. H., DaCosta, K.-A., Franklin, P. D., Alexander, E. A., Lamont, J. T., Sheard, N. F., and Beiser, A., Choline, an essential nutrient for humans, *FASEB J.*, 5, 2093, 1991.
157. Lieber, C. S., Leo, M. A., Ki, M., DeCarli, L. M., and Sato, S., Choline fails to prevent liver fibrosis in ethanol-fed baboons but causes toxicity, *Hepatology*, 5, 561, 1985.
158. Rushmore, T. H., Lim, Y. P., Farber, L. E., and Goshal, A. K., Rapid lipid peroxidation in the nuclear fraction of rat liver induced by a diet deficient in choline and methionine, *Cancer Lett.*, 24, 251, 1984.
159. Perera, M. I. R., Betschart, J. M., Virji, M. A., Katyal, S. L., and Shinozuka, H., Free radical injury and liver tumor promotion, *Toxicol. Pathol.*, 15, 51, 1987.
160. Patek, A. J., Jr., Kendael, F. E., de Fritsch, N. M., and Hirsch, R. L., Cirrhosis-enhancing effect of corn oil, *Arch. Pathol.*, 82, 596, 1966.
161. Patek, A. J., Jr., Bowry, S. C., and Anuras, A., Alcohol and sucrose in choline deficiency cirrhosis in the rat, *Arch. Pathol.*, 96, 377, 1973.
162. Takada, A., Ohara, N., Matsuda, Y., Sawae, G., and Takeuchi, J., Effects of long-term alcohol administration on the development of fatty cirrhosis in choline-deficient rats, *Digestion*, 6, 83, 1972.
163. Mezey, E., Potter, J. J., and Brandes, D., Effects of a choline-deficient diet on the induction of drug- and ethanol-metabolizing enzymes and on the alteration of rates of ethanol degradation by ethanol and phenobarbital, *Biochem. Pharmacol.*, 24, 1975, 1975.
164. Barak, A. J., Tuna, D. J., and Sorell, M. F., Relationship of ethanol to choline metabolism in the liver: a review, *Am. J. Clin. Nutr.*, 26, 1234, 1973.

165. Thompson, J. A. and Reitz, R. G., A possible mechanism for the increased oxidation of choline after chronic ethanol ingestion, *Biochem. Biophys. Acta,* 545, 381, 1979.

166. McClain, C. J., Van Thiel, D. H., Parker, S., Badzin, L. K., and Gilbert, H., Alteration in zinc, vitamin A, and retinol-binding protein in chronic alcoholics: a possible mechanism for night blindness and hypogonadism, *Alcoholism,* 3, 135, 1979.

167. Majumdar, S. K., Shaw, G. K., and Thompson, A. D., Vitamin A utilization status in chronic alcoholic patients, *Int. J. Vitam. Nutr. Res.,* 58, 273, 1983.

168. Bell, H., Nilsson, A., Norum, K. R., Pedersen, L. B., Raknerud, N., and Rasmussen, M., Retinol and retinyl esters in patients with alcoholic liver disease, *J. Hepatol.,* 8, 26, 1989.

169. Ray, M. B., Mendenhall, C. L., French, S. W., and Gartside, P. J., Serum vitamin A deficiency and increased intrahepatic expression of cytokeratin antigen in alcoholic liver disease, *Hepatology,* 8, 1019, 1988.

170. Mendenhall, C., Seef, L., Diehl, A. M., Nelles, M. J., Aigius, C., Ghosn, S., and French, S. W., Antibodies to hepatitis B and C virus in alcoholic hepatitis and cirrhosis; their prevalence and clinical relevance, *Hepatology,* 14, 581, 1991.

171. French, S. W., Wong, K., Nanji, A., Arseneau, R., and Mendenhall, C., The role of the Ito cell in fibrogenesis in alcoholic liver disease, in *Biomedical and Social Aspects of Alcohol and Alcoholism,* Kuriyama, K., Takada, A., and Ishii, H., Eds., Elsevier, Amsterdam, 1988, 767.

172. French, S. W., Nanji, A. A., and Mobarhan, S., Dietary fats modulate the effect of ethanol on hepatic vitamin A, *Hepatology,* 10, 702, 1989.

173. Leo, M. A., Lowe, N., and Lieber, C. S., Potentiation of ethanol-induced hepatic vitamin A depletion by phenobarbital and butylated hydroxytoluene, *J. Nutr.,* 117, 70, 1987.

174. Mobarhan, S., Layden, T. J., Friedman, H., Kunigk, A., and Donahue, P., Depletion of liver and esophageal epithelium vitamin A after chronic moderate ethanol consumption in rats: inverse relationship to zinc nutriture, *Hepatology,* 6, 615, 1986.

175. Mobarhan, S., Seitz, H. K., Russell, R. M., Mehta, R., Hupert, J., Friedman, H., Layden, T. J., Meydani, M., and Langenberg, P., Age-related effects of chronic ethanol intake on vitamin A status in Fisher 344 rats, *J. Nutr.,* 121, 510, 1991.

176. Sato, M. and Lieber, C. S., Hepatic vitamin A depletion after chronic ethanol consumption in baboons and rats, *J. Nutr.,* 111, 2015, 1981.

177. French, S. W., Miyamoto, K., Wong, K., Jui, L., and Briere, L., Role of the Ito cell in liver parenchymal fibrosis in rats fed alcohol and a high fat-low protein diet, *Am. J. Pathol.,* 132, 73, 1988.

178. Takahashi, H., Wong, K., Jui, L., Nanji, A. A., Mendenhall, C. S., and French, S. W., Effect of dietary fat on Ito cell activation by chronic ethanol intake and controls: a long-term serial morphometric study on alcohol-fed and control rats, *Alcoholism Clin. Exp. Res.,* 15, 1060, 1991.

179. Okanoue, T., Burbige, E. J., and French, S. W., The role of the Ito cell in pervenular and intralobular fibrosis in alcoholic hepatitis, *Arch. Pathol. Lab. Med.,* 107, 459, 1983.

180. Maher, J. J., Hepatic fibrosis caused by alcohol, *Semin. Liver Dis.,* 10, 66, 1990.

181. Minato, Y., Hasumura, Y., and Takeuchi, J., The role of fat-storing cells in Disse space fibrogenesis in alcoholic liver disease, *Hepatology*, 3, 359, 1983.

182. Mak, K. M., Leo, M. A., and Lieber, C. S., Alcoholic liver injury in baboons: transformation of lipocytes to transitional cells, *Gastroenterology*, 87, 188, 1984.

183. Horn, R., Junge, J., and Christoffersen, P., Early alcoholic liver injury: activation of lipocytes in acinar zone 3 and correlation to degree of collagen formation in the disse space, *J. Hepatol.*, 3, 333, 1986.

184. Mak, K. M. and Lieber, C. S., Lipocytes and transitional cells in alcoholic liver disease: a morphometric study, *Hepatology*, 8, 1027, 1988.

185. Kent, G., Gay, S., Inouye, T., Bahu, R., Minick, O. T., and Popper, H., Vitamin A-containing lipocytes and formation of type III collagen in liver injury, *Proc. Natl. Acad. Sci. U.S.A.*, 73, 3719, 1976.

186. Furr, H. C., Clifford, A. J., Smith, L. M., and Olson, J. A., The effect of dietary fatty acid composition on liver retinyl ester (vitamin A ester) composition in the rat, *J. Nutr.*, 119, 581, 1989.

187. Grummer, M. A. and Erdman, J. W., Jr., Effect of chronic ethanol consumption and moderate or high fat diet upon tissue distribution of vitamin A in rats fed either vitamin A or β-carotene, *Nutr. Res.*, 6, 61, 1986.

188. Senoo, H. and Wake, K., Suppression of experimental hepatic fibrosis by administration of vitamin A, *Lab. Invest.*, 52, 182, 1985.

189. Davis, B. H. and Madri, J. A., Vitamin A administration diminishes type I and III collagen production during carbon tetrachloride-induced hepatic fibrosis, *Hepatology*, 7, 1091, 1987.

190. Leo, M. A. and Lieber, C. S., Hepatic fibrosis after long-term administration of ethanol and moderate vitamin A supplementation in the rat, *Hepatology*, 3, 1, 1983.

191. Kim, C.-I., Leo, M. A., Lowe, N., and Lieber, C. S., Effects of vitamin A and ethanol on liver plasma membrane fluidity, *Hepatology*, 8, 735, 1988.

16 Protein-Calorie Malnutrition in Alcoholic Liver Disease

INTRODUCTION

For many years an association between protein-calorie malnutrition (PCM), chronic alcoholism, and alcoholic liver disease has been recognized.[1-3] In spite of this long-term recognition, the role of malnutrition in the development and progression of the disease is still unclear and controversial.

ETHANOL AND LIVER DISEASE

It is unequivocal that ethanol is hepatotoxic and capable of producing liver injury independent of nutrition deficiency. Epidemiologic studies[4,5] indicate that when alcohol intake is diminished, i.e., during Prohibition in the U.S. or wine shortages in France during World War II, the incidence of deaths from cirrhosis significantly decreased. In our own studies, linear regression analyses indicated that alcohol intake was a significant and independent factor in the development of alcoholic hepatitis either alone or combined with cirrhosis.[6] However, this relationship was not seen with other forms of the alcoholic disease, i.e., fatty liver or cirrhosis alone (not in combination with alcoholic hepatitis). In more controled animal studies, fatty liver was predictably produced in rats on a high-fat diet when ethanol was substituted for carbohydrate.[7] Some have suggested that this is the result of carbohydrate deficiency.[8,9] Others have shown that the amount[10] and type of dietary fat[11] are critical contributing factors in the severity of the fatty liver. Indeed, polyunsaturated dietary lipids in combination with ethanol appear to be more potent inducers of a fatty liver. On this regimen,

French and associates have produced in rats fat, fibrosis, and necrosis while maintaining good overall nutrition.[11]

In baboons, again on a high-polyunsaturated fat, low-carbohydrate diet, both fatty liver and cirrhosis was produced[12] without obvious changes in nutrition. Further, healthy human volunteers with and without a history of alcoholism all developed severe fatty liver after controlled heavy ethanol intake supplied as either a supplement to diet or as an isocaloric substitution for carbohydrate.[13,14] Hence, the evidence is very strong that ethanol is hepatotoxic and independent of nutrition in its ability to injure the liver. However, fatty liver is not typically a life-threatening disease like alcoholic hepatitis and cirrhosis.[6] Indeed, only about 20% of heavy drinkers develop cirrhosis and 8% get no pathology of any type.[15] Even in the baboon study, only about one third developed cirrhosis and none developed alcoholic hepatitis. This suggests that other cofactors contribute to the progression of the diseases to the more serious stages.

MALNUTRITION AND LIVER DISEASE

Malnutrition, independent of alcohol, has been linked to human liver disease. Significant loss of organ mass and protein content results from chronic starvation,[16] occurring in every organ of the body except the brain. However, clinically recognized liver failure is a late finding in starvation. In the early stages, enzyme systems are depleted, especially those of microsomal origin, resulting in a prolongation of the clearance of many drugs and toxins[17] and the inadequate synthesis of visceral proteins (i.e., albumin, transferrin, etc.).[18] As a result of inadequate lipoprotein synthesis, fat is inadequately transported from the liver and the severe fatty liver of Kwashiorkor results. However, cirrhosis is not a common feature of calorie and protein deprivation.

Starvation and protein deprivation are not the only types of malnutrition associated with liver pathology. Obesity may also be associated with liver disease.[19-21] Here the histology more closely resembles that seen in the alcoholic, i.e., moderate to severe fatty metamorphosis with necrosis, polymorphonuclear cellular infiltration, and in some instances "alcoholic" hyalin (Mallory bodies). Here, fibrosis of all types may be present, i.e., perivenular, centrolobular, periportal, and pericellular. In one recent study[23] in which sequential biopsies were obtained, the progression from fatty liver to inflammation to fibrosis and ultimately cirrhosis has been documented, but the progression was slow. Indeed, cirrhosis was seen in as many as

24% of the patients in one study.[20] Thus, the pathology may be identical to that seen in alcoholic hepatitis. To semantically differentiate the two diseases, the former has been termed "nonalcoholic steatohepatitis". In addition to the absence of alcohol, other apparent clinical differences are a greater predilection for females (approximately 80%) and an unusually high incidence of diabetes mellitus, up to 74% in one series.[21] Here the pathophysiology of the liver injury is unclear, but the histology suggests a similarity to that produced by alcohol excess. What has been established is that when jejunoileal bypass surgery is performed on such patients, the pathology progresses very rapidly during the period of weight loss.[22]

TECHNIQUES USED TO ASSESS NUTRITION STATUS

The biological response to calorie and protein deprivation is multifaceted. Just as liver injury may be associated with changes in bilirubin metabolism (i.e., serum bilirubin), enzyme leakage (i.e., serum alanine amino transferase (ALT) and aspartate amino transferase (AST)), protein metabolism of coagulation factors (i.e., prothrombin time), etc., so, too, a spectrum of physical findings and laboratory tests have been proposed to diagnose the presence and predict the severity of PCM. Many of these tests are more familiar to dieticians than clinicians. Therefore, before beginning a discussion of the nutritional changes in the PCM of the alcoholic, it is appropriate to establish the criteria used to assess this disease. The following are commonly used techniques in the diagnosis:

DIETARY RECALL HISTORY

The information obtained from dietary recall histories has been questioned. It is difficult for the normal individual to remember the types and amounts of foods consumed on a daily basis. This may be compounded by the presence of alcoholism. However, when performed by trained individuals the validity of these histories has been documented.[24] Eagles and Longman reported that the dietary recall histories taken from 28 alcoholics admitted to a metabolic ward correlated quite closely with their weighed and recorded food intakes, thus demonstrating that carefully performed histories do offer relatively accurate and useful information.

ANTHROPOMETRIC TESTS

Anthropometry is defined as the science of measuring the human body and its parts.

Percent ideal weight — The percent of ideal weight is derived from a table[25] based on the patient's height and weight. Because of the ease with which height and weight data can be obtained, the percent of ideal weight is a commonly used assessment for PCM. However, in the alcoholic with liver disease, caution must be exercised in the interpretation of such data. Fluid retention is a common clinical feature manifest as edema and/or ascites. In our series,[26] even with mild alcoholic hepatitis without cirrhosis, ascites was present in 24% of the patients. When present, such fluid retention can mask the severity of the weight loss. Although total body water can be measured by isotope dilution techniques, these are typically not performed except as sophisticated research tools. Simpler estimates, though less reliable, have been obtained by weighing the patient initially and after vigorous diuresis when dry weight has been achieved. This difference in observed weight represents the net change resulting from a loss of retained fluid plus a gain in dry weight associated with improved nutrition and abstinence from alcohol. The amount of weight gain associated with such nutrition therapy was approximated from the average weight increase in patients with alcoholic hepatitis who on initial examination demonstrated a reduced ideal body weight and gave a history of weight loss but were without ascites or edema. Such patients were observed to gain an average of 2.5 kg/month, which presumably represented an increase in dry weight. Calculations of initial bodyweight free of fluid are:

$$FW = IBW \ (wet) - FBW \ (dry) + (2.5 \times T)$$

$$IBW \ (dry) = IBW \ (wet) - FW$$

Where FW = fluid weight, IBW = initial body weight, FBW = final body weight, and T = time in months between IBW (wet) and FBW (dry). Based on these approximations, the presence of tense ascites contributed an average of 14.0 kg (30.9 lb) to the observed initial weight, moderate ascites contributed an average of 6.0 kg (13.2 lb), and minimal ascites contributed 2.2 kg (4.9 lb).

Skin-fold thickness — Skin-fold measurements are estimates of body-fat stores. They have been measured in a variety of locations, i.e., the fatty tissue over the biceps, triceps, or the subscapular, abdominal, or ileac area. The most commonly used measurement is the triceps skin-fold thickness. Problems in the interpretation of skin-fold data include the determination of an appropriate comparison population from which normal values are derived as well as lack of reproducibility of these techniques by individuals performing the procedure.[27] Nonetheless, significant correlations between the skin-fold measurements and clinical morbidity and mortality rate have been reported.[28,29]

Mid-arm muscle circumference and area — Mid-arm muscle circumference (MAMC) and area (MAMA) are indirectly estimates of skeletal muscle mass based on the direct measurement of mid-arm circumference and triceps skin-fold thickness (TSF). Using the following formula

$$MAMA\ (men) = \frac{(MAMC - \pi \times TSF)^2}{4\pi} - 10$$

$$MAMA\ (women) = \frac{(MAMC - \pi \times TSF)^2}{4\pi} - 6.5$$

the data obtained compares closely with those measured by direct computerized tomography[30] with an average error of 7.7%.

CREATININE: HEIGHT INDEX (CHI):

The CHI is another estimate of muscle mass. Unlike the anthropometric tests, this assessment is based upon the 24-h urine content of creatinine. Healthy muscle produces creatinine at a relatively constant rate in proportion to the muscle mass. Hence, as chronic muscle wasting decreases muscle mass, there is a proportional decrease in the daily (24-h) urine level of creatinine.[31-33] Values are expressed as percent of normal age- and sex-matched controls relative to the patients height. Hence, the name creatinine: height index. There are technical problems inherent in collecting a 24-h urine sample for this analysis. Usually, a 72-h collection is obtained to minimize the magnitude of error. Other factors affecting urinary creatinine excretion include large amounts of meat in the diet, altered renal function, and drugs such as steroids which alter muscle metabolism. Nonetheless, when properly performed, the CHI remains one of the better predictors of lean body skeletal mass.

VISCERAL PROTEINS

In addition to skeletal muscle protein there are also a large number of nonmuscle proteins, termed visceral proteins, whose body concentrations are decreased during PCM and have therefore been used to diagnose and monitor the course of the malnutrition. Those most commonly measured are transport proteins circulating in the blood; thus, they are easily obtained for measurement in the laboratory. They include albumin with a half-life of approximately 21 d, transferrin with a half-life of 8 d, prealbumin with a half-life of 2 d, and retinol-binding protein with a half-life of 0.5 d. Balance studies with albumin[35,36] reveal that low-protein diets result in almost immediate decrease in synthesis rate, but there is a concomitant or perhaps compensatory reduction in the rate of degradation which is already slow. In addition, a redistribution occurs from the intestinal tract to the intravascular space. Thus, the net observed reduction in serum albumin concentrations reflecting PCM is very slow to develop with a similarly long recovery time. This has led many to conclude that those visceral proteins with short half-lives are more sensitive and responsive to the changes in PCM and hence are better "tools" to monitor the state of nutrition. Unfortunately, changes in their serum concentrations reflect other abnormalities which have occurred either concomitant with or independent of the malnutrition.[34] These include micronutrient deficiencies such as zinc, iron (in the case of prealbumin and transferrin), of vitamin A (in the case of retinol-binding protein). Also, infections of any type, thyroid dysfunction, liver disease, and renal disease can each alter visceral protein synthesis and/or degradation resulting in marked changes in their serum concentrations independent of the state of nutrition. Yet, in spite of this lack of specificity, these tests are widely used as indicators of nutrition and have been shown to correlate well with both morbidity and mortality.[28,29] In the case of alcoholic liver disease, the reduction in visceral proteins may be as much a reflection of the inability of the liver to synthesize proteins after toxic injury as it is a result of shortages in the amino acid pool associated with malnutrition.

IMMUNE FUNCTION

Human immune function is maintained by a complex multifaceted system designed to protect the host from outside injurious agents (i.e., infectious organisms, exogenous "foreign materials"). To provide adequate protection, changes in the immune state must be capable of a rapid and sometimes massive response. This necessitates an energy source and an adequate amino acid pool capable of accommodating rapid cell replication as well as the synthesis of large amounts of proteinaceous materials such as antibodies and cytokines. It is not surprising then that protein and calorie deprivation are closely associated with immune dysfunction affecting almost every aspect, i.e., humoral response, phagocytosis, complement system, and especially cell mediated immunity.[43] It is beyond the scope of this chapter to detail all of the immunologic alterations associated with PCM. Some of the more common dysfunctions include loss of thymic, splenic, and lymph node mass,[37,38] decreased lymphopoiesis,[39,40] anergy,[39,42,45] depressed antibody responses to vaccination,[38] and at times an increased globulinemia.[41] This latter finding is usually attributed to past or present infections. For purposes of evaluating PCM, the two tests of immune status most commonly employed are the total lymphocyte count and skin test responsiveness (delayed cutaneous hypersensitivity (DCH)). Problems associated with tests of immune function are similar to those with most of the other parameters used to assess nutrition, i.e., lack of specificity. Some of the nonnutrition variables capable of altering immune responses, especially the DCH, include age, race, sex, geographic location, malignant diseases, and infections. A variety of clinically used drugs can also significantly influence the immune response. Shortcomings in the use of skin tests to assess PCM have been summarized in an excellent article by Twomey et al.[45]

ALCOHOLISM AND PROTEIN-CALORIE MALNUTRITION

WITHOUT LIVER DISEASE

Having established the five groups of tests used to assess PCM, let us now consider its relationship to chronic alcoholism. In the absence of liver disease, malnutrition is seen in the alcoholic at a much lower frequency compared to that observed in patients with alcoholic liver disease. It has been suggested by some that the prevalence of malnutrition in the alcoholic without liver disease is related to their socioeconomic status.[46] This was supported by Goldsmith et al.,[47] who carefully examined 100 patients admitted to an alcoholic rehabilitation program. They observed that in 50 patients with middle incomes, only 8% were moderately malnourished; while in 50 patients with low incomes, 24% were moderately malnourished and an additional 8% were severely malnourished. Perhaps this is related to differences in nutrient intake, i.e., as income decreases, funds normally used for food and necessities are diverted to provide for continued alcohol consumption. In our study,[48] evaluating Department of Veterans Affairs (DVA) medical center patients predominately of lower incomes, we observed a mean caloric intake of 3722 kcal/d, which was 144% of their estimated energy requirements. However, ethanol constituted 58% of their intake, with protein calories contributing only 8.1% of daily intake and

TABLE 1
Prevalence of Nutritional Abnormalities Among Patients with Alcoholic Liver Disease

Parameter	Severity of liver disease (%)				
	Overall (284)	Mild (129)	Moderate (83)	Severe (72)	Controls (21)
Skin-fold thickness	84.8	79	85	95	76
Creatinine: height index	81.6	76	83	90	57
Skin tests (DCH)	81.0	74	79	96	48
Transferrin	66.6	35	92	94	14
Albumin	66.3	46	79	88	5
% Ideal weight	62.7	51	66	80	25
Mid-arm muscle circumference	45.7	36	50	58	28
Lymphocytes	44.5	35	50	55	14

Note: Values indicate % occurrence; (n) = Number of patients studied at each level of disease severity. The severity of liver disease was based on the level of jaundice and degree of coagulopathy.[48] Controls were alcoholics matched for age, sex, and amount of alcohol consumed but were without evidence of liver abnormalities.

with approximately 1/2 of the patients consuming less than 1 g/kg/d of dietary protein. These values compare closely to those reported by others.[27] However, in spite of the high calorie intake, nutritional abnormalities were observed at a very high frequency. Indeed, 76% had evidence of PCM. In order of frequency, loss of fat stores (decreased skin-fold thickness) was the most frequently observed abnormality followed by CHI (57%), and skin test abnormalities (DCH) in 30%. The prevalence and severity of these abnormalities are shown in Tables 1 and 2 for both alcoholics without and with varying levels of liver injury. Note that the controls were very similar to patients with mild liver injury with the abnormal parameters related to marasmus being more frequent and of greater severity. However, as the liver disease progressed to the more severe stages, the prevalence (Table 1) and severity (Table 2) of parameters related to kwashiorkor predominated.

WITH LIVER DISEASE

When liver disease was present along with alcoholism, the incidence of one or more of nutritional abnormalities rose to 100%. All of the

TABLE 2
Alterations in Nutritional Parameters Used to Diagnose Marasmus and Kwashiorkor

	Severity of liver disease (%)			
	Mild	Moderate	Severe	Controls
Marasmus parameters				
% Ideal weight	98	92	89	100
Skin-fold thickness	71	68	60	73
Creatinine: height index	76	63	64	84
Mid-arm muscle circumference	97	92	91	100
Kwashiorkor parameters				
Albumin	100	77	66	100
Transferrin	100	73	63	100
Lymphocytes	100	100	91	100
Skin tests	77	58	54	70
Totals (mean)				
Marasmic	86.4	80.1	76.4	89
Kwashiorkor	94.2	77.0	68.6	93
Nutrition score	90.3	78.6	72.5	91

Note: Each of the values are expressed as percent of normal so that they can be combined into a total mean nutritional score. The lower the percent from normal (100%) indicates the greater degree of nutrition deficit.

parameters increased in frequency (Table 1) and severity (Table 2) as the severity of the liver disease increased. As in the alcoholic without liver disease, the most frequently observed abnormalities occurred in estimates of fat stores, CHI and DCH.

Shown in Table 3 are the prevalence of these eight parameters grouped according to their primary association with either calorie deprivation (marasmus) or protein deprivation (kwashiorkor). The diagnosis of marasmus required abnormalities in at least three of its four diagnostic parameters (i.e., percent ideal weight, skin-fold thickness, mid-arm muscle circumference, or creatinine: height index). The diagnosis of kwashiorkor required abnormalities in at least three of its four diagnostic parameters (i.e., albumin, transferrin, numbers of circulating lymphocytes, or skin test responsiveness). Isolated abnormalities are listed as abnormal but not diagnostic. All of the patients had complete prospective nutritional assessments. Because n varied between severity groups, prevalence is expressed as percent of total for each group.

TABLE 3
Prevalence of Kwashiorkor and Marasmus as Related to
Clinical Liver Disease

	Severity of liver disease (%)			
Classification of malnutrition	None (21)	Mild (129)	Moderate (83)	Severe (72)
Kwashiorkor	0	2.3	13.3	8.3
Marasmus	0	42.6	14.5	5.6
Both kwashiorkor and marasmus	0	4.6	47.0	72.2
Abnormal but not diagnostic	75.9	50.4	25.3	13.9
Normal	24.1	0	0	0

Note: (n) = Number of patients studied at each level of disease severity. To test the hypothesis that the prevalence of malnutrition was ordered with respect to disease severity, mild to moderate to severe, Bartholomew's test[49] for order was performed for total kwashiorkor (i.e., the sum of kwashiorkor alone and kwashiorkor and marasmus in combination) and total marasmus (the sum of marasmus alone and kwashiorkor and marasmus in combination). All were significant, p <0.005. Abnormal but not diagnostic changes showed a reverse order being highest in alcoholics without liver disease (None).

PROGNOSTIC RELATIONSHIP OF NUTRITION TO ALCOHOLIC LIVER DISEASE

Numerous mathematical analyses have been reported in the past to establish a means to predict the severity of the liver disease.[50-53] Most noted an association between acute mortality and the visceral protein albumin,[50,51,53] but attributed these changes to a failing liver which was injured too severely to synthesize the protein (a hypothesis not necessarily supported by studies related to albumin synthesis.[54] With one exception,[50] all failed to recognize the close association of the global nutritional status with severity of the liver disease and focused only on the clinical and biochemical features associated with the disease. Table 4 shows the relationship of each of the nutritional parameters to 30-d mortality in a group of 350 patients with varying degrees of alcoholic hepatitis and/or cirrhosis.[29] Note that the nutritional status utilizing all of the eight nutritional parameters had a much better predictive value for acute (30 d) survival

TABLE 4
Thirty-Day Mortality Associated with Nutritional Parameters

Nutrition parameters	Severity of PCM (%)			χ^2	$p \leq$
	Mild	Moderate	Severe		
Total nutrition	2	15	52	51	10^{-9}
	(100)	(209)	(33)		
Kwashiorkor (K)	0	17	31	37	10^{-8}
	(115)	(164)	(73)		
Marasmus (M)	5	13	40	35	10^{-8}
	(50)	(193)	(50)		
Albumin	5	23	23	24	10^{-5}
	(168)	(131)	(48)		
Creatinine: height index	2	6	21	22	10^{-5}
	(90)	(67)	(160)		
Transferrin	4	16	23	21	10^{-4}
	(144)	(60)	(125)		
DCH	4	2	23	18	10^{-3}
	(46)	(46)	(173)		
Fat stores	9	9	21	11	10^{-2}
	(94)	(101)	(157)		
Total lymphocytes	11	15	26	11	10^{-2}
	(224)	(48)	(75)		
Percent ideal weight	14	16	0	<1	NS
	(298)	(52)	(2)		
MAMC	15	14	0	<1	NS
	(299)	(52)	(1)		

Note: Values are expressed as percent mortality. (n) Indicates the number of patients evaluated with mild, moderate, or severe malnutrition. Parameters are listed according to the degree to which changes in each correlate with changes in mortality. Total nutrition is determined by the sum of all the parameters normalized to percent of lower limits ÷ number of parameters on which data is available. K is estimated from four parameters: albumin, transferrin, total lymphocytes, and DCH. M is estimated from five parameters: percent of ideal weight, fat stores, mid-arm muscle circumference (MAMC), creatinine height index, and DCH (delayed cutaneous hypersensitivity). Values for K and M are determined by the sum of the parameters ÷ number of parameters on which data is available. *p* Values are determined by chi square (χ^2). NS = not significant.

From Mendenhall, C. L. et al., *Am. J. Clin. Nutr.*, 43, 213, 1986. With permission. ©*Am. J. Clin. Nutr.* American Society for Clinical Nutrition.

TABLE 5
Acute and Long-term Mortality in Alcoholic
Hepatitis Associated with Varying Degrees
of PCM

Duration of follow-up (months)	Severity of PCM (%)			
	Mild (110)	Moderate (209)	Severe (33)	p
1	2	15	52	<0.001
6	7	31	67	<0.001
12	14	43	76	<0.001

Note: Values = percent mortality; (n) = number of patients; p at each time period is determined by chi square.

From Mendenhall, C. L., et al., *Am. J. Clin. Nutr.*, 43, 213, 1986. With permission. ©*Am. J. Clin. Nutr.* American Society for Clinical Nutrition.

($p = 10^{-9}$) than albumin alone ($p = 10^{-5}$), although admittedly both were highly sufficient.

Table 5 shows that this association between nutrition and survival persisted long term as well, being a highly significant predictor for 1-, 6-, and 12-month mortality.

PATHOPHYSIOLOGY

Although the accompaniment of PCM with alcoholic liver disease is a recognized phenomenon, the mechanism(s) responsible for the malnutrition is unclear. As with so many of the changes associated with alcoholism, it appears to be multifaceted.

Poor dietary intake is probably the predominant contributor. The addictive need for alcohol is strong, while available funds are limited. As a result, money needed for food is diverted for the acquisition of alcohol. This, in part, explains the close relationship between socioeconomic class and nutritional deficiency.[47] There may also be a striking loss of appetite as well as nausea and vomiting associated with the liver disease,[56] which contributes to the poor dietary intake. Leevy et al.[57] observed that 64% of 172 alcoholics gave dietary histories of inadequate food intake. Mezey and

Faillace[58] noted that 68% of 56 patients with minimal alcoholic liver injury (fatty liver) ate less than one meal a day prior to admission.

Other involved mechanisms include cytokine and endocrine regulation of nutritional status. Cachectin/tumor necrosis factor alpha has been observed to be increased during alcoholic hepatitis[79-81] and most likely accounts for some of the anorexia and ensuing malnutrition. We,[59] as well as others,[60] have observed a severe depression in insulin-like growth factor (IGF-1) in patients with varying degrees of alcoholic liver injury and PCM. In our studies,[59] serum concentrations were severely reduced in every patient with a mean concentration 77% below those observed in age-matched nonalcoholic controls. Of interest is the fact that a lesser reduction, 18.6%, was observed in alcoholics without clinical liver disease. Using partial correlation analysis, we were able to show that although the severity of liver dysfunction and the histopathologic alterations paralleled the plasma IGF-1 concentrations, IGF-1 alterations were most significantly and independently related to the level of malnutrition, thus suggesting a cause and effect relationship.

Energy wasting also occurs. In our patients,[48] caloric intake before hospitalization far exceeded estimated energy requirements, suggesting that energy wasting had occurred. The existence of PCM in the presence of high calorie intake is consistent with similar reported observations,[61,62] but has not been adequately explained. Presumably, it occurs from metabolic alterations associated with ethanol metabolism[63] and/or from altered metabolism of micro- and macronutrients.[64-67] Indeed, both acute alcohol toxicity and alcoholic liver disease increase the metabolic rate[63] and hence the energy requirements. Further, the "hardcore" alcoholic obtains 50% or more of daily caloric intake from ethanol,[27,48] but ethanol provides predominantely "empty" calories devoid of vitamins or minerals and squanders much of its derived energy as heat. Hence, levels of stored energy, adenosine triphosphate (ATP), are depleted, and multiple micronutrient deficiencies are frequent.[27,57]

Digestive abnormalities resulting from alcohol-induced intestinal and pancreatic injury have been reported. Intestinal malabsorption, as measured by Dy-xylose malabsorption, was observed in patients with alcoholic cirrhosis.[68,69] Others failed to confirm these findings.[70,71] Note that D-xylose testing in cirrhosis may be abnormal for reasons other than altered absorption, i.e., renal insufficiency, expanded extracellular space for D-xylose diffusion (ascites), and altered hepatic metabolism.[72] Histopathologic changes are also conflicting. Some[73] have described edema inflammation, fibrosis of the villi, and dilatation of the crypts of Lieber-kühn, while others observed little or no change.[74,75]

Alcoholic pancreatitis and/or pancreatic insufficiency may also be present and produce malabsorption. The reported prevalence of pancreatitis in this patient population varies from 10 to 50%,[76,77] but does not seem to correlate with either the occurrence or the severity of the malnutrition. None of our patients had symptomatology indicating pancreatitis or malabsorption and only 11.4% of the entire group had elevated serum amylase concentrations.[56]

Independent of intestinal or pancreatic pathology, malabsorption of lipids could result from poor micellar formation. Indeed, in one study[78] cirrhotic patients had a 63% reduction in the production and excretion of bile acids per day compared to comparable patients without cirrhosis. This mechanism appears to be more contributing to the steatorrhea seen in alcoholic cirrhosis than altered pancreatic function.[77]

Metabolic alterations associated either with alcohol excess or active liver injury could impair nutrient utilization and influence nutritional status. It is beyond the scope of this article to delineate all the reported metabolic changes associated with alcohol toxicity and/or cirrhosis except to say that they are numerous and involve protein, carbohydrate, lipids, vitamins, and minerals and that at times such metabolic abnormalities may have a significant effect on nutritional status. It would seem that all of these possibilities are contributing in varying degrees to the observed malnutrition in this population.

NUTRITION THERAPY IN ALCOHOLIC LIVER DISEASE

Because of the long-recognized association between alcoholic liver disease and PCM, reports of nutrition therapy have appeared in the literature for more than 50 years. One of the earliest and largest was by Dr. Patek and was initially reported in 1941[82] on 54 patients followed for 5 years. The study was expanded in 1948[83] to include ultimately 124 patients with alcoholic cirrhosis. Unfortunately, his control group of 486 similar patients were not randomized, but were treated at different hospitals around the city (Boston). Nonetheless, his results indicated a striking improvement in survival when a diet high in protein and supplemented by B vitamins was provided (controls, 61%, 296/486, mortality at 1 year vs. dietary treated patients, 35% mortality, 43/124). Since then, a large number of small or anecdotal reports have appeared,[84-97] ranging in numbers of patients studied from 4 to 52 and in duration of treatment from 3 d to 60 d. Most had no controls and were designed only to evaluate improvement in the nutritional status from pretreatment levels or to evaluate dietary protein tolerance in malnourished patients presenting with hepatic encephalopathy. Although individually they are of little value, collectively they strongly indicate that these patients do tolerate high-protein intake[92,94] and are capable of improving their nutritional status. Five of these reports give adequate acute survival data and have a comparable comparison group. These are summarized in Table 6.

By combining these reports, data can be obtained on a total of 174 patients (89 controls and 85 treated patients). Note that these results are not too different from those reported by Patek[82] 50 years ago, i.e., control mortality, 34% (30/89) vs. nutrition therapy treatment, 15% (13/85). These data would suggest that vigorous repletion of nutrition deficits was indicated in malnourished alcoholic liver disease patients.

TABLE 6
Acute Mortality in Patients with Protein-Calorie Malnutrition and Alcoholic Liver Disease

Lead author	Publication year	Treatment mode	Daily intake[a] (kcal/d)		Duration (d)	Mortality (%)	
			Treated	Controls		Treated	Controls
Nasrallah and Galambros[84]	1980	IV	3280–3340	1400	28	0/17 (0)	4/18 (22)
Mendenhall et al.[90]	1985	PO	3236 ± 102	2313 ± 121	30	3/18 (17)	7/34 (21)
Naveau et al.[94]	1986	IV	1110 ± 690 (PO) 40 kcal/kg (IV)	2124 ± 670	28	7/20 (35)[b]	7/18 (39)
Achord[95]	1987	IV	2000	1200	21	1/14 (7)	3/14 (21)
Cabre et al.[97]	1991	PO	2115	1320 ± 75	23–25	2/16 (13)	9/19 (47)
Total						13/85 (15)	30/89 (34)

a Values, when available, represent mean ± SEM or range of daily caloric intake (combined PO and IV). Values without SEM or range indicate a controlled intake with either IV or nasogastric intubation.

b 70% of patients developed sepsis during parenteral treatment, which may have altered outcome.

REFERENCES

1. Pateck, A. J., Toth, M. G., Saunders, G. A., et al., Alcohol and dietary factors in cirrhosis: an epidemiological study of 304 alcoholic patients, *Arch. Intern. Med.*, 135, 1053, 1975.
2. Korsten, M. A. and Lieber, C. S., Nutrition in the alcoholic, *Med. Clin. North Am.*, 63, 963, 1979.
3. Jacobs, R. M. and Sorrell, M. F., The role of nutrition in the pathogenesis of alcohol liver disease, *Semin. Liver Dis.*, 1, 224, 1981.
4. Lelbach, W. K., Cirrhosis in the alcoholic and its relation to the volume of alcohol abuse, *Ann. N.Y. Acad. Sci.*, 252, 85, 1975.
5. Lelbach, W. K., Epidemiology of alcohol liver disease, in *Progress in Liver Disease*, Vol. 5, Popper, H. and Schaffner, F., Eds., Grune & Stratton, New York, 494.
6. Chedid, A., Mendenhall, C. L., Gartside, P., French, S., Weesner, R. E., Roselle, G. A., Chen, T., Rabin, L., and the VA Cooperative Study Group, Prognostic factors in alcoholic liver disease, *Am. J. Gastroenterol.*, 86, 210, 1991.
7. Lieber, C. S., Jones, D. P., Mendelson, J., et al., Fatty liver, hyperlipemia and hyperuricemia produced by prolonged alcohol consumption despite adequate dietary intake, *Trans. Assoc. Am. Physicians*, 76, 289, 1963.
8. Rao, G. A. and Larkin, E. C., Fatty liver: a nutritional problem of carbohydrate deprivation and concomitant ethanol ingestion, *Nutr. Res.*, 4, 903, 1984.
9. Rao, G. A. and Larkin, E. C., Forum: role of nutrition in causing the effects attributed to chronic alcohol consumption, *Med. Sci. Res.*, 16, 53, 1988.
10. Lieber, C. S. and DeCarli, L. M., Quantitative relationship between dietary fat and the severity of the alcoholic fatty liver, *Am. J. Clin. Nutr.*, 23, 474, 1970.
11. Nanji, A. A., Mendenhall, C. L., and French, S. W., Beef fat prevents alcoholic liver disease in the rat, *Alcoholism Clin. Exp. Res.*, 13, 15, 1989.
12. Lieber, C. S. and DeCarli, L. M., An experimental model of alcohol feeding and liver injury in the baboon, *J. Med. Primatol.*, 3, 153, 1974.
13. Lieber, C. S., Jones, D. P., and DeCarli, L. M., Effects of prolonged ethanol intake: production of fatty liver despite adequate diets, *J. Clin. Invest.*, 44, 1009, 1965.
14. Lieber, C. S. and Rubin, E., Alcoholic fatty liver in man on a high protein and low fat diet, *Am. J. Med.*, 44, 200, 1968.
15. Christoffersen, P. and Nielsen, K., Histologic changes in human liver biopsies from chronic alcoholics, *Acta Pathol. Microbiol. Scand. Sect. A*, 80, 557, 1972.
16. Kriefer, M., Uber die Atrophie der menschlichen Orange bei Inanition, *Z. Agnes. Anat. Konstitutional.*, 7, 87, 1921.
17. Krishnaswamy, K. and Naidu, A. N., Microsomal enzymes in malnutrition as determined by plasma half-life of antipyrine, *Br. Med. J.*, 1, 538, 1977.
18. McFarlane, H., Adcock, K. J., Cooke, A., Ogbeide, M. I., Adeshina, H., Taylor, G. O., Reddy, S., Gurney, J. M., and Mordie, J. A., Biochemical assessment of protein-calorie malnutrition, *Lancet*, 1, 392, 395, 1969.
19. Attar, A. and Anuras, S., Spectrum of liver disease in obesity, *Hepatology*, 1, 1133, 1980.

20. Adler, M. and Schaffner, F., Fatty liver hepatitis and cirrhosis in obese patients, *Am. J. Med.*, 67, 811, 1979.
21. Itoh, S., Yougal, T., and Kawagoe, K., Comparison between non-alcoholic steatohepatitis and alcoholic hepatitis, *Am. J. Gastroenterol.*, 82, 650, 1987.
22. Holzbach, R. T., Wieland, R. G., Lieber, C. S., DeCarli, L. M., Koepke, K. R., and Green, S. G., Hepatic lipid in morbid obesity. Assessment at and subsequent to jejunoileal bypass, *N. Engl. J. Med.*, 290, 296, 1974.
23. Powell, E. E., Cooksley, W. G. E., Hanson, R., Searle, J., Holliday, J. W., and Powell, L. W., The natural history of nonalcoholic steatohepatitis: a follow-up study of 42 patients for up to 21 years, *Hepatology*, 11, 74, 1990.
24. Eagles, J. A. and Longman, D., Reliability of alcoholics reports of food intake, *J. Am. Diet Assoc.*, 42, 136, 1963.
25. Bray, G. A., Ed., Obesity in America, National Institutes of Health Publ. No. 79-359, U.S. Department of Health and Human Services, Washington, D.C., 1979.
26. Goldberg, S., Mendenhall, C., Anderson, S., et al., VA Cooperative Study on Alcoholic Hepatitis IV: The significance of clinically mild alcoholic hepatitis — describing the population with minimal hyperbilirubinemia, *Am. J. Gastroenterol.*, 81, 1029, 1986.
27. Antonow, D. R. and McClain, C. J., Nutrition and alcoholism, in *Alcohol and the Brain*, Tarter, R. E. and Van Thiel, D. H., Eds., Plenum Press, New York, 1985, 81.
28. Buzby, G. P., Mullen, J. L., Matthews, D. C., Hobbs, C. L., and Rosato, E. F., Prognostic nutritional index in gastrointestinal surgery, *Am. J. Surg.*, 139, 160, 1980.
29. Mendenhall, C. L., Tosch, T., Weesner, R. E., et al., VA Cooperative Study on Alcoholic Hepatitis II: Prognostic significance of protein-calorie malnutrition, *Am. J. Clin. Nutr.*, 43, 213, 1986.
30. Heymsfield, S. B., McManus, C., Smith, J., Stevens, V., and Nixon, D. W., Anthropometric measurement of muscle mass: revised equations for calculating bone free arm muscle area, *Am. J. Clin. Nutr.*, 36, 680, 1982.
31. Krause, M. V. and Mahan, L. K., Eds., Nutritional status of the individual. The assessment of nutritional status, in *Food, Nutrition, and Diet Therapy*, 7th Ed., W. B. Saunders, Philadelphia, 1984, 192.
32. Forbes, G. S. and Bruining, G. I., Urinary creatinine excretion and lean body mass, *Am. J. Clin. Nutr.*, 29, 1359, 1976.
33. Viteri, F. E. and Alvarado, J., The creatinine height index: its use in the estimation of the degree of protein depletion and repletion in protein calorie malnourished children, *Pediatrics*, 46, 696, 1970.
34. Golden, M. H., Transport proteins as indices of protein status, *Am. J. Clin. Nutr.*, 35, 1159, 1982.
35. James, W. P. T. and Hay, A. M., Albumin metabolism effect of the nutritional state and the dietary protein intake, *J. Clin. Invest.*, 47, 1958, 1968.
36. Hoffenberg, R., Black, E., and Brock, J. F., Albumin and γ globulin tracer studies in protein depletion states, *J. Clin. Invest.*, 45, 143, 1966.
37. Aschkenasy, A., Influence of alimentary proteins on the size of blood lymphocytes in the rat. The role of thymus in this effect, *Isr. J. Med. Sci.*, 1, 552, 1965.

38. Nalder, B. N., Mahoney, A. W., Ramakrishnan, R., and Hendricks, G. S., Sensitivity of the immunological response to the nutritional status of rats, *J. Nutr.*, 102, 535, 1972.

39. Smythe, P. M., Brereton-Stiles, G. G., Grace, H. J., Mafoyane, A., Schonland, M., Coovadia, H. M., Loening, W. E. K., Parent, M. A., and Vos, G. H., Thymolymphatic deficiency and depression of cell-mediated immunity in protein-calorie malnutrition, *Lancet,* 2, 939, 1971.

40. Aschkenasy, A., Dietary protein and amino acids in leucopoiesis, *World Rev. Nutr. Diet,* 21, 152, 1975.

41. Scrimshaw, N. S., Taylor, C. E., and Gordon, J. E., Interactions of nutrition and infection, *WHO Monogr. Ser.,* 57, 143, 1968.

42. Smith, N. J., Khadroui, S., Lopez, V., and Hamza, B., Cellular immune response in Tunisian children with severe infantile malnutrition, in *Malnutrition and the Immune Response,* Suskind, r. M., Ed., Raven Press, New York, 1977, 105.

43. Gross, R. L., Role of nutrition in immunologic function, *Physiol. Rev.,* 60, 188, 1980.

44. Cunningham-Rundles, S., Effects of nutritional status on immunological function, *Am. J. Clin. Nutr.,* 35, 1202, 1982.

45. Twomey, P., Ziegler, D., and Rombeau, J., Utility of skin testing in nutritional assessment: a critical review, *J. Parenter. Enter. Nutr.,* 6, 50, 1982.

46. Neville, J. N., Eagles, J. A., Samson, G., et al., Nutritional status of alcoholics, *Am. J. Clin. Nutr.,* 21, 1329, 1968.

47. Goldsmith, R. H., Iber, F. L., and Miller, P. A., Nutritional status of alcoholics of different socioeconomic class, *J. Am. Coll. Nutr.,* 2, 215, 1983.

48. Mendenhall, C. L., Anderson, S., Weesner, R. E., et al., Protein-calorie malnutrition associated with alcoholic hepatitis, *Am. J. Med.,* 76, 211, 1984.

49. Fleiss, J. L., Ed., Comparison of proportions from many samples, in *Statistical Methods for Rates and Proportions,* J. Wiley and Sons, New York, 1973, 92.

50. Conn, H. O., A peek at the Child-Turcotte classification, *Hepatology,* 1, 673, 1981.

51. Pugh, R. W. H., Murray-Lyon, I. M., Dawson, J. L., et al., Transection of the oesophagus for bleeding oesophageal varices, *Br. J. Surg.,* 60, 646, 1983.

52. Maddrey, W. C., Boitnott, J. K., Bedine, M. S., Weber, F. L., Jr., Mezey, E., and White, R. I., Jr., Corticosteroid therapy of alcoholic hepatitis, *Gastroenterology,* 75, 193, 1978.

53. Orrego, H., Israel, Y., Blake, J. E., et al., Assessment of prognostic factors in alcoholic liver disease: toward a global quantitative expansion of severity, *Hepatology,* 3, 896, 1983.

54. Mendenhall, C. L. and Wilkinson, P., Serum albumin turnover in normal subjects with cirrhosis measured by I[131] labelled human albumin, *Clin. Sci.,* 25, 281, 1963.

55. Rothschild, M. A., Oratz, M., Zimmon, D., Schreiber, S. S., Weiner, I., and Van Caneghem, A., Albumin synthesis in cirrhotic subjects with ascites studies with carbonate-^{14}C, *J. Clin. Invest.,* 48, 344, 1969.

56. Mendenhall, C. L. and the VA Cooperative Study Group on Alcoholic Hepatitis, Alcoholic hepatitis, *Clin. Gastroenterol.,* 10, 417, 1981.

57. Leevy, C. M., Baker, H., tenHove, W., et al., B-complex vitamins in liver disease of the alcoholic, *Am. J. Clin. Nutr.*, 16, 339, 1965.

58. Mezey, E. and Faillace, L. A., Metabolic impairment and recovery time in acute ethanol intoxication, *J. Nerv. Ment. Dis.*, 153, 445, 1971.

59. Mendenhall, C. L., Chernausek, S. D., Ray, M., Gartside, P. S., Roselle, G. A., and Grossman, C. J., The interactions of insulin-like growth factor I (IGF-I) with protein-calorie malnutrition in patients with alcoholic liver disease: VA cooperative study on alcoholic hepatitis VI, *Alcohol Alcoholism*, 24, 319, 1989.

60. Schrimpff, R. M., Lebrec, D., Donnadieu, M., and Repellin, A. M., Serum somatomedin activity measured as sulphation factor in peripheral hepatic and renal veins of patients with alcoholic cirrhosis, *Acta Endocrinol.*, 88, 729, 1978.

61. Bunout, D., Gattas, V., Iturriaga, H., Perez, C., Pereda, T., and Ugarte, G., Nutritional status of alcoholic patients: its possible relationship to alcoholic liver damage, *Am. J. Clin. Nutr.*, 38, 469, 1983.

62. Mills, P. R., Shenkin, A., Anthony, R. S., McLelland, A. S., Main, A. N. H., MacSween, R. N. M., and Russell, R. I., Assessment of nutritional status and *in vivo* immune responses in alcoholic liver disease, *Am. J. Clin. Nutr.*, 38, 849, 1983.

63. Pirola, R. C. and Liever, C. S., The energy cost of the metabolism of drugs, including ethanol, *Pharmacology*, 7, 185, 1972.

64. Leevy, C. M., Tamburro, C., and Smith, F., Alcoholism, drug addiction, and nutrition, *Med. Clin. North Am.*, 54, 1567, 1970.

65. Lindenbaum, J. and Leiber, C. H., Alcohol-induced malabsorption of vitamin B_{12} in man, *Nature*, 224, 806, 1969.

66. Halsted, C. H., Robles, E. A., and Mezey, E., Intestinal malabsorption in folate-deficient alcoholics, *Gastroenterology*, 64, 526, 1973.

67. Arky, R. A., The effect of alcohol on carbohydrate metabolism: carbohydrate metabolism in alcoholics, in *The Biology of Alcoholism*, Kissin, B. and Begleiter, H., Eds., Plenum Press, New York, 1977, 197.

68. Baraona, E., Orrego, H., Fernandez, O., et al., Absorptive function of the small intestine in liver cirrhosis, *Am. J. Dig. Dis.*, 7, 318, 1962.

69. Friedman, A. I. and McEwan, G., Small bowel absorption in portal cirrhosis with ascites, *Am. J. Gastroenterol.*, 39, 114, 1963.

70. Fast, B. B., Wolfe, S. J., Stormont, J. M., et al., Fat absorption in alcoholics with cirrhosis, *Gastroenterology*, 37, 321, 1959.

71. Sun, D. C., Albacete, R. A., and Chen, J. K., Malabsorption studies in cirrhosis of the liver, *Arch. Intern. Med.*, 119, 567, 1967.

72. Marin, G. A., Clark, M. L., and Senior, J. R., Distribution of d-xylose in sequestered fluid resulting in false positive tests for malabsorption, *Ann. Intern. Med.*, 69, 1155, 1968.

73. Astaldi, G. and Storsselli, E., Peroral biopsy of the intestinal mucosa in hepatic cirrhosis, *Am. J. Dig. Dis.*, 5, 603, 1960.

74. Summerskill, W. H. J. and Moertel, C. G., Malabsorption syndrome associated with anicteric liver disease, *Gastroenterology*, 42, 380, 1962.

75. Marin, G. A., Clark, M. L., and Senior, J. R., Studies of malabsorption occurring in patients with Laennec's cirrhosis, *Gastroenterology*, 56, 727, 1969.

76. Jacobs, R. M. and Sorrell, M. F., The role of nutrition in the pathogenesis of alcoholic liver disease, *Semin. Liver Dis.*, 1, 244, 1981.

77. Mezey, E., Liver disease and nutrition, *Gastroenterology*, 74, 770, 1978.

78. Vlahcevic, Z. R., Buhac, I., Farrar, J. T., et al., Bile acid metabolism in patients with cirrhosis. I. Kinetic aspects of cholic acid metabolism, *Gastroenterology*, 60, 491, 1971.

79. McClain, C. J. and Cohen, D. A., Increased tumor necrosis factor production by monocytes in alcoholic hepatitis, *Hepatology*, 9, 349, 1989.

80. Khoruts, A., Stahnke, L., McClain, C. J., Logan, G., and Allen, J. I., Circulating tumor necrosis factor, interleukin-1 and interleukin-6 concentrations in chronic alcoholic patients, *Hepatology*, 13, 267, 1991.

81. Bird, G. L. A., Sheron, N., Goka, A. K. J., Alexander, G. J., and Williams, R. S., Increased plasma tumor necrosis factor in severe alcoholic hepatitis, *Ann. Int. Med.*, 112, 917, 1990.

82. Patek, A. J., Jr. and Post, J., Treatment of cirrhosis of the liver by a nutritous diet and supplements rich in vitamin b complex, *J. Clin. Invest.*, 20, 481, 1941.

83. Patek, A. J., Jr., Post, J., Ralnoff, O. D., Mankin, H., and Hillman, R. W., Dietary treatment of cirrhosis of the liver, *J. Am. Med. Assoc.*, 139, 543, 1948.

84. Nasrallah, S. M. and Galambros, J. T., Amino acid therapy of alcoholic hepatitis, *Lancet*, 2, 1276, 1980.

85. Rudman, D., Kutner, M., Ansley, J., Jansen, R., Chipponi, J., and Bain, R. P., Hypotyrosinemia, hypocystinemia, and failure to retain nitrogen during total parenteral nutrition of cirrhotic patients, *Gastroenterology*, 81, 1025, 1981.

86. Smith, J., Horowitz, J., Henderson, M., and Heymsfield, S., Enteral hyperalimentation in undernourished patients with cirrhosis and ascites, *Am. J. Clin. Nutr.*, 35, 56, 1982.

87. Keohane, P. P., Attrill, H., Grimble, G., Spiller, R., Frost, P., and Silk, D. B. A., Enteral nutrition in malnourished patients with hepatic cirrhosis and acute encephalopathy, *J. Parenter. Enter. Nutr.*, 7, 346, 1983.

88. McGhee, A., Henderson, M., Millikin, W. J., Jr., Bleier, J. C., Vogel, R., Kassouny, M., and Rudman, D., Comparison of the effects of hepatic-aid and a casein modular diet on encephalopathy, plasma amino acids, and nitrogen balance in cirrhotic patients, *Ann. Surg.*, 197, 288, 1983.

89. Horst, D., Grace, N. D., Conn, H. O., Schiff, E., Schenker, S., Viteri, A., Law, D., and Atterbury, C. E., Comparison of dietary protein with an oral, branched chain-enriched amino acid supplement in chronic portal-systemic encephalopathy: a randomized controlled trial, *Hepatology*, 4, 279, 1984.

90. Mendenhall, C., Bongiovanni, G., Goldberg, S., Miller, B., Moore, J., Rouster, S., Schneider, D., Tamburro, C., Tosch, T., Weesner, R., and the VA Cooperative Study Group on Alcoholic Hepatitis, VA cooperative study on alcoholic hepatitis III. Changes in protein-calorie malnutrition associated with 30 days of hospitalization with and without enteral nutritional therapy, *J. Parenter. Enter. Nutr.*, 9, 590, 1985.

91. Christie, M. L., Sack, D. M., Pomposelli, J., and Horst, D., Enriched branched-chain amino acid formula versus a casein-based supplement in the treatment of cirrhosis, *J. Parenter. Enter. Nutr.*, 9, 671, 1985.

92. Diehl, A. M., Boitnott, J. K., Herlong, F., Potter, J. J., Van Duyn, M. A., Chandler, E., and Mezey, E., Effects of parenteral amino acid supplementation in alcoholic hepatitis, *Hepatology,* 5, 57, 1985.
93. Okita, M., Watanabe, A., and Nagashima, H., Nutritional treatment of liver cirrhosis by branched-chain amino acid-enriched nutrient mixture, *J. Nutr. Sci. Vitaminol.,* 31, 291, 1985.
94. Naveau, S., Pelletier, G., Poynard, T., Attali, P., Poitrine, A., Buffet, C., Etienne, J. P., and Chaput, J. C., A randomized clinical trial of supplementary parenteral nutrition in jaundiced alcoholic cirrhotic patients, *Hepatology,* 6, 270, 1986.
95. Achord, J. L., A prospective randomized clinical trial of peripheral amino acid-glucose supplementation in acute alcoholic hepatitis, *Am. J. Gastroenterol.,* 82, 871, 1987.
96. Bonkovsky, H., Jafri, I., Singh, R., Cotsonis, G., and Slaker, D., Treatment of alcoholic hepatitis with parenteral nutrition and oxandrolone: a randomized controlled train. II. Effects of nitrogen metabolism, *Hepatology,* 12(2), 978, 1990.
97. Cabre, E., Gonzalez-Huix, F., Abad-Lacruz, A., Esteve, M., Acero, D., Fernandez-Bañares Xiol, X., and Gassull, M. A., Effect of enteral nutrition on the short-term outcome of severely malnourished cirrhotics: a randomized control trial, *Gastroenterology,* 98, 715, 1990.

17 Nutritional Support in Alcoholic Liver Disease

INTRODUCTION

Although the majority of alcoholics without liver disease do not suffer from prominent malnutrition (especially protein calorie malnutrition),[1-6] alcoholics with liver disease regularly are malnourished.[7-11] For this reason, it seems reasonable that patients with alcoholic liver disease should benefit from nutritional support. The objective of this chapter is to review the topic of nutritional support in alcoholic liver disease.

MALNUTRITION IN ALCOHOLIC HEPATITIS

There is evidence demonstrating a correlation between the degree of severity of alcoholic hepatitis and the severity of malnutrition. In the Veterans Administration Cooperative Study on Alcoholic Hepatitis #119, 363 patients with this disorder were evaluated, and 284 patients had complete nutritional assessments. These patients had a mean ethanol consumption of 228 g/d and were categorized according to the severity of disease using the Maddrey's discriminant function and then analyzed separately. These patients had a mean age of approximately 50 years, and the alcohol consumption was similar in the patients with mild, moderate, or severe alcoholic hepatitis (222 to 234 g/d). All 3 groups had a drinking history of more than 20 years. Patients with mild disease took 45% of their calories as alcohol and had a creatinine: height index (CHI) of 76%, while patients with severe disease took 50% of their calories as alcohol and had a CHI of 64%. Dietary recall history also revealed that protein intake ranged from a mean of 7.0 to 7.9% of total calories in all three groups, but that nonalcohol calorie intake decreased stepwise from 2015 ± 98 in mild alcoholic hepatitis (AH) and 1809 ± 108 in moderate AH to 1552 ± 99 in severe AH cases. Similarly, albumin and transferrin were also depressed in a stepwise fashion (reflecting both liver disease and malnutrition). In general, the severity of alcoholic hepatitis correlated with the degree of malnutrition.[7] The stratification by severity of disease (that correlated well with the degree of malnutrition) was very accurate because the frequency of ascites and encephalopathy increased as the severity worsened. Of even more importance, the severity of disease (and the degree of malnutrition) correlated well with the morality, with a 1-year survival rate of 91% for the mild group, 75% for the moderate group, and 46% for the severe group. This study is the largest and most detailed study evaluating the nutritional status of patients with alcoholic hepatitis. This study and the topic of malnutrition in alcoholic liver disease are covered in greater detail in Chapter 16.

MALNUTRITION IN STABLE CIRRHOTICS

Malnutrition not only affects patients with alcoholic hepatitis, but also patients with stable alcoholic cirrhosis with ascites. Antonow and McClain evaluated 25 such patients and showed that while they had stable, adequate liver function as assessed by aminopyrine breath test (4.1 ± 0.6% vs. 7.5 ± 0.5% in controls), they had depleted visceral proteins when compared with normals (albumin, 3.1 ± 0.1 vs. 4.1 ± 0.2 mg/dl; prealbumin, 10.8 ± 0.9 vs. 26.0 ± 0.3 mg/dl; and retinol binding protein, 2.5 ± 0.4 vs. 6.8 ± 0.7 mg/dl). Anthropometric measurements of these stable cirrhotics were also depressed with arm muscle circumference of 51 ± 9% and triceps skin fold of 86 ± 6% when expressed as percent of normal. In addition, the CHI (indicators of muscle metabolism and lean body mass) was significantly depressed (71 ± 8% — normal 100%). Thus, even patients with well-compensated alcoholic cirrhosis have evidence of protein/calorie malnutrition.[12]

GOALS AND STRATEGIES FOR NUTRITIONAL SUPPORT IN ALCOHOLIC LIVER DISEASE

The goals of nutritional support in patients with alcoholic liver disease with or without portal-systemic encephalopathy are (1) maintenance of adequate nutrition, (2) enhancement of liver regeneration, and (3) prevention, amelioration, or correction of portal systemic encephalopathy.[13] In patients with alcoholic liver disease, who are already malnourished, it is not enough to maintain present nutritional status, but instead attempts should be made to initiate nutritional recovery.

The task of supplying nutrition for adequate nutritional recovery to patients with alcoholic liver disease is complicated because of the changes in the metabolism of carbohydrates, fats, proteins, vitamins, and minerals which usually accompany this disorder. These changes are fully described in previous chapters. In addition, chronic alcoholic patients can have marked electrolyte disturbances that can be life-threatening[14] and that frequently obligate the physician to modify the proportions of different nutrients, fluids, and minerals in the diet or formula provided. Because chronic alcohol ingestion followed by withdrawal is a dynamic process, active alcoholics with liver disease who are admitted to the hospital need careful monitoring of the serum electrolytes Na, K, Ca, P, and Mg during the initial course of therapy and at intermittent intervals thereafter.[14]

In general, it is better to postpone aggressive nutritional support in active alcoholics with liver disease for 3 or 4 d, because intense electrolyte disorders are likely to occur during this period. Indeed, hypokalemia, hypophosphatemia, and hypomagnesemia may be worsened by refeeding (commonly referred to as "refeeding syndrome"). In addition, it is better to have a complete assessment of the intravascular volume status of the patient, to correct any abnormalities and to control alcohol withdrawal syndrome if it is to occur. If the patient is alert, it is appropriate to offer a well-balanced diet *ad libitum* while avoiding overhydration and giving B vitamins, vitamin C, fat-soluble vitamins (if cholestasis is present or deficiency is suspected), and trace elements after evaluation for deficiency.

ELECTROLYTE DISTURBANCES IN ALCOHOLIC LIVER DISEASE

Real and apparent electrolyte disturbances are common in alcoholics and the most frequent causes are listed in Table 1. Hyponatremia is a frequent problem in patients with alcoholic liver disease.[15,16] When hyponatremia is detected, it is very important to search for evidence of intravascular depletion, to control the cause of depletion (vomiting, diarrhea, polyuria, perspiration, fever), and to restore the intravascular space with isonatremic IV fluids (the use of hypertonic saline or the increase of Na concentration in the total parenteral nutrition (TPN) solution is usually not necessary). Most hyponatremic patients have dilutional hyponatremia,

TABLE 1
Causes of Electrolyte Disturbances in Alcoholics

Hyponatremia
    Intravascular depletion (diarrhea, vomiting, polyuria, diuretics)
    Dilution (excessive water intake, increased ADH)
    K depletion
    Sequestration (ascites, edema)
    Artifactual (hyperlipemia)
Hypernatremia
    Extrarenal free water loss (lactulose, increased perspiration)
    Renal free water loss (osmotic diuresis, glucose, urea in GI bleeding)
    Iatrogenic (saline infusions)
Hypokalemia
    Potassium deficiency (poor intake, diarrhea, vomiting, diuretics)
    Repsiratory alkalosis
    β-Adrenergic stimulation (withdrawal syndrome)
    Insulin (glucose infusion)
Hyperkalemia
    K-sparing diuretics
    K supplements
    Azotemia
Hypophosphatemia
    Phosphorus deficiency (poor intake)
    Respiratory alkalosis
    Insulin (glucose or amino acid infusion)
    Renal tubular dysfunction with P loss
    Magnesium deficiency
Hypomagnesemia
    Magnesium deficiency (poor diet, diarrhea, ethanol, steatorrhea)
    Phosphorus deficiency
    Intracellular uptake (refeeding → ATP-Mg complex)
    Free fatty acid-Mg complex (secondary to alcohol withdrawal)
Hypocalcemia
    Hypoalbuminemia
    Mg deficiency (decreased parathyroid hormone (PTH) secretion, decreased response to PTH)
    Vitamin D deficiency (steatorrhea and poor liver activation)
    Steatorrhea (decreased Ca absorption with intestinal calcium soaps)
    Rhabdomyolysis (precipitation of Ca complexes)

which need to be managed with fluid restriction by decreasing the amount of free water given from the nutritional source or with medication administration.

Hypernatremia is a less common complication and is usually due to excessive loss of "free water"[15,16] that can be secondary to the use of lactulose,[17] to excessive perspiration, or to an inability to drink water in a patient receiving parenteral "iso-natremic" solutions. In this situation patients need to receive additional free water, either parenterally or enterally. Prompt recognition and treatment of hyponatremia and hypernatremia is important because both factors have been associated with increased mortality.[18,19]

Disturbances of serum potassium are also common. Alcoholics with liver disease are likely to have total body potassium depletion because of poor nutritional intake, decreased muscular mass, or excessive potassium loss (vomiting, diarrhea, diuretics). However, it is important to remember that some patients may have only minimal or no potassium deficiency and have mainly a shift of potassium from extracellular space into the cells, as may occur in respiratory alkalosis[20] or in patients with elevated epinephrine levels[21] due to alcohol withdrawal. Because of the potential catastrophic effects of hypokalemia, it is important to replace K by "IV runs" of 5 to 10 meq/h, at least during the acute phase, while obtaining frequent serum K levels in order to avoid dangerous hyperkalemia. After the patient stabilizes, it is adequate to give oral supplements, however, serum K must be monitored intermittently in all patients, but especially in those on K-sparing diuretics; in addition intravascular depletion and azotemia must be avoided.

Hyperkalemia is infrequent unless the patient develops kidney failure or is receiving potassium-containing salt substitutes and potassium-sparing diuretics. It is incumbent upon health care workers to stress to patients the potential danger of using potassium-containing salt substitutes (as many patients are on salt restriction) while taking potassium-sparing diuretics such as spironolactone.

Hypophosphatemia is a common,[22,23] multifactorial (see Table 1) and potentially life-threatening problem in the alcoholic. Many alcoholics are total-body phosphate deficient because of poor oral intake. Hypophosphatemia can worsen with refeeding because of insulin-mediated transfer of phosphorus to the intracellular space. Magnesium deficiency may also worsen this problem.[24,25] The serum phosphorus must be monitored carefully in alcoholic patients, and hypophosphatemia must be aggressively corrected.

Hypomagnesemia also is frequent in chronic alcoholics and may result from poor intake, poor absorption, excessive loss (in urine or diarrhea), phosphorus deficiency[26] or intracellular uptake. This disturbance can also worsen with refeeding because of shift to the intracellular space. Severe hypomagnesemia can cause alteration in mental status, tremor, convulsions, and even cardiac arrest. Therefore, magnesium deficiency with hypomagnesemia needs to be aggressively treated. In addition, low magnesium levels blunt the sensitivity of the parathyroid gland to low calcium and can cause hypocalcemia.[27] Other causes of hypocalcemia in alcoholics are also described in Table 1.

CAUSES OF MALNUTRITION IN ALCOHOLIC LIVER DISEASE

Alcoholics with liver disease have multiple reasons to be malnourished[28-36] including anorexia, altered taste sensation, diarrhea, nausea, vomiting (related to gastritis or pancreatitis), malabsorption, poor oral intake (in both quality and quantity), and metabolic disturbances (hypercatabolism, hypermetabolism, induction of microsomal ethanol-oxidizing system, etc.). In addition, because of the complications of liver disease (encephalopathy, ascites, GI bleeding) the patient may be offered unpalatable diets (low Na, low protein) or may be kept fasting for diagnostic or therapeutic procedures.

EFFECT OF NUTRITIONAL SUPPORT ON OUTCOME

The data is controversial suggesting that nutritional support improves survival in patients with alcoholic liver disease. However, a meta-analysis of the studies of therapy of patients with acute portal-systemic encephalopathy (mostly alcoholics) utilizing parenteral nutritional support including branched-chain amino acids (BCAA) showed a positive effect in survival for the patients receiving nonprotein plus protein calories (BCAA) when compared with those receiving nonprotein calories alone.[37] The rationale for the use of BCAA-enriched supplements was the observation that patients with alcoholic liver disease regularly have alterations on their plasma amino acid profile with an overall decrease in amino acids. The greatest reduction of these amino acids is at the expense of the BCAA leucine, isoleucine, and valine. At the same time, there is a mild increase in certain aromatic amino acids (AAA) like phenylalanine and tyrosine. These amino acid alterations have been postulated to contribute to the hepatic encephalopathy observed in some patients with alcoholic liver disease, and for this reason special amino acid formulations with high

BCAA and low AAA have been utilized to try to correct the amino acid profile, improve nutritional status, and improve mental status.

Theoretical advantage of BCAA supplements include:[28] (1) leucine-associated increased protein synthesis and decreased protein breakdown of skeletal muscle; (2) BCAA regulation of efflux of other amino acids across the myocyte membrane in conditions of catabolism and decreased insulin; (3) utilization of BCAA as an alternative energy source for skeletal muscle, brain, and heart; (4) increased metabolism of ammonia by muscle; (5) stimulation of hepatic protein synthesis when BCAA are given with other caloric sources; (6) decrease of plasma AAA due to increased protein synthesis and decreased proteolysis; (7) competition of BCAA with AAA for blood-brain transport; and (8) increase or norepinephrine synthesis in certain brain regions. Because of the increased cost of specialized amino acid formulations and because their advantage in clinical practice is not well documented, it is better to restrict their use to specific situations. One example would be their use as nutritional supplement for patients who develop portal systemic encephalopathy (PSE) without reaching optimal nitrogen intake despite the use of conventional therapy for PSE.

It is important to emphasize that to try to analyze the effect of nutritional support on encephalopathy, on nutritional status, and on outcome in patients with acute hepatic encephalopathy is very difficult. These studies involve patients who had different precipitating factors for their encephalopathy (volume depletion, sedatives, gastrointestinal bleeding, infection, etc.) and these factors have prognostic implications per se. Similarly, the management of these precipitating factors can affect the evolution of encephalopathy and the final outcome of the patient independently of any therapy directed at controlling the encephalopathy or malnutrition. Considering all these limitations, the suggestion that nutritional support has a positive effect on patient's survival, in the meta-analysis of these studies, is very encouraging, but not definitive proof. In addition, a study of total enteral nutrition (TEN) via tube feeding in severely malnourished cirrhotics (mostly alcoholics) with a BCAA-enriched balanced formula vs. encouraged ingestion of an equicaloric, equinitrogenous hospital diet, showed that tube-fed patients had a higher caloric intake (2115 vs. 1320 kcal) and that in-hospital mortality was lower in the tube-fed patients.[11] In all these studies[9,11,38-45] it is impossible to separate the beneficial effects of increased caloric and nitrogenous intake from those of the BCAA per se. Furthermore, the studies on parenteral nutrition include other confounding factors like the utilization of lipid emulsion as part of the nonprotein source of calories. This may be important because the study of Glynn et al. suggests that lipids per se may affect the course of PSE,[46] that is a factor that may be associated with final outcome. Another recent study exploring the effect of nutritional support in outcome is the VA Cooperative Study on Alcoholic Hepatitis.[53] The patients were divided in control group (34 patients) and treatment group (23 patients). The "controls" were given a 2500-kcal diet with protein content individualized for hepatic encephalopathy. The treatment group was given 2240 kcal as Hepatic Acid® (American McGaw, Irvine, CA) plus at least 1000 kcal as a hospital diet. Both groups were constantly encouraged to eat and had close medical and nursing supervision, and not surprisingly, caloric intake was excellent in both groups. However, the treatment group took a significantly greater amount of calories (3236 vs. 2313 kcal). Overall, mortality was similar in both groups. Because there was not a second control group with "not encouraged-*ad libitum*" diet intake, it is impossible to know if nutritional support per se is able to improve survival in alcoholic hepatitis (caloric intake in both groups was larger than what has been observed in patients outside nutrition studies). In the most recent VA Cooperative Study #275, "Protein-calorie therapy in combination with anabolic steroids in alcoholic hepatitis," preliminary, unpublished data shows a positive effect on survival utilizing nutritional support plus anabolic steroids in the subgroup of patients with moderate protein-calorie malnutrition.[64] In this study, all patients received a 2000-kcal, 75-g protein diet *ad libitum*. In addition, the treatment group was offered Hepatic Aid II® (American McGaw, Irvine, CA) to supplement 1600-kcal and 60-g protein equivalent a day plus oxandrolone 80 mg/d for 1 month followed by Hepatic Aid II® (1200 kcal plus 45-g protein equivalent) plus oxandrolone 40 mg/d for 56 additional days. The placebo controls were supplemented with 160 kcal plus 8 g of protein a day plus placebo pills. In this study, the mortality rate at 1 month was 22% in the placebo group vs. 9.5% in the treatment group ($p = 0.051$). The beneficial effect on mortality was maintained at 3 and 6 months with rates of 32 and 35% in the placebo group vs. 14 and 15% in the treatment group, at 3 and 6 months respectively ($p = 0.015$ and $p = 0.011$, respectively).

EFFECT OF NUTRITIONAL SUPPORT
ON HEPATIC ENCEPHALOPATHY
AND NUTRITIONAL STATUS

As mentioned before, interpretation of the effect of nutritional support in acute hepatic encephalopathy is very difficult because there are many factors that can affect the evolution of encephalopathy. The already mentioned meta-analysis of the controlled, randomized studies, published in the English language, of parenteral BCAA in patients with cirrhosis and acute portal systemic encephalopathy by Naylor and co-workers[37] showed that BCAA-enriched formulas were able to improve PSE. However, because there are many "noise factors" in the individual studies that were analyzed, this conclusion of the meta-analysis must be taken with caution (see Effect of Nutritional Support on Outcome).

Patients with latent (subclinical) and chronic stable portal systemic encephalopathy are the best ones to study with the effect of therapy on PSE because, when stable, they do not have the fluctuations in severity that are seen in acute PSE. Nonnutritional therapy like lactulose and liver transplant have been shown to be effective in chronic PSE. Nutrition intervention, in the form of pure vegetable diets or ornithine salts of branched-chain ketoacids also have been beneficial. We have summarized the effects of special diets and supplements on chronic stable PSE and found that current data suggest that BCAA supplementation, added to the maximal amount of protein tolerated by these patients (usually ≤ 40 g), may decrease the frequency of PSE decompensation.[28]

While the effects of nutritional support on mortality are controversial, it is clear that various modalities of nutritional support are able to improve nutritional status. Studies using high caloric density enteral feedings, BCAA supplementation, a "nutritious diet", standard TPN, and BCAA enriched TPN have shown that nutritional support improves the nutritional condition of patients having alcoholic liver disease with or without hepatic encephalopathy.[9,44,47-53]

One example of these studies is the VA Cooperative Study on Alcoholic Hepatitis. This study showed that nutritional status improved in patients with alcoholic hepatitis who abstained from alcohol and who received a high calorie, "nutritious diet". This study also showed that the CHI had further significantly greater improvement in the groups who received, in addition, a specialized supplement (BCAA-enriched formula) as compared with those on "nutritious diet" alone.

PROTEIN NEEDS FOR POSITIVE
NITROGEN BALANCE

The protein requirements needed in order to maintain positive nitrogen balance in patients with alcoholic liver disease are in the range of 60 to 80 g/d.[54,55] Chronic protein restriction below 60 g/d as treatment of chronic PSE is unacceptable because it leads to a negative nitrogen balance with progressive loss of muscular mass and worsening of overall nutritional status. Patients with diet-induced PSE can be treated with a short course of protein restriction of 40 g/d plus standard therapy with lactulose or similar agents, followed by prompt increase of protein intake to adequate amounts. In unusual circumstances when adequate amounts of nitrogen intake cannot be tolerated because of worsening of PSE, branched-chain amino acid supplements can be added to the maximal amount of protein that was tolerated without worsening PSE. This management is supported by the recent study by Weber et al.,[56] which demonstrated that leucine supplementation did not improve nitrogen balance or urinary 3-methyl-histidine in stable cirrhotics, but ammonia levels did improve. This suggested limited nutritional value of BCAAs, but a possible therapeutic role in chronic PSE.

PRACTICAL APPROACH TO
NUTRITIONAL SUPPORT

Many therapeutic modalities have been tried in patients with alcoholic liver disease; most of them have been directed at improving alcoholic hepatitis. Because the mechanism(s) of liver injury are unknown and the mortality is high in alcoholic hepatitis, limited benefit has been observed with these therapies. The most promising forms of therapy include methylprednisolone[57] (which seems helpful in the small group of patients with severe alcoholic hepatitis with spontaneous hepatic encephalopathy), propylthiouracil[58] (aimed to control the hypermetabolic state in alcoholic hepatitis), colchicine[59] (with the hope of inhibiting collagen synthesis and disease progression to cirrhosis), anabolic steroids,[60] and nutritional support. Of these forms of therapy, nutritional support is certainly the most available and the one that must be tried first, either alone or in combination with other therapeutic interventions.

A practical approach to the development of appropriate nutrition support for the patient with alcoholic hepatitis is outlined in Figure 1. In the

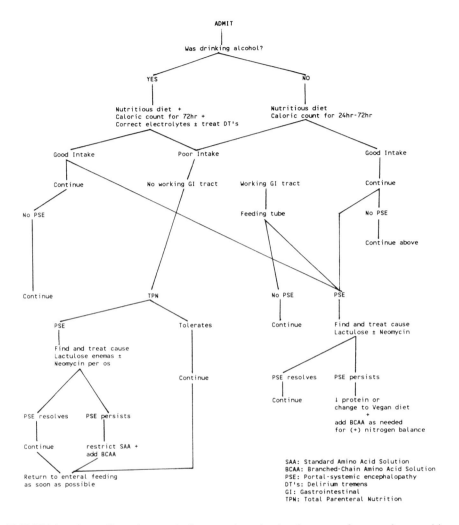

FIGURE 1.   An outline of a practical approach to the development of appropriate nutrition support for the patient with alcoholic hepatitis.

patient who has been actively drinking alcohol it is useful to first correct electrolyte disbalances and to treat and control withdrawal symptoms when present (this will facilitate control of electrolyte disorders and decrease the risk of having a feeding tube or TPN line pulled out). During this period (2 to 3 d), if the mental status of the patient is adequate, the patient can be offered a nutritious diet and a caloric count can be obtained. If the patient is able to ingest adequate amounts of calories and protein, this diet should be continued. If the patient develops encephalopathy and there is no evidence of other precipitating disorders (GI bleeding, sedatives, hypoxia, electrolyte or acid-base disturbances, volume depletion, infection, etc.), then protein could be restricted to as low as 20 g/d for 1 to 3 d and, as soon as mental status improves, protein intake must be increased to at least 60 g/d[54] and perhaps up to 1 to 1.5 g/kg/d[55,61] while giving lactulose and/or neomycin as needed. If, despite maximal medical therapy with lactulose/neomycin, an adequate protein intake cannot be obtained, the protein intake should be kept at the highest tolerated amount and then BCAA-enriched formula can be administered to supplement nitrogen intake (example: Hepatic-Aid®); another option is to use only vegetable protein.[62,63]

If the patient cannot eat adequate calories and has a functioning gastrointestinal tract, then a feeding tube should be placed and a standard isocaloric, isonitrogenous formula should be used following the guidelines already mentioned above. If the patient develops PSE without other precipitating factors, the amount of protein should be decreased until lactulose/neomycin controls the PSE and then protein must be increased to satisfy nitrogen requirements. If, despite medical therapy, standard feeding tube formula leads to the development of PSE, then the standard formula can be decreased until well tolerated and BCAA-enriched formula can be supplemented to meet nitrogen needs.

One infrequent problem in enterally fed patients with alcoholic liver disease is the development of steatorrhea secondary to pancreatic insufficiency. In this situation, supplementation with medium-chain triglycerides (MCT) while restricting long-chain triglycerides may be helpful. On the other hand, the use of pancreatic enzyme supplements, with or without control of gastric acidity (H_2-blockers or sodium bicarbonate), may correct most of the steatorrhea.

It is very important to emphasize the use of enteral nutrition over parenteral nutrition because of several factors like cost, risk of TPN line sepsis, preservation of the integrity of the gut mucosa and, theoretically, prevention of bacterial translocation and multiple organ failure.

If enteral nutrition is not possible, then TPN can be used, keeping in mind that it is important to return to the enteral route as soon as the small bowel shows evidence of recovered function. TPN can be started with a standard amino acid formula in increasing amounts until nitrogen needs are met. If the patients develops PSE, then standard therapy with lactulose/neomycin must be given. If the patient is still unable to tolerate the amount of amino acids needed to satisfy his nitrogen requirements, then the standard amino acids can be replaced by a BCAA-enriched solution specifically designed for liver disease (e.g., Hepatamine®). There is no reason to restrict lipid use in patients with alcoholic liver disease. Sometimes the patients are unable to "clear" triglycerides properly and for this reason triglycerides should be monitored weekly. If serum triglycerides are more than 250 mg/dl, then the lipid emulsion can be decreased, given over a longer period of time, or can be given every other day, every third day, or even once a week.

SUMMARY

There is a high rate of malnutrition in alcoholics with liver disease. In alcoholic hepatitis, the severity of malnutrition correlates with both the severity of liver disease and the mortality.

Nutritional support in active alcoholics with liver disease is complicated because these patients can have a wide range of electrolyte disturbances that may worsen because of the refeeding process, sometimes with life-threatening consequences. Also, the proportion of nutrients given may need to be modified according to complicating factors like electrolyte disturbances or concomitant disorders (pancreatic insufficiency, encephalopathy, ascites, etc.).

Nutritional support is able to improve nutritional status in patients with alcoholic liver disease. In some studies of severely malnourished alcoholic cirrhotics and in patients with alcoholic hepatitis (at least the ones with moderate protein calorie malnutrition), nutrition support has improved survival. Thus, it makes sense to give nutritional support to alcoholics with liver disease. Our current practice is to give these patients well-balanced diets or inexpensive enteral nutritional supplements, to meet their calorie and protein needs, and to secure nutritional recovery. If the patient develops PSE, we manage them by adding standard therapy with lactulose/neomycin. We reserve the use of BCAA supplements for those few patients who cannot achieve optimal calorie and nitrogen intake because of development of hepatic encephalopathy despite adequate therapy with lactulose/neomycin. We avoid parenteral nutrition as much as possible and when we use it, we do it for the shortest possible period of time and only when the small bowel is nonfunctioning.

REFERENCES

1. Neville, J. N., Eagles, J. A., Samson, G., et al., Nutritional status of alcoholics, *Am. J. Clin. Nutr.,* 21, 1329, 1980.
2. Tomaiolo, P. P. and Kraus, V., Nutritional status of hospitalized alcoholic patients, *JPEN,* 4, 1, 1980.
3. Hurt, R. D., Higgins, J. A., Nelson, R. A., et al., Nutritional status of a group of alcoholics before and after admission to an alcoholism treatment unit, *Am. J. Clin. Nutr.,* 34, 386, 1981.
4. Simko, V., Connell, A. M., and Banks, B., Nutritional status in alcoholics with and without liver disease, *Am. J. Clin. Nutr.,* 35, 197, 1982.
5. Goldsmith, R. H., Iber, F. L., and Miller, P. A., Nutritional status of alcoholics of different socioeconomic class, *J. Am. Coll. Nutr.,* 2, 215, 1983.
6. Dickson, B. J., Delaney, C. J., Walker, R. D., et al., Visceral protein status of patients hospitalized for alcoholism, *Am. J. Clin. Nutr.,* 37, 216, 1983.
7. Mendenhall, C. L., Anderson, S., Weesner, R. E., et al., Protein-calorie malnutrition associated with alcoholic hepatitis, *Am. J. Med.,* 76, 211, 1984.
8. Patek, A. J., Post, J., Ratnoff, O. D., et al., Dietary treatment of cirrhosis of the liver: result in one hundred and twenty-four patients observed during a ten year period, *J. Am. Med. Assoc.,* 138, 543, 1948.
9. Smith, J., Horowitz, J., Henderson, M., et al., Enteral hyperalimentation in undernourished patients with cirrhosis and ascites, *Am. J. Clin. Nutr.,* 35, 56, 1982.
10. Soberon, S., Pauley, M. P., Duplentier, R., et al., Metabolic effects of enteral formula feeding in alcoholic hepatitis, *Hepatology,* 7, 1204, 1987.
11. Cabre, E., Gonzales-Huix, F., Abad-La Cruz, A., et al., Effect of total enteral nutrition on the short-term outcome of severely malnourished cirrhotics: a randomized control trial, *Gastroenterology,* 98, 714, 1990.
12. Antonow, D. R. and McClain, C. J., Nutrition and alcoholism, in *Alcohol and the Brain,* Tarter, R. E. and Thiel, D. H., Eds., Plenum Press, New York, 1985, 81.
13. Fisher, J. E. and Bower, R. H., Nutritional support in liver disease, *Surg. Clin. North Am.,* 61, 653, 1981.
14. Marsano, L. and McClain, C. J., Effects of alcohol on electrolytes and minerals, *Alcohol Health Res. World,* 13, 255, 1989.
15. Fraser, C. L. and Arieff, A. I., Fluid and electrolyte disorders and the central nervous system, in *Clinical Disorders of Fluid and Electrolyte Metabolism,* 4th ed., Maxwell, M. H., Kleeman, C. R., and Narins, R. G., Eds., McGraw-Hill, New York, 1987, 1153.
16. Arieff, A. and Papadakis, M. A., Hyponatremia and hypernatremia in liver disease, in *The Kidney in Liver Disease,* 3rd ed., Epstein, M., Ed., Williams and Wilkins, Baltimore, MD, 1988, 73.
17. Nelson, D. C., McGrew, W. R. G., and Hoyumpa, A. M., Hypernatremia and lactulose therapy, *J. Am. Med. Assoc.,* 249, 1295, 1983.
18. Warren, S. E., Mitas, J. A., and Swerdlin, A. H. R., Hypernatremia in hepatic failure, *J. Am. Med. Assoc.,* 243, 1257, 1980.
19. Arroyo, V., Rodes, J., Gutierrez-Lizarraga, M. A., et al., Prognostic value of spontaneous hyponatremia in cirrhosis with ascites, *Am. J. Dig. Dis.,* 21, 249, 1976.

20. Burnell, J. M., Villamil, M. F., Uyeno, B. T., et al., The effect in humans of extracellular pH change on the relationship between serum potassium concentration and extracellular potassium, *J. Clin. Invest.*, 35, 935, 1956.
21. Mendelson, J. H., Biologic concomitants of alcoholism (part I), *N. Engl. J. Med.*, 283, 71, 1970.
22. Stein, J. H., Smith, W. O., and Ginn, H. E., Hypophosphatemia in acute alcoholism, *Am. J. Med. Sci.*, 252, 78, 1966.
23. Knochel, J. P., Derangements of univalent and divalent ions in chronic alcoholism, in *The Kidney in Liver Disease*, 3rd ed., Epstein, M., Ed., Williams and Wilkins, Baltimore, MD, 1988, 132.
24. Cronin, R. E., Ferguson, E., Shannon, W. A., et al., Skeletal muscle injury after Mg depletion in the dog, *Am. Physiol. (Renal Fluid Electrolyte Physiology)*, 243, F113, 1982.
25. Whang, R. and Welt, L. G., Observations in experimental magnesium depletion, *J. Clin. Invest.*, 42, 305, 1963.
26. Fuller, T. J., Carter, N. W., Barcenas, C., et al., Reversible changes of the muscle cell in experimental phosphorus deficiency, *J. Clin. Invest.*, 57, 1019, 1976.
27. Estep, H., Shaw, W. A., Watlington, C., et al., Hypocalcemia due to hypomagnesemia and reversible parathyroid hormone unresponsiveness, *J. Clin. Endocrinol. Metab.*, 29, 842, 1969.
28. Marsano, L. and McClain, C. J., Nutrition in alcoholic liver disease, *JPEN*, 15, 337, 1991.
29. Van Goidsenhoven, G. E., Henke, W. J., Vacca, J. B., et al., Pancreatic function in cirrhosis of the liver, *Am. J. Dig. Dis.*, 8, 160, 1963.
30. Baker, H., Frank, O., and Ziffer, H., Effect of hepatic disease on liver B-complex vitamin titers, *Am. J. Clin. Nutr.*, 14, 1, 1964.
31. Losowsky, M. S. and Walker, B. E., Liver disease and malabsorption, *Gastroenterology*, 56, 589, 1969.
32. Mezey, E., Jow, E., Slavin, R. E., et al., Pancreatic function and intestinal absorption in chronic alcoholism, *Gastroenterology*, 59, 657, 1970.
33. Leevy, C. M., Tamburro, C., Smith, F., et al., Alcoholism, drug addiction and nutrition, *Med. Clin. North Am.*, 54, 1567, 1970.
34. Halsted, C. H., Robles, E. A., and Mezey, E., Intestinal malabsorption in folate deficient alcoholics, *Gastroenterology*, 64, 526, 1973.
35. Pirola, R. C. and Lieber, C. S., Hypothesis: energy wasting in alcoholism and drug abuse: possible role of hepatic microsomal enzymes, *Am. J. Clin. Nutr.*, 29, 90, 1976.
36. Arky, R. A., The effect of alcohol on carbohydrate metabolism: carbohydrate metabolism in alcoholics, in *The Biology of Alcoholism*, Vol. 1, Kissin, B. and Begleiter, H., Eds., Plenum Press, New York, 1971, 197.
37. Naylor, C. D., O'Rourke, K., Detsky, A. S., et al., Parenteral nutrition with branded-chain amino acids in hepatic encephalopathy: a meta-analysis, *Gastroenterology*, 97, 1033, 1989.
38. Strauss, E., Santos, W. R., Cartapatti Da Silva, E., et al., A randomized controlled clinical trial for the evaluation of the efficacy of an enriched branched-chain amino acid solution compared to neomycin in hepatic encephalopathy (abstr.), *Hepatology*, 3, 862, 1983.

39. Gluud, C., Dejgaard, A., Hardt, F., et al., Preliminary treatment results with balanced amino acid infusion to patients with hepatic encephalopathy (abstr.), *Scan. J. Gastroenterol.,* 18(Suppl. 86), 19, 1983.

40. Wahren, J., Denis, J., Desurmont, P., et al., Is intravenous administration of branched-chain amino acids effective in the treatment of hepatic encephalopathy? A Multicenter Study, *Hepatology,* 3, 475, 1983.

41. Fiaccadori, F., Ghinelli, F., Pedretti, G., et al., Branched chain amino acid enriched solutions in the treatment of hepatic encephalopathy: a controlled trial, in *Hepatic Encephalopathy in Chronic Liver Failure,* Capocaccia, L., Fischer, J. E., and Rossi-Fanelli, F., Eds., Plenum Press, New York, 1984, 323.

42. Michel, H., Bories, P., Aubin, J. P., et al., Treatment of acute hepatic encephalopathy in cirrhosis with a branched-chain amino acids enriched versus a conventional amino acids mixture: a controlled study of 70 patients, *Liver,* 5, 282, 1985.

43. Cerra, F. B., Cheung, N. K., Fischer, J. E., et al., Disease specific amino acid infusion (F080) in hepatic encephalopathy: a prospective, randomized, double-blind, controlled trial, *JPEN,* 9, 288, 1985.

44. Rossi-Fanelli, F., Cangiano, C., Capocaccia, L., et al., Use of branched chain amino acids for treating hepatic encephalopathy: clinical experience, *Gut,* 27, 111, 1988.

45. Caballeria, E., Arago, J. V., Masso, R. M., et al., Tratamiento de la encefalopatia hepatica con aminoacidos de cadena ramificada (BCAA) por via oral. I. Encefalopatia aguda, *Rev. Esp. Enferm. Apar. Dig.,* 72, 116, 1987.

46. Glynn, M. J., Powell-Tuck, J., Reaveley, D. A., et al., High lipid parenteral nutrition improves portasystemic encephalopathy, *JPEN,* 12, 457, 1988.

47. Patek, A. J., Post, J., Ratnoff, O. D., et al., Dietary treatment of cirrhosis of the liver: results in one hundred and twenty-four patients observed during a ten year period, *J. Am. Med. Assoc.,* 138, 543, 1948.

48. Nasrallah, S. M. and Galambos, J. T., Amino acid therapy of alcoholic hepatitis, *Lancet,* 2, 1276, 1980.

49. Rudman, D., Kutner, M., Ansley, J., et al., Hypotyrosinemia, hypocystinemia and failure to retain nitrogen during total parenteral nutrition of cirrhotic patients, *Gastroenterology,* 81, 1025, 1981.

50. Achord, J. L., A prospective randomized clinical trial of peripheral amino acid-glucose supplementations in acute alcoholic hepatitis, *Am. J. Gastroenterol.,* 82, 871, 1987.

51. Naveau, S., Pelletier, G., Poynard, T., et al., A randomized clinical trial of supplementary parenteral nutrition in jaundiced and alcoholic cirrhotic patients, *Hepatology,* 6, 270, 1986.

52. Keohane, P. P., Attrill, H., Grimble, G., et al., Enteral nutrition in malnourished patients with hepatic cirrhosis and acute encephalopathy, *JPEN,* 7, 346, 1983.

53. Mendenhall, C., Bongiovanni, G., Goldberg, S., et al., VA cooperative study on alcoholic hepatitis III: Changes in protein-calorie malnutrition associated with 30 days of hospitalized with and without enteral nutritional therapy, *JPEN,* 9, 590, 1985.

54. Horst, D., Grace, N. D., Conn, H. O., et al., Comparison of dietary protein with an oral branched chain-enriched amino acid supplement in chronic portal-systemic encephalopathy: a randomized controlled trial, *Hepatology*, 4, 279, 1984.

55. Millikan, W. J., Henderson, J. M., Warren, W. D., et al., Total parenteral nutrition with F080 in cirrhotics with subclinical encephalopathy, *Ann. Surg.*, 3, 294, 1983.

56. Weber, F. L., Bagby, B. S., Licate, L., et al., Effects of branched-chain amino acids on nitrogen metabolism in patients with cirrhosis, *Hepatology*, 11, 942, 1990.

57. Carithers, R. L., Herlong, H. F., Diehl, A. M., et al., Methylprednisolone therapy in patients with severe alcoholic hepatitis: a randomized multicenter trial, *Ann. Intern. Med.*, 110, 685, 1989.

58. Orrego, H., Blake, J. E., Blendis, L. M., et al., Long-term treatment of alcoholic liver disease with propylthiouracil, *N. Engl. J. Med.*, 317, 1421, 1987.

59. Kershenobich, D., Vargas, F., Garcia-Tsao, G., et al., Colchicine in the treatment of cirrhosis of the liver, *N. Engl. J. Med.*, 318, 1709, 1987.

60. Mendenhall, C. L., Anderson, S., Garcia-Pont, P., et al., VA cooperative study on alcoholic hepatitis I: Acute and long-term survival in patients treated with oxandrolone and prednisolone, *N. Engl. J. Med.*, 311, 1464, 1984.

61. Rombeau, J. L., Rolandelli, R. H., and Wilmore, D. W., Nutritional support, in *Care of the Surgical Patient. Vol. 2 Care in the CCU*, Wilmore, D. W., Ed., Scientific American, New York, 1988, 10-1.

62. Greenberger, N.J., Carley, J., Schenker, S., et al., Effect of vegetable and animal protein diets in chronic hepatic encephalopathy, *Dig. Dis.*, 22, 845, 1977.

63. Jeppsson, B., Kjallman, A., Aslund, U., et al., Effect of vegan and meat protein diets in mild chronic portal-systemic encephalopathy, in Hepatic encephalopathy in chronic liver failure, Capocaccia, L., Fischer, J. E., Rossi-Fanelli, F., Eds., Plenum Press, New York, 1984, 359.

64. Mendenhall, C. L., personal communication, November, 1991.

18 Alcohol Malnutrition and the Gastrointestinal Tract

INTRODUCTION

Chronic alcoholism is assumed to be the leading cause of malnutrition in developed countries. A large intake of alcohol may cause primary malnutrition by displacing other nutrients and micronutrients from the diet or by reducing intake of them due to associated medical disorders and socioeconomic disturbances. In addition, malnutrition may result from either maldigestion or malabsorption of nutrients caused by gastrointestinal damage associated with alcoholism.

The gastrointestinal (GI) tract is particularly important for the influence of alcohol on nutrition for two reasons. In the first place, it is the site of alcohol absorption and also the site of the start of alcohol breakdown (first-pass metabolism[1]). Furthermore, the direct contact of alcoholic drinks with the mucosa of the upper GI tract leads to numerous functional changes that extend to marked mucosal damage capable of exerting a long-term effect on the digestion and assimilation of nutrients. In addition, alcohol-induced functional disorders and mucosal damage in the GI tract, together with diseases of the liver and pancreas, give rise to a loss of appetite and a multitude of complaints in alcoholics, such as nausea, vomiting, flatulence, and abdominal pain (Table 1).[2-4] Quantitatively, these disorders are probably of greater importance than maldigestion and malabsorption for the nutritional disturbances found in alcoholics (Figure 1).

In the present review, use will be made of data on alcohol and the GI tract published, for the most part, over the last ten years. Details of developments in this field up to the late 1970s are summarized in several earlier works.[5-9]

ISBN 0-8493-7933-4

TABLE 1
Incidence of Abdominal Complaints in Alcoholics with Various Types of Liver Disease

Symptom	A			B
	Alcoholic fatty liver (%)	Alcoholic hepatitis (without cirrhosis) (%)	Alcoholic cirrhosis (%)	Alcoholic hepatitis (with or without cirrhosis) (%)
	(n = 103)	(n = 61)	(n = 118)	(—)
Anorexia		51	47	67–75
Nausea, vomiting		49	45	20–50
Abdominal pain	19	41	66	45–70
Flatulence	23	26	33	—
Any of the symptoms 1 through 4	51	49	82	—

Note: A, Patients from a German study;[2] B, data from 7 series from the U.S.[3]

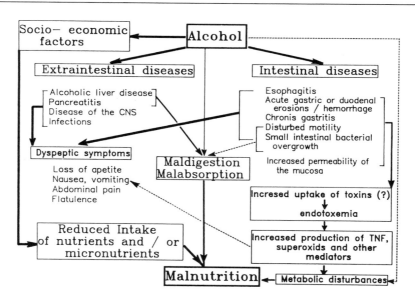

FIGURE 1. Alcohol-induced malnutrition: schematic representation of the role of the gastrointestinal tract including the liver and pancreas.

GASTROINTESTINAL ABSORPTION, METABOLISM, AND PRODUCTION OF ALCOHOL

ABSORPTION

Alcohol can be absorbed through the mucosa of the entire GI tract by simple diffusion; there is no evidence that alcohol is actively transported across the intestinal membrane. The rate of diffusion of ethanol across the intestinal mucosa is determined by the concentration gradient between the intestinal lumen and the subepithelial capillaries, regional blood flow, and the permeability of the mucosa in question.[6]

In both man and the dog there is a direct linear correlation between the concentration of alcohol ingested and the amount absorbed.[6,10] In studies on the significance of the stomach for alcohol absorption in man and the influence of meals on alcohol absorption,[6] the first-pass metabolism of alcohol in the stomach recently demonstrated[1] was not taken into account, so that the interpretation of the results of these studies is uncertain.

Many other factors affect the absorption of alcohol, including the type of alcoholic beverage drunk, certain drugs, body temperature, the temperature of the beverage, added spices, and the presence of magnesium and calcium ions. Most of these factors probably inhibit or enhance the absorption of ethanol by virtue of their effects on gastric motility and/or small intestinal blood flow.

METABOLISM

In mammals, alcohol is oxidized mainly in the liver.[11] The main enzyme involved in the first stage of oxidation is alcohol dehydrogenase. In both humans and the rat, alcohol dehydrogenase is also found in the stomach and in the upper small intestine.[6] The isoenzyme pattern of alcohol dehydrogenase in the intestinal mucosa differs from that found in the liver.[6,12] A microsomal ethanol oxidizing system has also been described in the mucosa of the small intestine of the rat,[13] but its physiological role within the gut still remains to be elucidated.

Recently, it has been reported that in both rats[14] and humans[1] a significant fraction of an intragastrically administered dose of ethanol never reaches the systemic circulation. This first-pass metabolism of ethanol correlates significantly with gastric ADH activity. First-pass metabolism of alcohol in women has been shown to be less efficient than in man, so blood ethanol concentrations are higher.[15] However, this difference seems to apply only to younger women (<50 years of age).[16] The first-pass effect was greater in fed, nonalcoholic volunteers than in those who fasted.[17] Of interest is the observation that alcohol-dependent men and women have less efficient gastric first-pass metabolism of alcohol than do nonalcoholic subjects[17] (the reverse of the hepatic response to regular alcohol intake[18]). Alcohol-dependent women have hardly any gastric mucosal ADH-activity and, therefore, first-pass metabolism of alcohol is virtually absent.[15] Diminished gastric oxidation and the resulting increase in alcohol bioavailability in women may contribute, along with other factors such as volume of distribution, to the increased vulnerability of women to the toxic effects of alcohol. Drugs, such as cimetidine and ranitidine, that inhibit gastric ADH, also affect the ability of the gastric mucosa to metabolize alcohol.[19,20] Studies on famotidine suggest that it does not share this effect.[21]

Bacterial ethanol oxidation may also have a role to play in the intestinal first-pass metabolism of ethanol.[22]

PRODUCTION

In a number of animal species significant amounts of ethanol are produced in the GI tract as a result of bacterial action on ingested carbohydrate.[6] Alcohol is also formed in the human stomach, and concentrations as high as 50 mmol/l may be found in patients with disturbed gastric emptying.[23]

CONCLUSION 1

Alcohol is absorbed mainly in the stomach and the upper small intestine. The rate of absorption of alcohol is influenced by many factors, predominantly its effects on gastric motility and/or small intestinal blood flow. A significant fraction of ingested alcohol is oxidized by first-pass metabolism in the stomach. This first-pass metabolism seems to be quantitatively important at low alcohol concentrations. Women have been shown to have less efficient first-pass metabolism than men. This difference might play a role in the increased vulnerability of women to the toxic effect of alcohol.

EFFECTS OF ALCOHOL ON THE ORAL CAVITY AND THE ESOPHAGUS

ORAL CAVITY

Individuals abusing alcohol may suffer from glossitis and/or stomatitis.[24] It is not clear whether these changes result from poor nutrition or whether they reflect a direct effect of alcohol on the mucosa. It has repeatedly been reported that alcoholics have an increased incidence of caries and periodontitis,[6] but no information is available on the exact frequency of their occurrence. Both inflammatory changes of the oral mucosa and chewing difficulties caused by defective dentures may have a major influence on nutrition in alcoholics. For this reason, more detailed information on the frequency of these changes would be desirable.

ESOPHAGUS

Esophageal Motility

Acute alcohol ingestion impairs the competence of the lower esophageal sphincter[6,9] and hence may induce gastroesophageal reflux. Thus in 11 out of 12 healthy individuals the mean gastroesophageal reflux rate increased fivefold when alcohol was given.[25] In addition, alcohol ingestion significantly reduced the acid-clearing capacity of the esophagus in normal subjects.[26]

In chronic alcoholics with peripheral neuropathy, peristalsis in the distal two-thirds of the esophagus is reduced.[6,9] Thus, when these individuals swallow, there is either no motor response in the esophagus or else only nonperistaltic contractions. However, despite the profound motor disturbance in the lower esophagus, both upper and lower sphincters are intact and function normally, and the individuals concerned do not experience dysphagia or other esophageal symptoms. In a recent manometric study, an abnormality known as a "nutcracker esophagus" was observed in a number of alcoholics within 3 d of alcohol withdrawal.[27] These manometric changes were reversible within one month of abstinence from alcohol.

Esophagitis

There is a widespread clinical impression that subjects who abuse alcohol are more likely to suffer from chronic esophagitis.[9] Only a few studies on the relationship between alcohol abuse and esophagitis have been undertaken. In a recent study a significantly higher incidence of esophagitis was found in alcoholics without liver disease compared with controls without alcohol abuse.[28] In other studies alcoholic individuals showed an increased incidence of histological abnormalities of the esophageal mucosa,[6] and there is a high incidence of alcoholism among patients with Barrett's esophagus.[9,29]

EFFECTS OF ALCOHOL ON THE STOMACH

GASTRIC MOTILITY

In man, beverages containing alcohol at concentrations of between 5 and 30% are said to delay gastric emptying.[6,30] In normal subjects, 1 g/kg of body weight of ethanol taken with food causes a marked delay in the gastric emptying of solids, but less of a delay in the emptying of liquids.[31] In other studies, very little difference was seen in the gastric emptying rates for liquids and solids in healthy male subjects fed wine or diluted wine.[32] It is possible that differences in the rate of gastric emptying and in the gastric first-pass metabolism of ethanol might explain, at least in part, the distinct intra- and inter-individual variations observed in blood ethanol concentration-time curves following standard doses of alcohol.[18]

Increased gastric pressure due to repeated retching and vomiting following acute alcohol excess is assumed to be a major causative factor in the development of the Mallory-Weiss syndrome.[33,34]

GASTRIC SECRETION

Acute Effects of Alcohol

Alcohol stimulates gastric acid secretion in several animal species whether given orally, intragastrically, or intravenously.[5,6,10] In healthy, nonalcoholic volunteers, intragastric instillation of 250 to 500 ml of pure ethanol at concentrations of between 1 and 10% (v/v), causes an increase in gastric acid secretion as measured by intragastric titration.[35,36] Beer and wine are potent stimulants of gastric acid secretion, while alcoholic beverages with a high alcohol content such as whisky or cognac have no effect on gastric acid secretion.[35,36]

The results of several studies indicate that alcohol-induced stimulation of gastric secretion is, at least in part, mediated via the nervous system. It is assumed that alcohol acts centrally and that the stimulus to gastric acid secretion is mediated through the vagus nerve.[5,6] The results of other studies suggest that alcohol may also stimulate gastric secretion indirectly via the release of histamine.[37] A number of alcoholic beverages contain significant amounts of histamine;[6] red wines and sherries may contain as much as 1.5 mg/100 ml. Alcohol increases the permeability of the intestinal mucosa to histamine,[6] thus, gastric secretion may be further stimulated by the effects of exogenous histamine. Furthermore, it has recently been shown that beer and wine cause a marked increase in plasma gastrin concentrations in healthy volunteers.[35,36] Oral ingestion of pure ethanol at concentrations of between 4 and 40%, or of whisky do not increase plasma gastrin levels, suggesting that ethanol per se may not be responsible for the gastrin release induced in man by the ingestion of beer and wine.[35,36]

In high concentrations alcohol may also decrease gastric acid output by inducing back-diffusion of hydrogen ions into the gastric mucosa,[38] thereby breaking the gastric mucosal barrier, an effect which might facilitate the development of mucosal damage.[6]

Chronic Effects of Alcohol

If large daily doses of ethanol are given over a prolonged period of time to dogs fed a nutritious diet, the mean daily secretion of acid increases 2.4-fold during the first month, and remains elevated thereafter.[5] In man, chronic alcohol abuse does not appear to lead to increased acid output. In alcoholics, mean basal and maximal stimulated gastric acid outputs were significantly lower than in healthy control subjects of comparable age and sex.[5,39] However, no significant difference was observed between the mean maximal acid output in male alcoholics abstinent for 4 to 8 weeks and a group of age-matched controls.[40]

ACUTE GASTRIC MUCOSAL INJURY

Ethanol increases the permeability of the gastric mucosa in various animal species.[5,10] Concentrations of 15% and more disrupt the gastric mucosal barrier in rats,[41] dogs,[10] and man,[42] thereby increasing hydrogen, sodium, and potassium ion fluxes. These and other findings, such as changes in transmural gastric potential difference brought about by alcohol ingestion,[43] suggest that disruption of the gastric mucosal barrier precedes the development of morphological changes in the gastric mucosa.[6]

Ultrastructural changes, such as widening of the intercellular spaces between epithelial lining cells, focal separation of cell junctions, and disruption of the apical membrane of the surface epithelial cells, progressively develop in the gastric mucosa of dogs as the concentration of alcohol applied increases.[44] Alcohol solutions of 20 to 40% lead to severe hemorrhage and erosions of gastric mucosa in animal experiments.[5,6] Alcohol is also an important cause of hemorrhagic erosive gastric lesions in man.[6,45,46] In a prospective study, gastric subepithelial hemorrhages were seen in 20 out of 125 actively drinking alcoholic patients with a mean daily ethanol use of 330 g.[47] Histologic evaluation of biopsy specimens of the hemorrhagic lesions revealed only mild inflammatory cell infiltration.[47] No relation seems to exist between the subepithelial hemorrhages and the presence of Helicobacter pylori.[48] In one study, 90% of a group of cirrhotic patients bleeding from acute hemorrhagic gastritis were found to chronically abuse alcohol.[49]

Low or moderate doses of alcohol cause neither erosive nor hemorrhagic lesions of the gastric mucosa in healthy subjects and do not increase fecal blood loss.[5,6] However, in patients with preexisting gastritis, alcohol ingestion may lead to gastric mucosal lesions, which may bleed.[6] Agents such as aspirin and congeners in certain alcoholic beverages such as acetaldehyde and acetic acid may also favor the development of acute gastric lesions in individuals consuming alcohol.[6] The acute gastric lesions induced by alcohol are localized mainly in the body and/or the fundus of the stomach, but they may be diffusely distributed throughout the entire organ.[47,50]

PROSTAGLANDINS AND LEUKOTRIENES IN ALCOHOL-INDUCED GASTRIC MUCOSAL INJURY

Prostaglandins have been shown to protect the gastric mucosa from damage by agents known to break the gastric mucosal barrier other than by inhibiting acid secretion ("cytoprotection").[51] Recently it has been reported that the acute ingestion of a 12% (v/v) ethanol solution, in a dose of 1 g/kg of body weight, significantly reduces the prostaglandin E_2 output in gastric juice in healthy subjects.[52] The results of studies performed in rats suggest that this effect of ethanol is due to an inhibition of microsomal synthesis of prostaglandin E_2.[53] The results of a number of other studies support the hypothesis that decreased prostaglandin formation might play a role in the mucosal injury induced by alcohol.[54,55] The mechanism by which prostaglandins protect against the effects of ethanol on the gastric mucosa remains unknown; luminal factors such as an increase in mucus or bicarbonate release might play a role.[56]

Other studies have shown that intraintestinal administration of 6% ethanol[57] or intragastric instillation of 20 to 50% ethanol[58] enhances mucosal production of leukotrienes. In the same experiments, prevention of leukotriene formation by inhibiting 5-lipoxygenase ameliorated the ethanol-induced mucosal injury. From these observations it was assumed that increased leukotriene production might play a role in the development of alcohol-induced mucosal injury.

TABLE 2
Incidence of Atrophic Gastritis in Heavy Drinkers and in Control Subjects[40,59]

	Subjects studied	Other potentially important factors	n	Mean age	Part of the stomach	Atrophic gastritis (%)
I (a)	Chronic alcoholics	1 to 2 months after cessation of alcohol intake and nutritious diet	62	52	Body Antrum	24.2 65.6
(b)	Healthy controls	Comparable in age to group (a)	28	38	Body	3.5
II (a)	Chronic alcoholics	Admitted because of alcoholism	28	34	Body	47
(b)	Heavy drinkers	Admitted because of non-ulcer dyspepsia	27	26		23
(a) + (b)			55		Body	35
(c)	Controls without alcohol abuse	27 Admitted because of non-ulcer dyspepsia	42	25[a]		19

Note: I: Chronic or intermittent malnutrition, 69%; II: chronic or intermittent malnutrition, 24%.

[a]   Extrapolated value.

CHRONIC GASTRIC MUCOSAL INJURY

In dogs, chronic feeding of alcohol in high concentrations resulted in the development of chronic gastritis.[5] After alcohol feeding for up to 2 years, repeated mucosal biopsy specimens obtained from the body of the stomach revealed glandular atrophy and increased fibrosis in the glandular portion of the mucosa. Controversy exists as to the effects of chronic alcohol on the gastric mucosa in man.[5,6,9] Several studies have suggested that the incidence of superficial and/or atrophic gastritis is increased in individuals chronically abusing alcohol (Table 2).[39,40,59,60] Heavy alcohol use was documented in 17 (85%) out of 20 males under the age of 30 with atrophic gastritis.[60] Other investigators have found that the incidence of more severe types of gastritis is comparable in alcoholics and nonalcoholic

TABLE 3

Incidence of Peptic Ulcer (PU) Disease in Patients with Alcoholic Liver Disease[6]

Diagnosis	n	Age (x ± SD)	Incidence of PU n (%)
All patients	282	49 ± 12	58 (20.6)
Subgroup with cirrhosis	118	52 ± 12	29 (24.6)
Fatty liver	103	48 ± 15	24 (23.3)

subjects.[61] Alcoholics may be malnourished, and this may play a role in the development of chronic gastritis. However, male alcoholics who had received a nutritionally balanced diet in the hospital for 1 to 2 months still showed a much higher incidence of superficial and atrophic gastritis than age- and sex-matched control subjects (Table 2).[40]

ALCOHOL AND PEPTIC ULCERATION

In several studies, no association has been documented between alcohol consumption and the prevalence of peptic ulceration.[62-64] In these studies, however, persons with relatively low levels of alcohol consumption were included in the group of alcohol consumers. Alcohol-induced acute gastritis and gastric erosions are only observed when excessive quantities of alcohol are ingested; thus it is possible that the risk of developing peptic ulceration may only be increased in heavy drinkers (alcohol consumption >80 to 100 g/d). In a recent controlled study in males, alcohol ingestion was associated with an increased risk of developing duodenal ulceration during the year before the first symptoms, and an increased lifetime risk.[65] Peptic ulcers were found in more than 20% of individuals with alcoholic liver disease (Table 3).[6] Further controlled studies on the frequency of ulcer disease in heavy drinkers in comparison with adequate control groups are needed.

CONCLUSION 2

Acute ingestion of alcohol leads

1. To changes in motility of the esophagus and stomach that favor gastroesophageal reflux and probably also the development of reflux esophagitis. In addition, they may promote nausea and vomiting and thus contribute to the development of Mallory-Weiss tears.

2.   To damage to the gastric mucosa that may extend to hemorrhagic-erosive gastritis.

Acid secretion in the stomach is stimulated by certain alcoholic drinks (beer, wine). The increase in acid secretion can favor the development of gastroesophageal reflux. Chronic abuse of alcohol probably favors the development of chronic gastritis, with a tendency to mucosal atrophy in the fundus and reduced acid secretion, and presumably also the development of esophagitis.

The already mentioned motility disturbances and mucosal damage can, for the most part via changes in appetite and such complaints as abdominal discomfort, nausea, and heart burn, lead to reduced food intake, thereby favoring the development of malnutrition (Figure 1).

EFFECTS OF ALCOHOL ON THE SMALL INTESTINE

SMALL INTESTINAL MOTILITY

Oral or intravenous alcohol decreases Type I (impeding) wave motility in the jejunum, but has no effect on Type III (propulsive) wave motility, in either chronic alcoholics or in healthy volunteers.[6] The suppression of impeding waves in the jejunum and the stimulation of propulsive waves in the ileum may contribute to the increased sensitivity to osmotic loads, shortened transit time, and tendency to diarrhea frequently observed in alcoholics.[66]

SPLANCHNIC BLOOD FLOW

Conflicting results have been reported for the action of alcohol on the splanchnic or hepatic blood flow. Small doses of alcohol infused intravenously lead to a slight decrease in estimated splanchnic blood flow, while increases in splanchnic blood flow in man were observed at relatively high doses of alcohol.[6] An increase in portal vein blood flow was also measured in rats following 2 g of ethanol per kilogram administered by gavage.[67]

SMALL INTESTINAL ABSORPTION

Monosaccharides

Alcohol given acutely partly inhibits glucose transport across the small intestine in various animals.[68,69] Although at present the mechanism by which ethanol reduces intestinal glucose transport is not fully understood,

TABLE 4
Malabsorption of Carbohydrates, Fat, and Protein in
Alcoholics[6]

Substance tested	Number of studies	Clinical findings	Abnormal results (%)
D-xylose	1	Cirrhosis	10
	5	No liver disease	18–76
Fat[a]	1	Cirrhosis	50
	2	No liver disease	35–56
Protein[b]	1	No liver disease	52

[a]   Fecal fat excretion.
[b]   Fecal nitrogen excretion.

it has been assumed to interfere with active transport across the brush border membrane.[7] In more recent studies it has been suggested that the inhibition of glucose transport is due to an effect of ethanol on passive diffusion, which results in a more prompt equilibration of the Na^+-gradient and a consequent reduction in the uptake velocities of Na^+-dependent transport systems.[70]

Alcoholics may malabsorb d-xylose, but there is little agreement as to the frequency with which this occurs; thus figures of from 0 to 76% are quoted (Table 4). This variation may reflect differences in the nutritional status of the individuals studied, in their mean daily alcohol intake, or in the severity or even the presence of any accompanying alcohol-related liver disease.[6]

Amino Acids

In animals and in man, alcohol in concentrations of 2% or more will inhibit the absorption of several amino acids from segments of the small intestine,[6,7] probably because of effects on their active transport. However, chronic alcohol consumption does not affect intestinal leucine absorption from the entire small intestine in rats fed a normal diet.[71,72]

Lipids

Some chronic alcoholics exhibit an elevated lipid excretion (Table 4). The frequency and extent of this steatorrhea varies considerably, depending upon the selection of the patients examined. Marked steatorrhea occurs in patients with exocrine pancreatic insufficiency and/or chronic liver disease.[73] Functional disturbances of the exocrine pancreas have been found in 50 to 60% of alcoholic individuals.[73,74] Changes in the composition of the bile, in particular a reduction in bile acid secretion in cholestasis and advanced liver diseases, can lead to a disturbance in micelle formation, and thus to a reduction in the absorption of fat. While earlier studies provided no direct evidence that ethanol interferes with the transport of fat across the intestinal mucosa,[6] the results of more recent studies have shown that ethanol ingestion affects intestinal lipid absorption.[75] In human biopsies from the upper small intestine, ethanol markedly inhibited triglyceride synthesis and secretion without affecting fatty acid uptake.[76]

Vitamins

Folic acid — Alcoholic individuals recently imbibing alcohol show significantly lower serum folate levels than alcoholics recently abstinent.[77,78] Folic acid deficiency results in megaloblastic anemia and in enlarged and presumably dysfunctional enterocytes and shortened villi in the jejunal mucosa.[78] The combination of alcohol ingestion and a folate-deficient diet decreases jejunal uptake of fluid, electrolytes, glucose, and folic acid, implying a mechanism for diarrhea and malabsorption.[78] There are several reasons why alcoholics become folate deficient. Poor nutrition with inadequate dietary folate intake appears to be of major importance.[77,79] Other etiologic factors are poor absorption,[78] decreased hepatic uptake and retention, and increased urinary excretion.[77]

Vitamin B_{12} — Chronic ingestion of large amounts of alcohol may cause malabsorption of vitamin B_{12}.[6,78] However, despite the fact that alcohol may interfere with vitamin B_{12} absorption, very few alcoholics show clinical evidence of vitamin B_{12} deficiency.

Thiamine — In earlier studies the prevalence of subclinical thiamine deficiency in alcoholics was estimated at between 30 and 80%.[6,77,80] In these studies thiamine status was estimated indirectly through the assay of erythrocyte transketolase activity, making interpretation of the results difficult. In more recent studies using direct assays, blood levels of thiamine in alcoholics were found to be normal,[22,81] suggesting that the frequency of thiamine deficiency in alcoholics has probably been exaggerated. Intestinal absorption of thiamine was shown to be reduced in alcoholics, and also in healthy subjects following acute ethanol ingestion in one study (Table 5).[83] However, in jejunal perfusion studies 5% ethanol had no effect on thiamine absorption in volunteers.[84] Alcohol administration has no effect on the absorption of high concentrations of thiamine, suggesting that it

TABLE 5
Effects of Acute or Chronic Alcohol
Administration on Intestinal Absorption of
Vitamins and Trace Elements[6,77,79,91]

Substance	Acute alcohol administration		Chronic alcohol administration	
	Rats	Humans	Rats	Humans
Thiamine	↓	nc or ↓	—	nc or ↓
Folic acid	nc or ↓	nc	nc	nc or ↓
Vitamin B_{12}	—	—	↓	nc or ↓
Vitamin D	—	—	—	nc
Vitamin A	—	nc or ↓	—	nc
Iron	nc or ↓	nc or ↑	nc or ↑	nc or ↑
Manganese	↑	—	—	—
Zinc	↓	—	↓	nc or ↓

Note: Decreased, ↓; increased, ↑; nc, no change; —, not studied. Changes in active transport only.

inhibits active transport but has no effect on passive diffusion of the vitamin.[85]

Vitamin B_6 — Pyridoxal-5-phosphate deficiency is observed in a high proportion of alcoholics.[77,79] Vitamin B_6 deficiency appears to be caused by factors other than malabsorption.[6,79]

Vitamin C — It has been assumed that ascorbic acid deficiency occurs in alcoholics.[79] Although it has been suggested that alcohol may impair absorption of this vitamin,[79] it seems more likely that inadequate intake is the more important cause.

Vitamin D — Alcoholics have decreases in bone density and increased susceptibility to fractures.[79,86] Plasma concentration of 25-hydroxychole-calciferol may be low in alcoholic individuals with or without liver disease.[79,87] Vitamin D appears to be absorbed normally in these individuals, although absorption may be impaired in the presence of pancreatitis or cholestasis.

Water and electrolytes — In man, acute administration of alcohol (2 to 10%) into the jejunum or into the ileum (2%) has no significant effect on water and sodium absorption.[88] Chronic alcohol ingestion affects both water and electrolyte absorption. Thus, in healthy subjects, the ingestion of a diet containing 36% of the calories as alcohol for 2 weeks results in a marked reduction in water and sodium absorption in the jejunum and ileum;[88] similar results are obtained in drinking alcoholics.[89] The reduced water absorption may contribute to diarrhea in alcoholics.

Minerals — Acute alcohol ingestion does not influence calcium absorption in healthy subjects, although decreased absorption of [47]Ca has been found in patients with alcoholic cirrhosis.[6] It has been suggested that the reduction in calcium uptake might reflect vitamin D deficiency.[87] Alcoholics may frequently have hypomagnesemia or low exchangeable magnesium.[79] Hypomagnesemia is caused mainly by increased magnesium excretion in the urine or as a result of diarrhea. Magnesium absorption seems to be normal.[6]

Iron — Hepatic siderosis may be observed in alcoholics with liver disease,[6,79] but the effects of alcohol on iron transport have not been clearly delineated. In man, whisky enhances the absorption of ferric chloride, but does not affect the uptake of the more readily absorbed ferrous ascorbate or hemoglobin iron.[6] No significant differences are observed in the mean percentage absorption of non-heme ferric chloride from a test meal in alcoholics with liver disease of varying severity who are not anemic and control subjects.[90]

Zinc — Hypozincemia and hyperzincuria are frequent findings in patients with alcoholic liver disease.[77,91] Low liver zinc concentrations have been found in patients with alcoholic cirrhosis[91,92] and also in alcoholics with fatty liver or alcoholic hepatitis.[92] Decreased zinc absorption was assumed to contribute to zinc deficiency in alcoholics (Table 5).[93] Zinc absorption was also reported to be low in alcoholic cirrhosis, while it was normal in cirrhosis of other etiologies.[94] However, normal or even increased zinc absorption was found in patients with alcoholic cirrhosis by other authors.[95] To date, it has not been possible to resolve the question as to whether zinc deficiency in alcoholics is in the first instance a consequence of alcohol consumption or of the liver disease frequently presenting at the same time. A reduction in zinc absorption has also been reported in patients with nonalcoholic cirrhosis.[96] Over and beyond this, marked reductions in the zinc content of the liver[92] and reduced plasma zinc levels[79,96] have also been described in patients with mild to marked chronic liver diseases with a nonalcoholic etiology. In view of the particular biological importance of this trace element, zinc supplementation would appear justified, irrespective of the actual pathomechanism of the zinc deficiency.[77]

CONCLUSION 3

The absorption of a number of nutrients, in particular those that are assimilated by an active transport mechanism, is inhibited by alcohol. The importance of these absorption disorders for the development of nutritional disturbances in alcoholics, however, is not clear. In alcoholics with exocrine pancreatic insufficiency, cholestasis or advanced diseases of the liver, maldigestion has a greater quantitative and qualitative significance. Together with motility disorders, maldigestion and malabsorption can favor the occurrence of such abdominal complaints as feelings of fullness, pain, and nausea in alcoholics (Figure 1). The resulting loss of appetite may, in turn, be one of the causes for the reduced uptake of nutrients.

ACUTE INTESTINAL MUCOSAL INJURY

In various animal species, administration of alcoholic solutions at concentrations corresponding to those of commonly available alcoholic beverages leads to mucosal damage that extends to pronounced exfoliation of the tips of the villi and hemorrhage.[7] Our present understanding of the development and pathogenesis of these mucosal injuries has been obtained exclusively in experimental studies in animals. The results of some studies lead to the assumption that ethanol has a direct effect on the integrity of the mucosal epithelium.[85,97] On the basis of very elegant and painstaking studies, other authors have proposed an indirect effect via alterations in the mucosal microcirculation that leads to enhanced transcapillary fluid filtration and subsequent rupture of the epithelial lining or a combination of these two events (for a review see Reference 7). In more recent studies the same group provided convincing evidence supporting their hypothesis that the mechanism of the injury of the intestinal mucosa by alcohol may be the induction of villus contraction that leads to villus-tip bleb formation, lymphatic obstruction, and eventually to exfoliation of the tips of the villi when the blebs rupture.[98] From the results of additional experiments, these authors assumed that the initial event in response to alcohol is the release of noxious mediators such as histamine[99] and leukotrienes,[58] which cause microvascular injury. The assumption that similar mucosal injury occurs in man is supported by the observation that marked duodenal erythema with subepithelial bleeding develops following a single large oral dose of alcohol.[100] Furthermore, alcohol in quantities similar to those ingested during moderate drinking significantly increases the number of damaged duodenal and jejunal villi observed in suction biopsy specimens obtained from healthy volunteers.[101]

CHRONIC INTESTINAL MUCOSAL INJURY

In rats chronically fed an ethanol-containing diet, the jejunal villi become shorter, the number of villous cells decreases, and regenerative activity in the crypts increases.[6] In alcoholics with folate deficiency, profound histological abnormalities such as shortening of the villi, decreased mitosis in the crypts, enlarged epithelial cells, and a reduction in epithelial surface area can be observed in biopsy specimens from the duodeno-jejunal junction.[6] However, in most earlier studies in unselected alcoholics the mucosa appeared normal, although minor histological changes were found in patients with alcoholic cirrhosis.[6] On the other hand, in a quantitative morphometric study, a significant decrease was observed in the calculated mean total mucosal surface in well-nourished chronic alcoholics as compared with normal subjects.[102] The latter observation has recently been confirmed.[103]

INTESTINAL PERMEABILITY TO MACROMOLECULES

The mucosal barrier in normal mammals is incomplete so that small amounts of antigens or similar macromolecules may pass through the intestinal wall.[104] In different animal species alcohol feeding resulted in an increased permeability of the intestinal mucosa to macromolecules like hemoglobin and horseradish peroxidase.[6] Permeability of the small intestine was also found to be increased in nonintoxicated alcoholic patients.[105] The enhanced permeability of the mucosa of the small bowel following acute or chronic alcohol ingestion could result in the absorption of toxic compounds such as endotoxin and other bacterial toxins which would not normally be absorbed and which might play a role in the development of alcohol-related damage to the liver and other organs.[106] This assumption is supported by the observation of endotoxemia in patients with early forms of alcohol-related liver damage, such as fatty liver,[107] or the transient endotoxemia observed following acute alcohol consumption in subjects with no evidence of alcoholic liver disease.[108] Endotoxins are powerful stimulants of the release of tumor necrosis factor (TNF)[109] and other mediators such as leukotrienes and interleukins[110,111] by macrophages. In fact, increased TNF production has recently been reported in monocytes from patients with alcoholic hepatitis.[112] TNF has been assumed to be a major mediator of the manifold noxious effects of endotoxin.[109] The term ''cachectin'' is employed as a synonym for TNF.[109] As the name implies, the

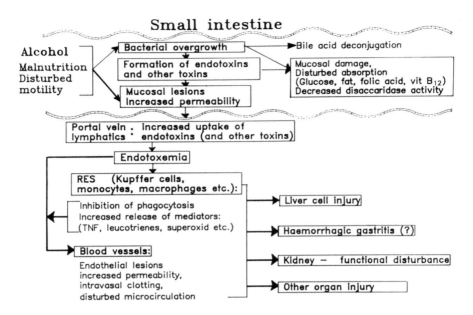

FIGURE 2. Schematic representation of the possible causes and consequences of an increased permeability of the mucosa of the small bowel to macromolecules such as bacterial toxins (especially endotoxin) and of bacterial overgrowth in the small intestine in individuals chronically abusing alcohol.

sequelae of its multifarious effects on the metabolism includes the development of a catabolic situation, with loss of muscle mass and body weight.

The above-mentioned findings lend support to the hypothesis, sketched in Figure 2, of the significance of intestinal changes for the development of alcoholic organic damage, with the following sequence: alcohol-induced mucosal damage in the (upper) small bowel, increased permeability of the mucosa for large-molecular substances, increased passage of endotoxins and/or other toxins into the blood or lymph, release of potentially toxic mediators by macrophages, through such mediators as TNF and leukotrienes, a multitude of disorders of the metabolism, of the microcirculation and membranes, and cellular damage extending to cell necrosis (liver and other organs).

INTESTINAL BACTERIAL MICROFLORA

Marked qualitative and quantitative changes are observed in the microflora in the small intestine of recently imbibing chronic alcoholics.[114] The most significant finding is the increase in the number of facultative and obligate anaerobic bacteria and/or the number of bacteria per unit volume of jejunal juice. Evidence of an increased incidence of bacterial overgrowth in alcoholics also stems from studies using the lactulose H_2-breath test.[115] Bacterial overgrowth in the small intestine might contribute to functional and/or morphological abnormalities of the small intestine in patients chronically abusing alcohol (Figure 2). Furthermore, it might lead to an increased production of endotoxin and other bacterial toxins, which can more readily pass through the mucosa as a result of the alcohol-induced mucosal damage (Figure 2).

CONCLUSION 4

Acute alcohol ingestion leads to mucosal damage in the upper gastrointestinal tract extending to exfoliation of the tips of the villi. A number of observations made in animal experiments and investigations in humans suggest that these mucosal defects favor an increase in the permeability of the mucosa for large molecular substances, such as endotoxin and other bacterial toxins. According to this hypothesis, the increase in endotoxin concentration in the blood results in a powerful stimulation of the release of potentially toxic mediators (TNF, interleukines, leukotrienes) from phagocytes. These mediators, in particular TNF, may be responsible for the development of a multitude of metabolic disturbances and organic damage, and thus have a major indirect effect on the nutritional status of alcoholics (Figure 2).

REFERENCES

1. Julkunen, R. J. K., DiPadova, C., and Lieber, C. S., First pass metabolism of ethanol — a gastrointestinal barrier against the systemic toxicity of ethanol, *Life Sci.*, 37, 567, 1985.
2. Bode, J. C., Kruse, G., Mexas, P., and Martini, G. A., Alkoholfettleber, Alkoholhepatitis und Alkoholzirrhose — Trinkverhalten und Häufigkeit klinischer, klinisch-chemischer und histologischer Befunde bei 282 Patienten, *Dtsch. Med. Wochenschr.*, 109, 1516, 1984.
3. Galambos, J. T., Alcoholic hepatitis, in *The Liver and Its Diseases*, Schaffner, F., Sherlock, S., and Leevy, C. M., Eds., Thieme, Stuttgart, 1974, 255.
4. Vasudeva, R., Verhulst, S., Colliver, J., Skinner, H., and Holt, S., Alcohol and smoking as determinants of dyspeptic symptoms, *Am. J. Gastroenterol.*, 84, 1172, 1989.
5. Chey, W. Y., Alcohol and gastric mucosa, *Digestion*, 7, 239, 1972.
6. Bode, J. C., Alcohol and the gastrointestinal tract, *Adv. Intern. Med. Ped.*, 45, 1, 1980.

7. Beck, I. T. and Dinda, P. K., Acute exposure of small intestine to ethanol. Effects on morphology and function, *Dig. Dis. Sci.*, 26, 817, 1981.

8. Mezey, E., Effect of ethanol on intestinal morphology, metabolism, and function, in *Alcohol Related Diseases in Gastroenterology*, Seitz, H. K. and Kommerell, B., Eds., Springer-Verlag, Berlin, 1985, 342.

9. Wienbeck, M. and Berges, W., Esophageal and gastric lesion in the alcoholic, in *Alcohol Related Diseases in Gastroenterology*, Seitz, H. K. and Kommerell, B., Eds., Springer-Verlag, Berlin, 1985, 361.

10. Davenport, H. W., Ethanol damage to canine oxyntic glandular mucosa, *Proc. Soc. Exp. Biol. Med.*, 126, 657, 1967.

11. Lieber, C. S., Alcohol and the liver, in *The Liver Annual*, Vol. 5, Arias, I. M., Frenkel, M., and Wilson, J. H. P., Eds., Elsevier, Amsterdam, 1986, 116.

12. Pestalozzi, D. M., Bühler, R., von Wartburg, J. P., and Hess, M., Immunohistochemical localization of alcohol dehydrogenase in the human gastrointestinal tract, *Gastroenterology*, 85, 1011, 1983.

13. Seitz, H. K., Garro, A. J., and Lieber, C. S., Enhanced pulmonary and intestinal activation of procarcinogens and mutagens after chronic ethanol consumption in the rat, *Eur. J. Clin. Invest.*, 11, 33, 1981.

14. Julkunen, R. J. K., Tannenbaum, L., Baraona, E., and Lieber, C. S., First pass metabolism of ethanol: an important determinant of blood levels after alcohol consumption, *Alcohol*, 2, 437, 1985.

15. Frezza, M., DiPadova, C., Pozzato, G., Terpin, M., Baraona, E., and Lieber, C. S., High blood alcohol levels in women: the role of decreased gastric alcohol dehydrogenase activity and first-pass metabolism, *N. Engl. J. Med.*, 322, 95, 1990.

16. Seitz, H. K., Egerer, G., and Simanowski, U. A., High blood alcohol levels in woman, *N. Engl. J. Med.*, 323, 58, 1990.

17. DiPadova, C., Worner, T. M., Julkunen, R. J., and Lieber, C. S., Effects of fasting and chronic alcohol consumption on the first-pass metabolism of ethanol, *Gastroenterology*, 92, 1169, 1987.

18. Bode, J. C., Factors influencing alcohol metabolism in man, in *Alcool et Tractus Digestif*, INSERM Colloques Vol. 95, Stock, C. and Sarles, H., Eds., INSERM, Paris, 1980, 65.

19. Caballeria, J., Baraona, E., Rodamilans, M., and Lieber, C. S., Effects of cimetidine on gastric alcohol dehydrogenase activity and blood ethanol levels, *Gastroenterology*, 96, 388, 1989.

20. Roine, R., DiPadova, C., Frezza, R., Hernández-Munoz, E., Baraona, E., and Lieber, C. S., Effects of omeprazole, cimetidine and ranitidine on blood ethanol concentrations (abstract), *Gastroenterology*, 98, A 114, 1990.

21. Holtmann, G. and Singer, M. V., Histamine H2-receptor antagonists and blood alcohol levels, *Dig. Dis. Sci.*, 33, 767, 1988.

22. Baraona, E., Julkunen, R. J. K., Tannenbaum, L., and Lieber, C. S., Role of intestinal bacterial overgrowth in ethanol production and metabolism in rats, *Gastroenterology*, 90, 103, 1986.

23. Bode, J. C., Rust, S., and Bode, C., The effect of cimetidine treatment on ethanol formation in the human stomach, *Scand. J. Gastroenterol.*, 19, 853, 1984.

24. Larato, D. C., Gewebeveränderungen in der Mundhöhle bei chronischen Alkoholikern, *Quintessenz,* 12, 131, 1973.
25. Kaufmann, S. E. and Kaye, M. D., Induction of gastrooesophageal reflux by alcohol, *Gut,* 19, 336, 1978.
26. Kjellen, G. and Tibbling, L., Influence of body position, dry and water swallows, smoking, and alcohol on esophageal acid clearing, *Scand. J. Gastroenterol.,* 13, 283, 1978.
27. Keshavarzian, A., Iber, F. L., Ferguson, Y., and Dangleis, M., Alcoholic nutcracker esophagus: a reversible manometric change with variable radio-nuclide clearance (abstract), *Gastroenterology,* 90, 1491, 1986.
28. Ederle, A., Franzini, G., Bulighin, G., Musola, R., Formentini, G., and Zamboni, G., Relationship between non-acute upper digestive tract diseases, alcohol intake and liver diseases (abstract), *Eur. J. Gastroenterol. Hepatol.,* 2 (Suppl. 1), S 24, 1990.
29. Messian, R., Hermos, J. A., Robbins, A. H., Friedlander, D. M., and Schimmel, E. M., Barrett's esophagus. Clinical review of 26 cases, *Am. J. Gastroenterol.,* 69, 458, 1978.
30. Barboriak, J. J. and Meade, R. C., Effect of alcohol on gastric emptying in man, *Am. J. Clin. Nutr.,* 23, 1151, 1970.
31. Jian, R., Cortot, A., Ducrot, F., Jobin, G., Chayvialle, J. A., and Modigliani, R., Effect of ethanol ingestion on postprandial gastric emptying and secretion, biliopancreatic secretions, and duodenal absorption in man, *Dig. Dis. Sci.,* 31, 604, 1986.
32. Moore, J. G., Christian, P. E., Datz, F. L., and Coleman, R. E., Effect of wine on gastric emptying in humans, *Gastroenterology,* 81, 1072, 1981.
33. Bodin, F., Delage, Y., Lichtenstein, H., Denez, B., and Conte, M., Le syndrome de Mallory-Weiss, *Gastroenterol. Clin. Biol.,* 1, 637, 1977.
34. Kerlin, P., Bassett, D., Grant, A. K., and Paull, A., The Mallory-Weiss lesion. A five-year experience, *Med. J. Aust.,* 1, 471, 1978.
35. Lenz, H. J., Ferrari-Taylor, J., and Isenberg, J. I., Wine and five percent ethanol are potent stimulants of gastric acid secretion in humans, *Gastroenterology,* 85, 1082, 1983.
36. Singer, M. V., Leffmann, C., Eysselein, V. E., Calden, H., and Goebell, H., Action of ethanol and some alcoholic beverages on gastric acid secretion and release of gastrin in humans, *Gastroenterology,* 93, 1247, 1987.
37. Dinoso, V. P., Chuang, J., and Murthy, S. N. S., Changes in mucosal and venous histamine concentrations during instillation of ethanol in the canine stomach, *Am. J. Dig. Dis.,* 21, 93, 1976.
38. Kuo, Y.-J., Shanbour, L. L., and Sernka, T. J., Effect of ethanol on permeability and ion transport in the isolated dog stomach, *Am. J. Dig. Dis.,* 19, 818, 1974.
39. Segawa, K., Nakazawa, S., Tsukamoto, Y., Goto, H., Yamao, K., Hase, S., Osada, T., and Arisawa, T., Chronic alcohol abuse leads to gastric atrophy and decreased gastric secretory capacity: a histological and physiological study, *Am. J. Gastroenterol.,* 83, 373, 1988.
40. Dinoso, V. P., Chey, W. Y., Braverman, S. Pl., Rosen, A. P., Ottenberg, D., and Lorber, S. H., Gastric secretion and gastric mucosal morphology in chronic alcoholics, *Arch. Int. Med.,* 130, 715, 1972.

41. Bailey, R. E., Levine, R. A., Schwartzel, E. H., Nandi, J., Beach, D. H., Borer, P. N., and Levy, G. C., Sensitivity of NMR to assess ethanol effects on gastric epithelial cells (abstract), *Gastroenterology*, 90, 1785, 1985.

42. Stern, A. I., Hogan, D. L., and Isenberg, J. I., A new method for quantitation of ion fluxes across in vivo human gastric mucosa: effect of aspirin, acetaminophen, ethanol, and hyperosmolar solutions, *Gastroenterology*, 86, 60, 1984.

43. Caspary, W. F., Einfluß von Aspirin, Antacida, Alkohol und Gallensäuren auf die transmurale elektrische Potentialdifferenz des menschlichen Magens, *Dtsch. Med. Wochenschr.*, 100, 1263, 1975.

44. Dinoso, V. P., Ming, S. C., and McNiff, J., Ultrastructural changes of the canine gastric mucosa after topical application of graded concentrations of ethanol, *Am. J. Dig. Dis.*, 21, 626, 1976.

45. Pötzi, R., Minar, E., Pesendorfer, F. X., Ferenci, P., and Meryn, S., Notfallendoskopie bei Patienten mit chronischem Alkoholabusus, *Z. Gastroenterol.*, 20, 722, 1982.

46. Sarfeh, I. J., Tabak, C., Eugene, J., and Juler, G. L., Clinical significance of erosive gastritis in patients with alcohol liver disease and upper gastrointestinal hemorrhage, *Ann. Surg.*, 194, 149, 1981.

47. Laine, L. and Weinstein, W. M., Histology of alcoholic hemorrhagic "gastritis": a prospective evaluation, *Gastroenterology*, 94, 1254, 1988.

48. Laine, L., Marin-Sorensen, M., and Weinstein, W. M., Campylobacter pylori in alcoholic hemorrhagic "gastritis", *Dig. Dis. Sci.*, 34, 677, 1989.

49. Glass, G. B. J. and Khodadoost, J., Erosive gastritis and acute gastroduodenal ulcerations as source of upper gastrointestinal bleeding in liver cirrhosis, *Arch. Fr. Mal. Appar. Dig.*, 61, 439, 1972.

50. Lo, S., Paulsen, G., and Guth, P. H., Ethanol-induced gastric antral and corpus injury in the rat (abstract), *Gastroenterology*, 90, 1524, 1986.

51. Robert, A., Prostaglandins: effect on the gastrointestinal tract, *Clin. Physiol. Biochem.*, 2, 61, 1984.

52. Bode, C., Ganzhorn, A., Brauner, B., and Bode, J. C., Effect of acute ethanol ingestion on human gastric luminal prostaglandine E_2, prostaglandin F_{2alpha} and 6-keto-prostaglandin F_{1alpha}, *Alcohol Alcoholism*, 24, 35, 1989.

53. Bode, C., Ito, T., Rollenhagen, A., and Bode, J. C., Effect of acute and chronic alcohol feeding on prostaglandin E_2 biosynthesis in rat stomach, *Dig. Dis. Sci.*, 33, 814, 1988.

54. Domschke, A., Dembinski, A., and Domschke, W., Partial prevention of ethanol damage of human gastroduodenal mucosa by prostaglandin E_2 in vitro, *Scand. J. Gastroenterol.*, 18, 113, 1983.

55. Stern, A. I., Hogan, D. L., Kahn, L. H., and Isenberg, J. I., Protective effect of acetaminophen against aspirin and ethanol-induced damage to the human gastric mucosa, *Gastroenterology*, 86, 728, 1984.

56. Robert, A., Lancaster, C., Davis, J. P., Field, S. O., Sinha, A. J. W., and Thornburgh, B. A., Cytoprotection by prostaglandin occurs in spite of penetration of absolute ethanol into the gastric mucosa, *Gastroenterology*, 88, 328, 1985.

57. Kvietys, P. R., Twohig, B., Danzell, J., and Specian, R. D., Ethanol-induced injury to the rat gastric mucosa. Role of neutrophils and xanthine oxidase-derived radicals, *Gastroenterology*, 98, 909, 1990.

58. Beck, I. T., Boyd, A., and Dinda, P. K., Evidence for the involvement of 5-lipoxygenase products in the ethanol-induced intestinal plasma protein loss, *Am. J. Physiol.*, 254, G 483, 1988.

59. Roberts, D. M., Chronic gastritis, alcohol and non ulcer dyspepsia, *Gut*, 13, 768, 1972.

60. Göbel, D., Die chronische-atrophische Gastritis aus klinischer Sicht, *Med. Klin.*, 72, 1246, 1977.

61. Cheli, R., Giacosa, A., Marenco, G., Canepa, M., Dante, G. L., and Ghezzo, L., Chronic gastritis and alcohol, *Z. Gastroenterol.*, 19, 459, 1981.

62. Østensen, H., Gudmundsen, T. E., Østensen, P. G., Burhol, P. G., and Bonnevie, O., Smoking, alcohol, coffee, and familial factors: any associations with peptic ulcer disease?, *Scand. J. Gastroenterol.*, 20, 1227, 1985.

63. Piper, D. W., McIntosh, J. H., Greig, M., and Shy, C. M., Environmental factors and chronic gastric ulcer. A case control study of the association of smoking, alcohol, and heavy analgesic ingestion with the exacerbation of chronic gastric ulcer, *Scand. J. Gastroenterol.*, 17, 721, 1982.

64. Würsch, T. G., Hess, H., Walser, R., Koelz, H. R., Pelloni, S., Vogel, E., Schmidt, P., and Blum, A. L., Die epidemiologie des Ulcus duodeni. Untersuchung an 1105 Patienten in Zürich, *Dtsch. Med. Wochenschr.*, 103, 613, 1978.

65. Piper, D. W., Nasiry, R., McIntosh, J., Shy, C. M., Pierce, J., and Byth, K., Smoking, alcohol, analgesics, and chronic duodenal ulcer. A controlled study of habits before first symptoms and before diagnosis, *Scand. J. Gastroenterol.*, 19, 1015, 1984.

66. Keshavarzian, A., Iber, L., Dangleis, M. D., and Cornish, R., Intestinal transit and lactose intolerance in chronic alcoholics, *Am. J. Clin. Nutr.*, 44, 70, 1986.

67. Verma-Ansil, B., Carmichael, F. J., Saldivia, V., Varghese, G., and Orrego, H., Effect of ethanol on splanchnic hemodynamics in awake and unrestrained rats with portal hypertension, *Hepatology*, 10, 946, 1989.

68. Cobb, C. F., Van Thiel, D. H., and Wargo, J., Ethanol inhibition of glucose absorption in isolated, perfused small bowel of rats, *Surgery*, 94, 199, 1983.

69. Dinda, P. K. and Beck, I. T., Ethanol-induced inhibition of glucose transport across the isolated brush-border membrane of hamster jejunum, *Dig. Dis. Sci.*, 26, 23, 1981.

70. O'Neill, B., Weber, F., Hornig, D., and Semenza, G., Ethanol selectively affects Na^+-gradient dependent intestinal transport systems, *FEBS Lett.*, 194, 183, 1986.

71. Hajjar, J. J., Tomicic, T., and Scheig, R. L., Effect of chronic ethanol consumption on leucine absorption in the rat small intestine, *Digestion*, 22, 170, 1981.

72. Martines, D., Morris, A. I., and Billington, D., The effect of chronic ethanol intake on leucine absorption from the rat small intestine, *Alcohol Alcoholism*, 24, 525, 1989.

73. Sarles, H. and Johnson, C. D., Alcoholic pancreatitis, *Eur. J. Gastroenterol. Hepatol.*, 2, 422, 1990.

74. Bode, J. C., Alcohol and the digestive system — effects on the pancreas, in *Topics in Gastroenterology*, Vol. 12, Jewel, T. P. and Gibson, P. R., Eds., Blackwell Scientific, Oxford, 1985, 39.

75. Mansbach, C. M., Effect of ethanol on intestinal lipid absorption in the rat, *J. Lipid Res.*, 24, 1310, 1983.

76. Zimmermann, J., Gati, I., Eisenberg, S., and Rachmilewitz, D., Ethanol inhibits triglyceride synthesis and secretion by human small intestinal mucosa, *J. Lab. Clin. Med.*, 107, 498, 1986.

77. Halsted, C. H. and Keen, C. L., Alcoholism and micronutrient metabolism and deficiencies, *Eur. J. Gastroenterol. Hepatol.*, 2, 399, 1990.

78. Lindenbaum, J., Folate and vitamin B_{12} deficiencies in alcoholism, *Semin. Hematol.*, 17, 119, 1980.

79. Lieber, C. S., The influence of alcohol on nutritional status, *Nutr. Rev.*, 46, 241, 1988.

80. Hell, D. and Six, P., Thiamin-, Riboflavin- und Pyridoxin- Versorgung bei chronischem Alkoholismus, *Dtsch. Med. Wochenschr.*, 102, 962, 1977.

81. Poupon, R., Gervaise, G., Riant, P., Houin, G., and Tillement, J.-P., Blood thiamine and thiamine phosphate concentrations in excessive drinkers with or without peripheral neuropathy, *Alcohol Alcoholism*, 25, 605, 1990.

82. Tallaksen, C., Bøhmer, T., and Bell, H., Thiamin and thiamin phosphate esters in patients with alcohol dependence syndrome before and after 24 hours thiamin injection (abstract), *Alcohol Alcoholism*, 25, 605, 1990.

83. Thomson, A. D., Baker, H., and Leevy, C. M., Patterns of ^{35}S-thiamine hydrochloride absorption in the malnourished alcoholic patient, *J. Lab. Clin. Med.*, 76, 34, 1970.

84. Breen, K. J., Buttigieg, R., Iossifidis, S., Lourensz, C., and Wood, B., Jejunal uptake of thiamin hydrochloride in man: influence of alcoholism and alcohol, *Am. J. Clin. Nutr.*, 42, 121, 1985.

85. Wilson, F. A. and Hoyumpa, A. M., Jr., Ethanol and small intestinal transport, *Gastroenterology*, 76, 388, 1979.

86. Spencer, H., Rubio, N., Rubio, E., Indreika, M., and Seitam, A., Chronic alcoholism frequently overlooked cause of osteoporosis in men, *Am. J. Med.*, 80, 393, 1986.

87. Luisier, M., Vodoz, J. F., Donath, A., Courvoisier, B., and Garcia, B., Carence en 25-hydroxyvitamine D avec diminution de l'absorption intestinale de calcium et de la densité osseuse dans l'alcoolisme chronique, *Schweiz. Med. Wochenschr.*, 107, 1529, 1977.

88. Mekhjian, H. S. and May, E. S., Acute and chronic effects of ethanol on fluid transport in the human small intestine, *Gastroenterology*, 72, 1280, 1977.

89. Krasner, N., Cochran, K. M., Russel, R. I., Carmichael, H. A., and Thompson, G. G., Alcohol and absorption from the small intestine. 1. Impairment of absorption from the small intestine in alcoholics, *Gut*, 17, 245, 1976.

90. Chapman, R. W., Morgan, M. Y., Boss, A. M., and Sherlock, S., Acute and chronic effects of alcohol on iron absorption, *Dig. Dis. Sci.*, 28, 321, 1983.

91. McClain, J. and Su, L.-C., Zinc deficiency in the alcoholic: a review, *Alcoholism*, 7, 5, 1983.

92. Bode, J. C., Hanisch, P., Henning, H., Koenig, W., Richter, F.-W., and Bode, C., Hepatic zinc content in patients with various stages of alcoholic liver disease and in patients with chronic active and chronic persistent hepatitis, *Hepatology*, 8, 1605, 1988.

93. Dinsmore, W., Callender, M. E., McMaster, D., Todd, S. J., and Love, A. H. G., Zinc absorption in alcoholics using zinc-65, *Digestion,* 32, 238, 1985.

94. Valberg, L. S., Flanagan, P. R., Ghent, C. N., and Chamberlain, M. J., Zinc absorption and leukocyte zinc in alcoholic and nonalcoholic cirrhosis, *Dig. Dis. Sci.,* 30, 329, 1985.

95. Milman, N., Hvid-Jacobsen, K., Hegnhøj, J., and Sølvsten Sørensen, S., Zinc absorption in patients with compensated alcoholic cirrhosis, *Scand. J. Gastroenterol.,* 18, 871, 1983.

96. Karayalcin, S., Arcasoy, A., and Uzunalimoglu, O., Zinc Plasma levels after oral zinc tolerance test in nonalcoholic cirrhosis, *Dig. Dis. Sci.,* 33, 1096, 1988.

97. Hunter, C. K., Treanor, L. L., Gray, J. P., Halter, S. A., Hoyumpa, A., and Wilson, F. A., Effects of ethanol in vitro on rat intestinal brush-border membranes, *Biochim. Biophys. Acta,* 732, 256, 1983.

98. Ray, M., Dinda, P. K., and Beck, I. T., Mechanism of ethanol-induced jejunal microvascular and morphologic changes in the dog, *Gastroenterology,* 96, 345, 1989.

99. Dinda, P. K., Leddin, D. J., and Beck, I. T., Histamine is involved in ethanol-induced jejunal microvascular injury in rabbits, *Gastroenterology,* 95, 1227, 1988.

100. Gottfried, E. B., Korsten, M. A., and Lieber, C. S., Alcohol-induced gastric and duodenal lesions in man, *Am. J. Gastroenterol.,* 70, 587, 1978.

101. Millan, M. S., Morris, G. P., Beck, I. T., and Henson, J. T., Villous damage induced by suction biopsy and by acute ethanol intake in normal human small intestine, *Dig. Dis. Sci.,* 25, 513, 1980.

102. Bode, J. C., Knüppel, H., Schwerk, W., Lorenz-Meyer, H., and Dürr, H. K., Quantitative histomorphometric study of the jejunal mucosa in chronic alcoholics, *Digestion,* 23, 265, 1982.

103. Persson, J., Berg, N. O., Sjölund, K., Stenling, R., and Magnusson, P.-H., Morphologic changes in the small intestine after chronic alcohol consumption, *Scand. J. Gastroenterol.,* 25, 173, 1990.

104. Walker, W. A. and Isselbacher, K. J., Uptake and transport of macromolecules by the intestine. Possible role in clinical disorders, *Gastroenterology,* 67, 531, 1974.

105. Bjarnason, I., Ward, K., and Peters, T. J., The leaky gut of alcoholism: possible route of entry for toxic compounds, *Lancet,* 1, 979, 1984.

106. Fukui, H., Brauner, B., Bode, J. C., and Bode, C., Plasma endotoxin concentrations in patients with alcoholic and non-alcoholic liver disease: reevaluation with an improved chromogenic assay, *J. Hepatol.,* 12, 162, 1991.

107. Bode, C., Kugler, V., and Bode, J. C., Endotoxemia in patients with alcoholic and non-alcoholic cirrhosis and in subjects with no evidence of chronic liver disease following acute alcohol excess, *J. Hepatol.,* 4, 8, 1987.

108. Beutler, B. and Cerami, A., Cachectin: more than a tumor necrosis factor, *N. Engl. J. Med.,* 316, 379, 1987.

109. Chadwick, V. S. and Anderson, R. P., Inflammatory products of commensal bacteria and gastro-intestinal disorders, *Dig. Dis.,* 8, 253, 1990.

110. Keppler, D., Hagmann, W., Rapp, S., Denzlinger, C., and Koch, H. K., The relation of leukotrienes to liver injury, *Hepatology*, 5, 883, 1985.
111. Nolan, J. P., Intestinal endotoxins as mediators of hepatic injury — an idea whose time has come again, *Hepatology*, 10, 887, 1989.
112. Bode, J. C., Bode, C., Heidelbach, R., Dürr, H.-K., and Martini, G. A., Jejunal microflora in patients with chronic alcohol abuse, *Hepato-gastroenterology*, 31, 30, 1984.
113. Bode, C., Kolepke, R., Schäfer, K., and Bode, J. C., Hydrogen breath test in patients with alcoholic liver disease: evidence for bacterial overgrowth in the small intestine (abstract), *J. Hepatol.*, 11 (Suppl. 2), S 9, 1990.

19 Nutrition and Alcohol-Induced Immunomodulation

INTRODUCTION

Chronic alcoholism is considered to be the most common cause of malnutrition in affluent societies of the western world.[1] Malnutrition is a major extrinsic factor which impairs the efficiency of the immune system to recognize and eliminate pathogens from the body.[2,3] Chronic alcoholics are at high risk of suppressing their immune response by direct and indirect mechanisms: as a nutrient, alcohol has a direct toxic effect on cells and organs of the host defense system[4] and alcohol consumption affects dietary intake, impairs absorption, utilization, storage, and excretion of nutrients and thereby may induce malnutrition, which in turn modulates immunocompetence.

In the U.S., 9% of all adults can be considered as heavy drinkers with at least 80 g of alcohol consumed per day.[5] However, combined data from various surveys indicate that chronic alcoholics consumed an estimated mean of 193 g/d of alcohol or 43% of their calorie intake was in the form of alcohol.[6-10] Alcohol-induced malnutrition together with the direct immunotoxic effects of alcohol may reduce the effectiveness of the host defense system against infections. This hypothesis is supported by epidemiological data showing that infectious and contagious illnesses are the most common cause of death in alcoholics.[11,12]

DIRECT EFFECTS OF ALCOHOL ON HOST DEFENSE

Interference of alcohol with mechanical host defenses and alteration of immune mechanisms are important factors that predispose alcohol abusers to an increased risk of infections. The main function of the gastrointestinal tract as a mechanical barrier in the host defense system is to control the intestinal flora and to prevent antigens from entering the system. Gastric acid secretion is an important regulator of the growth of the intestinal flora. Chronic alcoholics have a reduced secretion of gastric acid, which could contribute to the increased incidence of jejunal bacterial overgrowth found in chronic alcohol abusers.[13-15] An elevated intestinal permeability to a number of substances including bacterial endotoxin has been shown in chronic alcoholics.[13-15] The increased permeability causes a high endotoxin exposure of cytokine-producing cells of the liver, which might result in the induction of enhanced monokine secretion. Elevated serum levels of interleukin-1, interleukin-6 and tumor necrosis factor are normally found in chronic alcoholics with liver disease.[16] The deterioration of the intestinal mucosal barrier may promote absorption of immunogenic substances into the systemic circulation. At the same time, the clearance of antigens from circulation by Kupffer cells is impaired, which could explain in part the increased concentration of serum immunoglobulins found during alcoholic liver disease.[4]

Chronic alcohol consumption appears to depress the production of polymorphonuclear leukocytes in the bone marrow. Up to 8% of alcoholics admitted to hospitals have granulocytopenia, which disappears after several days of abstinence. Bone marrow examinations showed a decreased number of mature granulocytes and a decreased reserve capacity for these cells in alcoholics.[17] The absence of a bone marrow reserve and the inability to produce large numbers of new leukocytes expose alcohol users to increased risk when challenged by a severe bacterial infection. However, the release of leukocytes from the bone marrow is not inhibited by acute and chronic alcohol exposure of humans.[17]

Animal studies demonstrated that chronic alcohol feeding induces atrophy of thymus and spleen.[18] There is evidence that the majority of the cells lost from the thymus after short-term alcohol ingestion are of an immature phenotype (CD4$^-$/CD8$^-$).[19] In rats, 13 months of alcohol feeding reduced the total number of T lymphocytes from the spleen significantly. However, the percentage of lymphocytes with markers for T_H cells was higher in spleens from alcohol-fed rats.[20] So far, there are no data available about alcohol-induced thymus and spleen atrophy in humans.

Alcohol also exerts direct effects on immunocompetent cells. Since chronic alcoholics are often malnourished and have liver disease and underlying infections, their data about the immunotoxic effects of alcohol have to be analyzed very carefully as they may reflect nutritional and physiological changes. Acute and chronic alcohol ingestion prevent the normal delivery of neutrophilic granulocytes to sites of bacterial invasion and impair the ability of these cells to adhere to cell surfaces.[4] Moreover, chronic alcohol abuse results in a decreased chemotaxis of these cells, which contributes to the frequency and severity of infections in drinkers.[4] The mononuclear phagocytizing system is another component of the immune system, which is impaired by the toxic effects of alcohol. Phagocytosis, bactericidal activity, and adhesion are reduced in these cells after *in vitro* exposure to alcohol.[21] Alcohol further modulates the cytotoxic activity of natural killer cells, but the published data are very contradictory. Natural killer cells from nonalcoholic volunteers showed a decreased cytotoxicity in the presence of alcohol.[22] However, alcoholics without liver disease demonstrated a normal natural killer cell activity.[23,24] Mice given alcohol for 1 to 4 weeks showed a normal[25] and decreased[26,27] natural killer cell activity. Antibody-dependent cellular cytotoxicity,[28] lymphocyte proliferation responses,[29] and B lymphocyte functions[30] are also impaired by alcohol. The first metabolite in the metabolism of alcohol, acetaldehyde, is further known to affect various immune functions.[31,32]

INDIRECT EFFECTS OF ALCOHOL ON IMMUNOCOMPETENCE: ALCOHOL-INDUCED MALNUTRITION

The nutritional status of chronic alcoholics is influenced by a variety of factors, primarily by the amount and duration of alcohol intake, and the amount and quality of diets consumed. Further factors are the gastrointestinal and hepatic condition, diarrhea, vomiting, loss of appetite, and the socioeconomic status of the alcoholic. High alcohol intake correlates with a high frequency of missed or partly eaten meals, which results in an inadequate and imbalanced intake of nutrients, probably the most important cause of alcoholic malnutrition. Data from various surveys about the macronutrient intake in chronic alcoholics indicate that alcohol provided nearly half of the total calories.[6-10] The mean protein intake of the alcohol abuser exceeded 50 g/d, which would be adequate according to the RDA. However, it is possible that protein requirements are increased. Of heavy alcohol abusers without liver disease and RDA-adequate protein intake, 62% showed signs of protein malnutrition.[10]

Even with an adequate intake of macronutrients, the addition of empty calories from alcohol may cause vitamin and mineral deficiencies. The social status of the alcohol abuser correlates with the frequency of vitamin and mineral deficiencies. According to the results of several studies, lower-socio-economic class alcohol users have generally a higher chance to be malnourished (13 to 100%) than middle class ones (0 to 29%).[33] Besides the social class, the amount and duration of alcohol consumption influences the micronutrient intakes in alcoholics. Intakes of various micronutrients in chronic alcohol users are below the RDA, and up to 78% did not reach the recommendation for vitamin A, vitamin C, thiamin, folic acid, or niacin.[7,9,34-36]

The nutrient intake alone, however, is not sufficient for the evaluation of the nutritional status of alcohol abusers. Biochemical and anthropometric measurements are needed additionally, because alcohol has an impact on the absorption, utilization, storage, and excretion of micronutrients. Alcohol has direct effects on the structure, function, and motility of the small intestine.[13,15] These effects vary depending on the concentration of alcohol that is consumed. As a consequence, malabsorption of water-soluble vitamins is common to a moderate degree in alcohol abusers. Acute alcohol intake reduces the active absorption of folic acid, while in chronic alcoholics folic acid absorption was only impaired by alcohol in malnourished individuals.[13] Acute alcohol use further inhibits the uptake of thiamin and ascorbic acid, while chronic alcohol abuse decreases the absorption of thiamin and vitamin B-12.[15] There are no data published showing an impairment of the absorption of fat-soluble vitamins with alcohol abuse in humans. In adult rats, however, chronic alcohol consumption reduced the rate of vitamin A absorption.[37]

Alcohol interferes with the metabolism and utilization of various nutrients. For example, the conversion of thiamin to its active form thiamin pyrophosphate, as well as the utilization of the active form, are affected by alcohol.[38] Further, the hepatic formation and the release of 5-methyltetrahydrofolic acid, the conversion of pyridoxine to its active form, and the hepatic activiation of vitamin A are all impaired by alcohol.[38] Alcoholics with fatty liver demonstrated decreased hepatic concentrations of water-soluble vitamins and of vitamin A.[39] Hepatic vitamin A levels progressively decrease with increasing severity of alcoholic liver injury.[40] Alcohol induces hepatic microsomal enzymes for the oxidation of retinol to polar metabolites, which increases the hepatic vitamin A depletion.[40] In addition, alcohol promotes vitamin A mobilization from the liver.[41]

Alcoholic subjects without cirrhosis excrete abnormally large amounts of zinc in the urine.[9] Increased urinary losses of calcium, magnesium, and phosphate have also been reported following alcohol ingestion.[39]

The combination of reduced nutrient intake, decreased absorption, utilization and storage, and increased excretion as well as the increased requirements affect the antioxidant status in alcohol abusers. Several studies have shown that the serum antioxidant status (α-tocopherol, retinol, β-carotene, selenium, zinc) in alcoholics is significantly decreased compared with controls.[42-44] All of these antioxidants exert a strong impact on immunocompetence and the reduced serum concentrations of these micronutrients may contribute to the nutritional immunosuppression observed in heavy alcohol abusers. Clearly, the multiple effects of alcohol abuse on the nutritional status may result in malnutrition in these subjects with its known effect on immune functions.[2,3] In experimental studies, vitamin A and E supplementation resulted in normal T-lymphocyte response in guinea pigs, which was suppressed by chronic alcohol treatment.[45]

COMBINED EFFECT OF ALCOHOL AND MALNUTRITION ON IMMUNOCOMPETENCE

So far, very few controlled studies have investigated the combined effects of alcohol-induced malnutrition and heavy alcohol consumption on the immunocompetence in alcohol abusers. In one study with six non-cirrhotic alcoholics who were fully restored in nutrition, subjects were supplied with 320 ml/d of pure alcohol for 20 d.[46] Immunological tests were performed before and after that period. This study revealed remarkably little alteration of immune responses in well-nourished alcoholics given a large amount of alcohol. Chemotaxis was the only function found to be diminished with the high alcohol intake. The data from this and another similar study[47] support the hypothesis that severe alcohol-mediated immune cell damage only occurs in malnourished alcoholics.

The cytotoxic activity of natural killer cells from alcoholics with liver disease is reduced compared with healthy controls and with alcoholics without liver disease.[23,24] The poorer the nutritional status of the alcoholics with liver disease, the more severe was the deficit in natural killer cell activity. Response to standard skin testing in alcoholics without liver disease was also impaired.[10] Of the alcoholics tested, 29% showed anergy to the skin testing, while 62% of them were malnourished, which again emphasizes the combined immunotoxic effects of malnutrition and alcohol. These few studies indicate that especially the combination of heavy alcohol intake and malnutrition in humans results in significant immunosuppression.

The role of nutrition in alcohol-induced immunomodulation in animal studies is also not well defined. Malnutrition alone can be associated with immunological abnormalities similar to those observed in alcohol-treated animals. Despite the information about malnutrition in alcohol abusers and the synergistic immunosuppressive effect of malnutrition and heavy alcohol intake, animal studies in this area tend to neglect the nutritional component of immunosuppression in alcohol abuse. While heavy alcohol abusers often have an inadequate dietary intake and show signs of malnutrition,[48] animals used in alcohol studies are fed superoptimal diets which contain micronutrients in concentrations up to 46 times higher than the recommended amount.[49] Such diets interfere intensively with the objectives of these studies and potentially mask the immunosuppressive effects of alcohol-induced malnutrition.

NUTRITION IN EXPERIMENTAL ALCOHOL STUDIES

A variety of animal models of alcoholism exists using different techniques to administer alcohol.[50] For long-term animal studies (more than 2 weeks), however, the incorporation of alcohol in a liquid diet[51] or in the drinking water of the animals are the two most common models.[20,25-27,52-54] In the latter model, animals are fed a "natural ingredient", regular lab chow and alcohol is administered as part of the drinking water. Compared with the requirements of rodents,[55] these lab chows are high in protein and low in fat (animal and plant sources). Especially the content of fat-soluble vitamins significantly exceeds the requirements (Table 1). The liquid diet introduced by Lieber et al.[56] to study the pathological mechanism of alcoholic hepatitis contains a high amount of fat (35% of the calories, only plant source) and an extremely high concentration of vitamin A (Table 1). The high level of fat-soluble vitamins in such diets might confound the immunological data obtained in alcohol studies, since alcohol abuse has a severe impact on the status of fat-soluble vitamins[40,41] and especially vitamin A affects immunocompetence in various ways.[57-61] Therefore, most animal models of alcoholism do not resemble the immunosuppressive conditions in human alcoholics, since they exclude the

TABLE 1
Vitamin Allowances for Mice and Vitamin Content of Various Diets (Per kg Diet)

Vitamin	Unit	Requirement (NRC)	Mouse chow	Mouse chow/ requirement	Lieber-DeCarli liquid diet	Mouse chow/ requirement
A	IU	500	13,400	26.8	22,800	45.6
D	IU	150	5000	33.3	1520	10.1
E	IU	20	65	3.2	114	5.7
Niacin	mg	10.0	80	8.0	28.5	2.8
Pyridoxine	mg	1.0	9	9.0	6.7	6.7
Thiamin	mg	5.0	16	3.2	5.7	1.1
Folic acid	mg	0.5	4	8.0	1.9	3.8
Pantothenic acid	mg	10.0	33	3.3	15.2	1.5

TABLE 2
Composition of the
Experimental Diets

	Diet 1	Diets 2 and 3
Protein	18	12.5
Fat	35	30.0
Carbohydrate	17	27.5
Ethanol	30	30.0

Note: Values shown are %.

combination of the direct immunotoxic effects of alcohol with the alcohol-induced malnutrition.

The lack of animal models with appropriate diets prompted us to investigate the immunomodulating effects in mice of various alcohol-containing diets under controlled conditions.[49] We compared three liquid diets in which 30% of the calories were derived by alcohol: Diet 1, the Lieber-DeCarli diet (Table 2); Diet 2, a diet which supplied micronutrients at the amount recommended by the NRC[55] without additional safety margins for any kind of nutrient losses; Diet 3, this diet supplied only 60% of the micronutrients of Diet 2 in order to simulate the malnutrition occurring in heavy alcoholics. Protein and fat content were lower and the carbohydrate content was higher than in Diet 1, and all of the three liquid diets provided 1 kcal/ml. For each diet, animals were assigned to one of these groups: control group (*ad libitum*-fed diet, in which alcohol was isocalorically replaced by dextrin-maltose), alcohol group (*ad libitum*), and a pair-fed group (in which mice were fed the control diet at the average amount consumed in the alcohol group).

After 7 weeks on these diets, mice were sacrificed and immunological parameters were measured. Since no comparable study has been published so far, we describe the results of this study in more detail then it is usually done in such monographs.

Food intake and body weight — Food and alcohol intake did not differ between mice fed the three diets. The introduction of ethanol into the diets significantly reduced the calorie intake independent of the composition of the diets (Table 3). Ethanol in Diet 1, which supplied the highest concentration of micronutrients, resulted in the highest body weight, and decreasing micronutrient concentrations in Diets 2 and 3 reduced body

TABLE 3
Food Intake and Body Weight of Mice Fed Various Ethanol Diets

	Diet 1			Diet 2			Diet 3		
	C	A	P	C	A	P	C	A	P
Food intake[a] kcal/d/mouse	13.63 ± 1.21	9.88 ± 0.89	9.88 ± 0.89	13.51 ± 0.93	10.25 ± 1.59	10.25 ± 1.59	13.39 ± 1.50	10.00 ± 1.50	10.00 ± 1.50
Ethanol intake kcal/d/mouse	—	2.96 ± 0.27	—	—	3.07 ± 0.48	—	—	3.00 ± 0.45	—
Body weight g	22.12 ± 3.39	19.97[b,c,e] ± 1.50	18.08[f] ± 1.15	21.68 ± 1.79	17.30[b,d,e] ± 1.23	17.84[f] ± 0.70	21.65 ± 1.43	15.94[c,d,e] ± 0.94	18.92[f,g] ± 0.72

Note: C = Control diet; A = ethanol diet; and P = pair-fed control diet (matched with consumption of ethanol diet).

[a] Average daily food intake during the 7-week period.
[b] $p < 0.05$, Diet 1 vs. Diet 2.
[c] $p < 0.05$, Diet 1 vs. Diet 3.
[d] $p < 0.05$, Diet 2 vs. Diet 3.
[e] $p < 0.05$, Control vs. Ethanol within diets.
[f] $p < 0.05$, Control vs. Pair-feeding within diets.
[g] $p < 0.05$, Ethanol vs. Pair-feeding within diets.

weights significantly (Table 3). Diet 3 revealed that alcohol as part of an inadequate diet reduced body weight beyond the margin which could be explained by the decreased calorie intake in alcohol and pair-fed mice. Body weight was significantly different between alcohol and pair-fed mice only with this diet.

Spleen and thymus weight — Spleen and thymus weight were not different between control mice fed the three diets (Table 4). However, with Diet 1, spleen and thymus weight were comparable in alcohol and pair-fed mice, and in both groups the weights were significantly lower than in mice fed the control diet. With this diet it seems that the calorie restriction alone affects the weights of lymphoid organs and alcohol has no effect. In contrast to Diet 1, diets with lower concentrations of micronutrients demonstrate a significant alcohol effect. With Diets 2 and 3, spleen and thymus weight of alcohol and pair-fed mice were also significantly reduced compared with control mice, but the alcohol treatment reduced the weight beyond the margin which could be explained by the calorie restriction in pair-fed animals. Several investigators using Diet 1 (with 36% of calories derived from alcohol) also observed no differences in spleen weight between alcohol and pair-fed animals,[20,53,54] presumably due to the dietary composition of this diet. Spleen cell number was independent of the dietary treatment and was significantly affected by alcohol (Table 4).

Cytokines and natural killer cell activity — The lymphokine interleukin-2 (IL-2) is another parameter of the immune response which is very sensitive to alcohol, but is insensitive toward dietary modifications. In the three different diets, alcohol significantly increased the capacity of mitogen-activated splenocytes to produce IL-2 *in vitro* (Table 5). To our knowledge, this is the first report of an increased IL-2 secretion by splenocytes from alcohol-treated animals. So far, most studies showed no effect of alcohol on IL-2 secretion.[16] Preliminary data from a recent study also demonstrated with Diet 1 an increased responsiveness of murine splenocytes to various mitogens and an enhanced mixed lymphocyte response.[62] The secretion of interferon-τ (IFN) by splenocytes did not differ between controls fed the 3 different diets. Alcohol treatment together with Diet 1 did not change the capacity of splenocytes to secrete this cytokine, while alcohol treatment together with Diets 2 or 3 significantly enhanced the IFN release (Table 5). With Diet 2, calorie restriction by pair-feeding also resulted in significantly increased IFN secretion. No other studies are published reporting an effect of alcohol *in vivo* on IFN secretion.[16] Several

TABLE 4
Weight and Cell Number of Lymphoid Organs of Mice Fed Various Ethanol Diets

	Diet 1			Diet 2			Diet 3		
	C	A	P	C	A	P	C	A	P
Spleen weight mg	73.06 ± 10.81	52.32[b,d] ± 12.48	58.01[c] ± 8.56	72.64 ± 15.12	47.18[c,d] ± 15.81	65.23[f] ± 14.68	71.12 ± 9.88	29.18[b,c] ± 5.63	68.79[b,f] ± 10.18
Spleen cell number $\times 10^7$	12.92 ± 2.08	6.54[d,f] ± 2.33	10.53 ± 5.17	11.18 ± 5.01	4.76[d,f] ± 1.78	10.04 ± 3.94	12.59 ± 4.68	5.13[d,f] ± 1.86	10.01 ± 3.29
Thymus weight mg	70.61 ± 14.19	49.53[a,b,c] ± 14.27	58.99[a,b] ± 10.62	67.52 ± 12.73	35.92[d] ± 19.29	74.27[f] ± 7.97	66.87 ± 10.85	26.90[b,d] ± 4.95	73.40[b,f] ± 8.10

Note: C = control diet; A = ethanol diet; and P = pair-fed control diet (matched with consumption of ethanol diet).

[a] $p < 0.05$, Diet 1 vs. Diet 2.
[b] $p < 0.05$, Diet 1 vs. Diet 3.
[c] $p < 0.05$, Diet 2 vs. Diet 3.
[d] $p < 0.05$, Control vs. Ethanol within diets.
[e] $p < 0.05$, Control vs. Pair-feeding within diets.
[f] $p < 0.05$, Ethanol vs. Pair-feeding within diets.

TABLE 5
Immunological Activity of Splenocytes from Mice Fed Various Ethanol Diets

Cytokines	Diet 1			Diet 2			Diet 3		
	C	A	P	C	A	P	C	A	P
Interleukin-2 ng/ml	3.40 ± 0.69	6.06^[d,f] ± 1.34	2.75 ± 1.62	3.68 ± 1.26	7.50^[d,f] ± 3.76	3.08 ± 1.49	2.82 ± 1.34	6.30^[d,f] ± 2.35	2.98 ± 1.14
Interferon-γ ng/ml	8.71 ± 1.85	8.79^[a,b] ± 3.12	5.96^[a] ± 2.80	9.29 ± 3.16	17.43^[a,d] ± 5.29	20.67^[a,c] ± 7.94	7.08 ± 1.99	20.67^[b,d] ± 7.94	6.49^[c,f] ± 1.39
TNFα ng/ml	2.24 ± 0.96	1.26^[d] ± 0.53	1.62^[a] ± 0.48	1.83 ± 0.46	0.88^[d,f] ± 0.28	2.34^[a,e] ± 0.62	1.77 ± 0.78	1.27 ± 0.59	1.93 ± 0.48
NK activity %^[g]	16.97^[b] ± 4.11	28.61^[d,f] ± 9.68	20.24 ± 7.05	20.39 ± 5.57	23.55 ± 3.95	18.31 ± 6.41	23.04^[b] ± 6.40	24.39 ± 9.42	16.34 ± 7.36

Note: C = control diet; A = ethanol diet; and P = pair-fed control diet (matched with consumption of ethanol diet).

[a] $p < 0.05$, Diet 1 vs. Diet 2.
[b] $p < 0.05$, Diet 1 vs. Diet 3.
[c] $p < 0.05$, Diet 2 vs. Diet 3.
[d] $p < 0.05$, Control vs. Ethanol within diets.
[e] $p < 0.05$, Control vs. Pair-feeding within diets.
[f] $p < 0.05$, Ethanol vs. Pair-feeding within diets.
[g] E/T ratio, 100:1.

studies investigated the effects of chronic alcohol on tumor necrosis factor (TNF) secretion in rats. The injection of the mitogen lipopolysaccharide (LPS) resulted in increased serum TNF concentrations.[62,63] In our study, the chronic alcohol treatment reduced TNF secretion by LPS-activated murine splenocytes with all three diets, but differences were only significant with Diets 1 and 2. In an earlier study, we also observed in rat Kupffer cells a reduced TNF secretion after chronic alcohol treatment.[64]

The lytic activity of natural killer (NK) cells against YAC-1 cells was significantly enhanced with the alcohol-containing Diet 1 (Table 5). The control group for Diet 1 showed the lowest NK cell activity, while the NK cell activity of controls of Diets 2 and 3 were higher (significant differences between Diet 1 and 3). Pair-feeding obviously reduces NK cell activity compared with alcohol treatment (Diets 1 to 3) and with controls (Diets 2 and 3). An earlier study already reported that pair-feeding reduces NK cell activity,[65] which indicates that either the calorie restriction itself or the neuroendocrinological mechanisms related to such stress may have caused this reduction. Our data suggest that the extent of reduction is related to the composition of the dietary regimen, since NK cell activity is the highest in animals pair-fed with Diet 1 and the lowest with Diet 3. Other studies have also reported an enhanced NK cell activity with chronic alcohol treatment. Low concentrations of alcohol administered to mice for 2 to 6 weeks increased NK cell activity.[66] Chronic alcohol further stimulated hepatic lymphocytes (Pit cells) with NK cell activity to lyse YAC-1 cells.[67]

CONCLUSIONS

In summary, the above data clearly show that some immunological parameters are mainly influenced by the alcohol in the diet and not by the nutritional quality of the diets. To this group of nutrition-independent parameters belong spleen cell number and the capacity of mitogen-activated splenocytes to secrete IL-2 and TNF. In another group of immunological parameters, the effect of alcohol on these parameters varies with the nutritional quality of the diet. Alcohol administered in nutritionally inadequate diets decreases body, spleen, and thymus weight and enhances IFN secretion and NK cell activity when compared with commonly used, nutritionally superoptimal diets. The intensive interaction between alcohol consumption and nutritional status on one side and between nutritional status and immunocompetence on the other side creates many ways whereby nutrition affects alcohol-induced immunomodulation. It is apparent from animal and human studies in the absence of alcohol that single and multiple nutritional deficiencies suppress immune functions.[75] Especially vitamin A, the nutrient whose concentration in Diet 1 extremely exceeds the requirement, modulates the immune response in various ways. Vitamin A deficiency in rats decreased NK cell activity and interferon-α/β production,[59] and it impairs the antibody response to pneumococcal polysaccharides.[60,61] Further, it is suggested that vitamin A and retinoic acid are required for the release of cytolytic factors including TNF by human peripheral blood monocytes.[68] High concentrations of vitamin A in murine peritoneal macrophages induced increased phagocytic ability, tumoricidal activity, and interleukin-1 production.[57] In addition, high dietary intakes of vitamin E (100 to 2500 IU/kg diet) stimulate splenic NK cell activity and phagocytic activity of alveolar macrophages.[69] The quality of fatty acids used in Diet 1 to 3 might have also modified the effects of alcohol on the immune response, as it has been demonstrated in recent studies.[70-74] Further studies are necessary to devise animal diets which are as close as possible in their dietary composition to the actual requirement of the animals and resemble in a closer way the nutritional condition in chronic alcoholics. Based upon such diets, research in this area should obtain more conclusive data about the immunomodulating effects of alcohol and about the mechanisms which lead to the high risk of infectious diseases in chronic alcoholics. Finally, nutritional supplementation of alcohol or alcohol abusers may help compensate for alcohol-induced malnutrition.

ACKNOWLEDGMENT

Supported by the NIH Grant AA 08037.

REFERENCES

1. Thomson, A. D., Jeyasingham, M. D., and Pratt, O. S., Possible role of toxins in nutritional deficiency, *Am. J. Clin. Nutr.*, 45, 1351, 1987.
2. Watson, R. R., Ed., in *Nutrition, Disease Resistance, and Immune Function*, Marcel Dekker, New York, 1984, 404.
3. Chandra, R. K., Ed., in *Nutrition and Immunology*, Alan R. Liss, New York, 1988, 342.
4. McGregor, R. R., Alcohol and immune defense, *J. Am. Med. Assoc.*, 256, 1474, 1986.

5. Seventh Special Report to the U.S. Congress on Alcohol and Health, U.S. Department of Health and Human Services, Washington, D.C., 1987.

6. Patek, A. J., Toth, E. G., Saunders, M. G., Castro, A. M., and Engel, J. J., Alcohol and dietary factors in cirrhosis, *Arch. Intern. Med.*, 135, 1053, 1975.

7. Hurt, R. D., Higgins, J. A., Nelson, R. A., Morse, R. M., and Dickson, R. E., Nutritional status of a group of alcoholics before and after admission to an alcoholism treatment unit, *Am. J. Clin. Nutr.*, 34, 386, 1981.

8. Simko, V., Connell, A. M., and Banks, B., Nutritional status in alcoholics with and without liver disease, *Am. J. Clin. Nutr.*, 35, 197, 1982.

9. Mills, P. R., Shenkin, A., Anthony, R. S., McLelland, A. S., Main, A. N. H., MacSween, R. N. M., and Russell, R. I., Assessment of nutritional status and in vivo immune responses in alcoholic liver disease, *Am. J. Clin. Nutr.*, 38, 849, 1983.

10. Mendenhall, C. L., Anderson, S., Weesner, R. E., Goldberg, S. J., and Crolic, K. A., Protein-calorie malnutrition associated with alcoholic hepatitis, *Am. J. Med.*, 76, 211, 1984.

11. Cooper, B. and Maderazo, E. G., Alcohol abuse and impaired immunity, *Infect. Surg.*, March, 94, 1989.

12. Adams, H. G. and Jordan, C., Infections in the alcoholic, *Med. Clin. North Am.*, 68, 179, 1984.

13. World, M. J., Ryle, P. R., and Thomson, A. D., Alcoholic malnutrition and the small intestine, *Alcohol Alcoholism*, 20, 89, 1985.

14. Kozol, R. A. and Elgebaly, S. A., Ethanol and its effects on mucosal immunity, in *Drugs of Abuse and Immune Function*, Watson, R. R., Ed., CRC Press, Boca Raton, FL, 1990, 19.

15. Persson, J., Alcohol and the small intestine, *Scand. J. Gastroenterol.*, 26, 3, 1991.

16. Watzl, B. and Watson, R. R., Alcohol and cytokine secretion, in *Alcohol, Immunology and Cancer*, Yirmiya, R. and Taylor, A. N., Eds., CRC Press, Boca Raton, FL, 1992, in press.

17. Liu, Y. K., Effects of alcohol on granulocytes and lymphocytes, *Semin. Hematol.*, 17, 130, 1980.

18. Tennenbaum, J. I., Ruppert, R. D., St. Pierre, R. L., and Greenberger, N., The effect of chronic alcohol administration on the immune responsiveness of rats, *J. Allergy Clin. Immunol.*, 44, 272, 1969.

19. Jerrells, T. R., Smith, W., and Eckardt, M. J., Murine model of ethanol-induced immunosuppression, *Alcoholism Clin. Exp. Res.*, 14, 546, 1990.

20. Mufti, S. I., Prabhala, R., Moriguchi, S., Sipes, I. G., and Watson, R. R., Functional and numerical alterations induced by ethanol in the cellular immune system, *Immunopharmacology*, 15, 85, 1988.

21. Rimland, D., Mechanisms of ethanol-induced defects of alveolar macrophage function, *Alcoholism*, 8, 73, 1983.

22. Nair, M. P. N., Kronfol, Z. A., and Schwartz, S. A., Effects of alcohol and nicotine on cytotoxic functions of human lymphocytes, *Clin. Immunol. Immunopathol.*, 54, 395, 1990.

23. Charpentier, B., Franco, D., Paci, L., Charra, M., Martin, B., Vuitton, D., and Fries, D., Deficient natural killer cell activity in alcoholic cirrhosis, *Clin. Exp. Immunol.*, 58, 107, 1984.

24. Ledesma, F., Echevarria, S., Casafont, F., Lozano, J. L., and Pons-Romero, F., Natural killer cell activity in alcoholic cirrhosis: influence of nutrition, *Eur. J. Clin. Nutr.,* 44, 733, 1990.

25. Abdallah, R. M., Starkey, J. R., and Meadows, G. G., Alcohol and related dietary effects on mouse natural killer-cell activity, *Immunology,* 50, 131, 1983.

26. Meadows, G. G., Blank, S. E., and Duncan, D. D., Influence of ethanol consumption on natural killer cell activity in mice, *Alcoholism Clin. Exp. Res.,* 13, 476, 1989.

27. Blank, S. E., Duncan, D. A., and Meadows, G. G., Suppression of natural killer cell activity by ethanol consumption and food restriction, *Alcoholism Clin. Exp. Res.,* 15, 16, 1991.

28. Walia, A. S., Pruitt, K. M., Rodgers, J. D., and Lamon, E. W., In vitro effect of ethanol on cell-mediated cytotoxicity by murine spleen cells, *Immunopharmacology,* 13, 11, 1987.

29. Mutchnick, M. G. and Lee, H. H., Impaired lymphocyte proliferative response to mitogen in alcoholic patients. Absence of a relation to liver disease activity, *Alcoholism,* 12, 155, 1988.

30. Aldo-Benson, M., Ethanol and the B-cell: humoral immunity, in *Drugs of Abuse and Immune Function,* Watson, R. R., Ed., CRC Press, Boca Raton, FL, 1990, 175.

31. Levallois, C., Mani, J. C., and Balmes, J. L., Sensitivity of human lymphocytes to acetaldehyde: comparison between alcoholic and control subjects, *Drug Alcohol Depend.,* 20, 135, 1987.

32. Walia, A. S., Pruitt, K. M., Dillehay, D. L., Marshall, G. M., and Lamon, E. A., In vitro effect of acetaldehyde on cell-mediated cytotoxicity by murine spleen cells, *Alcoholism Clin. Exp. Res.,* 13, 766, 1990.

33. Derr, R. F., Porta, E. A., Larkin, E. C., and Rao, G. A., Is ethanol per se hepatotoxic, *J. Hepatol.,* 10, 381, 1990.

34. Hillers, V. N. and Massey, L. K., Interrelationships of moderate and high alcohol consumption with diet and health status, *Am. J. Clin. Nutr.,* 41, 356, 1985.

35. Rissanen, A., Sarlio-Lahteenkorva, S., Alfthan, G., Gref, C. G., Keso, L., and Salaspuro, M., Employed problem drinkers: a nutrition risk group?, *Am. J. Clin. Nutr.,* 45, 456, 1987.

36. Bunout, D., Gattas, V., Iturriaga, H., Perez, C., Pereda, T., and Ugarte, G., Nutritional status of alcoholic patients: its possible relationship to alcoholic liver damage, *Am. J. Clin. Nutr.,* 38, 469, 1983.

37. Leichter, J., Hornby, A. P., and Dunn, B. P., The influence of chronic ethanol ingestion on the absorption of vitamin A in adult male rats, *FASEB J.,* 4, A1438, 1990.

38. Darnton-Hill, J., Interactions of alcohol, malnutrition and ill health, *World Rev. Nutr. Diet,* 59, 95, 1989.

39. Morgan, M. Y. and Levine, J. A., Alcohol and nutrition, *Proc. Nutr. Soc.,* 47, 85, 1988.

40. Leo, M. A. and Lieber, C. S., Hepatic vitamin A depletion in alcoholic liver injury in man, *N. Engl. J. Med.,* 307, 597, 1982.

41. Leo, M. A. and Lieber, C. S., New pathway for retinol metabolism in liver microsomes, *J. Biol. Chem.,* 260, 5228, 1985.

42. Bjorneboe, G. E. A., Johnsen, J., Bjorneboe, A., Marklund, S. L., Skylv, N., Hoiseth, A., Bache-Wiig, J. E., Morland, J., and Drevon, C. A., Some aspects of antioxidant status in blood from alcoholics, *Alcoholism Clin. Exp. Res.*, 12, 806, 1988.

43. Ward, R. J., Jutla, J., and Peters, T. J., Antioxidant status in alcoholic liver disease in man and experimental animals, *Biochem. Soc. Trans.*, 17, 492, 1988.

44. Girre, C., Hispard, E., Therond, P., Guedj, S., Bourdon, R., and Dally, S., Effect of abstinence from alcohol on the depression of glutathione peroxidase activity and selenium and vitamin E levels in chronic alcoholic patients, *Alcoholism Clin. Exp. Res.*, 14, 909, 1990.

45. Davydova, T. V., Pletsityi, K. D., and Fomina, V. G., Further study of immunocorrecting properties of vitamins A and E in experimental chronic alcohol intoxication, *Vopr. Pitan.*, 3, 45, 1988.

46. Gluckman, S. J., Dvorak, V. C., and MacGregor, R. R., Host defenses during prolonged alcohol consumption in a controlled environment, *Arch. Intern. Med.*, 137, 1539, 1977.

47. Ericsson, C. D., Kohl, S., Pickering, L. K., Davis, J., Glass, G. S., and Faillace, L. A., Mechanisms of host defense in well nourished patients with chronic alcoholism, *Alcoholism Clin. Exp. Res.*, 4, 261, 1980.

48. Watzl, B. and Watson, R. R., Role of alcohol abuse in nutritional immunosuppression, *J. Nutr.*, 122, March suppl., 1992.

49. Watzl, B., Lopez, M., Shabazian, M., Chen, G., Colombo, L. L., Way, D., and Watson, R. R., Dietary factors in the study of alcohol-induced immunomodulation, *J. Nutr.*, in press.

50. Keane, B. and Leonard, B. E., Rodent models of alcoholism: a review, *Alcohol Alcoholism*, 24, 299, 1989.

51. Lieber, C. S. and DeCarli, L. M., Liquid diet technique of ethanol administration: 1989 update, *Alcohol Alcoholism*, 24, 197, 1989.

52. Morland, B. and Morland, J., Effects of long-term ethanol consumption on rat peritoneal macrophages, *Acta Pharmacol. Toxicol.*, 50, 221, 1982.

53. Grossman, C. J., Mendenhall, C. L., and Roselle, G. A., Alcohol and immunoregulation: I. In vivo effects of ethanol on concanavallin A sensitive thymic lymphocyte function, *Int. J. Immunopharmacol.*, 10, 187, 1988.

54. Mendenhall, C. L., Grossman, C. J., Roselle, G. A., Ghosn, S., Gartside, P. S., Rouster, S. D., Chalasani, P. V. R. K., Schmitt, G., Martin, K., and Lamping, K., Host response to myobacterial infection in the alcoholic rat, *Gastroenterology*, 99, 1723, 1990.

55. National Research Council, Nutritional requirements of the mouse, in *Requirements of Laboratory Animals*, 3rd rev. ed. (no. 10), National Academy of Sciences, Washington, D.C., 1978, 38.

56. Lieber, C. S., Jones, D. P., Mendelson, J., and DeCarli, L. M., Fatty liver, hyperlipemia and hyperuricemia produced by prolonged alcohol consumption, despite adequate dietary intake, *Trans. Assoc. Amer. Phys.*, 76, 289, 1963.

57. Moriguchi, S., Werner, L., and Watson, R. R., High dietary vitamin A (retinyl palmitate) and cellular immune functions in mice, *Immunology*, 56, 169, 1985.

58. Chandra, R. K. and Vyas, D., Vitamin A, immunocompetence, and infection, *Food Nutr. Bull.*, 11, 12, 1989.

59. Bowman, T. A., Goonewardene, I. M., Pasatiempo, A. M. G., Ross, A. C., and Taylor, A. C., Vitamin A deficiency decreases natural killer cell activity and interferon production in rats, *J. Nutr.*, 120, 1264, 1990.

60. Pasatiempo, A. M. G., Kinoshita, M., Taylor, C. E., and Ross, A. C., Antibody production in vitamin A-depleted rats is impaired after immunization with bacterial polysaccharide of protein antigens, *FASEB J.*, 4, 2518, 1990.

61. Pasatiempo, A. M. G., Taylor, C. E., and Ross, A. C., Vitamin A status and the immune response to pneumococcal polysaccharide: effects of age and early stages of retinol deficiency in rats, *J. Nutr.*, 121, 556, 1991.

62. Honchel, R., Rhoads, C. A., Fitzpatrick, E. A., McClain, C. J., Kaplan, A. M., and Cohen, D. A., Immune enhancement during chronic ethanol feeding in mice — autoimmune phenomena?, *FASEB J.*, 5, A782, 1991.

63. Hansen, J., McClain, C. J., Cherwitz, D., Schlater, J., Stahnke, L., and Allen, J., Induction of tumor necrosis factor and interleukin-6 message in rats by ethanol administration and endotoxin, *Hepatology*, 12, 261, 1990.

64. Watzl, B., Abril, E., Abbaszadegan, M. R., Scuderi, P., and Watson, R. R., Effects of ethanol in vivo on TNF secretion by cultured rat Kupffer cells, in *Cells of the Hepatic Sinusoid*, Vol. 3, Wisse, E., Knook, D. L., and McCuskey, R. S., Eds., Kupffer Cell Foundation, Leiden, The Netherlands, 1991, 480.

65. Abdallah, R. M., Starkey, J. R., and Meadows, G. G., Toxicity of chronic alcohol intake on mouse natural killer cell activity, *Res. Comm. Chem. Pathol. Pharmacol.*, 59, 245, 1988.

66. Saxena, Q. B., Saxena, R. K., and Adler, W. H., Regulation of natural killer activity in vivo: Part IV. High natural killer activity in alcohol drinking mice, *Indian J. Exp. Biol.*, 19, 1001, 1981.

67. Alboronoz, L., Jones, J. M., Crutchfield, C., and Veech, R. L., Natural killer activity of pit cells perfused from livers of rats treated with ethanol, *FASEB J.*, 5, A2753, 1991.

68. Turpin, J., Mehta, K., Blick, M., Hester, J. P., and Lopez-Berestein, G., Effect of retinoids on the release and gene expression of tumor necrosis factor-α in human peripheral blood monocytes, *J. Leuk. Biol.*, 48, 444, 1990.

69. Moriguchi, S., Kobayashi, N., and Kishino, Y., High dietary intakes of vitamin E and cellular immune functions in rats, *J. Nutr.*, 120, 1096, 1990.

70. Barone, J., Hebert, J. R., and Reddy, M. M., Dietary fat and natural-killer-cell activity, *Am. J. Clin. Nutr.*, 50, 861, 1989.

71. Lokesh, B. R., Sayers, T. J., and Kinsella, J. E., Interleukin-1 and tumor necrosis factor synthesis by mouse peritoneal macrophages is enhanced by dietary n-3 polyunsaturated fatty acids, *Immunol. Lett.*, 23, 281, 1990.

72. Olson, L. M. and Visek, W. J., Kinetics of cell-mediated cytotoxicity in mice fed diets of various fat contents, *J. Nutr.*, 120, 619, 1990.

73. Stewart-Phillips, J. L., Lough, J., and Phillips, N. C., The effect of a high fat diet on murine macrophage activity, *Int. J. Immunopharmacol.*, 13, 325, 1991.

74. Kor, H. and Scimeca, J., Influence of dietary fat replacement on immune function, *FASEB J.*, 5, A1130, 1991.

75. Delafuente, J. C., Nutrients and immune responses, *Nutr. Rheumatic Dis.*, 17, 203, 1991.

INDEX

P